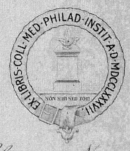

ANNUAL MEETING APRIL 24, 25, 26 . . . MAYO HOTEL . . . TULSA, OKLA.

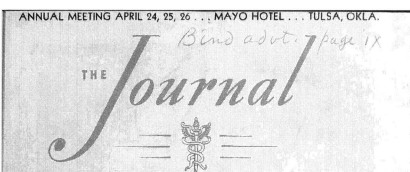

Bind advt. page IX

THE *Journal*

OF THE OKLAHOMA STATE MEDICAL ASSOCIATION

VOLUME XXXVII   OKLAHOMA CITY, OKLAHOMA, JANUARY, 1944   NUMBER 1
★ *Published Monthly at Oklahoma City, Oklahoma, Under Direction of the Council*

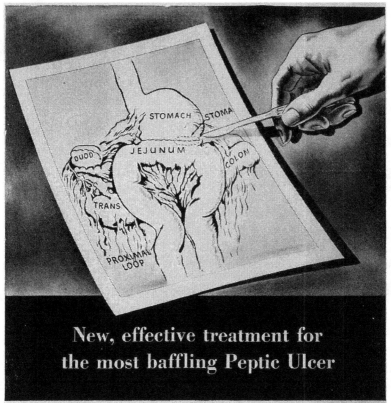

New, effective treatment for the most baffling Peptic Ulcer

Gastrojejunal ulcer is described as the type most difficult to treat satisfactorily. 1.

A new preparation, Phosphaljel, is effective in treating these highly resistant lesions. 2.

Phosphaljel is antacid, astringent, demulcent, pleasantly flavored. It is indicated in those cases associated with pancreatic juice deficiency, diarrhea, or low phosphorus diet.

Available in 12-fluidounce bottles. A pharmaceutical of John Wyeth & Brother, Division WYETH Incorporated, Philadelphia.

1. MARSHALL, S. F., and DE-VINE, J. W., Jr.: Gastrojejunal Ulcer, S. Clin. North America, 743-761 (June) 1941.

2. FAULEY, G. B.; FREEMAN, S.; IVY, A. C.; ATKINSON, A. J., and WIGODSKY, H. S.: Aluminum Phosphate in the Therapy of Peptic Ulcer, Arch. Int. Med. 67: 563-578 (March) 1941.

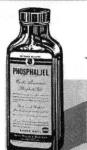

PHOSPHALJEL *Wyeth's* ALUMINUM PHOSPHATE GEL

THE JOURNAL
OF THE
OKLAHOMA STATE MEDICAL ASSOCIATION

| VOLUME XXXVII | OKLAHOMA CITY, OKLAHOMA, JANUARY, 1944 | NUMBER 1 |

Some Observations Relative to Surgery of the Thyroid*

H. M. McCLURE, M.D., F.A.C.S.

CHICKASHA, OKLAHOMA

Seeing patients daily in the clinic and in surgery gives one an opportunity to test theories and practices. Our theories are not always right and most of our practices may be improved. It is of our theories and practices that I propose to speak and I ask your indulgence while I give you our present opinion regarding disease of the thyroid gland and its surgical management.

The thyroid is a gland of internal secretion whose chief function, so far as is known, is the elaboration and storage of its own peculiar hormone or secretion which we call thyroxin. Originally it was a gland taking part in digestion, but in the course of evolutionary changes, it has lost its connection with the alimentary tract. As Means[1] aptly said, "For a role in digestion it has substituted a role in metabolism." In man, the thyroid attains its relative maximum size just prior to puberty, corresponding to the time of the greatest load on the organs, from factors of growth and development. Simple colloid goiter, so common in this age, is a clinical manifestation of this physiological fact.

Mangus-Levy[2] first recognized that the thyroid plays a role in the regulation of heat production or its equivalent, metabolism. Just how the thyroid controls these oxidation processes is not absolutely certain. We have definite clinical evidence that the condition we describe as myxedema, in which there is retention in the body tissues of water, salts and proteins[3], can be relieved by the administration of thyroxin. In a state of scarcity of the hormone, the patient lives at a low emotional level, reacts sluggishly, and cerebrates slowly. Conversely, the giving of large amounts of thyroxin to a normal individual will produce the symptoms and findings of hyperthyroidism. The action of an excess of the hormone causes emotional instability and increased irritability.

Coggeshall and Greene[4] have shown that thyroid hormone not only depletes hepatic glycogen but if in excess, can injure the liver so that it is unable to store glycogen. On the contrary, thyroidectomy leads to excessive storage of glycogen in the liver.

The hormone can produce changes in the muscular system varying from myasthenia to advanced muscular atrophy and hypotonicity.

The blood supply of the thyroid is abundant as the blood volume of man goes through the thyroid about once an hour. There is also a rich lymph plexus in close proximity to the follicles, and it is supplied by a rich network of autonomic nerve fibers, but we do not as yet know whether these fibers are secretory or vaso-motor.

If, in discussing pathology of the thyroid, one must give a classification in order to be didactic, the one below is brief and clinically workable:

1. Inflammation.
2. Tumors.
3. Goiters.

Briefly, the inflammatory diseases can be designated as acute or chronic. The acute conditions are rare and the treatment is conservative, unless suppuration develops. This

---

*Read before the Annual Meeting held in Oklahoma City, May 11-12, 1943.

requires drainage. The chronic inflammatory changes are commonly known as Hashimoto's disease and Riedel's struma. The treatment for Hashimoto's disease is total thyroidectomy, but insofar as I know, there is no treatment for Riedel's struma; perhaps the roentgenologists can aid us.

The tumors of the thyroid are the fetal adenomas and malignancies. The first are amenable to removal; the latter, total thyroidectomy followed by radium or x-ray.

The most common deviation from the normal is a symmetrical enlargement of the gland noticed most frequently around puberty. If the enlargement is gradual or slow, the gland will probably return to normal, or at least so far as we can tell, it is normal, but I am beginning to believe these adoles, cent goiters return to haunt us in later years, especially if they are neglected and forgotten.

There are two definite states to be discerned in goiters; one, overactivity characterized by epithelial hypertrophy and hyperplasia, and the other, degeneration of cells and colloids and quite often we see a mixture of the two. When stimulation to hyperplasia occurs, the stage is set for all the processes that follow. When can we know that hyperplasia is occurring? Only when the patient shows symptoms which we associate with toxicity. These may develop early or late, insofar as the enlargement of the thyroid is concerned. We feel the development of these symptoms depends on two things, namely, the degree of toxicity, and the ability of the body to withstand toxicity up to a given point. What starts the hyperplasia? The work of Marine is outstanding in this respect. He believes that the normal demands on a subefficient gland, whether it is due to lack of iodine or due to an originally substandard gland, is the beginning of a hyperplasia. Occasionally an emotional frustration, business anxieties, accidents, infections and vitamin deficiencies seem to be the inciting factors. As you know, the majority of goiters, or perhaps I should say goiter symptoms, develop after the third decade of life. Clinically, the only suggestion I can offer is that the thyroid gland is able to bear the stress and strain for years before its secretions become increased or altered, and that the body can perhaps withstand this increase or alteration of the secretions for a length of time.

In goiters occurring in the young, usually the stimulation is supplied to a gland which has had to bear the stress of life for only a few years, therefore, nothing hinders it from responding and, due to the youthfulness of our bodies, we are able to tolerate the toxicity unless it is unusually severe. The

heart races but does not fibrillate. The nervous system is "on fire" but seldom do the patients lose their mental faculties. As the toxicity persists, nervousness increases, pulse becomes more rapid, pulse pressure increases, there is loss of weight, muscular weakness, the eye signs become more prominent and exophthalmos may develop. These symptoms may subside, only to return as age progresses and degeneration begins, and is characterized by fibrillations, muscular weakness, hypertension, signs of cardiac and liver failure. This, I think, can be clinically explained by persistent toxicity with changes in the body tissues due to age. ˙ If time permitted, I could show you intervening stages with clinical and pathological findings, linking up the two extremes. What we are trying to determine is whether or not all goiters are toxic. We have been able to prove clinically that the removal of a so-called adenoma will lower the metabolic rate and reduce irritability and nervousness, although no cardinal symptoms of toxicity were present clinically. Who was wrong, the examiner or the thyroid?

Recognition of toxicity is dependent on the acuity of the patient and the doctor. A high-strung individual is likely to make a fuss about anything, while a hard-working, busy housewife may have toxic symptoms but never makes known her complaints until she has run the entire gamut of the disease and is dying of a toxic goiter. The doctor must recognize the early nervous symptoms. This can be done only by careful studying of the patient and making a meticulous examination of the thyroid gland. Many of the doctors that I have seen, are able to palpate and examine a thyroid within a period of ten to fifteen seconds, naturally nothing is ascertained. ˙

The basal machine must not be used as a yard-stick with reference to the amount of activity in hyperthyroidism. Neither should it be used to determine the amount of thyroid extract one should give in cases of hypothyroidism. It has been shown by Broda Barnes[5] that basal temperature is a better index for the amount of thyroid to be given .

In other diseases, we take great pride in striving for an early diagnosis. No one can question the good results that are obtainable through surgical procedures, yet few goiter patients come to surgery until their toxicity is severe. We have no hesitancy in eradicating an infected cervix or pre-cancerous lesion of the skin, still we are prone to allow our patients to run the entire range of hyperthyroid symptoms before surgery is advised. We insist that stones be removed from the kidney before the organ is damaged too severely; likewise do we insist that infected gall bladders be removed before serious liver damage develops. Why should not goiters be removed before invalidism develops? An early diagnosis can be made if we do a good physical examination, carefully studying our patient relative to nervous symptoms and the physical condition of the thyroid and then advise a therapeutic test with iodine. I can mention no laboratory procedures that are of any benefit. When the thyroid is removed and the symptoms having been eradicated, the patient is most grateful.

Once the diagnosis is made we strive to get the patient in the best preoperative condition, which not only includes a stabilization of the patient's mental, nervous and cardiac system, by whatever therapeutic measures are necessary, usually Lugol's solution and phenobarbital, but also includes large amounts of glucose and insulin, which we think has a direct bearing on the liver function. The gland is palpated frequently. When it softens and becomes movable, when the pulse rate lessens, when the patient gains or at least maintains his weight, then the time for surgery is ripe.

Criles dictum for the choice of operative procedure, whether it be polar ligation, lobectomy, partial or total thyroidectomy, depends on the age, physical condition, the duration of the disease, and emotional state of the patient. If this dictum were still observed in the severe cases in which a late diagnosis has been made more satisfactory results would be obtained.

Keep the original clinical picture of your patient in mind while planning surgery, as occasionally the preoperative reaction is so pleasing that the patient is scurried off to surgery before the patient or the gland is operable. Naturally, poor results follow.

We do all of our thyroidectomies under local and I assure you this is a most ideal anesthetic. Our technique is the one advocated by Hertzler, the anesthesia is excellent, the dissection is easy, there is little bleeding, and the structures are easily identified. In young patients, we remove at least 80 per cent of the gland. In patients past 30 years of age we do a total thyroidectomy. We wonder how many total thyroidectomies have been done unknowingly, as the usual technique is to ligate the superior, middle and inferior thyroid vessels, then leave a strip of gland along the trachea and in many instances this is sutured by a running stitch, which we think will produce necrosis or fibrosis of the remaining thyroid tissue. All of our operative wounds are closed with gauze drainage but they can be closed without any drainage whatsoever. Postoperatively, they are given large amounts of glucose and insulin intravenously for three days and then, if there is an increase in temperature or pulse rate, it is continued. This is done even if the patient is able to retain fluids by mouth, and we feel that we can see a distinct improvement in our postoperative reactions.

It is well known that partial thyroidectomy may be followed by exophthalmos, and that exophthalmos may become worse after partial thyroidectomy. This has not been our experience in any of our total thyroidectomies and no case of tetany has followed any of our operative procedures. We have had two cases of mild myxedema which followed total throidectomy. These two cases developed in elderly women with hard, enlarged thyroids, and who had hypertension for which no other cause could be found. If a patient has signs of toxicity which include any or all of the common symptoms and findings such as irritability, increased pulse, loss of weight, fatigue, eye signs or symptoms referable to cardiac disturbances, and has an enlargement of the thyroid especially if it be hard or nodular, and is relieved by rest and iodine, thyroidectomy is advised and the results have been gratifying. Caution must be exercised lest we regard a slow enlargement or firmness of the thyroid gland as normal, and assume that the associated symptoms are primarily idiopathic.

I would like to interject here a brief history of one of our most interesting cases which, clinically and pathologically, had symptoms and findings of both hyperthyroidism and hypothyroidism:

Mrs. D., age 52, was first seen by Dr. L. E. Woods in June, 1941. Her complaint was of swelling of both lower extremities which had been present for some ten months. He elicited a history of nervousness, palpifation, and the loss of 30 pounds of weight in six months. The findings at that time were: pulse 110, blood pressure 166/68, flabbiness of the skin, marked digital tremor, lid lag and a firm, fixed, enlarged thyroid. The skin of both lower legs presented a bronzed appearance, and appeared tight and glistening, and did not pit with pressure. She was sent to the hospital; her weight was 126½ pounds, her BMR was plus 66, and the above findings were confirmed. A preoperative diagnosis was made of hyperthyroidism with localized myxedema. A total thyroidectomy was done and a biopsy was taken from the skin of each leg. The pathologist reported hyperthyroidism associated with localized myxedema. She made an uneventful recovery, all of her toxic symptoms subsided and the myxedma disappeared. She was last seen on January 6, 1943, at which time her weight was 145½ pounds, blood pressure 138/80, pulse was 72. She was feeling extremely well and had no complaints. Her BMR at that time was minus 5.

We began doing total thyroidectomies with caution, selecting our cases using as our criteria, extreme toxicity and cardio-toxic patients, who were past 40 years of age, doing this on the assumption that the thyroid had by this time completed its role in growth and that perhaps it has fulfilled its relationship with the other glands of internal secretion. Our results have been so gratifying that we are slowly lowering the age limit.

Apparently, the fear of myxedema is the one and only reason why surgeons have not done total thyroidectomies. Should this develop, it is easily and accurately controlled. Contrast this with the failure to remove enough of the toxic goiter; the symptoms persist, organic damage progresses and another operative procedure is usually necessary. At the present time, at least until the physiologists, research men or clinicians can offer something better, we believe total thyroidectomy is the solution to toxic goiter.

DISCUSSION

R. M. HOWARD, M.D.

OKLAHOMA CITY, OKLAHOMA

Dr. McClure has given us a good paper on this subject. His discussion of the cause and development of goiter are excellent, and his observation in regard to the relationship between the thyroid enlargement of adolescence, and goiter of later life deserves careful consideration. To the medical practitioner and pediatrician, this is of special importance, as the treatment of this condition offers much in the prevention of goiter. I think that goiter is now sufficiently prevalent in our locality that prophylaxis should be instituted in all children during the adolescent age.

Since goiter is the most frequent pathologic process with which we have to deal in surgery of the thyroid gland, I shall devote my discussion to that phase of the subject.

To keep in mind the clinical classification of goiter adopted by the "American Association for the study of Goiter" greatly simplifies ones conception of the subject, and indicates the management best used in the treatment of the condition.

Goiters, and this excludes inflammation and malignancy, are divided as follows:

1. Diffuse non-toxic goiter.
2. Diffuse toxic goiter.
3. Nodular non-toxic goiter.
4. Nodular toxic goiter.

The first is largely a medical problem, the others, in the light of our present knowledge, are surgical with surgery to be instituted at a proper time. The essayist's observation that too many of these cases are permitted to go on to a dangerous phase is an important point.

The early diagnosis of toxic goiter is of extreme importance, having a definite bearing not only on the safety of operation, but on the expectancy of life in those who are submitted to surgery. Too many of these cases are being treated, even after diagnosis has been made, by the continued administration of iodine, thus depriving the surgeon of an important adjunct in the preparation of these cases for safe surgery.

Most cases are easily diagnosed. The questionable case should be kept under observation until a diagnosis can, with greatest certainly, be made.

We doctors treating thyroid disease have many more patients consult us who do not have thyroid trouble, than those who do have it. All of these cases whether they have or do not have goiter, are entitled to a very careful examination before an opinion should be given. Operation on the thyroid is too serious a matter unless the patient has a definite diagnosis and can be assured of the expected benefit. I think Lahey has made an important observation when he says that when first seen, before preoperative preparation is begun, the gravity of the risk should be placed on record. Many of these toxic cases will be so improved on preparation for operation, that when they come to surgery it is easy to underestimate the postoperative reaction they will develop.

The death rate of thyroid surgery has reached the low percentage today of about one per cent and if we are to do this type of work every safeguard must be used.

An eminent authority recently expressed this in a way that brings the responsibility for mortality in thyroid surgery very close to the operator. He believes that mortality in thyroid surgery comes from the following three causes:

1. There is an unpredictable mortality that is incident to any major surgery, vascular, accidents, etc.

2. Error in judgment as to when to operate, or how extensive an operation to do.

3. Errors in technique.

The first is probably unavoidable, the other two can be minimized by careful preparation and observation of the patient during this time, and extreme care in doing the operation.

There is a mistaken idea that the diffuse toxic goiter, after the administration of Lugols Solution for ten or twelve days, is ready for surgery. In many of them a sufficient remission is secured in that time so that operation is permissible . In others and particularly in those of long standing, or in those who previously have had iodine, a much longer time is required. I have seen no case harmed, or any of the beneficial effects lost, by prolonging the time of preparation.

The nodular toxic goiter of severe degree, and all toxic cases with vascular degeneration require, in addition to iodine, digitalis and plenty of rest and carbohydrate food. We give almost all of our cases glucose intravenously for a day or two before operation. Salt solution subcutaneously is always given when the patient returns from surgery. Local anesthesia should always be used unless one has available an anesthetist trained in thyroid surgery. No anesthetic should be used that does not permit the patient to be awake before closing the wound.

I have great respect for Dr. Hertzler and his students. Some of their opinions have not been adopted by most of our great authorities. I have not felt that I could do a rather large number of thyroid operations as safely by attempting a complete thyroidectomy. We continue to do a sub-total thyroidectomy with about two per cent recurrences, and have more trouble with hypothyroidism than we like. It has been a long time since we have had any serious trouble with tetany or bilateral adductor paralysis. For either condition I have the utmost respect. I am not condemning total thyroidectomy. It unquestionably has advantages, but I do not believe, that in the hands of the majority of doctors of thyroid surgery, it will prove to be technically as safe as the sub-total procedure.

BIBLIOGRAPHY

1. Means, J. H.: The Thyroid and Its Diseases. J. B. Lippincott Company, Philadelphia. 1937.
2. Mangus and Levy: Berl Klin SCHNSCHA, Vol. 32, page 650. 1895.
3. Thomas, Henry M. Jr.; Proteins. Bulletin Johns Hopkins Hospital, Vol. 89, No. 2. 1936.
4. Coggeshall and Greene: Amer. Jour. Physiology, Vol. 105, page 103. July, 1933.
5. Broda Barnes: Basal Temperature vs. Basal Metabolism. Jour. A.M.A., Vol. 119, pages 1072-1074. August, 1942.
6. Lahey, F. H.: Sugr. Gyne. & Obst., Vol. 64, No. 2A. February 15, 1937.

Dermatomyositis

JOHN H. LAMB, M.D.

OKLAHOMA CITY, OKLAHOMA

Dermatomyositis is a nonpurulent, rare polymyositis of a multiform character in which there is associated inflammation and degeneration of many muscle groups. There is a marked erythema of the skin associated with an edema of the lardaceous type. The course of this condition is variable. It may begin insidiously with listlessness and headache later followed by various types of eruptions and muscular weakness. Some of the cases are ushered in with chills and severe symptoms, and are rapidly progressive with death ensuing in one or two months. This is known as the acute type.

The sub-acute types have comparatively mild symptoms and are subject to partial remissions. In 60 per cent of the cases the outcome is fatal due to inflammatory involvement of the myocardium and the muscles of deglutition, and respiration. Those cases which recover are usually marked by residual muscular atrophy and permanent cutaneous changes.

Wagner[1] in 1863, was the first to describe this condition as a muscular disease. Potain[2] in 1875 used the term atypical glanders in describing a similar case. In 1887, Wagner[3] gave a report of a like condition which he called acute polymyositis. It was Unverrichit[4], in 1891, who described it under it's present title—dermatomyositis. Weber and Gray[5] gave an excellent review of the disease and stressed the predominant involvement of the subcutaneous fat.

OCCURRENCE

Both men and women are affected with it but it is much more frequent in women. It is an affliction of early middle life and effects the white race only. About 15 per cent of cases are in children.

ETIOLOGY

Most authors believe this condition to be caused by an infectious agent. Various organisms have been isolated from the infected muscles, including streptococci, diplococci and staphylococci. In most cases, however, no organisms are recovered from the blood or tissue culture. Many cases followed acute infections such as tonsillitis, chronic abscess, sinusitis and other infectious diseases. O'Leary[6] suggests that it is a bacteremia in a transitory or passive sense in which there is a migration to the muscles through the lymph channels from the foci, rather than a frank infection of the blood stream. There is also the second possibility that the resultant changes in the skin and muscles are due to bacterial toxins.

SKIN ERUPTION

The eruption has great similarity in some instances to two of the light-sensitive dermatoses; that is, lupus erythematosus disseminata which is always fatal and which Lane[7] first diagnosed his reported case to be; pellagra, which is probably the most common early diagnosis made for these cases. The skin eruption may be a bright red like erysipelas originating on the eyelids and cheeks and spreading over the face and part of the neck. Other cases reported were deep red, more like lupus erythematosus. The lesions on the body are of many types—urticarial, morbilliform, eczematous, vesicular and petechial. Fever may be intermittent, sometimes associated with a large spleen. Quite a number of cases are afebrile for many months.

MUSCLES

Many groups of muscles may be affected. In O'Leary's[6] group of 40 cases he reported that fifteen of them had generalized muscle involvement. In 24 the extremities were involved first. In all of them the outstanding involvement was in the muscles of the shoulder girdle, arms and neck. Twenty-seven cases had involvement of the pharyngeal muscles. Thirteen had vocal cord changes. Pathologic examination of the muscles show intracellular edema and hemorrhage between the muscle bundles and waxy degeneration of the muscles proper which caused them to be pale staining. Many show loss of striation. There is also a perivascular infiltration of lymphocytes, plasma cells and mast cells.

REPORT OF CASE

Mrs. E. F., 30 years old white woman, was admitted to the hospital on September 10, 1942. Her chief complaints were swelling of her face and sore muscles of six month's duration. The eruption started around the eyes, on the upper and lower lids and gradually spread to the forehead and upper lip. At the first the skin would swell, become red, and itch and then partly clear. It finally became constantly swollen. The eruption spread over the anterior face and down the neck forming a definite "V" at the exposed area over the chest. A red papular eruption appeared on the dorsum of the hands along the prominence of the phalangeal metatarsal joints. The patient had not felt well since the delivery of her last child in February, 1942 and during the past two months, before entrance to the hospital, she had complained of considerable pain in her neck, shoulders, and arms and

felt weak with lack of energy. In March, 1942, she received intravenous treatment for sinus trouble and also consulted doctors who cauterized her cervix and said she had a chronic infection of the cervix.

The past history revealed fever and repeated maxillary sinusitis, also repeated attacks of sore throat; otherwise, very good general health. There was no family history of any similar skin trouble like scleroderma or dermatomyositis. This patient had had four deliveries, the first being six years ago and the last, nine months ago. There was no evidence of pelvic pain or history of trouble with female organs.

The examination revealed a rather small, undernourished, white woman who appeared weakened and void of energy. The face in the anterior portion, on the forehead and down across the cheeks was reddened and swollen, most of the swelling and redness being just beneath the eyes. The nose was swollen in the area of the bridge and there was a redness extending down over the neck and running in a "V" shape on the chest down to the breasts. This eruption was reddish-blue in color and had a thin, white scale in some areas over the surface, resembling very much that seen in disseminated lupus erythematosus. At the "V" of the neck there were white-gray areas resembling scleroderma. There was a beginning redness on the back and the knees and some on the flexor surfaces of the arms. The tongue was somewhat reddened in the lateral borders. On deep pressure over the biceps and muscle groups in her neck she cried out in pain.

Vaginal examination revealed a slight laceration of the cervix but no evidence of infection.

Examination of the locations of a possible focus of infection revealed:

Throat: Effect of tonsillectomy with small tonsil tag at left base.

Nose: Right-mild congestion, otherwise negative. Left-mild congestion, otherwise negative.

Ears: Negative.

Sinuses: X-Ray revealed no evidence of infection.

Muscle biopsy removed September 22, 1942, revealed the following: the microscopic examination showed skeletal muscle which showed an occasional small area of interstitial tissue intensely and diffusely infiltrated with lymphocytes and plasma cells. The most marked areas were about the smaller blood vessels. They were fairly well circumscribed areas. Some of the muscle fibres appeared moderately degenerated with absence of striations and in several areas the muscle fibres were frayed. There was no specific type of degeneration and trichinae were not found. The overlying fat and connective tissue was also infiltrated with a few scattered lymphocytes in some areas.

The patient was studied from a bacterial standpoint and the bacterial complement fixation tests were four plus in reaction for a number of diagnostic streptococcus strains, especially a hemolytic type of diplococcus, a non-hemolytic type of streptococcus and a hemolytic type of streptococcus viridans. A four plus reaction for a hemolytic type of bacillus of the colon group was also found. Cultures made from the nasal mucosa revealed a hemolytic type of streptococcus viridans of the short-chain variety and a diplo-streptococcus of the non-hemolytic type.

Agglutination tests, done with the autogenously isolated organisms, on her blood serum revealed three plus agglutination in dilutions of 1-100 against the hemolytic type of streptococcus viridans, and two plus in dilutions of 1-200. Blood cultures were repeatedly negative. The red cell sedimentation test gave a positive curve.

The blood count on entering the hospital revealed hemoglobin 73 per cent, rbc 3,690,000, color index, size normal, shape normal, wbc 5,500, neutrophiles 27 per cent, small lymphs 60 per cent, eosinophiles 3 per cent. After several transfusions, the blood count, on October 2, was as follows: hgb 80 per cent, rbc 4,180,000, color index 9, wbc 6,200, neutrophiles 64 per cent, lymphs 36 per cent. On October 20, even with transfusions, the red count reduced to 3,640,000 with a marked increase in white count to 23,750, neutrophiles 94 per cent and only 5 per cent lymphs and 1 per cent myelocytes. Urine was apparently normal on admission but towards the end showed trace of albumin. Blood chlorides were 395 mg. per cent, blood urea nitrogen 12.2 mg. 5 per cent and basal metabolism rate was plus 10.

On admission to the hospital the patient was given sulfathiazole, 30 grs. daily, vitamin B complex in large doses, and diathermy. She was also given prostigmin menthyl sulfate as recommended by Lane of St. Louis, which apparently gave no relief from the muscle pain after two or three day's trial. Because of the history of several remissions in other cases by fever therapy, the patient was given three successive fever treatments up to 105 F. by the use of typhoid vaccine intravenously. There was marked relief of edema and reduction in amount of erythema and pain in the muscles. The patient was given sulfathiazole in doses of 46 grains daily for two weeks with little change in general condition, so was then given neo-prontosil 40 grains daily. Repeated blood transfusions were given with little reaction and only slight improvement.

Through most of the early course the patient had remained afebrile but on October

10, the temperature curve remained a little above 99 F. From October 10 to October 19, the temperature ranged from 100 F. to 101 F. After the discontinuance of sulfanilamide once for 36 hours, there was a spiking of the temperature to 103 F. and immediately on resuming the sulfonamides, the temperature was reduced to around 100 F. From October 19 until death, there was an intermittent septic type fever ranging from 102 F. to 104 F. associated with chills. The last four days before death the temperature was rarely below 102 F.

Because of the light desensitizing effect of theelin in other dermatoses, large doses were tried for a week without any notice-

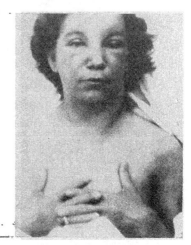

Fig. 1—Shows the marked larduceous type of edema of the face and neck.

able effect . In spite of supportive treatment, the patient became more debilitated, respiration and swallowing were more difficult and the day before her death, the breathing was entirely diaphragmatic in type. During the last week, the skin eruptions had spread over the entire back and over the breasts down to the umbilicus where there was a cleared area of normal skin in the shape of a large "V". The anterior surface of the legs was involved but the posterior aspect remained clear. She finally expired on October 31, 1942.

AUTOPSY

External Examination: The body was that of a fairly well developed and apparently slightly undernourished white woman of 25 to 35 years. The body was not embalmed. The skin of a greater portion of the arms, much of the anterior chest, some of the thighs and legs and other portions of the body were thickened, wrinkled, that is, to some extent, with considerable edema of the mid-portions of the arms. Sections were taken from the midsternal portions of the chest.

Internal Examination: The peritoneal cavity showed no free fluid, the peritoneum being smooth and glistening. The omentum was free. The pleural cavities showed no free fluid. Surfaces were smooth and glistening. Pericardial cavity contained an average amount of clear, straw colored fluid, and the pericardium was smooth and glistening. The lungs were pinkish gray and crepitant throughout except for rubbery, purple, atelectatic areas of the dependent portions. Considerable thick, mucoid fluid exudes from the larger bronchi. The heart was average size and shape except for extreme flabbiness of the entire right myocardium, the tricuspid valve being dilated. The left ventricle was contracted, waxy, red and moderately firm, and the greater vessels were grossly normal. The spleen was waxy, weighed roughly 300 grams, reddish-purple capsule, tense. Cut surface was purple, slightly bulging, pulp scraped easily. The liver was waxy, reddish-purple, surfaces smooth, regular, margins were slightly rounded. Cut surface was reddish brown, normal markings indistinct. Gallbladder and bile ducts were grossly normal. Left kidney was normal, average size, capsule stripped easily, surface was moderately pale, smooth. Cut surface showed poor differentiation between the cortex and the medulla. Peri-pelvic fat was slightly increased. Pelvis and ureter were grossly normal. The right kidney was similar to the left. Bladder was grossly normal; genitalia was normal; skeletal muscle showed intercostal and abdominal muscles waxy, reddish brown and moderately moist. Section was taken from intercostal muscles.

Gross Diagnosis:

1. Generalized dermatitis and myositis.
2. Dilated right heart.
3. Passive congestion of the spleen.
4. Liver degeneration.

MICROSCOPIC EXAMINATION

The skeletal muscle (intercostal) muscle fibers appeared slightly swollen and the individual cells were indistinct; interstitial tissue was unremarkable. There were no infiltrating leukocytes. Vessels were unremarkable.

Microscopic Diagnosis: Granular degeneration and cloudy swelling.

The myocardium showed granular degen-

eration; muscle fibers appeared smaller than the average. No remarkable changes were noticed in the nuclei.

Microscopic Diagnosis: Granular degeneration.

Anterior chest wall showed the epidermis almost completely desquamated. Superficial portions of the corium were dense and hyaline. Deeper portions of corium appeared denser than the average. There were no areas of infiltrating lymphocytes. Sweat glands appeared atrophic. Liver showed diffuse congestion and a moderate granular degeneration. Spleen showed moderate congestion but was otherwise apparently unremarkable. The lungs showed patchy areas intensely infiltrated with leukocytes. The surrounding structures were greatly congested. The vessels were larger than the average and were packed with red cells. Bronchioles filled with exudate.

Microscopic Diagnosis: Bronchitis, peribronchial pneumonia and congestion. Kidneys were unremarkable except for moderate congestion and slight granular degeneration.

DIFFERENTIAL DIAGNOSIS

Among the conditions to be differentiated from dermatomyositis, the most difficult is scleroderma which involves the skin and subcutaneous tissue. Histologic studies of scleroderma offer a differential diagnosis, particularly those of the muscle fibres, since there is usually no degeneration of the muscle fibres as in dermatomyositis. Scleroderma usually is more discreet and limited in extent, but there are many cases in which it is almost impossible to differentiate the diseases.

In lupus erythematosus disseminatus, the edema is not of the lardaceous type, the fever is much higher, and pain is not over the muscle groups but usually in the joints. There is nearly always a leukopenia and muscle biopsy does not show degeneration of muscle bundles. The skin manifestations as shown in our case and Lane's may resemble lupus erythematosus to a great extent.

Erysipelas is usually ushered in with more acute symptoms, with chills and the erythema of the face is a much brighter red. It usually starts with a small area and spreads very rapidly. Fever is high and there is no muscle swelling or pain.

Trichonosis, especially when the edema of the face is present, offers a difficult differential diagnosis. There is usually an accompanying gastrointestinal disturbance and the diaphragm and eye muscles are usually those affected by the Trichina. These are not usually early affected in dermatomyositis. Pathological examination of the muscle bundles reveals Trichinae.

Scleredema, adult form of Buske, may offer some difficulty in differentiation because the onset is somewhat similar to dermatomyositis. There is erythema of the face and neck and a tense edema of the skin over the upper extremities, chest, back and neck and face and sometimes generalized. The process may not only involve the dermis and subdermis but also the fascia and muscles. But, instead of progressing to the indurative and atrophic stages of scleroderma or the painful, destructive myositis of dermatomyositis, the process slowly regresses (8 to 18 months), leaving little or no residual changes.

Muscle biopsy does not show the infiltration and degeneration of dermatomyositis, but a looseness and swelling of the callogen with the interspaces filled with a homogenous mucin-like substance. The disease follows various infectious processes, i.e., whooping cough, influenza, scarlet fever, mumps, bronchitis, encephalitis and phyodermas.

REPORT OF A CASE

Mrs. C. J. reported to us complaining of redness and stiffness of the skin of the face, neck, breasts, upper abdomen, back and arms of four months duration. She complained of tenseness and rigidity of the neck and there was limitation of motion of the upper part of the body with particular emphasis on the mouth and jaws. She said that breathing was becoming most difficult and feared the tenseness would impede all respiration.

The redness and swelling was first noticed about the cubital fossae then the breasts and finally spread over the face and neck. She was placed on a limited diet, devoid of fats and was given small doses of thyroid without much improvement. Blood Wassermann test was negative and urinalysis was negative for albumin and sugar. Patient was chronically constipated and menses had been irregular since the onset.

The examination revealed a well-nourished white woman of 29 years of age who was not acutely ill. The temperature was 98.6° F. There was an erythema over the face, neck, breasts and arms which was not intense in type, the color not being bluish-red but pinkish-red. The skin appeared tense as though a substance had been injected beneath it. In the folds of the skin, at the cubital fossae, about the wrists and under the breasts, the color of the skin was blanched out by more induration. The creases of the skin were light red and were more depressed than normal although they were not fissured. The skin in these areas was rough, particularly on each side of the points of flexion . The general skin surface was not shiny and there was not the dryness of the myxedemous patient.

The tonsils were not enlarged and sinuses showed no signs of infection. The rest of the general examination was essentially negative. The basal metabolism rate was plus five. The blood count was, rbc 4,460,000, wbc 6,-250, neutrophilis 49 per cent, lymphocytes 48 per cent, monocytes 2 per cent and eosinophiles 1 per cent.

The patient was given thyroid extract grains one and one-half daily, and local massage with some improvement. Later, Dr. Paul O'Leary of the Mayo Clinic saw the patient and agreed with the diagnosis, suggesting use of typhoid vaccine intravenously to produce fever. She was subsequently given 5,000,000 typhoid organisms intravenously and suffered a marked exacerbation of all her symptoms, both erythema and edema, with a fever of 102 F. for five successive days. Following this reaction her skin improved about 80 per cent of normal. The difficulty in respiration was alleviated and motion was only slightly limited.

DISCUSSION

This case of dermatomyositis is of special interest first because of the history of several attacks of diseases of supposedly streptococcic origin, i.e., scarlet fever, sore throat and sinusitis. On the subsequent laboratory study, a high titre of the patients serum to an autogenous hemolytic streptococcus of viridans strain was found. Sulfanilamide seemed to counteract the toxicity of the bacterial toxin only to a certain extent. When the drug was discontinued for several days, the patient immediately became extremely toxic and a septic type of fever was produced. Toward the end, none of the sulfonamide drugs seemed to alter the extreme toxemia.

The stricking resemblance of this patient to disseminated lupus erythematosus early in the disease and the high degree of mortality

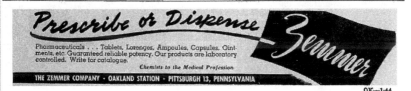

in both diseases suggests a similar etiology. Engman and Lane suggest that this clinical similarity of the two diseases may be due to an infectious or toxic agent or agents as yet unknown. Engman emphasized the point although the etiological agents might be closely related, the resultant infection could take one or two courses, either the lupus erythematosus way or the dermatomyositis way. O'Leary believes that in many cases only the data obtained at biopsy can be the means of distinguishing with accuracy between the two diseases.

Study of the muscles in fatal cases of lupus erythematosus revealed no pathologic alterations. Hazel[8] felt that a histamine-like substance was responsible for producing the destructive changes in the muscles. An attempt was made to desensitize our patient to histamine without success.

Treatment is comprised solely of empiric and symptomatic measures. General nursing care of the patient and a maintenance of a satisfactory nutritional state are essential. Concentrates of the vitamins should supplement the diet. Autogenous vaccines offer some encouragement if administered early but in the acute phase of the disease they are not practical. When dysphagia oc-

curs, frequent liquid feedings and use of the nasal tube feedings may be necessary. The sulfonamides should be tried in all cases because of the infectious history in nearly all cases and in many streptococcic in type.

Fever produced by typhoid vaccine has given remissions in several cases and caused a temporary improvement in this case.

Prostigmin as a muscle stimulant was of no benefit to our patient.

CONCLUSIONS

1. A case of dermatomyositis with autopsy is reported.
2. Sulfonamides and fever therapy seem to be of the greatest value in the treatment.

BIBLIOGRAPHY

1. Wagner, E.: Fall einer seltenen Muskelkrankheit. Arch. f. Heilkunde, Vol. 4, pages 282-283. 1863.
2. Potain: Morve chronique de forme, anormale. Bull. et mem. Soc. med. d. hop. de Paris, Vol. 12, pages 314-318. 1875
3. Wagner, E : Ein Fall Von Acuter Polymyositis. Deutsch. Arch. F. Klin. Med., Vol. 40, pages 241-266. 1886, 1887.
4. Unverricht, H.: Dermatomyositis Acuta. Deutsche. Med. Wchnschr., Vol. 17, page 41. 1891.
5. Weber, F. P., Gray, A. M. H.: Chronic Relapsing Polydermatomyositis with Predominant Involvement of Subcutaneous Fat (Panniculitus). Brit. Jour. Dermat., Vol. 36, pages 544-560. December, 1934.
6. O'Leary, Paul, Waisman, Morris: Dermatomyositis. Arch. Derm. & Syph. Vol. 41, pages 1001-1027. July, 1940.
7. Lane, Clinton: Dermatomyositis. Southern Medical Jour., Vol. 31, No. 3, 4, pages 287-294. 1938.
8. Hazel, Onis G., Hull, Wayne M.: Dermatomyositis in Children. A Report of Two Cases with a Fatal Termination. Southern Med Jour., Vol. 33, No. 8, page 809. Aug., 1940.

Cancer of the Breast[*]

GREGORY E. STANBRO, M.D.

OKLAHOMA CITY, OKLAHOMA

"Cancer is one of the most curable of diseases." To be curable, early diagnosis is essential, and prompt, proper, and adequate treatment is mandatory. Cancer is the most common cause of a definite lump in the breast of non-lactating women over 25 years of age. Each decade there is an increasing incidence of carcinoma of the breast in white civilized nulliparous women. Eleven per cent of all cancers occur in the breast, which is an external organ, and accessible to vision, palpation, and transillumination. One would expect a lump in the breast to be discovered early, investigated, receive treatment and be cured. Nevertheless the average woman of today who discovers a lump in her breast goes to her doctor only four weeks sooner than the women of the 1900's or about four to six months after discovering the lump. Consequently 50 per cent of carcinomas of the brest in large clinics already have axillary metastases.

*Read before the Annual Meeting held in Oklahoma City, May 11-12, 1943.

The breast is an organ which is never quiet. Even before birth it is active. From adolescence to senescence, the female breast is in a constant process of progression and regression. At puberty, during menses, and during pregnancy there is an active growth of the epithelial elements and a regression of the connective tissue elements. Epithelial cells grow, ducts grow and bud and branch until the breast is packed with epithelial lined ducts. This profuse epithelial hyperplasia pushes aside and necessitates a regression of the connective tissue. When lactation is interrupted the process is reversed and there is a regression of epithelial cells. Cloudy swelling, liquefaction, autolysis and degeneration follow and the interstitial tissue again grows. The breast never returns to the state of a virgin breast, but throughout life until the cessation of menses and senescence, this process of progression and regression is constantly taking place. If regression is not complete, small lumps, frequently painful, are present and so called chronic mastitis develops. A duct may become blocked or walled off and a galactocele or cyst result. Again two or more cysts may rupture into one and a blue domed cyst result from the hemorrhage of rupture. As a consequence the various tumors of the breast develop, their type and kind depending on the predominating cell and the stage of progression or regression in which the tumor grows.

Whenever cells are given the urge to multiply, the cell growth is physiologically controlled but too frequently that control is lost and the cellular hyperplasia over shoots its mark, is beyond all control, and malignancy may follow.

The growth urge in the breast is constantly present and the cells of the breast can multiply at any time during their life cycle. If the cellular hyperplasia overruns its normal control during the stage of early progression a carcinoma simplex may result. If normal hyperplasia is surpassed during the stage of high differentiation an adeno carcinoma may develop. Again the whole breast may explosively become malignant in a few weeks and a highly malignant diffuse duct carcinoma may be discovered. The normal unrest of the cells of the breast is therefore admittedly a factor in this problem.

The nulliparous breast is more susceptible to malignant change for the nulliparous breast is the unused breast. Failure to nurse results in incomplete secretion and drainage, and incomplete physiological function. The incidence of carcinoma of the breast therefore increases with each decade in nulliparous civilized women. There are 109 breast carcinoma deaths per 100,000 in single women and 44 breast carcinoma deaths in married women.

The average doctor sees only two cases of carcinoma a year. Be that as it may, early diagnosis by the physician is paramount. He should always be aware of the possibility of malignancy and the steps that are necessary for an early diagnosis of carcinoma of the breast is almost inexcusable. The responsibility involves the patient and the physician. There should be no delay on the part of the physician in diagnosing a tumor of the breast; an external and easily examined organ. In a series of 158 cases of carcinoma of the breast in the New Haven Hospital the physician was responsible for diagnosis delay in 17.5 per cent and the patient and physician in 28 per cent. Why? As above stated, the average doctor sees but two cases of cancer a year, and is not on the alert . Lack of thorough examination is a large factor. Failure to appreciate the curability of prompt adequate treatment may explain the delay in definite diagnosis.

Preventing exposure of the female breast is a phase of a routine physical examination. Exposure of the breasts is avoided by the patient, prevented by the well trained nurse and neglected by the doctor. If and when the patient complains of a lump in her breast the breast examination is made, casually or thoroughly, depending upon the individual doctor.

Primarily we should discard the classical signs and symptoms of cancer of the breast. Fixation of the tumor, pigskin or orangepeel skin, retraction of the nipple, bleeding from the nipple, palpable lymph nodes in the axilla, anemia and weight loss are all signs of advanced malignancy. Waiting and watching for the foregoing signs and symptoms may be compared to waiting for the signs and symptoms of general peritonitis before diagnosing appendicitis. Routine, systematic examination of both breasts should be carried out. First, the patient being in the sitting posture with both breasts and anterior chest uncovered, the breasts should be inspected. Observe the comparative shape, contour, asymmetry, dimpling or skin retraction. What is the relative position of the nipple? Is there fixation of the tumor, visible abrasions, ulcerations, and is there infra or supra clavicular fullness? Palpation should then be thoroughly carried out, not grasping sections of the breasts between the thumb and fingers, which is misleading, but by placing the palmar surfaces of the fingers against the breast. The foregoing having been done the same procedure should be repeated with the patient lying recumbent. A small tumor missed in the erect posture may become obvious in the recumbent position. Palpating the axillae with the arms adducted permits deep axillary examination while again axillary nodes and subpectoral metastases may become apparent when the patients arms are extended over the head. Always examine both breasts as 5 per cent of breast cancers are bilateral or become bilateral, and Handleys triangle at the sternal zyphoid should not be overlooked.

A tumor located, transillumination is a definite help in differentiation. The normal breast transilluminates well, while lactating breasts and galactocele are totally opaque. Chronic mastitis is less translucent than the normal breast. A cyst containing clear fluid is translucent, maybe clear cut and well defined. A cyst containing blood will be opaque clear cut and well defined. However, it may be a haematoma, an intra cystic papilloma or a carcinoma. Solid tumors are not as translucent as fluids and less opaque than blood.

"Any tumor or lump in the breast is malignant until proven otherwise." Therefore the tumor found should never be biopsied, but should be excised enbloc and a frozen or quick section made. The unnecessary loss of a breast is most unfortunate in any woman's life while incomplete diagnosis and the resultant inadequate treatment of a carcinomatous breast is a tragedy without comparison. Five thousand women die yearly of carcinoma of the breast. Theoretically this is unnecessary.

As before stated, when a lump or tumor is found in the breast, that lump is malignant until proven otherwise. The family history and particularly the breast history should be traced. Age is very important in the diagnosis of breast tumors.

Fibro ademenoma is one of the common benign tumors. It is a fibrous tumor, rounded, firm, freely movable, and transilluminates poorly. It occurs in young people in the 'teen age and may go on into the twenties. If not removed it may ultimately become a sarcoma. Sarcoma of the breast is always preceded by a tumor and that tumor is a fibro adenoma.

The second non malignant tumor to be considered is the cyst. Cysts rarely occur in women under 30. In Adair's series, cysts occurred between the ages of 30 and 52. They are, generally speaking, premenopausal, usually not solitary and are difficult diagnostic problems. The large cyst is encapsulated, freely movable, transilluminates in sharp outline and is non-adherent. Too frequently, however, what seems to be a solitary cyst is only a part of cystic disease of the breast and on section numerous minute cysts will be seen even microscopically. On microscopic examination chronic mastitis is associated with malignancy in 50 per cent of cases. Clinical diagnosis alone is therefore incomplete.

Localized mastitis must always be considered in early diagnosis of carcinoma of the breast. It is a most difficult differential problem. Within an area of localized mastitis there may be an early carcinoma. On the other hand the lumpy, shotty breasts of chronic diffuse mastitis infrequently become malignant.

Tuberculosis of the breast is a possibility and is always associated with a sinus (Adair). Syphilis of the breast in the form of gumma may be a rare confusing problem.

Traumatic fat necrosis is another problem which cannot be decided clinically with assurance. There is usually a history of trauma which frequently accompanies carcinoma. There is skin attachment and nipple retraction. The inflammatory signs are helpful but not diagnostic.

A haematoma following trauma may stimulate malignancy. Its progressive decrease in size, tenderness, associated with definite opacity on transillumination may rule out malignancy. On the other hand trauma to the breast may disrupt the equilibrium of a pre-cancerous lesion into active malignancy. Of clinically benign breast tumors, 11.2 per cent are malignant while 5 per cent of clinically malignant tumors are benign.

These and other benign lesions may become malignant or perhaps they were originally malignant. The only real evidence of cancer is the presence of living, growing, invading cells outside their normal boundaries. The average age incidence of carcinoma of the breast is 50. Anyone over 60 having a lump in the breast has a malignancy in 75 per cent of instances. However, this age incidence is in reality the end results of a process beginning years before and breast carcinoma is the most common cause of a lump in the breast of non lactating women over 25. Therefore, the greater frequency of mammary carcinoma in later life is of no diagnostic significance. By this same token, the infrequency of mammary carcinoma under 30, 9 per cent, is of no diagnostic significance.

Carcinoma originates at some minute point where it should be diagnosed before it invades or metastasizes. The growth spread is affected by the age of the patient, the presence of pregnancy or lactation and possible intercurrent disease such as diabetes mellitus.

A search should always be made for evidence of spread and metastases. The axillary space, infra and supra clavicular regions are routinely observed. The chest should be x-rayed, the spine examined and any pain or skeletal complaint investigated. In 423 autopsies following carcinoma of the breasts, 50 per cent had pleural involvement and 49.9 per cent showed lung involvement. Mammary carcinoma is the most common cause of bone metastases in women (26-74 per cent). The liver is the most frequently invaded organ and should be considered accordingly.

Prompt radical mastectomy is the treatment indicated following the microscopical diagnosis of malignancy. The most radical excision of the growth is alone productive of good results. Theoretically pre-operative irradiation has its place although breast cancers as a whole are radio resistant. Practically the necessary time loss of at least two months permits dissemination of the malignancy during this waiting period in addition to the increased surgical difficulty following irradiation. Pre-operative x-ray has not been used at the Mayo Clinic in nine years. Dr. Frank Lahey states, "We have not used pre-operative x-ray in our clinic." Adair says,

"To our mind this phase of this controversial problem of the value of pre-operative irradiation is definitely settled." Radical mastectomy is the treatment indicated and when radical mastectomy is designated it means fundamentally the Halstead operation. The tumor should occupy the center of the operative field regardless of the location of the tumor. Wide removal of skin and all the excised tissues should be removed in one block. Both pectoral muscles must be removed and unless the pectoralis minor is removed completely, adequate exposure of the axilla is hampered. The axillary contents are removed carefully but thoroughly as part of the complete block. An incomplete radical mastectomy is not a radical mastectomy.

When is carcinoma of the breast inoperable? When there is fixation of the mass to the ribs or sternum. Involvement of the supraclavicular nodes is evidence of spread beyond surgical control. Fixation of axillary nodes is a contraindication remembering that palpable axillary nodes may be inflammatory. The signs of acute fulminating disease contraindicate surgery and distant metastases make operability a false hope. Constitutional contraindications are of significance not to be neglected.

Irradiation of the ovaries should be done in all cases of inoperable and metastatic carcinoma when the patient has not passed the menopause.

To conclude this brief resume, the first statement is repeated—'Carcinoma is one of the most curable of diseases." Early diagnosis and prompt proper treatment is the only solution of this scourge on humanity. A most radical excision of the growth is alone productive of good results. X-ray and radium have their place as a phophylactic measure as post-operative irradiation, and in palliative administration. We must educate the patient. We cannot educate the patient unless we ourselves are persistently on the alert for the early and curable malignancy of the breast.

DISCUSSION

J. H. ROBINSON, M.D.

OKLAHOMA CITY, OKLAHOMA

Dr. Stanbro has given an up-to-date interpretation of the subject, "Carcinoma of the Breast." So far as I am concerned, I can think of no important points which he omitted. His line of thinking in general runs parallel to mine.

Early in his discussion he states that carcinoma of the breast is curable. There is just one way of curing this disease; that is, radical surgical removal. He makes the statement that 11 per cent of tumors that are benign clinically prove to be malignant after removal. This stimulates our feeling that any lump in the breast in a woman over 30 years of age may be serious.

He states that a biopsy should not be made. So far as I can remember I have never done a biopsy on the breast. By this I mean that I have never taken a section from a tumor and sent it to the laboratory for microscopic examination. I always enucleate the tumor, cutting widely around it, and sent the entire tumor to the laboratory.

I believe very much in his recommended method of examination; that is, as to posture. Any examination of the breast is not complete until the patient has been in at least a sitting and a lying position. Sometimes I am unable to find the tumor when the patient is sitting on the examining table, but when the patient lies down the skin will be bulging sufficiently that its position can be seen from across the room.

Dr. Stanbro has discussed the place of x-ray therapy in this disease and it seems to me it is not necessary to further discuss this subject. I note in the Lahey Clinic volume which was recently published that in discussing this subject they state they have never used x-ray therapy there, and for that reason are not prepared to discuss it. I am speaking of pre-operative irradiation. After operation is completed for a period of ten days to two weeks I am convinced that x-ray therapy should be used for the purpose of retarding the growth should any be left in the field. I believe it does retard the growth and has a definite beneficial result. At least it causes a delayed action and perhaps we may get an occasional cure that we would not get otherwise.

I was interested in the statement made in the Lahey Clinic volume that they figure the five-year cures only as survivals. In the checkup periods they speak of three, five and seven year survivals instead of the older way of three, five and seven year cures. This, I believe, is a more suitable way of speaking of the condition.

There is one important point that Dr. Stanbro made which I believe is not generally understood and that is that carcinoma is more frequent in nulliparous women than in women who have had pregnancies. I have the feeling that many physicians have indulged sense of security when the old maid school teacher, or the clerk in the dry goods store who has never had a pregnancy appeared with a tumor in the breast. According to statistics which Dr. Stanbro quoted this feeling was not justified.

The fact is that we should be more concerned when the single woman of the third or fourth decade presents herself with a tumor of the breast. Because the breast has not functioned as a lactating breast or has

not been physiologically active, seems to pave the way for malignant growth.

I thank you very kindly for an opportunity to discuss this paper.

The Child in the War Time Local Health Program*

GLIDDEN L. BROOKS, M.D.

CITY-COUNTY HEALTH DEPARTMENT

MUSKOGEE, OKLAHOMA

Attention to child health is recognized in general terms as an integral and important part of any well planned local health program. However, the shift of local health activities into wartime operation has in many units been accomplished by sufficient clashing of gears to obscure or confuse the precise place this function should occupy in the accelerated or decelerated program. This change in pace is alluded to advisedly, since Health Units in centers of war production or military contonments are confronted with a sudden influx of health problems whereas the districts not involved in large war enterprises find themselves faced with need for retrenchment occasioned by loss of departmental personnel and shrinkage of population. Obviously, the greatest adjustment needs be made in the former and it is with the children in communities feeling the impact of war activity that we are primarily concerned. We shall discuss the problem from the standpoint of a local health officer faced with such an adaption.

The attitude of the local health officer toward the child health phase of his work is one of respect and attention. The place of school children, pre-school children, and immunization procedures in a normal health department set up is well known and has been reasonably clearly defined in all Public Health texts. Its importance as an entering wedge into community cooperation has never been under-emphasized. Children, as a group, present a particularly significant base on which to build a general health program. First, because of all groups, they are the most susceptible to control, particularly through the medium of the schools. Second, they present a receptive and more or less organized target for educational projects and third, the results of health efforts are more readily perceptible and an increment of work in this group is apt to produce the most

measurable results. What, if any, revision of the health officer's attitude should take place in the altered situation?

It is well, as a starting point, to appraise, dispassionately, the status of the child in wartime. His "rights" like those of his elders, of necessity suffer curtailment and a transition from the ultimately ideal to the immediately practical. It is these latter practicalities that may be lost sight of in the face of more pressing needs. First, the fact remains that, although the physician health officer may view the child unemotionally, his parents can't and possibly should not. For this reason, the preventable illness, however slight, of a child constitutes a ponderable cause of lost man-hours on the part of his parents' war effort and, at the least, results in reduced efficiency. A worker with a sick child at home is only half a worker. Secondly, war effort is calling an increasing number of mothers away from home and is depriving the child of teachers, nurses, and other sources of care and security. Thirdly, (to be mentioned at the risk of being reviled as a dreamer) the place of todays child in the post-war world is one of unquestioned responsibility. Nothing is more short sighted than to talk of "winning the peace" as an inheritance without giving like consideration to insuring that the heirs will be capable of receiving it.

An illustration of the numerical status of children in one type of war community may be drawn from the population figures in Mayes County, site of the Oklahoma Ordnance Works, an active war industry employing some 6,000 workers which suddenly burgeoned in the midst of a quiet and predominantly agricultural section of the state. This area has absorbed the initial impact of thousands of construction workers engaged in building the plant and, for the three months prior to the date of these figures, had seen a shift from construction to operations work. This has meant a gradually diminishing pop-

*Read before the Annual Meeting held in Oklahoma City, May 11-12, 1943.

ulation from the construction peak and also a growing predominance of a relatively more stable and permanent population, who, unlike the migratory construction workers, tend to bring their families and function as a component of the community.

In the 1940 census, the population of the county was 21,668. In December 1942, the estimated population was 25,336. This included 6,276 school children and 2,658 of preschool age, a total of 8,934 children representing 35.3 per cent of the entire population. The bulk of the increase was absorbed by three towns adjacent to the plant. A further in-migration of operations personnel is anticipated with the completion of several large housing projects. An inkling as to the effect of this movement on the child population may be gained from the results of a questionnaire answered by a one-fourth sample of the Oklahoma Ordnance Works employees in which the ratio of preschool to school children in the families was found to be 1:1. This increase in the younger children might have been predicted from the fact that this productive labor element represents a relatively young group of adults. A similar trend might be expected wherever in-migration for war work is taking place. It must be pointed out that these figures are obtained by estimates and are accurate only as cross-sectional impressions of a group in a state of flux.

For these reasons, as soon as the urgent problems of environmental sanitation and emergency protection of the war-swollen population are brought under control, the child health program should occupy the paramount status. Its only possible rival (and this only in certain types of war areas) is the venereal disease control program.

An asset which the Health Officer has available in creating a constructive program is one which may also be a source of confusion unless firmly controlled. By this, I mean the multitude of agencies at the national, state and local level, which are interested in the whole problem of children or in its special phases. Examples of these are the Children's Bureau, Crippled Childrens Commission, Infantile Paralysis Commission, State Health Department, 4-H Clubs, Womens Clubs, Schools and Child Welfare

Agencies. Some of these work through the local health department while others carry on their activities independently. If carefully coordinated in a county, the sum of these forces constitutes a powerful influence. Uncoordinated, there is usually ample opportunity for duplication and waste of effort. Whether the health department should take the lead in this coordination or merely serve as a cooperating agency is a question which is obviously dependent on local conditions and involves, usually, the unregimentable factor of personality.

Probably the greatest single hurdle which is encountered in establishing a satisfactory child health program in a war-active community is the intense pre-occupation of the public, both as individuals and as a community, with the actual business of war production. Added to this is the inevitable concentration of effort in exploitation of newly found opportunities for launching and enlarging gainful commercial enterprises. This is especially conspicuous in areas frequented by military personnel. This trend often limits community support of a health program to lip service alone. Add to this the current transportation difficulties and the burden of overworked teachers, nurses, and welfare workers and the obstacle becomes more impressive. Here again, the adjustment lands squarely on the Health Officer's shoulders and needs to be made on an individual community level. As usual, the mothers in the community constitute the most available avenue of approach.

An effective child health program must of necessity be a long range program if results are to be commensurate with the efforts expended. This must be reconciled to the need for a certain volume of emergency activity involving the children of transients. Here an organization of reporting and recording on the state or national level which provides for transfer of children from clinic to clinic in a manner analogous to the present handling of venereal disease patients would perhaps be of value. This is particularly applicable to children in the process of being immunized against contagious diseases.

With these normal and abnormal factors in mind it is well to consider a broad outline of what might be deemed a reasonable wartime program for a county. This resolves itself under four general categories, listed in order of what might be their "emergency" significance.

PREVENTION OF CONTAGION

Concomitant with environmental sanitation, a massive immunization program is essential to minimize the increased possibilities of epidemics. Initially, this may be aimed particularly at the migratory group, but should be continued through the more stable community groups. Intensification of routine reporting and quarantine functions of the department is likewise called for. Additional support for this phase of the program is often available through the authorities responsible for the war production or military establishment concerned.

NUTRITION

The nationwide interest in nutrition which now exists provides an opportunity for the health officer to step beyond the usual "cod liver oil and orange juice" limitations of his efforts in this important field. Here the above mentioned function of cooperating with other agencies is especially applicable. In addition to assuring the provision of nourishing foods to children, it is also within the province of the Health Department to aid in securing a safe food supply. The logical starting point here seems to be in the field of milk and water sanitation.

HEALTH EDUCATION

Because of the preoccupation of adult groups with the more immediate business of war, the educational phases of a health department must be directed in increasing volume towards the child. Here the obstacle of overloaded school facilities looms large. The use of recreational and extra-school programs sponsored by 4-H clubs, Scouts ,and such organizations provides a means of partially bridging this gap. Even so, it is here that a wartime program is in the greatest danger of frustration. Obligatory inclusion of a workable health education scheme in school curricula is needed.

FINDING AND CORRECTING DEFECTS

This important category is mentioned last for two reasons. First, it is the most susceptible to postponement in the face of an emergency and second, only too often this comprises almost the sole child health activity of a local health department. The increased press of activity in a wartime situation magnifies the need for the Health Officer carefully to appraise the results of previous efforts in this category. He may then decide for himself whether the situation in his county lends itself better to wholesale examinations of children with the view to stimulating the maximum number of corrections or whether it is more productive to concentrate

on the groups of individuals most badly in need of attention and most likely to get it if sufficient energy is expended. On the whole, even in emergency situations, it seems better to concentrate on the child as a individual rather than to attempt wholesale methods, impressive in the annual report but questionable as to actual results.

A review of the four point program shows it to be applicable in many instances to the Health Program as a whole, including both children and adults. A fifth category is worthy of emphasis in the adult field and should be mentioned because of its ramifications in the sphere of child hygiene. This is the control of "Social Diseases" which may include venereal disease, tuberculosis and malaria.

These thoughts are presented not as an answer to the problem of child health in war time, but rather as a stimulus to more constructive attempts to integrate a predominant peace time pursuit into a wartime life. Most of our counties faced with the problem of boom conditions are just now approaching the status where the immediate control measures are under way and such a reorganization of thinking and effort may constitute the next step in the program. Indeed, changing trends may invalidate most of these preliminary impressions and call for more drastic revisions of policy. One fact, however, seems clear—that the normal local health program must be altered to fit the tempo of today's changes.

DISCUSSION
C. W. ARRENDELL, M.D.
PONCA CITY, OKLAHOMA

A careful study of Dr. Brooks' essay on "The Child in the Local War-Time Health Program" reveals a complete outline for a Public Health Program which is both timely and practical.

Dr. Brooks points out that children comprise more than one-third of the total population in a typical war industry area in Northeastern Oklahoma. Health officers as well as physicians in civilian practice should realize the importance of this figure and should be gratified to recognize the significance of schools as a medium of contact and control. Parents, particularly mothers, tend to cooperate better and to give more attention to the welfare of their children than to other phases of public health endeavors. Thus the schools, with the aid of teachers, nurses, and Parent-Teachers' Associations serve as an entering wedge into general community of "Environmental sanitation and emergency protection."

Many mothers are engaged at present in industrial work, but they nevertheless seek intelligent advice and help in the care of their children. Here physicians in civilian practice must cooperate with the health officer to obtain the optimum in physical and moral development.

Some of the difficulties which the health officer may encounter in establishing a child-health program are set forth:

First: A large per cent of the population in industrial areas is transient and therefore lacks civic pride.

Second: Crowded living conditions and transportation problems retard the program.

Third: Both industrial workers and the citizen population are over-burdened with additional work and responsibilities.

Dr. Brooks makes no mention of a fourth obstacle that is probably the most difficult with which he has to deal. Namely, the attitude of county medical organization as well as that of physicians in private practice, is often not only one of indifference but amounts sometimes to absolute rejection.

The four-point program suggested by Dr. Brooks as a "Reasonable war-time health program" is not only very practical, but may be used as the basis of the health program as a whole. His program consists of:

1. Prevention of contagion.
2. Nutrition.
3. Health education.
4. Finding and correcting defects.

A program for the prevention of contagious and infectious diseases in itself would require a wide application of knowledge and experience pertaining to sanitation in general. Nutrition and Health education provide the Health Officer an opportunity for teaching and stabilizing the various and confusing concepts that universally exist.

The finding of defects requires much time and great tact, especially in organizing the community facilities to better carry on this project. After defects have been found, a follow-up to explain and urge correction is extremely important. I would emphasize the addition of the control of Social Diseases to the Four-Point program, as it is so often an integral part of child hygiene.

Since the personality and ability of health officers varies and since the requirements of communities differ, the exact mode of procedure may follow only the broad outline as set forth. However, Dr. Brooks would have the health officer accept the entire responsibility of bringing into relative harmony all the factors necessary for the effective consummation of the program.

The RH Factor Its Relation to Erythroblastosis Foetalis and Transfusion Accidents*

DAVID J. UNDERWOOD, M.D.

TULSA, OKLAHOMA

This paper is presented as a review of some of the recent literature on the Rh Factor of human blood, showing its relationship to the cause of Erythroblastosis Foetalis and its bearing on some of the heretofore unexplained intra-group transfusion reactions—with such unhappy end results.

In 1940, Landsteiner and Wiener[1] reported on an agglutinin developed in rabbits by injecting blood from the Macacus Rhesus monkey. When tested with human bloods, this agglutinin demonstrated the presence of a new substance in human red blood cells—called the Rh Factor (Rhesus Factor). About 86 per cent of human bloods contain this factor (Rh-Positive) and 14 per cent do not (Rh-Negative).

Present knowledge[2] of the Rh Factor can be summed up as follows:

1. It is an antigenic substance in human blood cells similar in some ways to other previously discovered antigenic factors; the most important of which are those known as A, B, M, and N.

2. It is inherited as a Mendelian dominant, as are the others.

3. It occurs only in red blood cells, resembling in this respect the factors M and N, but differing from A and B, which occur in the tissues and secretions of some persons.

4. There are no normal agglutinins against the Rh Factor in man, again resembling in this respect the factors M and N, while such agglutions are present normally against A and B. On the other hand—when blood containing the Rh Factor (Rh-Positive) is introduced into a person without it, agglutinins may develop against it; while they never develop blood containing the M and N Factors is injected into persons without these factors in their blood.

5. The Rh Factor has isoimmunizing ability while M and N factors lack it. That is

*Read before the Annual Meeting held in Oklahoma City, May 11-12, 1943.

why the M and N factors are of no signifi-cance in blood transfusions.

Soon after the discovery of the Rh Factor, Wiener and Peters studied the blood of pa-tients who had hemolytic reactions after one or more previous uneventful transfusions of blood of the correct group. The serums of these patients contained atypical isoagglutin-ins which clumped blood with the Rh Factor. These serums behaved in a like manner as did the serums of the rabbits immunized with monkey blood. The blood of these patients did not contain the Rh Factor. They ex-plained the presence of the atypical agglutin-ins in the patients by assuming that Rh-Positive blood was given to them during one or several transfusions which they had re-ceived previously. The fact that they did not possess the Rh Factor in their own blood made it possible for the injected Rh-Posi-tive blood to act as an antigen and to stimu-late production of anti-Rh agglutinins. After these agglutinins developed, Rh-Positive blood was not suitable for these patients, even if the donors belonged to the identical blood groups. The administration of Rh-Positive blood was followed by a hemolytic reaction .

It was found that patients manifesting hemolytic reactions following one or several previous uneventful transfusion of blood of the correct group, were, as a rule, Rh-Neg-ative and that some of them had anti-Rh agglutinins in their blood, that the donors were Rh-Positive, and that Rh-Negative blood could be subsequently administered without untoward reactions.

The same mechanism was found to be re-sponsible for reactions after first transfu-sions given to pregnant women.

Here the development of the negative ag-glutinins (anti-Rh) was explained by the presence of the Rh Factor in the blood of the fetus, to whom it was transmitted by the father and by its passage through the pla-centa to the mother, who was thus immun-ized during pregnancy. Levine[3], et al, first suggested that erythroblastosis foetalis may be due to such a mechanism.

Here the cycle of events goes further than the production of anti-Rh agglutinins in the mother. These anti-Rh agglutinins formed in the blood of the mother pass through the placenta from the mother to the fetus; enter the fetal circulation and by their continued action on the Rh-Positive fetal red blood cells, produce erythroblastosis foetalis. The correctness of this hypothesis is based on the assumption of, at least, four conditions;

1. The father must have the Rh Factor in his blood, in order to trasmit it to the fetus.

2. The fetus must have the inherited Rh factor in his blood.

3. The mother must lack the Rh Factor in her blood in order to develop the anti-Rh ag-glutinins.

4. There must be a free exchange of anti-genic substances and of antibodies through the placenta from the fetus to mother and vice versa.

The fulfillment of the fourth condition can be taken for granted—the passage of protein substances from the fetus to the mother and of antibodies from the mother to fetus has been satisfactorily demonstrated.

Levine tested the first three conditions by a study of the blood of 153 mothers of in-fants with erythroblastosis, of whom only 7 per cent were Rh-Positive and 93 per cent Rh-Negative. This is almost the reverse from the findings of 1035 controls of random population, in which 86 per cent were Rh-Positive, and 14 per cent Rh-Negative. All husbands were Rh-Positive and 99 per cent of all the erythroblastosis infants were Rh-Positive. The absence of the Rh Factor in one infant with erythroblastosis and the presence of the Rh Factor in 8 per cent of mothers of erythroblastosis infants, indi-cated that there are other factors involved in the pathogenesis of erythroblastosis besides the Rh Factor, but these facts do not dis-prove the concept of isommunization as a cause of the disease.

Three types of Erythroblastosis Foetalis[4] are generally recognized, namely:

1. Hemolytic anemia, which is the mildest form.

2. Icterus gravis, which is more serious.

3. Universal fetal hydrops, which is sel-dom compatible with independent life.

These infants are often lethargic and ex-hausted, although early they may appear es-sentially normal. The symptoms may develop rapidly, depending on the rate of blood destruction. Petechial hemorrhages may oc-cur; the heart is often enlarged; the pulse rapid and weak; liver and spleen are en-larged in most cases. Deposition of blood pigment in localized areas of the brain may result in a nuclear jaundice, causing death in the first few days of life, or symptoms may appear later.

Henderson[5] has reported three cases which seem to belong to a fourth type not previous-ly described, in which hydramnios is common and intrauterine death occurs some time be-fore delivery.

Fetuses of this type show little or no edema; are severely macerated, and have diffuse hepatic cirrhosis and splenomegaly, This new type is the most severe manifesta-tion of the disease, with the possible ex-ception of cases of earlier intra-uterine death resulting in miscarriage.

Degenerative changes in the Parenchymal

cells of the liver, some times amounting to actual necrosis, are a common feature in icterus gravis and hydrops foetalis. Cirrhosis is also is common in infants with icterus gravis who die after a few weeks of life, but is only occasionally seen when death occurs earlier.

In two infants who died of icterus gravis within two days of birth, a fine diffuse intercellular cirrhosis was noted, and portal cirrhosis was observed in a few cases.

The pronounced degree of hepatic cirrhosis in the severely macerated fetuses proves that erythroblastosis may run a long intra-uterine course. This type of disease bears a close superficial resemblance to congenital syphilis, but closer examination of the fetus and placenta renders differentiation easy.

It is regrettable that such a common fetal and neo-natal disease as erythroblastosis is not generally recognized. The more severe types are still usually regarded as congenital syphilis, and the unfortunate mothers are condemned as syphilitics, despite negative serological reactions.

The Rh Factor and the isoimmunization theory has some very practical applications particularly as regards transfusions. Experience reveals that the Rh Factor is a good antigen in Rh-Negative individuals, i.e., either by repeated transfusions or in Rh-Negative women who may be immunized by the Rh-Positive fetus, and actually, pregnancy provides a far better antigen sitmulus than repeated transfusions do.

For the prevention of these reactions, the most important single measure is the selection of Rh-Negative donors for Rh-Negative patients. Special care should be exercised in transfusing women who have recently delivered erythroblastic infants, unexplained dead fetuses, past history of stillborns, neonatal deaths and transfusion reactions. Particularly in emergencies involving the recently delivered woman with a dead fetus, it is far safer to use pooled plasma, rather than blood transfusion unless the bloods can be thoroughly tested.

Once an Rh-Negative donor is selected for an Rh-Negative recipient, a direct cross matching test must be carried out. It is assumed, of course, that the blood groups of donor and patient are compatible. It is re-commended that the patient's serum be incubated with donor's cell suspension at 37° for fifteen to thirty minutes, and that the mixture then be centrifuged at low speed and the sediment re-suspended for the final reading.

It is well known that many afflicted infants with severe anemia recover following numerous blood transfusions. There is some theoretic basis for the suggestion that these infants preferably receive the blood of Rh-Negative donors. Obviously the infants own Rh-Positive, or any other Rh-Positive blood is subject to the hemolytic process which, for one or another reasons still continues in the early neo-natal period. In a small number of cases it was observed for longer intervals than Rh-Positive blood. Actually, the hemoglobin and red blood cells are maintained at higher levels and at the same time there is a remarkable improvement in the clinical condition of the infant. The anti-Rh agglutinins which might be still present in the baby's serum would hemolyze the Rh-Positive cells the baby recieved by transfusion. In at least one instance the use of mother's blood (of compatible blood group) which contained potent anti-Rh aggulutinins resulted in hemolysis of the infant's blood as evidenced by a rise in temperature, increased jaundice and hemoglobinuria.

A third example of the practical application of this principle is in the Rh-Negative patient (any Rh-Negative patient—about 14 per cent of the population) who must receive repeated transfusions over a period of weeks or months. Such patient must be protected from possible isoimmunization through receiving blood repeatedly from Rh-Positive donors. Any early transfusion might stimulate anti-Rh agglutinins and these in turn would hemolyze Rh-Positive blood cells given the patient in subsequent transfusions. It is probable that these anti-Rh agglutinins are responsible for about 90 per cent of all intra-group transfusion accidents after repeated transfusions, or in pregnancy at the first transfusion.

From these findings, one may conclude that the cause of most cases of erythroblastosis foetalis can be explained by the isoimmunization of the mother by the Rh-Positive fetus, and that 90 per cent of the transfusion accidents in the heretofore compatible group may be avoided by the practical application of the isoimmunizing theory.

BIBLIOGRAPHY

1. Landsteiner, Karl and Weiner, Alexander S.: Studies on an Agglutinogen (Rh) in Human Blood Reacting with Anti-Rhesus Sera and with Human Isobodies. Journal of Experimental Medicine, Vol. 74, page 309. October 1, 1939.
2. Davidson, I. and Toharsky, B.: The Blood Factor on Antigenic Analysis, American Jour. of Clinical Path., Vol. 12, page 454. August, 1942.
3. Levine, Phillip: The Pathogenesis of Fetal Erythroblastosis. N. Y. State Jour. of Med., Vol. 42, page 1928. October 15, 1942.
4. Abt, Isaac: Yearbook of Pediatrics, page 207. 1942.
5. Henderson, J. L.: A Fourth Type of Erythroblastosis Foetalis showing Hepatic Cirrhosis in the Macerated Fetus. Report of Three Cases. Archives of Diseases in Childhood, Vol. 17, page 49. March, 1942.
6. Sinclair, F. D.: Transfusion Accidents and Isoimmunization Rh Factor. Jour. Okla. State Med. Ass'n., Vol. 85, page 286. July, 1942.

A SALUTE TO PHYSICIANS IN WAR-TIME*

In this world struggle for the freedom and happiness of mankind there are many factors that are having a part in bringing victory to the Allies—the farmer, the factory worker, the engineer, the sailor, the marine and the nurse, the administrator, the transporter of men and material, the morale builder and the news reporter.

Without detracting one iota from the glory that all these and others are entitled to, this is a salute to the physicians of America, for their names should be placed high on the war-time service roll of honor.

Among the 130 million citizens of the United States, there are around 150,000 physicians who are battling disease, repairing human damage and saving life. To-day these physicians are meeting their responsibilities to the public as never before they have gone out in large numbers as a part of our military forces to the four corners of the world. They are doing their job in the front lines, in the air, on the sea, under the water and on the land. They are meeting the medical problems of the frozen north and of the tropical jungle. They are working relentlessly at the casualty stations, in the hospitals and in the military camps. At home, besides their usual work, they are filling in the gaps made by their comrades who have joined the military forces. These physicians are crowding the production of new doctors; they are in public health work, in industry; they are manning the reception hospitals; they are guiding medical research; they are general practitioners, and specialists. They are community servants of the highest order.

These physicians are carrying on successfully with whatever equipment and supplies are at hand. They are applying the new knowledge in medicine with astonishing results. The hours of service of the physician are limited only by his strength to carry on. Many of these physicians are young, catapulted into situations that involve grave responsibilities; others are at an age when they deserve a reduction in their professional load, but they are all carrying on in a fashion that brings pride and joy to everyone.

These professional men and women are doing a grand job, from the home front to the outposts of this world conflict. They are keeping our fighting forces up to par, salvaging the injured, and staving off epidemics. They are saving life and preserving mental strength.

Again, we salute them!

*Bulletin of Lederle Laboratories. Volume XI, No. 1, November, 1943. Page 3.

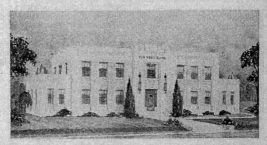

• THE PRESIDENT'S PAGE •

The annual meeting of The Oklahoma State Medical Association will be held in Tulsa, April 24-26, at the Mayo Hotel. The exhibit space was all sold a few days after announcement of the meeting date was made. This shows the interest that the pharmaceutical firms, the medical book publishers, the supply houses and others have in our Association and in the medical profession generally. Their interest is not all selfish—they are genuinely our friends and necessary partners in our duty to best serve the health needs of our people. Take time enough to adequately inspect the exhibits of these friends of ours and to become acquainted with the representatives of our exhibitors.

The scientific program is nearly complete at this writing, and promises to be an outstanding one. So many of us are now interested in learning more of industrial medicine, and more of tropical diseases which may concern us in the post-war era. These subjects may be fully discussed at this meeting.

The Tulsa County Medical Society is proud to act as host to our Association and is planning to make your visit a personal pleasure as well as scientifically beneficial. Its offices, including a medical library worth crossing the State to see, will be open for your inspection. The hospitals of the city will be more than pleased to have you visit them. Those interested in the recent epidemic of acute anterior poliomyelitis may inspect the facilities used to combat this malady in the acute stage.

To those of you who are close to physicians in the Armed Forces, please extend the sincere desire of our Association that they attend as guests. Many of these men are members of other state associations but would welcome the opportunity of being with us.

We all have a duty to attend this Convention—a duty to ourselves, our patients and to our members in the Armed Forces who expect us to keep intact, until they return, the practice of medicine as they knew it.

James Stevenson

President.

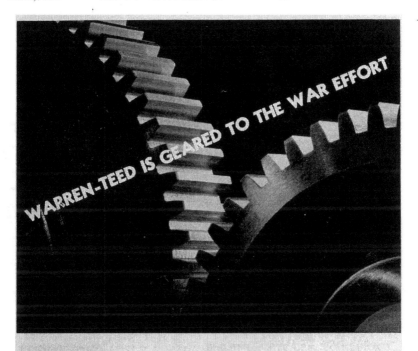

The JOURNAL Of The
OKLAHOMA STATE MEDICAL ASSOCIATION

EDITORIAL BOARD
L. J. MOORMAN, Oklahoma City, Editor-in-Chief
E. EUGENE RICE, Shawnee   NED R. SMITH, Tulsa
MR. R. H. GRAHAM, Oklahoma City, Business Manager
(Serving in the Armed Forces)

CONTRIBUTIONS: Articles accepted by this Journal for publication including those read at the annual meetings of the State Association are the sole property of this Journal.

The Editorial Department is not responsible for the opinions expressed in the original articles of contributors.

Manuscripts may be withdrawn by authors for publication elsewhere only upon the approval of the Editorial Board.

MANUSCRIPTS: Manuscripts should be typewritten, double-spaced, on white paper 8½ x 11 inches. The original copy, not the carbon copy, should be submitted.

Footnotes, bibliographies and legends for cuts should be typed on separate sheets in double space. Bibliography listing should follow this order: Name of author, title of article, name of periodical with volume, page and date of publication.

Manuscripts are accepted subject to the usual editorial revisions and with the understanding that they have not been published elsewhere.

NEWS: Local news of interest to the medical profession, changes of address, births, deaths and weddings will be gratefully received.

ADVERTISING: Advertising of articles, drugs or compounds unapproved by the Council on Pharmacy of the A.M.A. will not be accepted. Advertising rates will be supplied on application.

It is suggested that members of the State Association patronize our advertisers in preference to others.

SUBSCRIPTIONS: Failure to receive The Journal should call for immediate notification.

REPRINTS: Reprints of original articles will be supplied at actual cost provided request for them is attached to manuscripts or made in sufficient time before publication. Checks for reprints should be made payable to Industrial Printing Company, Oklahoma City.

Address all communications to THE JOURNAL OF THE OKLAHOMA STATE MEDICAL ASSOCIATION, 210 Plaza Court, Oklahoma City. (3)

OFFICIAL PUBLICATION OF THE OKLAHOMA STATE MEDICAL ASSOCIATION
Copyrighted January, 1944

EDITORIALS

A GOOD EXAMPLE:
GOVERNMENT MEDICINE A FAILURE

Since it is the editorial policy of this Journal to oppose government control of medicine to the last ditch, it seems fitting that we should call attention to the government's failure in one particular field of medical management. This is an exceedingly sad story not only because of much unnecessary suffering, with morbidity and mortality rates excessively high when compared with private management, but because the free movement of the patient, under the rules and regulations, created centers of infection which never should have existed, thus greatly increasing the incidence of disease and causing untold suffering and sorrow. Though the spiritual and physical values greatly outweigh all other considerations, the financial loss to the tax-payers and private individuals is stupendous. We refer to the tuberculous veterans of World War No. I who were provided for by the government through the Veterans' Bureau, later the Veterans' Administration.

Good doctors and every facility for adequate care plus generous pensions were made available. But as often happens, good intentions were thwarted because of the complicated set-up with varied interests and divided authority. Instead of a simple, effective partnership with mutual understanding and a vital spirit of cooperation which tends to hold the most thoughtless and unruly in line, there was a lack of authority on the part of physicians and administrators which, coupled with the patients freedom to go and come at will, often created a spirit of antagonism.

No doubt everyone connected with the Veterans' Administration wanted to do as much as possible for the tuberculous veterans. The laws, rules and regulations governing the care of these veterans have made proper discipline and cooperation virtually impossible; the provisions for pensions and payments for home care often causes the patient to consider it financially advantgeous to turn to home no matter how adequate the institutional care provided by the government may be.

In the December issue of The American Journal of Public Health[1], Louis I. Dublin, has presented this subject with convincing authority. We quote his figures in order that the true situation may be clearly understood.

"In spite of the extraordinary development of the services for tuberculous veterans, the experience of the veterans' hospitals has been unfavorable. Thus, in 1942, of the 9,854 cases discharged from these hospitals, only 1.9 per cent were designated 'arrested' at discharge; only 0.3 per cent 'apparently arrested,' and only 0.8 per cent 'quiescent.' If we combine these three categories, the fact emerges that only 3 per cent of the patients discharged during the year were medically rehabilitated. The remainder of the cases were discharged as 'condition improved' 32.7 per cent; 'condition unimproved' 28.9 per cent; 'dead' 19.5 per cent; and 'condition not stated' 16.0 per cent. It is clear that the vast majority of the patients discharged were not yet ready to be released to civilian life. The so-called 'improved' cases represent, for the most part, patients with unstable lesions. As a matter of fact, a very large proportion of them left without authorization or consent. Thus, the Veterans' Administration itself classified the hospitalization of 58 per cent of the cases as 'incomplete'. The 1942 figures on condition at discharge from the Veterans' hospitals are rather typical, somewhat worse but not greatly different from those of earlier years. At no time since 1929, when the present type of report of the Veterans' Administration began, has the total for the 'arrested', 'apparently arrested' and 'quiescent' reached 6 per cent.

"Admittedly, one cannot make exact comparisons among various sanatoria as to results of treatment on the basis of crude figures of this type. This is particularly true now, for with the passage of the years, the usual case admitted to the veterans' hospitals is of the chronic type common among middle aged and older persons. Thus, of recent admissions, only 4 per cent were 'incipient' cases, 22 per cent were 'moderately advanced', and 74 per cent were 'far advanced'. With all due allowance for this fact, there is a painful contrast between these recent figures (as well as those of earlier years) and the results obtained in well managed state, municipal, and private sanatoria. Thus, in a country-wide survey of tuberculosis hospitals and sanatoria in the United States during 1933-1934, made by the American Medical Association, patients with tuberculosis 'arrested', 'apparently arrested', or 'quiescent' on discharge, accounted for 29 per cent of the total discharged. A survey of discharges from the Michigan State sanatoria from 1930 to 1934, also showed a high proportion of cases in these three categories— 61 per cent of the total discharged. The experience of the Mount McGregor Sanatorium of the Metropolitan Life Insurance Company for males discharged between 1919 and 1936, and excluding incipient cases, showed that

48 per cent, or practically half of the cases, were 'arrested', 'apparently arrested', or 'quiescent' on discharge; and even for the cases far advanced on admission, this proportion was 34 per cent."

Dr. Dublin points out the fact that legislators and others interested in the welfare of the veterans were not apprised of the fundamental requirements for effective management and did not provide for the necessary hospital restrictions but permitted them to make their own decisions regardless of medical advice. It is stated that there are cases on record showing 24 different admissions for institutional care and that 6 to 8 admissions of the same patient are common. This could not happen in any well managed institution with the proper patient-doctor relationship.

Note that the American Medical Association's country-wide survey, including veteran hospitals showed a total for arrested, apparently arrested and quiescent approximately five times that of the highest figure for the duration of the Veterans' Administration. Certain private and state institutions show percentages which more than double the general average reported by the American Medical Association.

Obviously the record would be better if the tuberculous veterans of World War No. 1 had returned to their family physicians and followed the usual channels for care through local agencies, private, county and state sanatoria.

1. Dublin, Louis I.: Function of the Health Officer in the Control of Tuberculosis Among Veterans. Amer. Jour. Public Health, Vol. 33, No. 12, December, 1943.

NOW IS THE TIME

Repeatedly in these columns doctors have been urged not only to write to their representatives protesting the Wagner-Murray-Dingell Bill but to induce their patients and their friends to do the same. This is most important at this time because the political ear at the base of administrative antennae now has a wide range of receptivity. Waves of unrest are being picked up all along the way from the grass roots up to the realm of big business. The law makers are ready to respond to public opinion.

American individualism which was born in '76 and safeguarded by the American Constitution is now accorded an opportunity to retrieve some of its recent losses. If our patients and friends are not concerned about the present trend toward the socialization of medicine, it may be our fault. The layman must depend upon available knowledge for the formulation of his opinion. If we have not presented the benefits of American Medicine in an impressive manner, he may find it necessary to depend upon the one-sided publicity which has been coming out of Washington for the past ten years. It is readily admitted that no profession is perfect and that medicine, with all its virtues, cannot stand a sustained inquisition with its alleged imperfections paraded before the public year after year with never a word of credit or commendation for its good qualities.

How can we expect the people to know that, in spite of its faults, American Medicine is the best in the world. Idly we have sat with folded hands and permitted an unfavorable psychological build-up through unfavorable publicity from Washington in anticipation of political control of medicine. Perhaps it is not too late to tell the people what medicine has done for them and to show them what political medicine will mean in the sacrifice of freedom, in the inferior quality of medical care and the relative increase in cost.

If we are forced to accept some form of socialized medicine it will not be because the people are dumb, but because they are not informed as to the relative value of what Arthur C. Jacobs has designated as "medical humanism and the new medical collectivism". If we do not inform our people and fight for their freedom we may count on medical bondage which is bad for the doctor but worse for the patient.

Medical Collectivism means coercive cooperation. Medical humanism means voluntary cooperation with spiritual values which thrive only in an atmosphere of free initiative. This is still the land of the Pilgrim's Pride; the land where our fathers died; we still love its rocks and rills, its woods and templed hills; it must continue to be our sweet land of liberty. With all our might, let us hold high the torch of freedom's holy light. Now is the time.

WE WANT OPPORTUNITY—NOT FREEDOM FROM WANT

Though this discussion is not strictly medical, we must admit that it is within the doctor's province to consider the spiritual and economic values of life. While the average doctor is willing to do and die for his country it is natural for him to stop and reason why, when he hears so much about proposed social legislation, apparently designed to discourage initiative, to destroy individual industry and thus to threaten personal integrity.

Are we planning to bring our hearty American stock to a state of impotency through governmental paternalism; are we forgetting the principles of evolution, which include the primitive urge for individuality, growth and development through instinctive effort? Let us resolve that in our America, man-made slavery in the guise of administrative benefactions shall not replace our God-given freedom.

The following story from *Christ in the Camp*[1] by J. William Jones, who followed the fortunes of the Army of Northern Virginia from Harper's Ferry in '61 to Appomattox Court House in '65, as a private soldier and as Lee's famous chaplain, supplies a striking illustration of what we want. "In the summer of 1865, I was traveling one day along a country road in Virginia, when I saw a young man plowing in the field, guiding the plow with one hand, while an empty sleeve hung at his side . . . And so I said to the friend who was with me: 'We must stop. I must speak to that young man.' . . . I knew his history. Raised in the lap of luxury he had resisted its temptations, and when the war broke out he was about to bear off the highest honors of one of our colleges, and seemed destined to shine in his chosen profession, for which his tastes and talents fitted him. He was one of the first to step to the front when Virginia called on her sons to rally to her defense, and was one of the best of her noble soldiers.

"To see him thus, then, his hopes blighted, his fortune wrecked, and his body maimed for life, deeply touched my heart, and my words of greeting and sympathy were right warm. I shall never forget how the noble fellow, straightening himself up, replied, with a proud smile: 'Oh, Brother Jones, that is all right. *I thank God that I have one arm left and an opportunity to use it for the support of those I love'*."

No matter what we suffer, God grant that we may come out of this war with the will to work and the "opportunity to use it for the support of our loved ones." If the lawmakers of our America do anything to stifle this will or to rob us of opportunity, may they be prepared for the deepest pit in Inferno where Dante placed the designing sinners of Florence.

1. Jones, J. William: Christ In The Camp. B. F. Johnson & Company. Richmond, Virginia, 1887.

GOOD MEDICINE IN SPITE OF OPPOSITION

The development of public health and sanitation has grown out of medicine's laborous efforts to safeguard physical well being in the face of the mounting hazards consequent upon the course of civilization. The past century of mechanization with its inevitable urbanization has presented stupendous public health problems. That these problems have been well met by the medical profession is evident in the shining streets and the creditable health records of the world's great cities where people live in cleanliness, comfort and safety above the scientifically submerged filth of their composite existence. This physical security has been achieved in spite of the immediate material and political obstacles so often encountered. In the past, medical opinion ultimately commanded popular support and in the end, the people pursued the course of public welfare.

In the United States we are now threatened with a serious break in the sound continuity of the established medical service which has so adequately encompassed private and public needs. If the political vultures who would take advantage of the unstable national psychology arising through our present world crisis to foist upon the people the Wagner-Murray-Dingell Bill, could have three months in Washington under present conditions without sanitary engineering and preventive medicine, they would be so busy dodging the shadows of carrion crazed vultures they would be glad to preserve the present method of medical practice which unobstrusively has given them the life saving security they now enjoy without a moment's thought as to its source and its true significance.

Doctors have never considered it good taste to talk about their accomplishments but the time has come when the people should know the facts in order that they may act accordingly.

ROBERT·KOCH

In the first quarter of the 19th century, the death rate from tuberculosis in London was approximately 700 per 100,000. On December 11, 1843, Robert Koch was born in Hanover, Germany. In 1866 he received his medical degree from Gottingen. In 1871, while still a struggling country doctor, his wife gave him a microscope as a birthday gift. Behind a curtain which partially partitioned his otherwise one room office, he studied bacteriology at the expense of his already unprofitable practice. In 1876 he startled the world by his remarkable investigations of anthrax. In 1880 he was called from his country practice to the Imperial Health Office in Berlin. In 1882 he discovered the tubercle bacillus and in 1890 he prepared tuberculin, which, though disappointing as a therapeutic agent, has become a valuable aid to diagnosis. In 1900 the death rate in the United States was 200 per 100,000, today it is less than 45 per 100,000.

What would Robert Koch think of Germany's present policies with reference to life and death and human welfare. Noteworthy is the fact that the phenominal personal initiative having to do with the development of laboratories, research and clinical procedure in Germany was well under way before Bismarck initiated his program of social legislation.

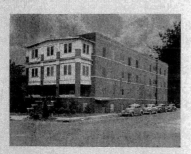
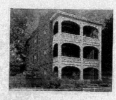

ASSOCIATION ACTIVITIES

DATE SET FOR FIFTY SECOND ANNUAL STATE MEETING

The Oklahoma State Medical Association will hold its 52nd Annual Meeting in Tulsa at the Mayo Hotel on April 24, 25 and 26, 1944.

At a recent meeting of the Annual Session Committee it was decided to hold a three-day meeting again in 1944 rather than a two-day, streamlined session as in 1943. The prospectus and floor plan was recently mailed to technical exhibitors, and all available booth spaces were immediately reserved by many of the companies who have previously exhibited as well as several who will be with the State Association at its Annual Meeting for the first time.

The program for the scientific session is well under way. The Scientific Work Committee has recently announced that several out-of-state Guest Speakers will be invited to participate in the General Session, and the various Section Officers are in the process of securing local physicians to participate in the Sectional Meetings. Additional details will be published as soon as available.

It is suggested that every member of the Association begin his plans now to attend the meeting as it is only through this means that we, as physicians, are able to keep abreast of present scientific knowledge.

SESSION OF NATIONAL CONFERENCE ON MEDICAL SERVICE TO BE HELD FEBRUARY 13 IN CHICAGO

The 1944 Session of the National Conference on Medical Service will be held February 13 at the Palmer House in Chicago on the day preceding the Annual Congress on Medical Education and licensure. This meeting comes at a critical time in the life of the nation and of medicine. The Secretary, Dr. C. L. Palmer of Pittsburgh and other officers of the conference are hoping to make the program vital and comprehensive and will greatly appreciate any suggestions you can make.

It is felt advisable that as many as possible should plan to attend the meeting because if ever an exchange of ideas, looking toward wise and public-spirited planning for health of the nation was needed it is now; and this meeting provides the one opportunity of the year for an informal exchange on the subject between representatives of organized medicine all over the country. The national conference is an independent body, as you know, without practical discussion of issues which may make or break our system of medicine in the United States.

POSTGRADUATE MEDICAL FELLOW-SHIPS AVAILABLE THROUGH THE COMMONWEALTH FUND

Dr. Grady F. Mathews of the Public Health Department, has received word that through the Commonwealth Fund's Division of Public Health, a number of postgraduate medical fellowships for practicing physicians will be available during 1944. Work under these fellowships will be offered at Tulane University Medical School at New Orleans and Harvard School in Boston. The courses thus far announced at Tulane include pediatrics January 24-27; surgery, February 21-26; medicine, March 20-25. The courses set up at Harvard include obstetrics, one month, available during any calendar month throughout the year; internal medicine, one month in September; and pediatrics, two weeks the early part of August.

Each of the fellowships mentioned above carries, as in the past, provision of refund of necessary travel expense from the physician's home to the school at the beginning of the course and for the return trip when the course is completed, plus tuition, and a daily stipend of $10.00 for the short courses, and a monthly stipend of $250.00 for the courses of a month's duration.

Applications from physicians who are graduates of a grade A medical school who have not yet attained the age of 60 will be given consideration, although preference will be given to applications from physicians located in the smaller communities in the state and to those who have not yet attained the age of 50. As in the past, inquiries and applications should be sent directly to the Division of Public Health of the Commonwealth Fund, 41 East 57th Street, New York City 22. It is obvious that those interested in the course in pediatrics at Tulane in January must make application promptly so that the necessary personal interview can be had with them and their credentials cleared at least a week before the course begins.

WESTERN OKLAHOMA HOSPITAL AT SUPPLY IS ACCREDITED BY AMERICAN COLLEGE OF SURGEONS

On January 7, word was received that the Western Oklahoma Hospital at Supply had been accredited by the American College of Surgeons. Dr. John L. Day, Superintendent of the Hospital, said that few mental hospitals have been so accredited.

Dr. Paul Ferguson, of the American College of Surgeons, made the inspection of the Hospital. It was suggested that a trained dietitian and trained nurses be employed. It has been very difficult to obtain the necessary, trained personnel.

THREE OKLAHOMA PHYSICIANS ACCEPTED INTO FELLOWSHIP IN AMERICAN COLLEGE OF SURGEONS

The following three physicians are initiates from Oklahoma who were accepted into Fellowship in the American College of Surgeons in 1943:

Andre B. Carney, M.D., Tulsa;
Denman C. Hucherson, M.D., Oklahoma City;
John M. Parrish, Jr., M.D., Oklahoma City.

PHYSICIANS RECENTLY LICENSED IN OKLAHOMA

Word has been received from J. D. Osborn, M.D., Secretary of the State Board of Medical Examiners that the following physicians have been licensed since July, 1943 to practice medicine in Oklahoma:

Applegate, Albert Earl, Oklahoma City; Bell, Ben, Washington, D. C.; Cain, James Henry, Tulsa; Cales, John Othal, Ralston; Cassidy, Charles Anthony, Oklahoma City; Colyar, Ardell Benton, Des Moines, Iowa; Cochran, Joseph E., Byars; Darden, Paul Martin, Oklahoma City; Dudley, Albert Webb, Oklahoma City; Davis, John Paul, Jr., Frenso, Cal.; Ellis Leonard Jas., Jr., Oklahoma City; Faulkner, Mortimer Sharpe, Orange, N. J.; Fite, Marcia, Tulsa; Howard Herbert Hardin, Ft. Worth, Tex.; Huff, Thos. Jefferson, Walters; Hughes Barbara Jean, Oklahoma City; Hallendorf, Leonard Chas., Des Moines, Iowa.

Hartig, Otto Joseph, Tulsa; Jones, James Earl, Frederick; Jones, Nathaniel A., Oklahoma City; Kennedy,

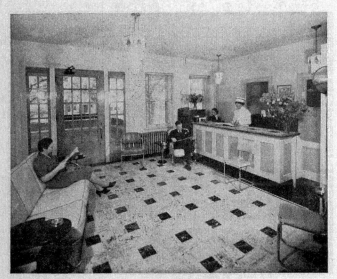

James Ralph, Oklahoma City; Lucan, Boyd Vance, Oklahoma City; McCellan, James Thomas, Rochester, Minn.; McGill, Joseph John, Oklahoma City; Maxwell, Thos. Meredith, Vinita; Orr, Herbert Stokes, Jr., Tulsa; Robinson, Lillian Harris, Helena; Schaff, Hartzell V., Holdenville; Sims, Harry James, Richmond, Cal.; Taylor, Robert Leroy, Tulsa; Williams, Byron Edward, Oklahoma City; Walden, Dewey Hobson, Evansville, Ind.; Zager, Warren Jack, Tulsa.

SURGICAL DIAGNOSIS COURSE TO OPEN FEBRUARY 14

In the November Journal physicians will remember the Postgraduate Committee announced the appointment of A. G. Fletcher, M.D., F.A.C.S., as instructor for the coming course in Surgical Diagnosis. Announcement letters containing the outline of Dr. Fletcher's course were mailed December 11 to the first circuit which includes the centers of Bartlesville, Claremore, Vinita, Pryor and Miami. The course will open the week of February 14.

The following are the past teaching and clinical connections of Dr. Fletcher:

Date of Birth: August 16, 1882.
1905: Graduated from University of Illinois, Medical Department.
1905-1909: Internship, Residency in Surgery, Methodist Hospital, Sioux City, Iowa.
1909-1914: Surgical Staff of Presbyterian and Good Hope Hospitals, Taiku, Korea, Japan.
1914: London School of Tropical Medicine, London, England.
1915-1918: Surgical Staff of Presbyterian and Good Hope Hospitals, Taiku, Korea, Japan.
1919: Graduate Study in Phipps Institute of University of Pennsylvania.
1920: Research Work in Johns Hopkins Hospital.
1921-1941: Surgeon in Chief Presbyterian and Good Hope Hospitals, Taiku, Korea, Japan.
1942-1943: Surgical Section of the Graduate School, University of Pennsylvania.

The following is the outline of the course which will be taught by Dr. Fletcher:

Lecture No.

1. FRACTURES
Principles of Repair: Rate of Repair: Classification; Treatment: First Aid, Six R's; (a) Recognition, (b) Roentgen Ray, (c) Relaxation, (d) Reduction, (e) Retention, (f) Restoration; Delayed or non-union— 6 causes; Indications for operative treatment (five); Operative methods (six); Craniocerebral injuries; Diagnosis; Differential Diagnosis; Treatment; Treatment of compound Fractures.

2. SHOCK
Types of Shock not under discussion; (1) Shell Shock, (2) Spinal Shock, (3) Gravity Shock, (4) Anaphylactic Shock, (5) Toxic Shock, (6) Anesthetic Shock, (7) Hemorrhage Shock. Surgical or Trumatic Shock; Primary Surgical Shock; Secondary Surgical Shock; Symptoms: (1) Blood Pressure, (2) Pulse, (3) Respiration, (4) Temperature, (5) Characteristic appearance of the patient. Etiology; Pathology of Shock; The present understanding of Shock; Measurement of Shock; Treatment of Shock.
The Principal Functions of the Blood, Hemorrhage

3. A. BURNS
(1) Severity and (2) Extent; First degree, Second degree, Third degree, Fourth degree; Pathology; Treatment; Plasma; Fluid Balance; Chemotherapy; Surface Treatment of Burns; (1) Koch Method, (2) Tanning Agents; Skin Grafting.
B. INFECTION OF THE HAND
(a) Felon, (b) Paronchyia, (c) Subcutaneous Infections. Treatment. Major Infections: (a) Tenosynovitis, (b) Fascial Space Infections.
4. THE SURGICAL PATIENT
A. Preparation for Operation

B. Postoperative care including,
C. Fluid Balance
5. A. CERVICAL SWELLINGS
B. THYROID ENLARGEMENTS
C. BREAST DISEASES
6. A. CHEST INJURIES
B. CHEST DISEASES
C. DIFFERENTIAL DIAGNOSIS OF CHEST CONDITIONS, PHRENIC AND LIVER ABSCESSES
7. DISEASES OF THE PERITONEAL CAVITY
A. Peptic Ulcer
B. Gall Bladder Diseases
C. Appendicitis
D. Intestinal Obstruction
8. DIFFERENTIAL DIAGNOSIS OF THE ACUTE ABDOMEN
9. DISEASES OF THE FEMALE GENITALIA
10. NEOPLASMS
A. Classification
B. Characteristics
C. Diagnosis, Prevention and Treatment

RESOLUTION

While the physicians of Northwestern Oklahoma have always known and appreciated the work and outstanding character of Doctor O. C. Newman of Shattuck, we are gratified that other parts of the State and other peoples now know of it also. We are also gratified that finally the Medical Profession has been recognized for its work and devotion to duty.

THEREFORE, BE IT RESOLVED that the members of the Woodward County Medical Society commend the Trustees of the Hall of Fame for recognizing the Medical Profession, and especially Northwestern Oklahoma in the person of Doctor O. C. Newman.

Signed by the Committee

NEW LEDERLE REPRESENTATIVE

M. K. Dodgen, formerly associated with Southwestern Drug Co., Dallas, Texas, is now with Lederle Laboratories in Eastern Oklahoma with headquarters in Tulsa. Mr. Dodgen is replacing Mr. L. J. Ebeling who has recently accepted a position as Kansas City Office Manager for Lederle.

• OBITUARIES •

Isaac Sylvester Hunt, M.D.
1861-1943

Isaac Sylvester Hunt was born in Skulfork County, Ohio, March 19, 1861 and passed away at Freedom, Oklahoma, October 15, 1943, age 82 years. He grew up in his home county and secured his primary education in the village school.

Dr. Hunt attended the Ohio Eclectic College but was compelled to quit before graduation on account of economic conditions. He moved to Oklahoma at the time of the opening and practiced for many years at Curtis. He moved to Old Freedom in 1918 and moved with the town when the railroad was built through. He continued there in practice until the time of his final illness.

"Doc" Hunt, as he was known to most of the people of western Woods County, was a typical country doctor. He practiced in Woodward County and later in Woods County, using a saddle horse with saddle bag, then a team and buggy before the days of the automobile. Through day and night, sunshine or storm, snow or sleet, he carried the gospel of healing into many a home dark from clouds of illness of saddened by

death. He would spend hours with severely ill and comfort the bereaved when death overcame his medical skill.

Dr. Hunt was active in work of the church and was a member of the Masonic and Odd Fellow Lodges. He belonged to the Woods County Medical Society, of which he was a regular attendant, and the Oklahoma State Medical Association, being an honorary member at the time of his death.

Jeff T. Parks. II. M.D.
1909-1943

Dr. Jeff T. Parks, II, Oklahoma City, died November 11 in Wesley Hospital. He had made his home in Oklahoma City for the last fourteen years.

Dr. Parks was born in Tahlequah where he lived until his graduation from the State Teachers College there in 1928. At that time he entered the University of Oklahoma School of Medicine and graduated in June, 1943. At the time of his death, Dr. Parks was serving an internship at Wesley Hospital.

Services were conducted in Oklahoma City at the Smith and Kernke Funeral Home. The body was then taken to Tahlequah where services were held at the First Methodist Church. He is survived by his widow, Mrs. Mary Parks of Oklahoma City, his father, Judge Jeff T. Parks of Tahlequah, and three sisters.

James R. McLauchlin. M.D.
1884-1943

Dr. James R. McLauchlin, Oklahoma City, pioneer state physician, died on December 7, in St. Anthony hospital after a brief illness. Dr. McLauchlin was County Physician, in which capacity he served for eight years. Prior to that time he was in private practice in Oklahoma City and Norman.

In 1907, Dr. McLauchlin came to Oklahoma where he entered the Oklahoma University School of Medicine, graduating in 1911. Following his graduation he began practice in Denver, Oklahoma, near Norman, moving to Norman within five years. After a short time in Norman, Dr. McLauchlin joined the staff of the Central State Hospital, where he served three years. In 1921, when the State Tuberculosis Sanitarium was established at Clinton, he became its first superintendent, and served two years. Dr. McLauchlin came to Oklahoma City in 1923 and remained until the time of his death.

Dr. Lauchlin is survived by his widow, three daughters, Mrs. J. Gunter Johnson, Delphine Margaret McLauchlin and Mrs. M. E. Trapp, all of Oklahoma City, and three sons, Dr. James R. McLauchlin, Jr., Oklahoma City, Pfc. Robert Allen McLauchlin, a student at the University of Chicago, and Rex Vincent McLauchlin, seminary student at Oconomowoc, Wisconsin.

Funeral services were held December 30 by the Capitol Hill funeral home.

Benjamin W. Slover. M.D.
1873-1944

Dr. Benjamin W. Slover, Blanchard, died January 8 in an Oklahoma City Hospital after an illness of one month. Dr. Slover was president of the McClain County Medical Society and very active in all civic affairs.

Dr. Slover graduated from Barnes Medical College, St. Louis, Missouri, in 1901. Shortly afterward he came to Oklahoma where he took up private practice. Retiring from active practice several years ago, he had devoted most of his time to farm and ranch interests.

Surviving Dr. Slover are his widow, Mrs. Lucy Slover, Blanchard, a daughter, Mrs. E. B. Collingsworth, El. Paso, Texas, and one brother, Dr. G. W. Slover, Sulphur. Burial will be in Durant where Dr. Slover lived for thirteen years.

RESOLUTION

The following resolution was passed at the October 18 meeting of the Members of the Oklahoma State Medical Board:

In honor of Dr. C. E. Bradley, a Member of the Oklahoma State Board of Medical Examiners, who passed

away in July, Dr. Leslie submitted the following resolution for adoption:

WHEREAS, Dr. C. E. Bradley, who died at his home in Tulsa, July 6, 1943, was an active Member of the State Board of Medical Examiners, and a very efficient worker to the best interest of Organized Medicine in Oklahoma; therefore,

BE IT RESOLVED, That the State Board of Medical Examiners, in extra session held in Oklahoma City, October 18, 1943, wish to express our sincere regrets over the passing of our friend and colaborer;

THEREFORE, BE IT FURTHER RESOLVED, That a copy of this resolution be sent to his wife, Mrs. Bradley, and a copy spread on the minutes of our Board.

Motion by Dr. Johnson, seconded by Dr. Weber, that we accept the resolution, that it be made a matter of record on our minute book, and that it be published in the Journal. Motion carried.

University of Oklahoma School of Medicine

Seven (7) students in the School of Nursing were granted the Diploma of Graduate Nurse at the Commencement Exercises. They were:

    Billy Hutchison Bell
    Margaret Barlow Byrd
    Maxine Norman Dickson
    Evelyn Green
    Effie Agnes Hughes
    Evelyn Norman
    Loveda May Scharnhorst

On January 1, 1944, the following men will have completed a nine-months internship at the University of Oklahoma Hospitals:

    John H. Ademetz, M.D., University of Wisconsin
    Frank A. English, M.D., University of Syracuse, N. Y.
    Harold R. Henstorf, M.D., University of Iowa.
    Albert E. James, M.D., University of Colorado
    Franklin G. Osberg, M.D., University of Colorado

Dr. George N. Barry, Medical Director, was recently injured by a "hit and run driver" and spent several days in the Polyclinic Hospital.

Dr. Tom Lowry, Dean, recently spent two weeks in New York City.

Dr. H. A. Shoemaker, Assistant Dean, attended a conference for the selection of medical and dental Army Specialized Trainees at Dallas, Texas, December 9, 1943.

Dr. Arthur A. Hellbaum has been named Professor of Pharmacology and Acting Chairman of the Department of Pharmacology. Dr. Hellbaum has for several years served as Associate Professor of Physiology.

Dr. John F. Haekler has been appointed Professor of Hygiene and Public Health. He recieved his A.B. Degree from Northeastern State College, Tahlequah, Oklahoma, his B. S. in Medicine from the University of Oklahoma in 1931, and the Degree of Doctor of Medicine from the University of Oklahoma School of Medicine in 1933. He did special work in Public Health at Vanderbilt University School of Public Health and at Johns Hopkins School of Hygiene and Public Health, where he received the Degree of Master of Public Health in 1940. Recently Dr. Hackler has been associated with the Oklahoma State Health Department.

Dr. John W. Cavanaugh has been appointed full-time Professor of Surgery at the School of Medicine and the University of Oklahoma Hospitals. He is a graduate of the University of Iowa College of Medicine, having received the degree of Doctor of Medicine in June, 1939. He was a member of the Alpha Omega Alpha Honorary Medical Society. He served a two-year rotating internship at the University of Oklahoma Hospitals, after which he was appointed Assistant Resident in Surgery and later as Resident in Surgery. Since July, 1943, he has been associated with Dr. M. M. Mills, Topeka, Kansas.

———

Dr. Turner Bynum, Visiting Lecturer in Medicine, has

been granted a leave of absence for the duration of the War, effective November 15, 1943.

———

Dr. H. J. Binder, Associate in Pediatrics, has been granted a leave of absence for the duration, as he has been ordered to active duty with the Armed Forces as of November 16, 1943.

———

Dr. Mary V. S. Sheppard has recently been appointed Instructor in Medicine.

Commencement Exercises were held at the University of Oklahoma, Norman, Oklahoma on Thursday, December 23. The following students were granted the degree of Doctor of Medicine and will serve internships as indicated:

NAME	INTERNSHIP	LOCATION
Adams, George Mullins	U. S. Naval Hospital	San Diego, California
Alexander, James Leon	Jefferson Davis Hospital	Houston, Texas
Anderson, Thomas Page	St. Paul's Hospital	Dallas, Texas
Archer, Homer Vincent	New Rochelle Hospital	New Rochelle, N. Y.
Arrendell, Eugene Hamlin	U. S. Naval Hospital	(Not Designated)
Ballard, Jack Duane	U. S. Naval Hospital	(Not Designated)
Bell, Joseph Price	University Hospital	Oklahoma City
Bodine, Charles David	Mercy Hospital	Chicago, Ill.
Brown, Clifford Alton	St. Anthony Hospital	Oklahoma City
Brown, George MacMillan, Jr.	U. S. Naval Hospital	Bainbridge, Md.
Carter, Herschel Gray	U. S. Naval Hospital	(Not designated)
Cohen, Samuel Lewis	French Hospital	San Francisco, Calif.
Conn, Julia Harold	St. Luke's Hospital	Cleveland, Ohio
Cooke, Everett Ellis	Jersey City Medical Center	Jersey City, N. J.
Cosby, Glenn Wendelle	St. Anthony Hospital	Oklahoma City
Cullen, Marvin LeRoy	Jersey City Medical Center	Jersey City, N. J.
Dawson, Clarence Benton	Augustana Hospital	Chicago, Ill.
Donnell, John	Jersey City Medical Center	Jersey City, N. J.
Farr, Louise Kinkead	University Hospital	Oklahoma City
Fife, Phillips Raymond	Wesley Hospital	Oklahoma City
First, Safety Reuel	Hillcrest Memorial Hospital	Tulsa, Oklahoma
Flanigin, Herman Floyd, Jr.	University Hospital	Oklahoma City
Fluhr, William Forrest	Presbyterian Hospital	Los Angeles, Calif.
Gastineau, Clifford Felix	Colorado General Hospital	Denver, Colo.
Gerard, Rene Gabriel	St. Paul's Hospital	Dallas, Texas
Holt, Robert Perry	Aucker Hospital	St. Paul, Minn.
Hough, Jack Van Doren	U. S. Naval Hospital	Farragut, Idaho
Huff, Dick H. P.	(Not definite as yet)	
Kincy, Kenneth B.	Hollywood Presbyterian Hospital	Los Angeles, Calif.
Klebanoff, Milton	University Hospital	Oklahoma City
Knight, William Ewart	University Hospital	Oklahoma City
McIntyre, John Aubrey	U. S. Naval Hospital	Norman, Oklahoma
Macrory, Paul David	Wesley Hospital	Oklahoma City
Meis, Armon M.	Mercy Hospital	Denver, Colo.
Meis, Donna Lea Hammer	Mercy Hospital	Denver, Colo.
Neal, James Hal	St. Luke's Hospital	Duluth, Minn.
Rector, William Lee, Jr.	Iowa Lutheran Hospital	Des Moines, Iowa
Robinson, Earl Moore	Wesley Hospital	Oklahoma City
Rockett, Louis Stong	Iowa Lutheran Hospital	Des Moines Iowa
Sanders, Harold Ray	St. Anthony Hospital	Oklahoma City
Stickle, Arthur Waldo	University Hospital	Oklahoma City
Strong, Clinton Riley	U. S. Naval Hospital	Long Beach, Calif.
Taylor, Fred Wilbur	U. S. Naval Hospital	Farragut, Idaho
Thompson, William Best	New Rochelle Hospital	New Rochelle, N. Y.
Toibert, Jack Burgess	Good Samaritan Hospital	Portland, Oregon
Trzaska, Henry Constantine	St. Mary's Hospital	Chicago, Ill.
Turner, Edwin Charles	Swedish Hospital	Seattle, Wash.
Walker, Ethan Allen, Jr.	U. S. Naval Hospital	Bainbridge, Md.
Whiteneck, Ronald Alven	University Hospital	Oklahoma City
Winn, George Louis	U. S. Naval Hospital	Bethesda, Md.
Witcher, Jones E.	Baptist Memorial Hospital	Memphis, Tenn.

OFFICERS SELECTED FOR OKLAHOMA COUNTY SOCIETY AND OKLAHOMA CITY CLINICAL SOCIETY

Dr. William E. Eastland has been chosen president of the Oklahoma County Medical Society succeeding Dr. Walker Morledge. Dr. Gregory E. Stanbro was named president-elect and automatically will become president in 1945.

Other officers of the Medical Society include Dr. W. Floyd Keller, vice-president; and Dr. Elmer R. Musick,

re-elected secretary-treasurer and also named treasurer of the Oklahoma City Clinical Society. Members of the Society Board of Directors are: Dr. Eastland; Dr. Keller; Dr. F. M. Lingenfelter; Dr. Walker Morledge; Dr. Musick; Dr. C. R. Rountree; Dr. Gregory Stanbro; Dr. W. K. West and Dr. J. H. Robinson.

The Oklahoma City Clinical Society selected as its president, Dr. D. H. O'Donoghue. Other officers are: Dr. C. P. Bondurant, director of clinics; Dr. Clark H. Hall, vice-president and Dr. L. Chester McHenry, secretary.

MEDICINE AT WAR

IMMEDIATE NEED FOR ADDITIONAL MEDICAL PERSONNEL MADE EVIDENT BY REVISED FEDERAL ACT

The Directing Board, Procurement and Assignment for Physicians, War Manpower Commission, recently issued a directive citing an immediate need of several thousand additional medical personnel. All State Chairmen are re-appraising physicians of military age as it is felt that those who have been rejected may now be able to meet the physical standards now in effect. Names of those who are classified as available but who have not as yet accepted a commission are certified as available to the State Director of Selective Service for any action which may be taken.

One important change in the status of physicans was approved on December 10. The recently enacted law includes the following provision: "Provided, That no individuals shall be called for induction, ordered to report to induction stations, or be inducted because of their occupations, or by occupational groups, or by groups in any plant or institution, except pursuant to a requisition by the land or naval forces for persons in needed medical, professional and specialist categories." This provision is taken to mean that special quotas for physicans may be established and those classified as available for military service may be inducted under special procedure regardless of order number in the event that the Armed Forces make special requisition for medical officers.

The following is a list of questions, with the answers, which are frequently asked by physicians. These have been prepared by the Washington Office for Procurement and Assignment Service.

Q. *What are the present age limits for service in the Medical Corps of the Armed Forces?*

A. The upper limit in the Army is, in general, the 45th birthday, but for specific position vacancies men up to 60 are eligible. The limit in the Navy is, in general, the 50th birthday.

Q. *What is the present status of physical requirements?*

A. The Navy at the present time still has the highest standards, although they are lower than they were. The Army is next, and those who are physically disqualified for Army service may be eligible for commission in the United States Public Health Service.

Q. *What ranks are being offered by the services at the present time?*

A. The Army is limiting those under 38 to first lieutenancies and those above 38 and over, to captaincies and above if they meet special requirements of the Surgeon General. The latter rank depends upon special qualifications. The Navy is limiting those 34 and under to lieutenancies, jr. gr., those from 34 to 38 lieutenancies, sr. gr., and those from 38 to 44 lieutenant commanderships. For specific position vacancies requiring special qualifications higher commissions may be offered. The Public Health Service has commissioned ranks similar to those in the Army.

Q. *What are the present needs of the services?*

A. All three branches of the Armed Forces are in immediate dire need of several thousand additional medical personnel. This immediate period of need is between now and January 1st.

Q. *Why is the Public Health Service classed as one of the branches of the Armed Forces as far as medical officers are concerned?*

A. For many reasons, among them the fact that they supply the medical personnel for the U. S. Coast Guard. Physically qualified eligible officers are assigned by the Public Health Service for active duty with the Coast Guard and may be assigned anywhere the American flag flies.

Q. *Why have so many practitioners who are capable of serving long hours in civilian practice been disqualified for military service?*

A. The exigencies of service in combat areas are such that civilian practice is no criterion of physical qualification. The services at the present time have a full quota of those that they can accept for limited duty. They are being forced to discharge some at present. Certain individual physicians who still will be able to undertake heavy civilian duties are no longer able to cope with the needs of combat troops.

Q. *Why is it necessary for a physician to take an indoctrination course after entering the Medical Corps?*

A. The reason for this is that a physician becomes a medical officer, which means that he is at all times an officer subject to the duties of other officers of other branches of the service. He must be responsible for those under his command and must be entirely capable of meeting any situation which confronts such personnel as is under his direct supervision whether it be in open field duty requiring the setting up of field hospitals or the maintenance of food suppy and shelter for his personnel, as well as a correlation of the activities of his group with the other services under the same command.

Q. *Is it true that the Armed Forces are not making efficient use of their medical personnel?*

A. There have been many occasions in the past when appearances would lead anyone to believe that they were not. At present time efficient use is being made of such personnel, and it must always be remembered in this connection that a reserve supply of such personnel must be maintained for immediate assignment to duty. Such a group must have been trained to meet the situations it will face immediately after assignment and cannot be gathered together at the last minute to be assigned to some specific post. Furthermore, the planning of any military campaign requires a complete line-up of all services. If reverses are suffered such men who are in preparation of projected positions may not be able to fill such positions and must be held for further plans. War, by its very nature, is not essentially efficient, but the lack of medical personnel in the various branches of the Armed Forces has resulted in a high increase in their efficient use.

Q. *On the basis of present ratios of physicians to individuals, which service has the greatest need at the present time?*

A. The Army ratio is slightly over 6 per 1,000, whereas the Navy is somewhat under 4 per 1,000. Therefore, the Navy needs men somewhat more than the Army.

Q. *Why is any man under 38 ever classified as essential?*

A. He is only essential if he were to leave his community or his institution and there were no replacement for him. No man under 38 is, as a general rule, considered permanently essential, but only essential until he can be replaced by another physician who is not eligible for service with the Armed Forces.

Q. *Has not the civilian population been endangered by the number of physicians who have entered the Armed Forces?*

A. Not for the Nation at large. There are various problems of redistribution which have been partially or complete solved and some which will be difficult to solve, but if such distribution is equitable there is no shortage at present for minimal adequate civilian care.

Q. Will not the needs of the services continue and require that additional personnel leave civilian life?

A. To some extent, yes, but primarily the services will be able to meet their own needs for replacement from the students they are training at present. The Navy may need some additional personnel even though they are also training students. The Public Health Service will continue to have needs since they do not have any students in training.

Q. Why do not the Armed Forces adopt the liberalizations that exist in England and elsewhere?

A. Because it is essential that American standards be maintained for the men in the Armed Forces as well as on the home front. Comparisons with the Armed Forces of other Nations are not in order any more than comparisons of physician-population ratios on the home front are with those of other Nations. The mortality in the Armed Forces at the present time is astoundingly low and every effort will be made to keep them at that level. This will obviously require further sacrifices on the part of those on the home front, but the Procurement and Assignment Service is constantly aware of the fact that supplies of all kinds must continue to flow to those who are on active duty and that, therefore, the health of the home front is as much a part of the war effort as is the health of the soldier.

Q. What action does Selective Service take on physicians?

A. Although local boards differ somewhat in their actions, in general, no action is taken at present on physicians or others over 38. Reclassificatoin of those under 38 is going on constantly and dependency is not considered to the same extent as it was in the past.

Implications of Waivers for Physical Defects

The following is a release from the War Manpower Commission dated January 8, 1944:

"What are the implications of waivers for known physical defects which physicians sign upon being appointed for limited service in the Army Medical Corps?

The answer to this recurrent question is clarified in a recent opinion on the subject by the Office of The Judge Advocate General of the Army. The opinion, released by the Procurement and Assignment Service of the War Manpower Commission, is as follows:

"Response is made to your oral inquiry whether acknowledgment, on the accompanying form, of existing physical defects would preclude a person from thereafter claiming benefits to which he would otherwise be entitled on account of the service connected aggravation of such defects. As to the defects acknowledged, the execution of such an instrument merely provides additional evidence of their existence, and to that extent would operate to preclude the person involved from thereafter claiming benefits on account of them. It is the opinion of this office, however, that the mentioned form does not support to be a waiver of possible future benefits to which the individual might become entitled by reason of any service-connected aggravation of such defects, and would not operate to deprive the individual of any possible benefits on account of such aggravation."

NEW COMMITTEE CHAIRMEN APPOINTED BY PRESIDENT STEVENSON

The resignation of Dr. Fannie Lou Leney as Chairman of the Committee on Pediatrics occassioned the elevation of Dr. Luvern Hays, Tulsa, former Secretary, to the position of Chairman. Dr. James Stevenson, President, has appointed Dr. G. R. Russell, Tulsa, to the position of Secretary.

Dr. Stevenson has appointed Dr. W. S. Larrabee, Tulsa, as the new Chairman of the Committee on Dermatology and Radiology to succeed Dr. Leon H. Stuart, who has resigned the position.

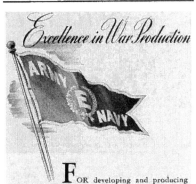
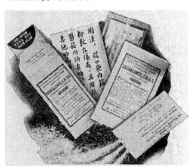

★ FIGHTIN' TALK ★

Lt. David Norman Trimble, Tulsa has been ordered to active duty. The following have received recent promotions: From Lieutenant to Captain; *Clifton Felts*, Seminole; *William R. Lytle*, Seminole; *Eric McLain White*, Tulsa; *Willard Dennis Holt*, Altus; *Jack Francis Parsons*, Cherokee; *Frank Thomas Joyce*, Chickasha. From Captain to Major: *William Harrell Webster*, Ada; *O. H. Cowart*, Bristow; *Tom Hall Mitchell*, Tulsa; *George Thomas Allen*, Oklahoma City.

Lt. Dick Graham, former Executive Secretary of the Oklahoma State Medical Association, arrived from his station in the Surgeon General's Office in Washington to spend a few days in Oklahoma City. *Dick's* main objective was to see Mrs. Graham and the new son, Richard, Jr., who was born December 28, at Wesley Hospital in Oklahoma City. Both mother and baby are reported as doing fine.

All of *Dick's* many friends were glad to see him and look forward to another visit in the future.

Lt. Elmer Ridgeway, Jr., Oklahoma City, returned to the states recently from the Southwest Pacific Area where he has been Naval Surgeon at a secret base. *Lt. Ridgeway* brought the good news to relatives and friends of fighting men in that area that they are being well taken care of and that the "mortality rate in the hospital was less than one-tenth of 1 per cent." Casualties are brought by air to the hospitals and arrive within a short time after they are wounded.

Romance found *Lt. Ridgeway*, or vice-versa, in the Southwest Pacific. Miss Virginia Boling of Terre Haute, Ind., a member of the first nursing contigent to arrive in the South Seas Hospital, and *Lt. Ridgway* were married upon their return to the States.

Dr. Virgil F. Doughtery, medical missionary from Oklahoma City, graduate of the Oklahoma University School of Medicine in 1923, recently acted as his own physician in Saye, Ethiopia, and narrowly escaped death. After an encounter with a thief who had entered his home, Dr. Doughtery was seriously injured by several stab wounds in the back and abdomen. Although nearing an unconscious condition, he was able to instruct his wife and an Amharic doctor to administer adrenalin and morphine and to sew up his wounds. He is recovering nicely.

Dr. Doughtery has been a medical missionary in Iran, Sudan and Ethiopia for several years. He has recently had to leave Gere because of the Italian invasion.

Major James O. Hood, Norman, and his regimental medical detachment in Italy, in recognition of their heroism, have recently received well-deserved recommendations and decorations. *Major Hood* says that the glory goes to the detachment and not to himself.

In a letter to his wife, *Major Hood* says that his men have seen plenty of action and that many of them had been decorated and other decorations will be presented soon. So far, he has escaped without a scratch. *Major Hood*, is the birth on December 16, of his second son, ilized in September, 1940, left the States June 1, 1943, landing in Africa. They were there only a few days; then took part in the capture of Sicily before going on to Salerno, Italy. The heroic deeds of *Major Hood* and his detachment will long live in the minds of Oklahoma physicians and citizens.

Another important happening in the life of *Major Hood*, is the birth on December 16, of his second son,

Robert Sidney. It is not known whether this news has reached him or not, although he has been notified by cable and V-Mail.

Captain Ralph Phelan, Wanrika, is close to the scene of fighting on the battlefields of Italy. *Captain Phelan's* untiring efforts to care for the wounded have made him an admirable figure to his men. Night and day, with little rest, he and his men are on the battle front with their litter squads, braving fire to evacuate the wounded.

Major M. M. Appleton, Oklahoma City, writes from England where he is stationed that he is "well-fed, busy and reasonably happy." *Captain T. A. Ragan*, Fairfax and *Captain R. E. Roberts*, Stillwater, are in the same unit and he sees them often.

Lt. Hayes R. Yandell, Tulsa, is now stationed on a tropical island 'some-where in the South Pacific.' *Lt. Yandell* says that it gives the men 'over there' a feeling of security to know that someone is fighting the Wagner Act at home.

Lt. Col. James G. Hughes, formerly instructor for the Postgraduate Committee, is stationed 'somewhere in Italy.' His recent letter reads in part: "Our hospital is highly interesting . . . we get the boys here and they are the salt of the earth. Never a whimper and always a smile. We have air raids now and then and I've crouched in fox holes in the best infantry style and heard the bombs whistle down nearby but the Red Cross of a hospital is well respected and nearby bombs are merely interesting accidents."

The following interesting letter was received from *Major H. B. Shorbe*, Oklahoma City. "My unit is composed of general surgeons and specialists divided into teams and these teams are sent where needed. It so happened that I led a number of teams on the Invasion of Italy. We arrived with the infantry ahead of the tanks. I was once between German and American tanks when a duel started—I retreated!

"We set up and operated in a clearing station on the beach for three days before the evacuation hospitals could be set up. Then we assisted the hospitals. I assure you that there was no trouble with doctors grabbing another's patients. Unfortunately, there was enough for all.

"We have followed the troops in our push up Italy. Now I am working in an evacuation hospital 'some-where on the front'. I have seen a number of Oklahoma doctors the past few months and I know our State is doing more than its share in this theater. All we want is to get this mess over and return to our homes and practices—this is no picnic!"

Lt. (jg) R. E. Schnoebelen, Mooreland, is stationed at the Navy Recruiting Station in Tulsa. Lt. Schnoebelen reports that he is now 'proud papa' of baby Renee Margaret.

We send our sympathy to *Lt. Comdr. Johnny A. Blue*, Guymon, who recently lost his mother, Mrs. Dannie Josephine Blue, State poineer. Lt. Comdr. *Blue* is stationed at the Navy medical center, Bainbridge, Md., where he is Chief of the Allergy Department of a 1,700 bed Naval Hospital and has received an appointment for further postgraduate work in Allergy in the near future.

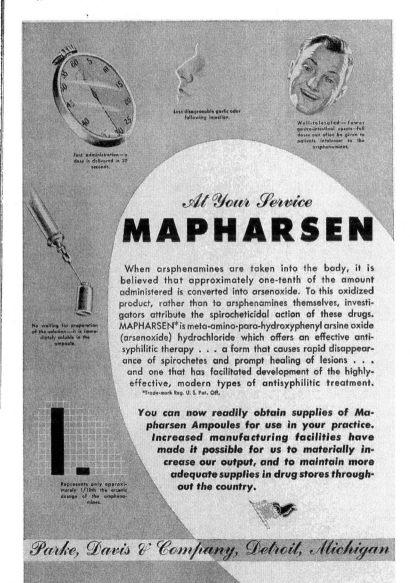

Woman's Auxiliary

HOW THE WOMAN'S AUXILIARY CAN HELP IN THE U. S. CADET NURSE CORPS PROGRAM*

LUCILE PETRY, R.N.

*Director, Division of Nurse Education,
U. S. Public Health Service*

This nation faces a wartime shortage of nurses, so acute as to impair not only the structure of nursing service but the successful prosecution of total war itself.

Recognizing the dangers of this condition, both Houses of Congress last June unanimously passed the Bolton Act establishing the U. S. Cadet Nurse Corps, and appropriated funds to be allotted to accredited nursing schools for the nation-wide operation of the Cadet Nurse Corps program. The basic purpose of the program, which is being administered by the Division of Nurse Education, U. S. Public Health Service, is to supply a larger number of nurses more quickly than ever before. This year's recruitment goal for the Corps is 65.000 new student nurses.

As of the end of October, almost 900 of the nation's 1300 nursing schools had been accepted for participation in the Corps program, with additional schools being approved each day. The estimated enrollment at that time was approximately 83,000 students—of whom 41,-000 are expected to be new recruits.

All kinds of help, both individual and collective, are needed to recruit additional students. The members of the Woman's Auxiliary to the American Medical Association have indicated that they would aid in the recruitment drive to the total extent of their ability and close relationship with the medical nursing professions. It is the purpose of this article to outline—specifically and in some detail—what form which aid might take.

First, let us review briefly the basic details of the Cadet Nurse Corps program. Cadet Nurses receive free tuition and fees, living expenses, uniforms, and a graded monthly allowance. Under the Bolton Act, Federal funds are provided for these purposes, but schools participating in the Corps carry out their own programs in accordance with their own policies and traditions. There are no government schools of nursing.

Recruits must be between the ages of 17 or 18 (depending on state of school regulation) and 35. They must be in good health and graduates of accredited high schools. Students already in training at approved nursing schools may become members of the corps in their school, entering at the stage of advancement at which they then find themselves.

In what way can the Woman's Auxiliary be of service to the U. S. Cadet Nurse Corps? There are at least four ways in which you—both as individuals and as members of an organization—can be of great help:

1. By recruiting additional student nurses.
2. By helping interested girls choose the right school.
3. By holding—and strengthening—the interest of candidates for the Corps between the time they seek information and the time they are admitted.
4. By assisting local nursing councils and local hospitals in staffing hospital Information Centers for the Corps.

This is volunteer work of high importance.

The wives of physicians are in a particularly advan-

*Reprinted from Bulletin of the Woman's Auxiliary, February, 1944,, page 56.

tageous position to recruit nurses. To begin with, you are interested in and acquainted with the details of that profession; you are well-equipped to present the most convincing arguments for nursing as a wartime service and as a lifetime asset.

Then, too, young women who are considering entering the nursing profession—as well as the parents of such young women—generally come to a physician or to members of his family for advice. You are in a position to meet and talk with girls who you think would make good nurses—and with the parent's of these girls. Your husband may have a number of women patients who, with the proper encouragement, might easily become interested in a nursing career for themselves or their sisters or daughters. You can make sure that your husband understands fully the Corps program, and you can suggest that he try to encourage those patients—and those advice-seekers—whom he considers suitable to enter the field of nursing.

You can help also by assisting girls to choose the right school. What do we mean by the "right school?" We mean, first of all, a school that has been approved and that offers experience and instruction in a variety of services. Besides the four essential services offered, medical, surgical, pediatric, and obstetric, good schools usually offer experience in a combination of any of the following: psychiatric nursing, community or public health nursing, communicable disease nursing, out-patient nursing, and experience in a nursery school with well children. Also to be recommended is a school which gives emphasis to social and preventive aspects of nursing care.

Auxiliaries may also be of assistance by holding the interest of candidates for the Corps between the time they first seek information and the time they enter nursing school. Youthful ardor is sometimes quickly quenched, especially with so many wartime distractions and competitions. Frequent talks with interested girls, informal discussions about their future in nursing, a little encouragement once in a while—all this will help to keep the flame of interest alive. The advantages of nursing as a profession with great career possibilities, a profession which can be easily re-entered after a period of inactivity, or practiced on a part-time basis, should be discussed. Nursing as a preparation for homemaking, motherhood, and intelligent citizenship should be emphasized to the girl who wants to be of maximum service to her country in war time but does not wish a career. Perhaps you can suggest certain activities that the candidate might engage in, or certain courses that she might take with advantage. She might, for example, make up certain deficiencies in her educational background by taking evening courses in biology or chemistry. A senior in high school might enter a well planned pre-training program provided in some hospital and health agencies. In any case, your interest and moral support will be more than valuable.

Every accredited hospital in the United States—6,500 of them—has been asked to act as an Information Center for the Corps program. Staffing these centers for most of the day with volunteer workers presents a problem. You will be making a substantial contribution to the Corps and to the war if you arrange to devote a few hours of your time each day or each week to serving as attendant at the Information Center in your local hospital. You may offer your services to your local Nursing Council for War Service or directly to any hospital in your town.

These, briefly, are the ways in which you can help us. Your country urgently needs that help. We call upon you for assistance now—in bringing the right young woman into the field where character and capacity count for so much, a field in which they learn living as well as working, helping their country as well as helping themselves.

BOOK REVIEWS

"The chief glory of every people arises from its authors."—Dr. Samuel Johnson.

BIOCHEMISTRY AND MORPHOGENESIS. Joseph Needham, F.R.S. (Gonville and Caius College). XVI—785 pp., 328 figs., 35 plates. Cambridge University Press. Macmillan Co., New York, 1942. $12.50.

This monumental treatise deals in Part I with the developing embryo and its raw materials, in Part II with morphogenetic stimuli or embryonic inductions, in Part III with morphogenetic mechanisms. Only sampling methods can be employed here. In Part I the hen's egg is for obvious reasons much discussed. As to the vitelline membrane the Schreinemakers' equations are found inapplicable, and the distribution of ions in yolk and white is different from that required by the Donnan equilibrium theory (only 2-3 mV instead of the 130 mV required for such equilibria). The yolk of avian eggs contains all vitamins but C, the white only B2; the Fe of yolk is inorganic, probably adsorbed on to proteins or lipoprotein complexes (0.045 per cent). In the relation of egg to environment are discussed the evolution of the cleidoic egg, the metabolic properties of the cleidoic state and the transition from the non-cleidoic state to ovoviviparity. Embryonic nutrition is considered first in the light of the chick embryo's three "scaffoldings," the yolk-sac, amnion and allantois. The amount of material retained each day for construction of yolk-sac and that passed on for maintenance of the embryo are calculated by defining the Membrane Absorption Rate as $\frac{y_i + a_i + e_i + c_i}{y + a} \times 100$, and the Membrane Transit Rate as $\frac{a_i + e_i + c_i}{y} \times 100$, where y_i, a_i and e_i are daily increments (wet weights) respectively of yolk-sac, allantois and embryo, c_i daily increment of material combusted and lost from the egg, y wet weight of yolk, a wet weight of allantois. Hereby it is found that before the 9th day, the high Absorption Rate is almost exclusively concerned with construction of yolk-sac; thereafter the Transit Rate indicates that almost all absorbed material goes to the embryo. Further discussion of embryonic nutrition deals with yolk utilization in lower vertebrates and invertebrates, "pigeon milk" and mammalian colostrum; nidicolous and nidifugous birds are compared, as are epithelio-chorial and haemo-chorial types of placenta. Part I closes with consideration of maternal diet and embryonic constitution in mammals, the mammalian placentation, its constitution and metabolism.

Part II reviews the large field of experimental morphology, with attention centering on the organizer effect of the dorsal lip of the blastopore in amphibian embryos, as studied by Spemann et al. The classical experiment of Spemann was to transplant presumptive mesoderm (dorsal lip) to epidermis or elsewhere, the result being that the transplant invaginated and organized the surrounding tissue to form a secondary embryo. A routine test, the *Einsteckung* method of O. Mangold, is to make a slit in the roof of the blastocele and introduce into the cavity a fragment of tissue or chemical: when the blastocele cavity disappears the test fragment lies between yolk-endoderm and ectoderm, thus testing its power to induce neural plate formation. Many living fragments show no such power, but if they are killed by heat or other means of denaturation, they do show this power very strongly; so do bits of killed adult tissues of all phyla indiscriminately (Holtfreter); so do many chemicals. The "evocator" or chemical in such tissues is said to be unmasked by killing, apparently a release from combination with some specific protein. This chemical appears to be a steroid; in fact, Waddington and Needham obtained fine neural tube inductions by implanting polycyclic hydrocarbons (1:9-dimenthylphenanthrene, and 9:10-di-n-butyl-9:10-dihydro-1:2:5:6-dibenzanthracene). And significantly Waddington obtained similar inductions with the carcinogens methyl-chol anthrene, styryl blue and 3:4 benzpyrene, also with various estrogens. Comparing organizers and cancer, it is shown that the organizer has a relation to the whole body plan: it exists in an "individuation field" whose mechanism represents an interplay of evocators and competencies (reactivity states) of the tissues. In contrast a cancerous growth escapes from the controlling pattern of its individuation field. Similar results follow if evocators are unmasked; new fields or chaotic growths ensue. There is much overlap of various domains of chemical specificity. Thus primary evocators are overlapped by 4 carcinogens and 4 estrogens, with one chemical (3:4 benzpyrene) common to all three domains; estrogens overlap androgens and both overlap sterols and bile acids. As to the hierarchy of organizers: neural tube induction by notochord and somites is first grade, lens and ear-capsule inductions by eye-cup and ear-vesicle respectively are second grade, tympanic membrane by ear-capsule is third grade. A long section is devoted to genes and organizers, where the underlying assumption is that genes are catalysts or producers of catalysts (enzymes) or of inhibitors. Lethal genes are discussed in the following categories: those (1) causing death of the embryo before action of the primary organizer, (2) interfering with action of the primary organizer, (3) interfering with action of second or third grade organizers, (4) producing anomalies of the individuation field by changes in growth rates of parts, (5) producing anomalies of embryonic metabolism, (6) killing or deforming the embryo by unknown mechanisms. Many cases are shown to have their "phenocopies," these being similar but non-heritable changes produced by external chemical or physical agents. Part II closes with a critique of regeneration, determination, "fate maps" and organ districts, with special attention to determination in insects and echinoderms.

Part III, dealing with morphogenetic mechanisms, asserts that these mechanisms may become dissociated from one another. Dissociability is considered under the following heads: (a) Growth or increase in spatial dimensions and in weight; (b) Differentiation or increase in complexity and organization; (c) Metabolic changes in the organism. The relation of growth rate of a part of the developing organism to growth rate of the whole or of another part is termed *Heterauxesis*, the suggested equation for which is $\log y = \log b + k \log x$, where y is the magnitude of the differentially growing part, x the magnitude of the whole organism, b the fraction of x which y occupies when x is unity ("fractional coefficient"), and k the important constant representing the ratio of growth rate of the part to growth rate of the whole. The sections on metabolism deal with carbohydrates, proteins, nucleins, lipins, sterols and pigments. There is selected evidence of the organization of cell protoplasm. The transparent sea urchin egg examined in the ultra-violet spectrometer shows no absorption curve typical of protein; only when the egg is dead does the protein curve appear (Vles and Gex). The findings of Chambers and others by micro-manipulator methods are cited, as are those of Conklin on the possible "spongioplasmic framework" of eggs. Living systems are held to be in a paracrystalline state (liquid crystals), where the molecules pass through a succession of "mesoforms," having some liquid-like flow but also a definite and regular arrangement, as shown, e.g., in transplanted limb-bud discs, in which the antero-posterior axis remains determined whereas the other axes are labile (Harrison). The book closes with consideration of the mechanism of gastrulation, the fibers of mesoderm, and dynamic structure at the molecular level.

With all deference to old and honored strategies of approach, the present book reviews three other armies converging on the ivory citadel of the embryo, those of experimental morphology, endocrinology and genetics. The attack is still peripheral; no inner defenses have been breached. Yet withal we become convinced that only through such closing of ranks as may be effected by the biochemist can the citadel be reduced to a clear matter of fact.—C. F. DeGaris, M.D., Professor of Anatomy, University of Oklahoma School of Medicine.

THE PRINCIPLES AND PRACTICE OF OB-STETRICS. Joseph B. DeLee, A.M., M.D., formerly Professor of Obstetrics and Gynecology, University of Chicago; Consultant in Obstetrics, Chicago Lying-In Hospital and Dispensary; Consultant in Obstetrics, Chicago Maternity Center. J. P. Greenhill, B.S., M.D., attending Obstetrician and Gynecologist, Michael Reese Hospital; Obstetrician and Gynecologist, Associate Staff, Chicago Lying-In Hospital; Attending Gynecologist, Cook County Hospital; Professor of Gynecology, Cook County Graduate School of Medicine.

This eighth edition of the late Joseph B. DeLee's monumental volume, "Principles and Practices of Obstetrics," should be a 'must' in the library of every general practitioner and specialist in Obstetrics. Dr. Greenhill, the new editor, has made every effort to maintain Dr. DeLee's perfectionism in both presentation of the text, as well as in illustration. The text has its usual durable binding, is attractive in appearance and has 1,074 illustrations, 209 of which are in color.

Many major changes have been made, among these is the rearrangement of the material in the first third of the book. Dr. Greenhill made this change to avoid the slight confusion in the sequence of chapters in previous editions. The substitution of English terminology instead of Latin, in the designation of position and presentation is commendable.

Complete new sections, and in some instances, new chapters have been added, dealing with obstetrics and gynecologic endocrinology. The use of Vitamin K, vitamins and minerals, roentgenography in obstetrics, and sulfonamide drugs.

Particular mention should be made in reference to the new chapter on erythroblastosis fetalis, which is illustrated with beautiful colored plates, also the Water's Extraperitoneal Cesarean Section has been included.

Several chapters and sections have been completely rewritten, notably those on the toxemias of pregnancy in which the new classification proposed by the American Committee on Maternal Health has been followed.

The chapter on contracted pelvis is also notable, the older classification has been deleted and the new anatomic classification of Caldwell, Moloy, and d'Esopo and Thoms have been included.

The use of chemotherapy in the management of puerperal sepsis and the use of sulfonamides in the treatment of urinary tract infections in pregnancy has been emphasized. New developments in analgesic and anesthetic agents have been reviewed. The use of the oxytocics, namely pituitary extract, ergot and ergonovine is again discussed. One of the best written of the new sections is that on the indication for and the contraindications for Cesarean Sections.

A list of references at the end of each chapter has been limited to worthwhile contributions, chiefly to those of more recent articles dealing with the subject matter, although all the classic contributions have been listed.

It is the opinion of this reviewer that this new eighth edition will enjoy the universal acclaim that was accorded each of the preceeding editions throughout the English speaking world during the past thirty years. —Gerald Rogers, M.D.

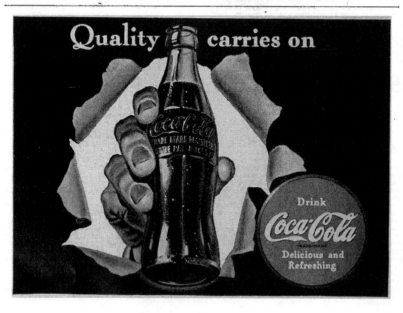

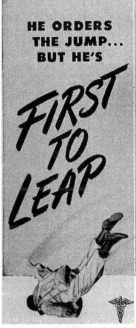
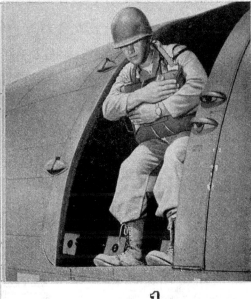
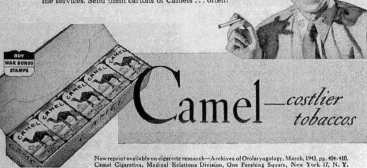

MEDICAL ABSTRACTS

"STUDIES ON 2-SULFANILAMIDE-4-METHYL-PYRIMI-DINE (SULFAMERAZINE, SULFAMETHYL-DIAZINE) IN MAN. THE TREATMENT OF PHEUMOCOCCIC PNEUMONIA." From the Committee for the Study of Pneumonia, which includes J. G. Reinhold, Ph.D., and S. B. Rose, M.D. By Harrison F. Flippin, M.D., William I. Geiter, M.D., Albert H. Domm, M.D. and Jefferson H. Clark, M.D. (From the Philadelphia General Hospital, Philadelphia, Pa.) _The American Journal of the Medical Sciences, page 498, June 11, 1943.

Therapeutic Results. The results of treatment in the two therapeutic groups are shown. Of the patients treated with sulfamerazine, six died, and in the sulfadiazine treated group, eight died, the mortality rates being 7.5 per cent and 10 per cent respectively. Eighteen patients with bacteremia were treated with sulfamerazine and six of these died, 33.3 per cent mortality. In the sulfadiazine treated group, four of the 22 bacteremic patients died, 18.2 per cent mortality.

In evaluating any therapeutic agent clinically, one must consider the effect of the agent on the course of the disease as well as its influence on the mortality incidence. A critical drop in temperatures occurred within 24 hours in 51.4 per cent of the patients treated with sulfamerazine, as compared with 30.6 per cent of the patients in the sulfadiazine treated group. Within 48 hours, 77.1 per cent of the patients receiving sulfamerazine and 66.7 per cent of those treated with sulfadiazine showed a critical drop in temperature. The temperature returned to normal within 24 hours in 17.5 per cent of the patients in the sulfamerazine treated group and in 15.3 per cent of the patients receiving sulfadiazine. Within 72 hours a return to normal temperature occurred in 72.9 per cent of patients in the sulfamerazine and sulfadiazine groups respectively.

Complications. The incidence of complications was low, 4.4 per cent. Three cases developed endocarditis and died. On case of empyema occurred in three sulfadiazine treated cases with no deaths.

Toxic Reactions. Out of the 160 patients, the incidence of toxic reactions attribute to the drug was small, being 9.4 per cent. Vomiting was noted in two patients in each group; hematuria in three patients receiving sulfamerazine and in four with sulfadiazine. Crystalluria was indicated in approximately 15 per cent of each group; toxic psychosis in one patient treated with sulfamerazine; drug fever in three patients, one with sulfamerazine and two with sulfadiazine. No skin lesions observed. No marked reduction or change in the blood count.

The average blood concentration in sulfamerazine was 12.7 mg. and with sulfadiazine 7.9 mg.

"*Comment.* Sulfamerazine and sulfadiazine are both effective drugs in the treatment of pneumococcic pneumonia. The mortality of 7.5 per cent in the sulfamerazine group and 10 per cent in the sulfadiazine group compare favorably when all the factors influencing fatality are considered. Clinical response, as manifested by a fall in temperature, was slightly more in evidence with sulfadiazine; and this, we believe, may be related to the more rapid rise and higher concentrations in blood attained by sulfamerazine as compared with sulfadiazine.

"In both therapeutic groups there was a low incidence of toxic manifestations, none of which was serious, following the use of these drugs. It is to be remembered, however, that the hazard of severe toxic reactions increases with the prolonged use of both sulfamerazine and sulfadiazine. In this series of pneumonia cases most patients required more than 20 to 30 gm. of either drug, extending over a short period of approximately six days. We believe that this explains in part the low incidence of toxicity encountered in this study.

SUMMARY

"1. Sulfamerazine was given to 80 adult patients with pneumococcic pneumonia and the response was compared with that of a control series of 80 adult patients treated with sulfadiazine.

"2. Mortality in the two therapeutic groups showed no significant difference (sulfamerazine 7.5 per cent, sulfadiazine 10 per cent.)

"3. Sulfamerazine tended to lower the temperature somewhat more rapidly than did sulfadiazine; however, the duration of chemotherapy and the incidence of complications were essentially the same for the two groups.

"4. The incidence of toxic reactions was low and comparable for both sulfamerazine and sulfadiazine. No serious reactions were encountered with either drug.

"5. The group treated with sulfamerazine showed higher plasma concentration of free drug than did the group receiving larger or equivalent amounts of sulfadiazine."—H.J., M.D.

"THE VALUE OF THE EXAMINATION OF GASTRIC CONTENTS FOR TUBERCLE BACILLI." John A. Foley, M.D., F.A.C.P., and John B. Andosca, M.D., Boston, Massachusetts. Annals of Internal Medicine, Vol. 19, Number 4, October, 1943.

In this the authors have again called to attention the fact that gastric lavage yields sputum valuable in the diagnosis of tuberculosis. This has been mentioned many times before, as is pointed out, various authors reporting as high as 20 to 80 per cent positive sputum findings in their cases of proven tuberculosis.

Six interesting cases are briefly reported; the mechanism of the sputum and bacilli being inadvertently swallowed, is explained; the technic of examination of the sputum is given and the results of 639 cases, in which such examinations were made, reported.

They summarize as follows:

1. The importance of gastric lavage for the detection of tubercle bacilli cannot be overestimated.

2. Out of 639 cases with negative sputum, 187 or 29.2 per cent were found to be positive by gastric lavage; 32 non-tuberculous cases employed as controls were all negative.

3. Guinea pig inoculation of the gastric contents definitely gives a higher percentage of positive results than direct microscopy.

4. Gastric lavage is an aid not only in establishing a diagnosis of pulmonary tuberculosis but also in its differential diagnosis, treatment and prognosis. It is in addition an accurate guage of the infectiousness of a patient and helps to determine his relationship to society.

5. We have attemped to show by case reports the reliability and importance of gastric lavage.—H.J., M.D.

"DERMATOLOGIC LESIONS ABOUT THE EYES." Oliver S. Ormsby. American Journal of Opthalmology. Series 3, Vol. 26, No. 8, pages 850-855, August, 1943.

The disease described under the title "essential shrinkage or shriveling of the conjunctiva" is considered synonymous with ocular pemphigus. It may occur independently or as a symptom of some other affection.

The early symptoms of the disease consist of a catarrhal inflammation of the conjunctiva associated with a thick mucoïd discharge. There is some burning and itching at this time. These symptoms may be recurrent over a period of years. Vesicles and bullae are early manifestations and may occur on any portion of the cornea and conjunctiva. In the late atrophic stage such vesicles will occur on other mucous membranes. At a later date the disease is characterized by xerosis, chronic inflammation of the subconjunctival tissue, causing shrinkage, formation of scar tissue and symblepharon. There may be associated phenomena on the cornea. The course of the disease varies. It usually is very slow, lasting over a period of years with remission and exacerbations. Blindness has ensued within two years in some cases.

Ectodermosis erosiva pluriorificialis is an affection resembling erythema multiforme. It is characterized by an acute onset with fever and constitutional symptoms and an eruption that involves the extremities chiefly, together with stomatitis, conjunctivitis, and sometimes involvement of the mucosa of the nose, urethra, vagina, and anus. The constitutional symptoms consists of chills and elevation of temperature ranging from 102 degrees to 104 degrees F. There is also headache and malaise. Stomatitis, which may be severe, begins with vesicular lesions; later, pseudomembranes will develop. The inflammation often extends to the throat and epiglottis. Profuse salivation is usually present. Ocular symptoms are always prominent and may be so severe as to cause partial or total blindness. They begin with a vesicular bilateral conjunctivitis. Inflammation of the nasal mucosa is also present and there may be a vesicular dermatitis in the anogenital region. After several days a multiform eruption, consisting of macules, vesicles, and purpuric lesions, develops on the hands and feet. The disease runs its course from three to six weeks as a rule. Relapses have been reported.

In 1940 Bencet described a new disease characterized by aphthous ulcers in the mouth, ulcerating lesions on the genitalia, and retinitis and iridocyclitis. In some cases lesions resembling erythema modosum were present. The syndrome is recurrent, runs an indefinite course, and varies in severity. A virus infection is possibly present.

The chief vitamin deficiencies with ocular and cutaneous symptoms are that of vitamin A and vitamin G or B2 (riboflavin.) The association of night blindness, keratomalacia and follicular hyperkeratosis is now a well recognized syndrome due to deficiency of vitamin A. Such condition can be corrected by prescribing the best sources of vitamin A in the diet, which are butter, cream, egg yolk, fish-liver oils, and green leafy vegatables.

In ariboflavinosis there is a perlechelike eruption at the angles of the mouth, a scaley inflammation of the vermilion portion of the lips, together with a mild, greasy, seborrhealike dermatitis in the nasolabial folds and at the inner and outer canthi of the eyes. Sometimes there may be also a vascularizing keratitis. This will cause photophobia, dimness of vision, circumcorneal injection, and burning sensations of the eyeball. Corneal opacities and iritis may occur. Keratitis and conjunctivitis are quite often associated with rosacea and are examples of a riboflavin deficiency. Riboflavin in the dosage of 5 mg .thrice daily is efficient in clearing up these lesions. Best sources of riboflavin are milk, eggs, liver, muscle, and yeast.

A dermatitis occurring on-the lids is one of the commonest affections seen by the dermatologist. The commonest cause of such dermatitis in women is the use of cosmetics, particularly nail polish. Very often due to nail polish, the face and the region around the ears may be involved in addition. Other sensitizing agents are present in proprietary hair dyes and hair lotions. When it has been proved that an external irritant is an exciting factor, the management of the case becomes simple. Sodium thiosulfate may be injected in the dosage of one gram intravenously every other day for a week,

together with a 10 per cent naftalan ointment applied locally.

Xanthelesma is limited to the eyes in many cases. In a size ranging from pinhead to pea, or larger, the lesion involves the upper lip at the inner canthus as chrome-yellow lesions that merge to form large plaques which sometimes interfere with vision. In about 70 per cent of the cases there is a moderate to marked elevation of blood lipoids. The management of xanthelesma is often unsatisfactory. If the skin is lax, complete surgical removal is efficient. Electric needling gives a fairly good result in some patients. In others refrigeration with carbon dioxide snow is efficient.—M.D.H., M.D.

"EAR, NOSE AND THROAT CASUALTIES IN A GENERAL HOSPITAL IN THE MIDDLE EAST." E. G. Collins. British Medical Journal, Volume 2, pages 366-389. September 25, 1943.

The present report covers the period from September 20, 1940 to February 20, 1941. During the months under review war injuries affecting the ear, nose and throat were few in number, and the type of disease bore a close resemblance to that found in any hospital in the British Isles.

There is no doubt that the frequency of otitis externa is increased by service in the Middle East. External and middle-ear otitis are approximately the same in number. It is in its acute form that the disease interferes with the efficiency of the soldier, but there is no sharp demarcation between the acute and the chronic stage. With the least provocation the latter is liable to flare up and become acute. The etiology still remains obscure. Dust, heat with its concimitant sweating, bathing, and, in the Western Desert, lack of water for personal ablution have all been mentioned as factors in its causation. Other possible causes are the high salt concentration of the water and an allergic origin due to focal sepsis. It seems possible that several factors, and not one factor alone, may be responsible, and that anything that favors the growth of organisms and the maceration of the skin may play a part. In a series of aural swabs examined the organisms found were diphtheroids, B. proteus, and B. pyocyaneus. The last named was very difficult to eradicate. Staphylococcus aureaus was present in a great proportion, while the Streptococcus was infrequent.

In acute otitis extrena the soldier experiences very severe pain in the ear, there is scanty aural discharge, and the meatus is greatly narrowed and often pin-hole. There is often a deficiency of true waxy secretion, and the return of normal soft wax was regarded as one of the signs of cure.

Many acute cases could be prevented or aborted if the soldier reported to the medical officer at the first sign of any aural discharge. Some protection was afforded by the use of vaselined cotton-wool plugs inserted in the ears while bathing. Great care should be taken in drying out the ears with any rough towel after bathing. It is better to use a pencil of cotton-wool. Bathing in swimming-baths appeared to be more harmful than bathing in the sea. Where there is an associated seborrheic dermatitis of the scalp it must be treated. Thorough cleaning of the external auditory meatus, and especially the recess near the anterior-inferior part of the tympanic membrane is an essential part of successful treatment. Ten per cent ichthyol in glycerin and 8 per cent solution of aluminum acetate are very valuable.

Acute otitis media did not form a large proportion of the cases during the period of review, but there was a definite increase during the summer months. This was probably due to the greater use of the swimming-baths. The prophylactic measures include the avoidance of diving and of swimming under water when the soldier has a cold. The use of dirty handkerchiefs and incorrect blowing of the nose are other obvious causes. Treatment was greatly influenced by the oral administration of sulfonamides, and it was necessary to submit only 6 patients out of a total of 47 cases of acute otitis media to a cortical mastoid operation. In local treatment it matters little whether the wet or dry method is used so long as the ear is cleaned out thoroughly before any drops are instilled. The otologist should bear in mind that radical mastoid cavities are slow to heal in the Middle East. The modified radical mastoid operation is, where possible, the method of choice.

The prophylaxis of acute tonsillitis consists essentially in isolation. Every effort should be made to carry this out near the front line; only cases of frequently recurrent attacks should be sent back. At a base hospital a special ward should be available for cases of tonsilitis only, even at the cost of empty beds. The infecting organism in the majority of cases in the Middle East was Streptococcus Viridans; but in spite of this fact the administration of sulfonamides decreased the length of stay in the hospital. Local treatment followed the usual lines. Operation by dissection of tonsils was undertaken in 17 per cent of cases. Only those patients who suffered from three or four attacks were considered suitable candidates for operation.

The figures for sinusitis strongly suggest that there is a high incidence of sinus infection in the Middle East. Part of this must be attributed to the infected dustladen atmosphere as there was a noticeable increase during a dust storm. Bathing in the swimming-pool appeared to have a deleterious effect, as even if the bacillary content was low, the heavy chlorination practiced had a harmful effect on ciliary activity in the nose. Conservative measures are recommended, such as inhalations with the use of ephedrine in saline sprays, headlight baths, shortwave diathermy, and repeated proof-puncture. It was found that 74 per cent were cured by these means, and later experience in the desert confirmed that operated cases did badly. Many patients with so-called vacuum sinus disease were improved by rest in bed and the ordinary conservation treatment of acute sinusitis.

It is the general opinion that during war the septum operation should be regarded as a luxury measure except in cases of gross nasal obstruction or where it forms a contributory factor in the causation of catarrhal deafness or sinusitis.—M. D. H., M.D.

"THE OCULAR MANIFESTATIONS OF SPONTANEOUS SUBARACHNOID·HAEMORRHAGE." A. J. Ballantyne. The British Journal of Ophthalmology. Volume 27, pages 383-414. September, 1943.

Subarachnoid hemorrhage may occur spontaneously or as a result of head injury. The traumatic and non-traumatic cases present many points of similarity, but important differences result from the physical factors attending their onset.

The author discusses the non-traumatic group, with pathological findings in five cases. Since the hemorrhage, in the majority of cases, comes from the vessels of the circle of Willis, being due to the rupture of either an aneurysm or a weakened portion of the vessel wall, cases occur in which the effusion of blood is relatively slight, but prone to recurrence. The leading symptoms are severe deep-seated pain often accompanied by paresis of one or other of the ocular muscles. Cerebral arteriography may reveal the presence of an aneurysm, and lumbar puncture discover blood staining of the cerebrospinal fluids.

In the severe cases the clinical picture·is entirely different. The patient is seen in a more or less comatose state, with a history of sudden onset, and with signs suggestive of cerebral compression and meningeal irritation: pupil anamalies, mystagmus, conjugate deviation of the eyes, and paralysis of cranial nerves, including the oculomotors, are often observed. These are not in themselves sufficient to justify a diagnosis of subarachnoid hemorrhage. The presence of retinal hemorrhages and papilledema, if these are found on ophthalmoscopic examination, strongly supports such a diagnosis, and a history of minor attacks adds to its

probability, but the matter is settled by the discovery of blood in the cerebrospinal fluid.

Such cases are usually terminated fatally, and it is not surprising that in the majority no record is obtained of the state of the vision. At post-mortem examination blood is found in large amounts in the subarachnoid spaces at the base of the brain, sometimes breaking through into the substance of the brain or into the lateral ventribles. The source of the blood is usually found in a ruptured aneurysm or a ruptured branch of the circle of Willis.

Immediately behind the optic canal, the optic nerves may show a bluish coloration owing to the presence of blood between the sheaths, and blood in this situation may be seen on the cut surface of the nerve. Even in cases where no blood is found in this region, exposure of the orbital part of the optic nerve often shows this to be expanded and discolored by the presence of blood between its sheath. In some cases this appearance affects the whole nerve from the optic foramen to the eyeball; but in the majority the ecchymosis is patchy and intermittent. It is usual to find some degree of bulbous distention of the optic nerve sheaths immediately behind the globe. Distension of the orbital veins, and hemorrhages amongst the orbital contents and on the surface of the sclera may also be observed.

In the five cases reported by the author there was a certain similarity: the history of sudden onset with severe pain, symptoms of cerebral irritation and compression, and coma preceding death. Blood-staining of the cerebrospinal fluid was present in all.

The discovery of hemorrhage in the subarachnoid space at the base of the brain, within the sheaths of the optic nerve, and in many cases in the retina and even in the vitreous, originally led to the belief that the blood passed in a continuous manner in the subarachnoid space through the optic canal into the orbit, and thence along the course of the central retinal vessels, or by lymph channels accompanying the optic nerve at the periphery of the lamia cribrosa into the retina.

It is now generally agreed that the blood in the cerebral subarachnoid space does not, as a rule, travel through the optic foramen into the subarachnoid space of the optic nerve. It is more generally assumed that hemorrhage occurs in the dural sheath at the apex of the orbit, and tracks forward into the subdural and subarachnoid spaces, and that blood in the latter situation, by putting pressure and tension on the central retinal vein where it crosses the space, causes stasis in the central retinal vein and thus accounts for the retinal and vitreous hemorrhages.

On the basis of the five cases described it is shown that hemorrhages occur over a much wider field than the optic nerve sheaths, the retina and the vitreous, and that these cannot be accounted for by the assumed pressure on the central retinal vein.

The hemorrhages varied in distribution from case to case, but were found in and between the sheaths of the optic nerve, among the orbital fat and orbital muscles, surrounding the posterior ciliary nerves, ciliary ganglion, ophthalmic and posterior ciliary arteries, and the vessels of the chiasma and optic tracts; as well as beneath the retina, in all its layers, in front of the retina and in the vitreous. Serial sections showed that these were not in continuity with one another, but were dicrete and independent hemorrhages, simultaneous in their occurence. The occurence of such multiple hemorrhages can only be explained by a sudden rise of intracranial pressure causing stasis in all the venous channels which drain the tissues of the eye and the contents of the orbit.—M.D.H., M.D.

KEY TO ABSTRACTORS

E. D. M. ....Earl D. McBride, M.D.
H. J. ....Hugh Jeter, M.D.
M. D. H. ....Marvin D. Henely, M.D.

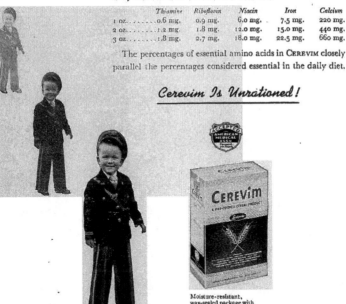
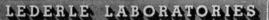

OFFICERS OF COUNTY SOCIETIES, 1944

★

COUNTY	PRESIDENT	SECRETARY	MEETING TIME
Alfalfa	H. E. Huston, Cherokee	L. T. Lancaster, Cherokee	Last Tues. each Second Month
Atoka-Coal	R. C. Henry, Coalgate	J. S. Fulton, Atoka	
Beckham	H. K. Speed, Sayre	E. S. Kilpatrick, Elk City	Second Tuesday
Blaine	Virginia Olson Curtin, Watonga	W. F. Griffin, Watonga	
Bryan	J. T. Colwick, Durant	W. K. Haynie, Durant	Second Tuesday
Caddo	F. L. Patterson, Carnegie	C. B. Sullivan, Carnegie	
Canadian	P. F. Herod, El Reno	A. L. Johnson, El Reno	Subject to call
Carter	J. R. Pollock, Ardmore	H. A. Higgins, Ardmore	
Cherokee	P. H. Medearis, Tahlequah	*James K. Gray, Tahlequah	First Tuesday
Choctaw	C. H. Hale, Boswell	E. A. Johnson, Hugo	
Cleveland	J. A. Rieger, Norman	Curtis Berry, Norman	Thursday nights
Comanche	George S. Barber, Lawton	W. F. Lewis, Lawton	
Cotton	A. B. Holstead, Temple	Mollie F. Scism, Walters	Third Friday
Craig	F. M. Adams, Vinita	J. M. McMillan, Vinita	
Creek	H. R. Haas, Sapulpa	C. G. Oakes, Sapulpa	
Custer	F. R. Vieregg, Clinton	C. J. Alexander, Clinton	Third Thursday
Garfield	Julian Feild, Enid	John R. Walker, Enid	Fourth Thursday
Garvin	T. F. Gross, Lindsay	John R. Callaway, Pauls Valley	Wednesday before Third Thursday
Grady	Walter J. Baze, Chickasha	Roy E. Emanuel, Chickasha	Third Thursday
Grant	I. V. Hardy, Medford	E. E. Lawson, Medford	
Greer	R. W. Lewis, Granite	J. B. Hollis, Mangum	
Harmon	W. G. Husband, Hollis	R. H. Lynch, Hollis	First Wednesday
Haskell	William Carson, Keota	N. K. Williams, McCurtain	
Hughes	Wm. L. Taylor, Holdenville	Imogene Mayfield, Holdenville	First Friday
Jackson	C. G. Spears, Altus	E. A. Abernethy, Altus	Last Monday
Jefferson	F. M. Edwards, Ringling	L. L. Wade, Ryan	Second Monday
Kay	Philip C. Risser, Blackwell	J. Holland Howe, Ponca City	Second Thursday
Kingfisher	C. M. Hodgson, Kingfisher	H. Violet Sturgeon, Hennessey	
Kiowa	J. William Finch, Hobart	William Bernell, Hobart	
LeFlore	Neeson Rolle, Poteau	Rush L. Wright, Poteau	
Lincoln	W. B. Davis, Stroud	Carl H. Bailey, Stroud	First Wednesday
Logan	William O. Miller, Guthrie	J. L. LeHew, Jr., Guthrie	Last Tuesday
Marshall	O. A. Cook, Madill		
Mayes	Ralph V. Smith, Pryor	Paul B. Cameron, Pryor	
McClain	B. W. Slover, Blanchard	R. L. Royster, Purcell	
McCurtain	A. W. Clarkson, Valliant	N. L. Barker, Broken Bow	Fourth Tuesday
McIntosh	Luster I. Jacobs, Hanna	Wm. A. Tolleson, Eufaula	First Thursday
Murray	P. V. Annadown, Sulphur		Second Tuesday
Muskogee-Sequoyah-Wagoner	H. A. Scott, Muskogee	D. Evelyn Miller, Muskogee	First Monday
Noble	C. H. Cooke, Perry	J. W. Francis, Perry	
Okfuskee	L. J. Spickard, Okemah	M. L. Whitney, Okemah	Second Monday
Oklahoma	Walker Morledge, Oklahoma City	E. R. Musick, Oklahoma City	Fourth Tuesday
Okmulgee	A. R. Holmes, Henryetta	J. C. Matheney, Okmulgee	Second Monday
Osage	C. R. Weirich, Pawhuska	George K. Hemphill, Pawhuska	Second Monday
Ottawa	W. B. Sanger, Picher	Matt A. Connell, Picher	Third Thursday
Pawnee	E. T. Robinson, Cleveland	R. L. Browning, Pawnee	
Payne	L. A. Mitchell, Stillwater	C. W. Moore, Stillwater	Third Thursday
Pittsburg	P. T. Powell, McAlester	W. H. Kaeiser, McAlester	Third Friday
Pontotoc	O. H. Miller, Ada	R. H. Mayes, Ada	First Wednesday
Pottawatomie	E. Eugene Rice, Shawnee	Clinton Gallaher, Shawnee	First and Third Saturday
Pushmataha	John S. Lawson, Clayton	B. M. Huckabay, Antlers	
Rogers	C. W. Beson, Claremore	C. L. Caldwell, Chelsea	First Monday
Seminole	Max Van Sandt, Wewoka	Mack I. Shanholtz, Wewoka	Third Wednesday
Stephens	W. K. Walker, Marlow	Wallis S. Ivy, Duncan	
Texas	R. G. Obermiller, Texhoma	Morris Smith, Guymon	
Tillman		O. G. Bacon, Frederick	
Tulsa	Ralph A. McGill, Tulsa	E. O.Johnson, Tulsa	Second and Fourth Monday
Washington-Nowata	K. D. Davis, Nowata	J. V. Athey, Bartlesville	Second Wednesday
Washita	A. S. Neal, Cordell	James F. McMurry, Sentinel	
Woods	Ishmael F. Stephenson, Alva	Oscar E. Templin, Alva	Last Tuesday Odd Months
Woodward	H. Walker, Buffalo	C. W. Tedrowe, Woodward	Second Thursday

*(Serving in Armed Forces)

OKLAHOMA STATE MEDICAL ASSOCIATION

Executive Office: 210 Plaza Court, Oklahoma City, Okla. Telephone: 7-0976.

Meeting Place: Tulsa, Okla., April 24-26, 1944.

OFFICERS

President, James Stevenson, M.D., Tulsa.

President-Elect, C. R. Rountree, M.D., Oklahoma City.

Vice-President, J. G. Edwards, M.D., Okmulgee.

Secretary-Treasurer, L. J. Moorman, M.D., Oklahoma City.

Executive Secretary, Mr. R. H. Graham, Oklahoma City.

Speaker, House of Delegates, George H. Garrison, M.D., Oklahoma City.

Vice-Speaker, House of Delegates, H. K. Speed, M.D., Sayre.

Delegates to the A.M.A., W. A. Howard, M.D., Chelsea, 1942-43; A. S. Risser, M.D., Blackwell, 1943-44.

Meeting Place, Tulsa, 1944.

SPECIAL COMMITTEES, 1943-1944

Conservation of Vision and Hearing: F. Maxey Cooper, M.D., Chairman, Oklahoma City; Charles H. Haralson, M.D., Tulsa; J. B. Hollis, M.D., Mangum.

Crippled Children: Ian MacKenzie, M.D., Chairman, Tulsa; Carroll M. Pounders, M.D., Oklahoma City; L. S. Willour, M.D., McAlester.

Industrial and Traumatic Surgery: J. S. Chalmers, M.D., Chairman, Sand Springs; D. H. O'Donoghue, M.D., Oklahoma City; C. E. Northcutt, M.D., Ponca City.

Malpractice Insurance: V. K. Allen, M.D., Chairman, Tulsa; John R. Walker, M.D., Enid; L. J. Starry, M.D., Oklahoma City; I. B. Oldham, M.D., Muskogee.

Maternity and Infancy: Edward N. Smith, M.D., Chairman, Oklahoma City; E. O. Johnson, M.D., Tulsa; J. T. Bell, M.D., Oklahoma City.

Medical Economics: McLain Rogers, M.D., Chairman, Clinton; H. M. McClure, M.D., Chickasha; L. R. Kirby, M.D., Okeene.

Military Affairs: Louis H. Ritzhaupt, M.D., Chairman, Guthrie; Ralph V. Smith, M.D., Pryor; P. P. Nesbitt, M.D., Tulsa.

Necrology: J. S. Fulton, M.D., Chairman, Atoka; O. S. Somerville, M.D., Bartlesville; John A. Walker, M.D., Shawnee.

Postgraduate Medical Teaching: Gregory E. Stanbro, M.D., Chairman, Oklahoma City; H. M. McClure, M.D., Chickasha; H. C. Weber, M.D., Bartlesville; D. B. Ensor, M.D., Hopeton; J. C. Matheney, M.D., Okmulgee; M. J. Searle, M.D., Tulsa.

Prepaid Medical and Surgical Service: John F. Burton, M.D., Chairman, Oklahoma City; V. C. Tisdal, M.D., Elk City; W. Floyd Keller, M.D., Oklahoma City; A. S. Risser, M.D., Blackwell; H. C. Weber, M.D., Bartlesville; Finis W. Ewing, M.D., Muskogee; A. W. Pigford, M.D., Tulsa; Ben W. Ward, M.D., Tulsa.

Public Health: Carroll M. Pounders, M.D., Chairman, Oklahoma City; E. H. Werling, M.D., Pryor; Philip C. Risser, M.D., Blackwell.

Study and Control of Cancer: Ralph A. McGill, M.D., Chairman, Tulsa; Joseph W. Kelso, M.D., Oklahoma City; Paul B. Champlin, M.D., Enid.

Study and Control of Tuberculosis: F. P. Baker, M.D., Chairman, Talihina; Floyd Moorman, M.D., Oklahoma City; R. M. Shepard, M.D., Tulsa.

Study and Control of Venereal Diseases: David V. Hudson, M.D., Chairman, Tulsa; John H. Lamb, M.D., Oklahoma City; E. Halsell Fite, M.D., Muskogee.

STANDING COMMITTEES, 1943-1944

Annual Session: James Stevenson, M.D., Tulsa; C. R. Rountree, M.D., Oklahoma City; L. J. Moorman, M.D., Oklahoma City.

Credentials: Finis W. Ewing, M.D., Muskogee; H. K. Speed, M.D., Sayre; J. V. Athey, M.D., Bartlesville.

Judicial and Professional Relations: S. A. Lang, M.D., Nowata; J. M. Bonham, M.D., Hobart; Claude S. Chambers, M.D., Seminole.

Medical Education and Hospitals: Tom Lowry, M.D., Oklahoma City; Roscoe Walker, M.D., Pawhuska; Sam A. McKeel, M.D., Ada.

Publicity: W. A. Tolleson, M.D., Eufaula; A. Ray Wiley, M.D., Tulsa; M. D. Carnell, M.D., Okmulgee.

Public Policy: J. D. Osborn, M.D., Frederick; J. T. Martin, M.D., Oklahoma City; Frank W. Boadway, M.D., Ardmore.

Scientific Work: W. A. Showman, M.D., Tulsa; Ben H. Nicholson, M.D., Oklahoma City; M. J. Searle, M. D., Tulsa.

SCIENTIFIC SECTIONS

General Surgery: Oscar White, M.D., Chairman, 1200 N. Walker, Oklahoma City; Gregory E. Stanbro, M.D., Vice-Chairman, Medical Arts Building, Oklahoma City; J. C. Perry, M.D., Secretary, Medical Arts Building, Tulsa.

Eye, Ear, Nose and Throat: Leo F. Cailey, M.D., Chairman, Medical Arts Building, Oklahoma City; Hugh J. Evans, M.D., Secretary, Medical Arts Building, Tulsa.

Dermatology and Radiology: Walter Larrabee, M.D., Chairman, Medical Arts Building, Tulsa; John Heatley, M.D., Secretary, Medical Arts Building, Oklahoma City.

Urology and Syphilology: Alfred R. Sugg, M.D., Chairman, Ada; J. W. Rogers, M. D., Secretary, Medical Arts Building, Tulsa.

General Medicine: Mary Sheppard, M.D., Chairman, 1200 N. Walker, Oklahoma City; H. A. Ruprecht, M.D., Vice-Chairman, 604 S. Cincinnati, Tulsa; Philip M. Schreck, M.D., Secretary, Medical Arts Building, Tulsa.

Neurology, Psychiatry and Endocrinology: C. T. Steen, M.D., Chairman, Norman; Charles E. Leonard, M.D., Vice-Chairman, 131 N. E. 4th St., Oklahoma City; Coyne Campbell, M.D., Secretary, 131 N. E. 4th St., Oklahoma City.

Pediatrics: Luvern Hays, M.D., Chairman, Medical Arts Building, Tulsa; G. R. Russell, M.D., Secretary, 604 So. Cincinnati, Tulsa.

Public Health: John W. Shackelford, M.D., Chairman, State Health Dept., Oklahoma City; Carl Puckett, M.D., Vice-Chairman, 22 W. Sixth Street, Oklahoma City; Charles W. Haygood, M.D., Secretary, Shawnee.

Obstetrics and Gynecology: Edward N. Smith, M.D., Chairman, 400 N. W. 10th St., Oklahoma City; Roy E. Emanuel, M.D., Secretary, Chickasha.

COMMITTEE ON STANDARDIZATION

Earl D. McBride, M.D., Chairman, 605 N. W. Tenth Street, Oklahoma City;

Maurice J. Searle, M.D., Vice-Chairman, Medical Arts Bldg., Tulsa;

Joe N. Hamilton, Secretary, 313 Franklin Bldg., Oklahoma City;

J. F. Park, M.D., McAlester, V. C. Tisdal, M.D., Elk City; E. Eugene Rice, M.D., Shawnee, and Dale D. Henry, D.D.S., Okemah.

STATE BOARD OF MEDICAL EXAMINERS

Dr. Sam A. McKeel, Ada, President; Dr. Finis W. Ewing, Muskogee; Dr. J. D. Osborn, Frederick, Secretary-Treasurer; Dr. O. C. Newman, Shattuck; Dr. H. C. Weber, Bartlesville; Dr. S. B. Leslie, Okmulgee; and Dr. Galvin L. Johnson, Pauls Valley.

STATE COMMISSIONER OF HEALTH

Dr. Grady F. Mathews, Oklahoma City.

OKLAHOMA REPRESENTATIVE AMERICAN SOCIETY FOR THE CONTROL OF CANCEER

Dr. Wendell Long, Medical Arts Bldg., Oklahoma City.

COUNCILORS AND THEIR COUNTIES

District No. 1: Alfalfa, Beaver, Cimarron, Dewey, Ellis, Harper, Texas, Woods, Woodward—O. E. Templin, M.D., Alva. (Term expires 1944.)

District No. 2: Beckham, Custer, Greer, Harmon, Jackson, Kiowa, Roger Mills, Tillman, Washita—V. C. Tisdal, M.D., Elk City. (Term expires 1945.)

District No. 3: Garfield, Grant, Kay, Major, Noble, Pawnee, Payne—C. W. Arrendell, M.D., Ponca City. (Term expires 1946.)

District No. 4: Blaine, Canadian, Cleveland, Kingfisher, Logan, Oklahoma—Tom Lowry, M.D., 1200 North Walker, Oklahoma City. (Term expires 1944.)

District No. 5: Caddo, Carter, Comanche, Cotton, Grady, Jefferson, Love, Murray, Stephens—J. I. Hollingsworth, M.D., Waurika. (Term expires 1945.)

District No. 6: Creek, Nowata, Osage, Rogers, Tulsa, Washington—J. V. Athey, M.D., Bartlesville. (Term expires 1946.)

District No. 7: Garvin, Hughes, Lincoln, McClain, Okfuskee, Pontotoc, Pottawatomie, Seminole—Clinton Gallaher, M.D., Shawnee. (Term expires 1944.)

District No. 8: Adair, Cherokee, Craig, Delaware, Mayes, Muskogee, Okmulgee, Ottawa, Sequoyah, Wagoner—Finis W. Ewing, M.D., Muskogee. (Term expires 1945.)

District No. 9: Haskell, Latimer, LeFlore, McIntosh, Pittsburg—L. C. Kuyrkendall, M.D., McAlester. (Term expires 1943.)

District No. 10: Atoka, Bryan, Choctaw, Coal, Johnston, Marshall, McCurtain, Pushmataha—J. S. Fulton, M.D., Atoka. (Term expires 1944.)

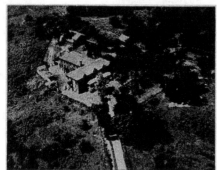

THE JOURNAL

OF THE

OKLAHOMA STATE MEDICAL ASSOCIATION

VOLUME XXXVII   OKLAHOMA CITY, OKLAHOMA, FEBRUARY, 1944   NUMBER 2

Fractional X-Ray Treatment of Skin Cancer*

MARQUE O. NELSON, M.D.

TULSA, OKLAHOMA

Until about 10 years ago, the treatment of cancer with x-rays was mainly by massive dosage, given in one or perhaps two or three treatments. The percentage of cures varied with the type of growth but in most types of deep-seated cancer, treatment was palliative only and cure was not to be expected.

Since the announcement of Coutard of his protracted practional method, the treatment of cancer by x-rays has been greatly improved and many cases that some years ago would have been hopeless, are now being cured. Coutard's method consists in giving comparatively small or moderate doses at frequent intervals continuing until a reaction, which he calls "radioepidermitis" on the skin and "radioepithelitis" on the mucous membrane, appears in the tumor or in the tissues overlying it.

It is interesting to note that at least in cancers of the skin a similar method of treatment was used and recommended by the American dermatologist Pusey as long ago as 1910 and even earlier but probably, owing to the crudity of dosage measurement at the time, it did not receive much attention. Except for the physicial factors used, Pusey's method very nearly coincided with Coutard's and if it had received due attention by radiologists, the possibilities of the fractional method of x-ray treatment of cancer would have been discovered much sooner than they were.

In Coutards method, the dosage varies with the size of the area being treated, small areas tolerating larger doses and more

*Read before the Annual Meeting held in Oklahoma City, May 11-12, 1943.

intensive treatment. It varies also with the type of the lesion, the rate of irradiation being more rapid with the embryonic forms and less rapid and larger total dosage with the more differentiated forms. It is his opinion that doses of at least 3,000 r to 4,000 r in the affected tissues are necessary for cure, requiring doses on the skin overlying the tumor of 6,000 to 8,000 r. Daily dosage varies from as little as 150 r to 700 r or even 800 r and are continued until the reaction appears. This consists of a destruction of the epithelial cells covering the irradiated surfaces and appears about two or three weeks after the beginning of treatment. When the treatment has been correct, the reaction lasts about 7 to 14 days. Healing of the ulcerated areas thus produced occurs in islands and also from the periphery. Contrary to what one would expect from experience with the usual x-ray ulcer, repair is rapid and satisfactory if treatment has been properly given. The factors used by Coutard were 200 K.V., 2 mm. zinc, 3 mm. aluminum, 3 cm. wood filter, 50 to 60 cm. or even 100 cm. distance and about 6 r per minute to the skin.

Since 1936 I have been using a method similar to Coutard's in the treatment of selected cases of cancer of the skin. Thirty-four of these cases were of the basal cell or rodent type, seven were of cancer of the lip, one was squamous cell epithelioma of the nose, and four were malignant melanomas. In the first group there have been 5 seven year cures, 4 six year cures, 2 five year cures, 3 four year cures, 1 three year cure, 5 in which there has been no recurrence in two years, and 11 in which there has been no recurrence in one year. One patient died of other causes after four years. Of the cases of epithelioma of the lip there is 1 six year cure, 1 five year cure, 2 in which there has been no recurrence in four years, 1 with no recurrence in two years and 1 with no recurrence in one year. One patient died after four years and one died of other causes after two years. In neither case was there any sign of recurrence of the cancer at the time of death. Of the cases of malignant melanoma, 2 had metastases when first seen and in 2 cases no metastases could be found. Of those with metastases, 1 died in 15 months and 1 is living and well after two years. The other two patients are in good health, one and two years respectively, after treatment. No metastases have been found in either case.

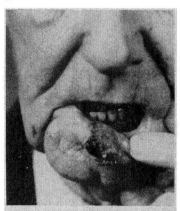

Fig. 1.—Epithelioma of the lip before treatment.

TECHNIC

The technic of treatment has varied with the individual case, depending on differing conditions, i.e., the location and size of the lesion, the type of skin, the age of the patient, the kind of underlying tissues and the type of neoplasm being treated. The total dosage of x-rays has varied from 300 r to 10,500 r, the individual doses being from 200 to 750 r and total number of treatments from 4 to 31. Tension was approximately 100 p.k.v., filtration varied from none to one-half mm. copper, plus 1 mm. aluminum, current 5 m.a., distance usually 8 to 10 inches.

TREATMENT OF METASTASES

Metastases in lymph nodes can be treated either by surgical removal, by the interstitial use of radium or by fractional x-ray treatment of the metastatic nodes, protecting adjacent tissues with lead. It seems unlikely that fractional irradiation of entire lymph node-bearing areas, with the hope of destroying all metastases in the area, can have more than a palliative effect. If used at all, irradiation of this kind must be thorough and carried to the point of ulceration of the skin in the irradiated area. Although treatment of large areas in this way is not likely to destroy metastases because of the impracticability of giving sufficiently large doses, I believe it is possible to check the growth of metastases in individual lymph nodes by fractional irradiation if the node is treated perseveringly and vigorously enough and proper dosage and other factors are used.

RESULTS

The results of treatment have been very encouraging. In fact, the outcome in several cases has been unexpectedly good and has made me enthusiastic about the possibilities of this method of treatment of cancer. In one case, that of a man 83 years old, a large irregular epithelioma measuring 3 x 6- x 9 cm, covered the entire nose. The lesion was so large that it interfered with vision in the left eye and prevented shaving the upper lip. On account of the patient's age and the location and type of the lesion, surgical removal was considered too dangerous, from the standpoint of possible hemorrhage and shock, consequently treatment with x-rays was undertaken more as a palliative measure than with the hope of cure. The patient was given a total of 5,600 r to each side of the nose, the first dose being given March 30, 1937 and the last on May 25, 1937. The tumor began to shrink within a week and in

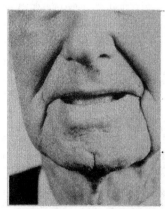

Fig. 2.—Appearance after fractional x-ray treatment. No trace of the epithelioma remains. Except for a thinning of the mucous membrane there is little change from the normal appearance.

two weeks was little more than half its original size. Four months after the beginning of treatment there was no trace of the epithelioma and the nose had returned to its normal size and appearance, except for an atrophic thinning of the skin in the irradiated area. The patient died two years later from nephritis and old age with no sign of recurrence of the epithelioma.

The fractional method of x-ray treatment is time-consuming and proportionally expensive to the patient and the question might be raised as to whether it has sufficient advantage to justify its use. The answer is that in some cases it has no great advantage. Many small epithelioma can be removed by less expensive methods, with very good chance of permanent cure and without too much subsequent disfiguration. The experience of different operators indicates that from 80 per cent to 98 per cent of these lesions can be cured by other methods. What percentage of cures will be obtained by fractional x-ray treatment of lesions of this kind is not yet known but I am convinced from experience it will be nearer 100 per cent than by any other method of treatment. However, in cases in which the cosmetic effect is of no great importance, other methods may be used with a saving of time and expense to the patient. In a good many of the cases the cosmetic result is of great importance and in these and in the case of lesions overlying tissues that might be damaged by massive irradiation, the fractional method of x-ray treatment represents a welcome advance. In the more serious cancers,

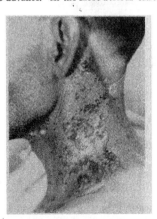

Fig. 3.—Cervical region after fractional irradiation for metastase, showing the so-called "radioepidermitis." The skin has been ulcerated but is healing rapidly.

such as extensive or recurrent lesions of the cancer, it is my belief that the fractional method of treatment will prove distinctly superior in the matter of permanency of cure and will obviate many undesirable irradiation sequelae that would be certain to occur if adequate doses of x-rays were given by the method of massive irradiation.

In closing, it should be emphasized that this method of treatment cannot be standardized and carried out in all cases with the same set of factors. It is no more feasible to use x-ray routinely than to perform all surgical operations in the same way. The observation and individual attention of the radiologist are all important and the success or failure of the treatment depends to a large extent upon his judgment and experience.

SUMMARY

The protracted fractional x-ray treatment of Coutard has opened great possibilities in the treatment of malignant neoplasms. The method of treatment can be used against cancer of the skin. It is especially suitable in cases in which treatment by other means would be either unsafe or likely to cause unsightly deformity and in cases of long standing, extensive or recurrent cancer. Fractional x-ray treatment cannot be standardized. Success or failure in its use depends to a very large extent on the individual attention and judgment of the radiologist.

DISCUSSION

W. A. SHOWMAN, M.D.
TULSA, OKLAHOMA

Dr. Nelson has presented a very interesting group of cases and a well recognized procedure, therefore any discussion of this particular paper and procedure will open many divergent views for treating skin cancer.

The selection of any one recognized standard procedure is based entirely upon the particular individual who has formulated a plan to meet his requirements, providing that the selected arrangement fulfills the general concept of adequate dosage. This, in my opinion, is of paramount importance, whether it be as presented today by a modified Coutard method, a single unfiltered massive dose, by fractionation of large doses of unfitered irradiation with moderate low voltage (85 k.V. to 100 K.V.), or the use of radium.

For the past several years, in selected cases, I have followed a plan similar to the one outlined by Dr. Nelson and find it to be a most excellent one, however, it is not without disadvantages and I agree with the author concerning the disadvantages enumerated. I am of the opinion that in most cases the time element should not enter into the selection of any one procedure but there are cases in which this is of extreme importance. I have used, more frequently, the massive single dose, or fractional large doses of unfiltered radiation where the tumor has not been too large, and I am sure that the end results are comparable to any other method providing adequate dosage has been given. In most instances, the bad results have been due to the failure to deliver sufficient irradiation to destroy the cancer cell.

The essential consideration in using rays with K.V. and 100 K.V. wave length range is the amount of radiation rather than its specific quality. The average target distance has been 20 cm., non shock proof type tube, giving a total dosage of 4,000 r to 6,000 r for basal cell lesion of 1 to 2 cm., in diameter. For the squamous type lesion, large doses are given, 4,000 r at first session, which is followed in a week by 2,000 r or 4,000 r additional. All lesions are shielded close with several layers of lead, and as shrinkage takes place, the aperture is closed to conform with the shrinkage.

Preference to the harder rays with 120 K.V. and filtration of 3 mm al., or one-half mm copper is done on the basis that a smaller skin dose is required in order to deliver an adequate dose to the tumor, however, because of the greater depth effect with the possibility of damage to the deeper healthy tissues, the quantity radiation given must be smaller than when unfiltered radiation is administered. The hard rays do not lend themselves readily to the principle of massive superfical caustic effect.

Examination of Foodhandlers . . . Findings In City of McAlester, Oklahoma

P. T. POWELL, M.D.
Director, Pittsburg County Health Department

HARRY LOWENS, P.A.
Surgeon, United States Public Health Service

This study covers the findings in 769 foodhandlers examined, a great majority of whom are migratory caused by the increase in employment due to the war industries in this vicinity. The constant turnover of workers made examination a continuous process, and the follow-up in many cases impossible. Thus, much of the data is not as complete as we would like it to be. This is especially true in the reports of stool examinations and x-rays. In the former instance, the patient had to obtain the stool at home and send it to the State Health Department Laboratory, and in the latter, x-rays were made by private physicians, which in many cases were refused because of the cost. However, the results should serve as a fairly typical example of what may be found in the examination of foodhandlers.

In the examination the following procedure was adhered to:

. History, both personal and family with reference to typhoid and tuberculosis. A special point was made to obtain the time elasped since typhoid affected either the foodhandler or his family.

2. Whether foodhandler or dairy worker.

3. Physical examination of lungs.

4. Blood: Wassermann, Brucellosis, agglutination test in dairy workers.

5. Sputum examination, where indicated.

6. Stool examination:
   (a) those having had either personal or family history of typhoid fever.
   (b) routine for dairy workers.

7. Tuberculin tests in those having had contact with cases of tuberculosis, and also in those found to have suspicious pulmonary signs of possible tuberculosis.

8. Chest x-ray in contacts and those showing physical signs of tuberculosis.

9. Smears: For gonorrhea, when indicated.

TUBERCULOSIS

The most important data with reference to this disease was the securing of information regarding family contacts. Twenty-four gave histories of being in contact with known cases of tuberculosis.

CHART No. 1
769 Foodhandlers Examined Pittsburg County, 1943

Disease	Cases Found	Rate per 100 examined
Tuberculosis	2	.3
Syphilis	72	9.4
Gonorrhea	12	1.7
Typhoid Fever	0	.0

A history and chest examination was done on each patient. If there were any symptoms or signs of respiratory involvement, they were classed with the contacts as 'suspects' and asked to have a chest x-ray made. These patients were referred to private physicians for the x-rays and out of 56 'suspects', 44 x-rays were made.

From the x-ray reports available, five were reported as suspicious, to be re-examined later; two cases were diagnosed as bronchiectases, and one far advanced tuberculosis.

There was also one colored male patient, 56 years of age, who showed some pulmonary signs, who died within a month following his examination, before a chest plate was made. The lesion, by physical examination, involved the upper two thirds of the right lung.

These findings compare favorably with the results of 114 x-rays taken by this department since January 1, 1943, on contacts in 23 families where tuberculosis was known to be present. No active cases of tuberculosis were found in this group.

VENEREAL DISEASE

Syphilis: Seventy-one cases of this disease were found among 769 persons examined. One case was in the secondary stage and 21 in the early latent stage. A detailed study of these cases is given in Chart No. 2.

There is probably a higher incidence of this disease among waitresses than in the population in general. To furnish comparative figures, a chart was prepared from the data furnished by the Federal Security Agency on their findings in the examination of the 611 from Pittsburg County and McAles-

ter among the first 2,000,000 Selective Service registrants. See Chart No. 3 .

CHART No. 3
First 2,000,000 Examinations for Selective Service Prevalence of Syphilis in Pittsburg County, Oklahoma, and City of McAlester

	Selective Service			Foodhandlers		
		Rate per 100			Rate per 100	
	Exam.	Pos.	exam.	Exam.	Pos.	exam.
Pittsburg County	611	35	5.73	546	53	9.7
McAlester	184	14	7.61			

Gonorrhea: Smears were not done routinely. In instances where there was strong suspicions, this disease was likely to be found in certain female foodhandlers, positive findings were reported in 100 per cent of all the cases examined.

Enteric Disease: Intestinal disease such as typhoid are undoubtedly spread by an occasional carrier and so may lead to local epidemics. Thus, all persons who gave a histroy of typhoid were asked to submit a specimen of their stool for examination. Ideally, stool specimens should have been obtained on all foodhandlers, but for practical purposes this was impossible because of the increased load it would have placed on the State Health Department Laboratory.

A total of 130 gave either a personal or family history of typhoid and of this number only 96 stools were obtained for examination. Of these, 14 were reported unsatisfactory. Negative results were given by 80 cases and two specimens showed the presence of S. alkalescens, an organism of the bacillary dysentery group.

The percentage of stools obtained for examination was low, but they were extremely difficult to obtain from a disinterested, apparently healthy individual. It is doubtful if an appreciable difference in the results would have occurred if 130 stools were submitted.

Out of 797 typhoid carriers in New York City in 1937, 23 had been found over an 11 year period of compulsory foodhandlers examination. Three hundred ninety seven were found by epidemiological investigation of typhoid cases and of this number 28 are foodhandlers who had been missed by the routine examination.

CHART No. 2
Syphilis in 769 Food Handlers by Age and Color, Pittsburg County, Oklahoma
1943

Age	Total			White			Other		
	Exam.	Pos.	Rate per 100 exam.	Exam.	Pos.	Rate per 100 exam.	Exam.	Pos.	Rate per 100 exam.
All ages	769	72	9.4	642	42	6.5	127	34	26.8
Under 21	193	7	3.6	167	3	1.8	26	4	15.4
21 - 30	195	19	9.8	158	10	6.3	37	9	24.3
31 - 40	158	27	17.1	123	12	9.3	35	15	42.9
41 and over	223	23	10.3	194	17	8.8	29	6	20.

Epidemiological study would then seem to be the method of choice in finding typhoid carriers. Two typhoid carriers were found in Pittsburg County as the result of epidemiological investigation of the four cases of typhoid reported so far this year. Forty-seven stools were examined in this investigation. This method of attacking the problem is not only more fruitful and thus of greater public health benefit but may also be done with less cost because of the small number of stool cultures required.

DAIRY WORKERS

This group was handled in a special way. Stool examinations were deemed advisable in all of them. Although each patient was given a stool container only 37 were sent to the State Laboratory. One case of shigella paradysenteriae (Flexner) and one of S. alkalescens was found. Two cases of brucellosis by agglutination test were found in one dairy. One case of eczema of both hands was found. See Chart No. 4.

CHART No. 4
Dairy Workers Examinations
Number examined 44

Typhoid Histories
Personal 5
Family 5
Stool Examinations
Negative 30
Positive
  Shigella
  Paradysenteriae
  Flexner 1
Unsatisfactory 6
Blood Examinations
Brucellosis
  Negative 43
  Positive 2
Tuberculosis Suspects
Contacts 1
Suspects, physical 3
Tuberculin tests
  Negative 2
  Positive 2
Skin Diseases
Occupational
One case of eczema of both hands.

CONCLUSION

There is some question whether foodhandlers should be singled out as a group and treated apart from all other members of the community. As had been noted, syphilis, gonorrhea, tuberculosis and enteric diseases were of paramount interest. All are impor-

tant as public health problems, but the possibility of transmitting any, other than enteric diseases, by foodhandling is rather remote. Thus the results obtained from the examinations are interesting as to incidence of public health problems among a particular group, but are discriminatory and do not justify the purpose for which they were done. They are more likely to form a false sense of security in the minds of the public as well as the foodhandlers. Assuming that all communicable diseases may be a public health menace through foodhandling, we have no assurance that the day following the issuance of the health certificate or any time during the period of its tenure that person will not contract a communicable disease. Cost, which has not been considered before, would not be commensurate with the results if thorough examinations were done. In addition to a physical examination, each individual should have a chest x-ray, a Wassermann, and a stool examination for typhoid, paratyphoid, emebic and bacillary dysentery, not to mention tuberculin tests, and sputum examination in special cases. If all the facilities were available to the Health Department for such an examination, the cost would be a conservative minimum of $4.00 per examination. This would mean an expenditure of $3,076.00 for the 769 examined which would not be justified in the evaluation of the public health benefits obtained; i. e., the reduction of sickness and death in the community.

Much more can be accomplished through education of the employer and employee in the necessity for personal cleanliness and the proper methods of handling food and utensils without contamination. Communicable disease should be reported promptly by the employer or employee. They should be held jointly responsible. These are the steps, rather than physical examination, which will reduce to a minimum the spreading of communicable disease by foodhandlers.

BIBLIOGRAPHY
1. Best: American Journal of Public Health. Vol. 27, page 1003. October, 1937.

When the tyrant has disposed of foreign enemies by conquest or treaty, and there is nothing to fear from them, then he is always stirring up some war or other, in order that the people may require a leader.—*Plato.*

Unusual Aspects of Coronary Thrombosis

HOMER A. RUPRECHT, M.D.

TULSA, OKLAHOMA

Like many other disease syndromes, coronary thrombosis presents a typical picture which has been so well publicized that it is familiar to physicians and laymen alike. Difficulties in diagnosis arise, however, from unusual or atypical patterns which tend to bear a greater resemblance to other entities in one or many respects than they do to the typical pattern of coronary thrombosis itself. It is such variations that I wish to direct your attention in order that the condition may be recognized and proper treatment instituted as soon as possible.

It might be well to first define what is meant by the term coronary thrombosis. Actually, reference is made to myocardial infarction, because all cases of thrombosis of the coronary arteries are not followed by infarction, because all cases of thrombosis without thrombosis, and occasionally even without complete occlusion of the artery. However, the term has become so widely used that it will in all probability continue to be used to describe this clinical entity.

Summarized briefly, the syndrome of coronary thrombosis is due to infarction of the myocardium following arteriosclertic alterations and their sequelae of the coronary arteries. It is a degenerative disease, occurs in the final third of the life span, has a strong familial tendency, affects males about three times as frequently as it does females, and has a most striking predilection for certain economic and occupational groups. It is fond of diabetics, of the obese, and of those who have hypertension, probably of those who smoke, and much less probably of those who do not drink. It occurs more commonly among physicians than any other occupational group.

It seems to be occurring or at least is being recognized more frequently, in the younger age group. Men of 38 to 40 are commonly affected. I· recently saw it in a young man of 30. It has been reported even in the teens. In a late compilation by the Journal of the American Medical Association approximately twenty per cent of the deaths of physicians in the armed services were due to coronary thrombosis. I have seen one woman develop this disease while still in the child-bearing age.

The familial incidence is sometimes quite striking. Three members of one family were seen in which the father died of coronary thrombosis at the age of 62, the mother developed angina at the age of 54, and a son had an attack of coronary thrombosis at the age of 38. Its occurrence in brothers is not at all uncommon.

PAIN

Undoubtedly the most striking characteristic of coronary thrombosis is pain. Typically this pain is located in the midline of the chest with symmetrical radiation to both sides, and radiation to the left or both upper extremities. This pain may vary from a dull ache to an excruciating feeling of compression about the chest. The typical pain of coronary thrombosis is unaffected by nitroglycerine, and its use is often suggested to differentiate it from simple angina. Frequently, however, the pain of coronary thrombosis is relieved more or less completely by nitroglycerine and this is not a reliable differential point. Occasionally the pain may be located in the upper abdomen and the condition confused with an acute abdomen. One patient was observed whose pain was confined to his lower jaw and who had first consulted a dentist thinking the cause of the pain lay in his teeth. Another patient, a chronic alcoholic, developed pain limited to a small area below his left clavicle. Previously he had had several attacks of an alcoholic peripheral neuritis and his physician thought that he was again dealing with the same thing. Consequently he was allowed to remain ambulant for two weeks before the condition was recognized.

Instead of the typically continuous type of pain usually present, we may have the anginoid type. This consists of separate and brief attacks of pain following either exertion or food intake. The latter will usually masquerade as indigestion. Frequently it is impossible to isolate one attack as more severe than any of the others and say that this is the one when the infarction occurred. A history of relief by alkalies or by consequent belching is frequently obtained.

Pain may be entirely absent—the so-called silent coronary. However, here a differentiation must be made from chronic coronary insufficiency and serial electrocardiograms may be necessary. One patient had been seen by a California physician and on the basis of an electrocardiogram a diagnosis of a silent coronary thrombosis was made. Six months later another electrocardiogram showed an identical pattern, indicating that we were dealing with chronic coronary insufficiency rather than an acute infarction. The sudden onset of congestive failure without other explanation should always suggest the possibility of a silent infarction.

Perhaps the most difficult aspect of the pain problem consists of pain in the left shoulder and back. This type of pain closely resembles and at times, at least in so far as I am concerned, is indistinguishable from the pain of arthritis. Furthermore, many if not most of these patients have radiological evidence of osteoarthritis and many of them will have had arthritis pain. Unfortunately, nitroglycerine may relieve either type of pain. In some patients a careful analysis of the history may be helpful: in doubtful cases only the frequent use of the cardiograph can make us certain that coronary thrombosis has or has not occurred. The problem of arthritis again obtrudes itself in the late recovery or post-recovery period. At this time about three out of four patients will develop joint symptoms varying from mild arthralgias to typical rheumatoid arthritis. This may be due either to an exacerbation of an old process or the development of a new one.

IMMEDIATE REACTION TO INFARCTION

The textbooks tell us that the patient who has had an infarction is acutely ill, anxious, dyspneic, cyanotic, in some degree of shock, with a cold clammy skin, fall in blood pressure, and a rapid thready pulse. The typical patient instinctively goes to bed and remains absolutely quiet.

However, this typical picture is by no means constant. Many patients feel entirely well after a brief attack of, what may seem to them, inconsequential pain. During the attack there is an occasional patient who prefers to stand still, perhaps in some peculiar position while others may prefer to walk about during the attack of pain.

The blood pressure instead of falling in an orthodox manner may rise abruptly and remain elevated until the pain subsides.

The pulse, usually rapid, may be normal or even present marked sinus bradycardia.

Fever of low grade is a usual accompaniment, but occasionally may be sufficiently high that together with pulmonary congestion, dyspnea, bloody sputum, and syanosis, may cause the condition to be mistaken for pneumonia.

A curious feature is how well some patients may feel after an attack. I saw one patient, a physician, who played a vigorous game of squash only a few days after an attack of acute coronary thrombosis. His only observation afterwards was that he felt somewhat more tired than usual.

PHYSICAL FINDINGS

The physical findings in so far as the heart itself is concerned are not as a rule extensive. Pericardial friction rub, gallop rhythm, and the arrhythmias cover the usual findings. Obviously any abnormalties which were previously present will probably continue to exist.

Systolic murmurs are quite common and are apparently due to dilation of the left ventricle. Diastolic murmurs are quite rare. They may, of course occur in patients who have had pre-existing valvular disease. I have seen a diastolic murmur occur in a patient with infarction and rupture of the septum with a communication between the ventricles. Another similar case, however, failed to show any murmur.

Another interesting murmur suddenly appeared in a 58 year old man about a week after his second attack of coronary thrombosis. It was a low rumbling diastolic murmur like that heard in mitral stenosis. At necropsy a ball thrombosis was found lodged underneath a leaflet of the mitral valve and producing a functional stenosis by preventing the valve from opening.

PROGNOSIS

The outlook following an attack is by no means the least varied and unpredictable feature. Death may occur instantaneously or the patient may live for many years. Recovery may be apparently complete or he may be an invalid the rest of his life. I have one patient who has gone on Army hikes and over obstacle courses without at least any immediately apparent reaction. Patients who appear to be recovering uneventfully may die suddenly and without warning, patients who remain critically ill for a long time may make a beatiful ultimate recovery.

SUMMARY

Today a constantly increasing number of men and women who have had attacks of coronary thrombosis are again leading useful lives. In order to give our patients their best chance to achieve this objective, it is necessary that the condition be recognized promptly and the most effective measures instituted. This paper has been written with the view that if some of the more unusual features of the disease are kept in mind more, cases will be recognized and proper care given.

Spontaneous Gastrocolic Fistula[*]
A Report of Two Cases

PETER E. RUSSO, M.D.

*Department of Radiology, State University
and Crippled Children's Hospitals*

OKLAHOMA CITY, OKLAHOMA

These two cases of spontaneous gastrocolic fistula, both due to malignancy of the digestive tract, illustrate the various aspects met with in this condition.

Spontaneous gastrocolic fistula are in most cases due to neoplasm arising either in the stomach or colon. Perforation at the site of origin occurs, forming a fistulous communication with another organ in its proximity whose wall and surrounding tissues are also invaded by malignant cells. Other lesions such as ulcers, leutic, tuberculosis and non specific infections may also produce this pathological anastamosis of the alimentary canal. Gastro jejunocolic fistula following gastroenterostomy occurs much more frequently than the spontaneous type.

McNealy and Hedin[6] in reviewing 3,289 cases of carcinoma of the stomach found that perforation occurred in 113 cases. Of these, 15 cases developed spontaneous gastrocolic fistula. Further these authors reported that in the cases with perforation approximately one half the patients presented a classical clinical picture of perforation, whereas in the remaining cases the signs and symptoms were of such an obscure nature that perforation was not even suspected clinically.

The typical case of gastrocolic fistula does not present a very difficult diagnostic problem. The cardinal symptoms are a foul fecal odor of the breath, fecal vomiting without other signs of intestinal obstruction, persistent diarrhea progressive weakness and rapid loss of weight. To confirm this diagnosis one may instill a harmless dye into the rectum which later may be recovered in the vomitus or gastric contents. A more satisfactory means of examination however is by the fluoroscopic and roentgenographic method using barium as the contrast medium. By this method the size, location and extent of the fistulous tract can be visualized. In addition, in most cases the underlying pathology may be identified. In the obscure cases, because of a ball valve mechanism, repeated examinations may be necessary

*Read before the Annual Meeting held in Oklahoma City, May 11-12, 1943.

before the true nature of the disease can be determined[3]. Ever since Handeck[2] first described the x-ray findings in these cases in 1912, examination by this method has been found to be most satisfactory.

Since carcinoma of the stomach and colon occurs much more frequently in the male than in the female, this explains why most cases of spontaneous gastrocolic fistula are most often reported in men. The location of the new growth will in most cases determine whether or not this complication develops. The most favorable sites appear to be the greater curvature or posterior surface of the pars media of the stomach and the left side of the transverse colon. Fusion of the layers of the gastrocolic ligament bringing these two organs in closer proximity would also be a favorable anatomical factor. Most of the cases reported in the literature are fairly evenly divided between those where the cancer started in the stomach or in the colon[8,9]. Williams[10] reported two cases, one a carcinoma of the colon producing a gastro jejunocolic fistula, the other developed from an ulcerative colitis. In Feldman's case[1], a cancer of the colon formed a duodenocolic fistula. Horner and Kenamore[4] reported a case of a carcinoma of the stomach perforating into the proximal portion of the jejunum forming a spontaneous gastroenerostomy. Hubeny and Delano[5] were able to demonstrate a gastro duodenocolic fistula due to a carcinoma of the transverse colon. Henzel[7] is reported as the first to perform an operation for a gastro colic fistula in 1905.

Since lesions other than malignancy may be responsible for this condition the first case presents this diagnostic problem. In addition it gave a classical picture of perforation and the presence of a gastrocolic fistula could be diagnosed clinically.

CASE NO. 1

J. W., a 67 year old white male, a barber, was seen in the outpatient clinic on December 5, 1940, because of failing vision. The Ear, Nose and Throat Department made a diagnosis of bilateral cataracts and advised extraction. A routine chest film was reported as showing some peribronchial mottling in both apices and left first costal interspace. A diagnosis of bilateral fibrous tuberculosis was made. The patient failed to return until October 10, 1941, at which time he was admitted into the hospital. His complaints at this time were severe vomiting and diarrhea of 10 days duration and sores of the tongue and mouth. The vomitus had been coffee ground in color, and the stools had been tarry. There had been a loss of 40 pounds in weight in the past year with the development of a tumor mass in the abdomen which had become progressively larger. This patient has had stomach trouble for 44 years following an attack of typhoid fever.

Physical examination revealed an acutely ill, markedly emaciated adult male. Lens of both eyes were gray and opaque. There were numerous excoriations of the mucous membranes of the buccal surfaces of the cheeks, tongue and palate. A foul, fecal odor could be detected emitting from the mouth. The abdomen was flat and a tumor mass about 5 x 6 cms. could be palpated in the upper abdomen just left of the midline. No enlarged lymph nodes could be detected anywhere in the body. Pulse 100, blood pressure 128/80, R. 24. Laboratory data: urine sp. gr. 1.016, no alb., no sugar. Hb 10 gms. R.B.C. 3,300,-000, W.B.C. 20,000, 88 per cent neutrophiles, 12 per cent lymphocytes. Sputum — stools: negative for acide fast bacilli: feces benzidine 4 —/—. Kahn negative. Gastric secretion—benzidine 4 —/—, total HCL 40 de-

grees, free HCL two degrees to ten degrees. Smears and cultures of mouth lesions; fusiform bacilli and spirilla.

On November 4, 1941, a fluoroscopic examination and radiograms revealed a large tumor mass, producing a filling defect along the greater curvature of the pars media of the stomach. Without any manual manipulation barium can be seen to leave this portion of the stomach through a large fistulous tract into the lumen of the left side of the transverse colon. Some of the barium left the stomach by way of the pylorus and duodenum when peristaltic movement along the lesser curvature of the stomach became active. The duodenum and proximal portion of the jejunum show a normal mucosal pattern.

A chest film revealed an extension of the fibrous tuberculosis process in both apices and subapical areas. A barium enema performed a few days later revealed essentially the same findings—the entire lumen of the stomach could be filled easily through the fistulous tract. The x-ray diagnosis of a gastrocolic fistula probably due to a perforated carcinoma of the stomach was made, although we were unable to rule out definitely a tuberculous infection.

On November 19, 1941, an operation was performed by Dr. J. P. Wolff, who resected about three-fourths of the stomach and 26 cm. of the transverse colon en masse including the fistulous tract. No gross evidence of any local or distant metastases were found. The patient got along well for about five

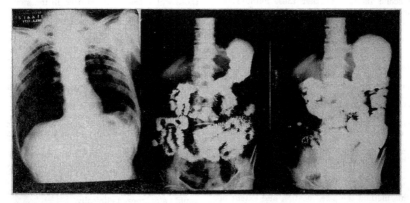

Case 1—Fig. 1
Infiltrations of both apices and left subapical lung fields: Bilateral fibrous tuberculosis.
Case 1—Fig. 2
Barium meal can be seen leaving the stomach by means of a large fistulous tract along the greater curvature communicating with the lumen of the colon. Barium

also passes through the pylorus and duodenum. Filling defect of the stomach can be clearly outlined along its greater curvature.

Case 1—Fig. 3
Barium enema also shows fistulous communications between left transverse colon and stomach.

days after the operation, but after that, developed signs of peritonitis and finally succumbed on the twentieth post-operative day.

Miscropic section of surgical specimen by Dr. Hugh Jeter was reported as adenocarcinoma of the stomach.

A necropsy performed on December 15, 1941 revealed that a generalized peritonitis had developed although the gastrojejunostomy showed evidence of complete healing with no leakage—no metastases were found in any of the other organs. Pulmonary tuberculosis in both apices as diagnosed on the x-ray film was confirmed.

The second case, due to a carcinoma of the colon, is representative of the obscure type of perforation and the final diagnosis was not made until repeated examinations had been performed. Also the underlying pathology could be identified by fluoroscopic and roentgenographic examination.

CASE NO. 2

This patient was a 50 year old white male first seen in the outpatient clinic on October 27, 1941, at which time he was complaining of an epigastric pain of 10 months duration. Large meals and emotional upsets seemed to aggravate the pain and there had been a loss of 35 pounds in weight within the past year. A physical examination including a G. I. series made at that time was essentially negative outside of a generalized pain on pressure over the entire abdomen. An Ewald meal gave the following data: Free Hcl 37 degrees and total acid 58 degrees. Blood

Wassermann was reported as negative. The patient was placed on an ulcer diet; sedatives and antispasmodic drugs were prescribed. He returned to the clinic for a check-up examination once a month for the next five months showing considerable improvement when he kept the ulcer regime but would get exacerbations of his former symptoms as soon as he abandoned his diet. On April 23, 1942, a 4 —/— benzidine test was reported on a stool specimen. The G. I. series was repeated which showed the stomach to be normal size, shape and position — mucosal pattern and peristalsis were normal. There was a persistent deformity of the duodenal cap. However at 5 hours there was no gastric residue; barium meal had reached the terminal ileum and cecum. A diagnosis of a peptic ulcer was made. The patient was again placed on an ulcer diet supplemented with alkalies. Although the patient improved within the next three months on this form of treatment—the epigastric pain and discomfort never did subside completely.

On July 21, 1942, the patient reported complaining of vomiting which on occasion contained some fresh blood. Although he did not appear critically ill at this time, he was admitted into the hospital for a suspected bleeding peptic ulcer. There was very little change in his general condition.

Laboratory date: urine, sp. gr. 1.033. No. alb., no sugar, occ. W.B.C.

Hb 12 gm. R.B.C. 4,700,000, W.B.C. 7,500. N.P.N. 20.4, Chlorides 442, Total Protein 5.07.

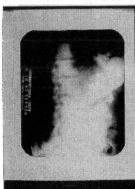 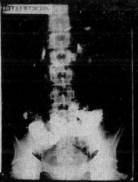 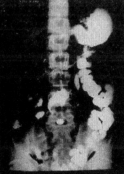

Case 2—Fig. 4

Examination on August 15, 1942—a fistulous tract along the greater curvature can be detected suggestive of perforation of the stomach.

Case 2—Fig. 5

Five hour film shows the fistulous tract somewhat indistinct, but barium within the lumen of the transverse

colon can be clearly seen. The remaining portion of the barium meal is in the terminal loops of the ileum.

Case 2—Fig. 6

Barium enema examination outlines more clearly the fistulous communication between the left portion of the transverse colon and the lumen of the stomach. The distortion of mucosal pattern of the colon at this site, and the annular constricted lumen gave evidence of a malignant neoplasm of the colon at this site.

Blood and C.S.F. negative for luetic infection.

The patient improved considerably so that he was discharged in two weeks as all his symptoms had practically subsided. However, he was re-admitted two weeks later because of return of all his former symptoms. Vomiting now became more frequent and the epigastric pain more severe. The G. I. examination was repeated and now revealed the true nature of his condition. Under fluoroscopic examination and immediate films a deformity of the duodenal cap was noted. On the 5 hr film however, a small fistulous tract between the stomach and left side of the transverse colon could be identified. Barium enema examination revealed a portion of the transverse colon with a narrow constricted lumen, with distortion of mucosal pattern involving approximately 5 cm. of the colon. A small fistulous tract allowing barium to enter into the lumen of the stomach could be seen. A tumor mass overlaying this area was palpable which did not appear to be firmly fixed to the surrounding structures. A diagnosis of carcinoma of the colon with a gastrocolic fistula was made.

An explanatory operation by Dr. C. M. O'Leary of the surgical staff was performed on August 25, 1942. The tumor mass was found to be formed by the adjoining portions of the greater curvature of the stomach and transverse colon. In the absence of local or distant metastases, the mass was deemed resectable. This consisted of removing about one-third of the stomach, the fistulous tract and surrounding tissues, about 12 cm. of transverse colon. A gastrojejunostomy and a double barrel colostomy completed the surgical procedure. The patient made an uneventful recovery and was discharged on the 30th post-operative day.

Microscopic report of the specimen was reported as columnar cell carcinoma of the colon with neoplastic invasion of the stomach wall.

A check-up five months after discharge showed that the patient had gained considerable weight and had gotten complete relief of his epigastric distress. When seen again in March 4, 1943, when the patient returned to have his colostomy closed it was found that there was evidence of recurrence of the malignancy of the abdominal wall around the colostomy opening and also of the gastric wall.

COMMENTS

Two cases of spontaneous gastrocolic fistula are presented. Both were due to malignancy of the digestive tract, one a carcinoma of the stomach, the other a carcinoma of the colon.

One case demonstrates the classical clinical picture of perforation, whereas the other is of the obscure type in which the condition was not suspected clinically. In the latter case reported G. I. examinations were necessary before a correct diagnosis could be made. In the first case because of active pulmonary tuberculosis there was some question as to whether or not the lesion of the digestive tract was neoplastic or tuberculous in nature.

DISCUSSION
RALPH E. MYERS

Dr. Russo has presented two very interesting cases. While gastrocolic fistulae are not very common, nevertheless, we must bear them in mind in all cases of severe digestive disturbances.

Since the majority of these conditions occur in the male, it is not strange that the two cases sighted here were both in men. For some reason the preponderance in the male is even greater than can be explained by the greater frequency of peptic ulcer and of cancer of the stomach and colon in the male over that of the female. While the ratio is more than two to one in the case of ulcer, the difference in the occurrence of malignancy is not very marked between the male and the female. It would appear that some other factor besides ulceration or malignancy must enter in to explain this discrepancy.

When two organs lie contiguous to each other, it is very easy for the malignancy to spread from one to the other. Since cancer outgrows its blood supply, the ensuing necrosis would naturally, now and then, make fistulous openings between hollow organs. Such cases are not very hard to diagnose. The failure to make the diagnosis in the beginning in the second case sighted by Dr. Russo, was probably due to the fact that the fistula had not as yet formed.

When the fistula is caused by perforation followed by a low grade infection, the fistulous tract may be rather long and the passage-way small. Furthermore, several organs may be matted together in a mass of inflamatory tissue. In such cases the diagnosis may be impossible to make by means of the Roentgen Ray.

BIBLIOGRAPHY

1. Feldman, M.: Amer. Jour. Digestive Diseases. Vol 9, pages 195-197. June, 1942.
2. Glickman, L. Grant: Radiology. Vol 23, pages 609-614. November, 1934.
3. Groeschel, L. B.: Amer. Jour. Roent, Vol. 8, pages 516-520. 1921.
4. Horner, J. L., Kenamore, B.: Radiology. Vol. 35, pages 493-495. October, 1940.
5. Hubeny, J. M., Delano, Percy J.: Amer. Jour. Roent. Vol. 43, pages 198-200. February, 1940.
6. McNealy, R. W., Hedin, R. F.: Jour. Surg, Gyn. & Obst. Vol. 67, pages 818-822. December, 1938.
7. Monroe, T. Robert: Amer. Jour. Med. Soc., Vol. 174, pages 599-609. 1937.
8. Ritvo, M. McDonald, E.: Radiology. Vol. 37, pages 269-276. September, 1941.
9. Comm, Thomas J. R.: Mil. Surg., Vol. 87, pages 232-243. September, 1940.
10. Williams, E. R.: British Jour. Radiology. Vol. 14, pages 36-40., January, 1941.

Hyperventilation Syndrome

ROBERT C. KIRK, M.D.
Captain, Medical Corps
FT. SILL, OKLAHOMA

Tetany from hyperventilation was first described by Vernon[1] in 1909. He experimented on himself with forced breathing and noted that after some time rigidity and paresthesias of the fingers set in. In 1920, Haldane[2] showed that prolonged hyperventilation would produce muscular spasms and changes in neuro-muscular excitability.

Physiologically this condition is similiar to primary alkali excess, arising from either of two causes, alkali retention or acid loss. The former may result from excessive alkali ingestion, and the latter from excessive vomiting. Such situations are frequently met with and are usually recognized. Tetany as a result of "primary carbon dioxide deficit"[3] is less well known but probably quite frequent. This deficit is caused by ventilation in excess of that required to maintain the usual relationship between the acid and the base in the blood. This hyperventilation has been noted as a result of oxygen deficit, hot baths, fevers, encephalitis[4], psycho-neuroses[5], pain[6], excessive exercise[6], anxiety and effort[7], spontaneous overbreathing[8], treatments in fever cabinets[9] and most recently under certain flying conditions[10]. Indeed the latter authors suggest that a common flying accident referred to as "frozen controls" as well as the extremely common swimmers' cramps may both be definitely attributed to hyperventilation tetany.

Peters states that when the Ph of the blood reaches 7.6, tetany results. There may be definite clinical symptoms earlier than this which are equally distressing, and it is my purpose to report one such case which has been called hyperventilation syndrome as distinguishing from two typical cases of tetany from overventilation.

CASE NO 1

The patient was a twenty-five year old, single, white girl, whose past history is not of significance except for a series of yawning attacks which are as follows. Following a laparotomy seven years ago, on the fifth or sixth post-operative day the patient developed an attack of yawning. She yawned for three or four days without stopping, day and night. Various procedures, the nature of which she was not aware, were tried, and finally a physician told her that her difficulty was "lack of oxygen" and gave her an injection into her antecubital which resulted in the relief of her symptoms in about twelve hours. The patient was in good health, worked every day, until about two years ago when she had a second recurrence of yawning. At this time she was seen by another physician and various procedures were again tried over a period of four or five days. Finally she was given some medication by vein which relieved her promptly. Her third attack began July 14, 1938, about two weeks after she had given the second of two 500 cc. blood donations, one week apart. This episode was much more severe than her previous attacks. She complained of numbness and tingling in her extremities; she was dizzy; she fainted at one time while attempting to work. Her mother states that she yawned in her sleep. She was given nembutal, phenobarbital, coramine and various other hypnotics and sedatives over a period of two weeks with no relief of her symptoms. She was rapidly becoming depressed, worried and anxious about her condition. She was seen in consultation on the fourteenth day of her illness. At this time her pulse and blood pressure were within normal limits. She had no fever. She was walking restlessly about her room, holding her arms high above her chest and complaining of an inability to take a deep breath. Her eyes were somewhat glazed. Her skin was warm and moist. The most striking abnormal physical finding, and the only one, was a very irregular type of breathing which was characterized by four or five rather deep breaths in rapid succession, followed by a very deep breath which was accompanied by a yawn. Following this yawn the patient would always state that she felt a little better, her respirations would become more shallow, and in about five more breaths she would go through this same cycle again. Her respiratory rate was about forty-five per minute. The patient was fluoroscoped and it was noted that aeration was equal on both sides. Her lungs filled well, and there was noticeable hyperaeration during the periods of her yawning. The Chvostek and Trousseau signs were negative. There was no carpopedal spasm; however, because of the numbness and tingling of her extremities and the deep and rapid respirations, it was felt that this condition was one of hyperventilation and alkalosis. Consequently 10 cc. of calcium gluconate were given intravenously. As the sixth cc. was introduced the patient had a definite and striking reduction in her respiratory rate, and at the end of the introduction of 10 cc. she was apparently breathing normally; however, she immediately rose to her feet and said that she would have to take a deep breath. It was urgently pointed out to her that to do so would be to undo the therapeutic procedure which had been tried and it was insisted that she not take a deep breath for at least fifteen minutes. At the end of this time, although it was somewhat of an effort for her not to take a deep breath, she was completely relieved of all her symptoms and yawning.

In the ensuing eight weeks she received 10 cc. of calcium gluconate nearly every evening to enable her to sleep because of the yawning. This amount afforded her relief for about twelve hours at the end of which time the rapid breathing and yawning recurred. During this time she had left the city upon one occasion and was unable to obtain any medication. She had "walked the floor for thirty-six hours" before she finally collapsed. The physician who saw her at this time diagnosed the case as "sub-sternal thyroid" and advised operation. Refusing this suggestion she continued to receive medication. On October 8, 1938, she received in addition to her calcium gluconate, morphine sulphate one-half grain, which gave her complete relief for three days before her hyperpnea recurred. A second injection October 18 accomplished the same results. A basal metabolic rate determination was minus one. This patient has continued to have intermittent attacks of hyperventilation up to the present time. The blood calcium on Ocober 8, 1940, was 11.2 mgms. An electrocardiographic tracing was physiologic. The attacks continued to respond to intravenous calcium

gluconate. It is the opinion of her present attending physician that she has recurrent hyperventilation on a psychogenic basis.

CASE No 2

The patient is a thirty-one year old, white, married woman with two children. The past history is of importance in that she had an appendectomy nineteen years ago for gangrenous appendix with drainage, and a bilateral salpingectomy and unilateral oophorectomy two years ago. Since that time she has had eight or ten intermittent attacks of subacute intestinal obstruction, characterized by vomiting, cramp-like pains in the abdomen, and prostration, which have been relieved in two or three days by various procedures. The patient was seen in January in such an attack which was relieved by one-fourth grain of Morphine sulphate and 1/150 grain of atropine, subcutaneously. The present illness was a recurrence of sub-acute intestinal obstruction which occurred on the fourth of August. The patient went to bed and was severely nauseated, vomiting at frequent intervals for nearly twenty-four hours before medical aid was sought. When seen at 11:00 P. M. the night of August 5, 1938, she was complaining of low, diffuse, abdominal cramping with vomiting. The vomitus was not fecal in character. The abdomen was relatively soft and no masses were felt. She was given one-fourth grain of morphine sulfate, 1/150 grain of atropine hypodermically, and in three hours was relieved sufficiently to fall asleep. The following day the patient's condition was not good and she seemed to be much worse in spite of the fact that her abdominal cramps were considerably less severe. When seen, this patient was lying almost in opisthotonus position, crying hysterically. She was held in bed by three women and her husband and was complaining bitterly of severe cramps in her arms and legs. She was not vomiting. She did not complain so severely of abdominal cramps as of muscular cramps. Examination disclosed a marked degree of carpopedal spasm which was so great as to almost prohibit unflexing of the fingers by forceful action. There was muscular cramping in both calves of her legs. She was perspiring freely, crying and breathing about fifty to sixty times a minute. Trousseau's and Chvostek's signs were positive. A quarter of a grain of morphine sulphate and 1/150 of a grain of atropine sulfate hypodermically were given immediately upon arrival and in ten minutes had produced no relief whatsoever. She continued to complain of these severe muscular cramps at which time the marked hyperventilation appeared to be of more significance. She was given 6 cc. of 20 per cent calcium gluconate by vein at which time she was so markedly relieved of her entire muscular cramps that the full ampule of 10 cc. was not given and she was completely relaxed in bed.

CASE No 3

F. P., male, age 45. This patient was seen in the medical out-patient department of the Ohio State University Medical School, November 15, 1938, complaining of tachycardia, palpitation and pain in the left chest which had its onset one year previously. At the time of his first severe attack he was ordered to bed by his local physician where he remained for two weeks receiving digitalis for "coronary spasm." Following this period of bed rest he had experienced numerous attacks similar in every detail having their onset after exertion. Rising from a chair induced an attack which could be relieved by lying down. Attacks did not occur when he was at rest. These episodes became so frequent as to necessitate stopping all gainful employment. On physical examination the blood pressure was 130/80, his height 6 feet 2 inches, weight 129 pounds, when seen in the dispensary. His physical findings were essentially negative except that he appeared to be about ten years older than his stated age. His heart was negative to auscultation and percussion, as well as to fluoroscopy. An electrocardiogram was normal. A chest plate showed a normal heart outline with a normal aorta and clear lung fields. His basal metabolic rate was plus 2 per cent. His blood count was not remarkable and his urinalysis was normal. A diagnosis of neurosis or neuro-circulatory asthenia was made. As a further test he was asked to hyperventilate freely for one minute. He was able to do this only for about fifty seconds before he became markedly exhausted; his face became pale; his pulse rate increased to 120; his eyes watered; his jaw trembled; he was unable to sit erect and he was forced to lie down on the examining table where he shook and trembled for nearly twenty minutes following this procedure. After he had regained his composure he said it was the worst attack he had had since his first attack one year before. A reproduction of his entire symptomatology by hyperventilating seemed to be a justifiable reason for considering this case as one of hyperventilation syndrome, which is in accord with the findings of Soley and Shock[7], which have been previously mentioned. The patient was placed on ammonium chloride, seven and one-half grains four times a day, but because of gastric distress this was changed to dilute hydrochloric acid, 15 drops three times a day. He had fewer attacks since that time and "it was expected that he should make a fairly satisfactory recovery from this syndrome." He was advised in case of severe attacks to rebreathe in a paper bag. The demonstration of his syndrome following hyperventilation was so dramatic to him that "it was felt that he will be extremely cooperative in avoiding recurrence of this hyperventilation." In October 1939, he returned complaining of weakness, loss of weight and a vague burning in his epigastrium. A cholecystogram on October 7, 1939, by the reinforced oral dye technique showed a questionable gall bladder shadow not seen after a fat meal and it was considered that he had a partial obstruction of his cystic duct. He was placed on a choleretic drug with some relief. On November 21, 1939 he was gastroscoped. Free hydrochloric acid was present and the gastroscopist reported a normal stomach. In February 1940, he returned complaining of pain in his back. An x-ray on January 18, 1940 was reported as showing "marked decalcification of the dorsal spine." He was placed on calcium gluconate and Brewer's yeast and has improved considerably since then although a repeat spine film on July 25, 1940 showed no changes. He was last seen December 28, 1940 at which time his chief complaint was inability to gain weight. His stomach complaints were relieved. He had returned to work as a night watchman and seemed to be doing very well. His blood pressure was 124/78 with a pulse rate of 78. He was asked to lie down and breathe deeply for one minute. After twelve deep breaths his blood pressure fell to 100/60, his pulse increased to 140, he had jerkings of his arms and sensation of impending death. All these alarming symptoms were relieved by holding his breath.

DISCUSSION

Forced breathing in a normal person will as a rule give rise to the following symptoms. After some minutes there will be humming in the ears, dizziness, vertigo, and now and then headache. Tingling of the skin, espec-

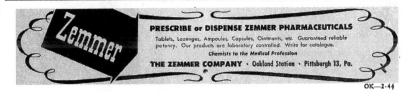

ially in the hands, feet and in the face, are often accompanied by cutaneous anesthesia. This will be followed by twitching of the facial muscles, a feeling of dryness in the throat, constriction of the throat, and strain about the chest. The pulse becomes rapid and small. Definite tetanic symptoms occur in about fifteen minutes. These symptoms are a result of the well known increase in muscle and nerve irritability resulting from alkalosis, as seen when patients suffering from petit mal attacks hyperventilate. This is associated with constriction of the capillary bed as discussed by Barach and his associates[11], which serve as an adequate explanation for the circulatory changes previously noted, particularly in the third patient.

That these three cases were manifestly obvious examples of hyperventilation seems unquestionable. Two of them are typical of the tetany produced by this state, similar in every way to the cases previously reported. Therapeutic response was identical. The first case of yawning is unusual. I was unable to find any similar case in text books or current medical literature. This was probably an unusual example of hyperventilation as a result of constant subconscious response to emotional stimuli and fatigue.

TREATMENT

Once these cases have been diagnosed the treatment is specific and rapidly effective. Attacks may be stopped by the administration of five per cent carbon dioxide inhalation, by rebreathing, and by holding the breath. All these have the effect of raising the carbon dioxide content of the plasma and thus simply reverses the changes produced by hyperventilation. The warding off of attacks in patients who are susceptible to this type of breathing may be accomplished by the administration of ammonium chloride, which decreases the Ph of the blood without necessarily altering the carbon dioxide content. Ammonium chloride was given to Case No. 1 to take home with her if she found that she was having a recurrence of her symptoms. The most rapidly effective and probably the most therapeutically useful method of stopping hyperventilation tetany is by the intravenous injection of a calcium salt more alkaline than the blood, such as was used in two of these cases reported. It is thus possible, as Harwood[5] states, that the decreased carbon dioxide content and the increased Ph of the plasma in hyperventilation produce some change in the blood calcium which causes tetany, although no one has been able to prove conclusively that the blood serum calcium is lowered in this condition. A psychotherapeutic approach with a careful explanation to the patient of the cause of his affection is most helpful in these cases with no demonstrable etiology.

SUMMARY

This report deals with the changes occurring in hyperventilation. Three cases of hyperventilation syndrome have been presented, two of which resulted in typical tetany and the other in a very unusual manifestation of yawning. In such individuals the hazards of swimming and aviation are greatly increased.

BIBLIOGRAPHY

1. Vernon, H. M.: The Production of Prolonged Apnoea in Man. Jour. Physio. Vol. XVIII, page 38. 1909.
2. Davies, H. W., Haldane, J.B.S., Kennaway, E. L.: Experiments on the Regulation of the Blood's Alkalinity. Jour. Physiol. Vol. 54, pages 32-45. 1920.
3. Peters, J. P., Van Slyke, D. D.: Quantitative Clinical Chemistry, Interpretation, Page 954. William & Wilkins Co. Baltimore. 1931.
4. Barker, L. F., Sprunt, T. P.: A Spontaneous Attack of Tetany during a Paroxysm of Hyperpnea in a Psychoneurotic Patient Convalescent from Epidemic Encephalitis. Endocrin. Vol. 6, pages 1-15. January, 1922.
5. Harwood, Reed: Hyperventilation Tetany. N.E.J.M. Vol. 218, pages 502-506. April 7, 1938.
6. Goldman, Arthur: Clinical Tetany by Forced Respiration. J.A.M.A. Vol. 78, pages 1193-1195. 1922.
7. Soley, M. H., Shock, N. W.: The Etiology of Effort Syndrome. Amer. Jour. Med. Science. Vol. 116, pages 840-851. December, 1938.
8. Schultzer, P., Lebel, H.: Spontaneous Hyperventilation Tetany. Acta. Med. Scand. Vol. 101, pages 302-313. 1939.
9. Dosn, C. A.: Personal Communication.
10. Hinshaw, H. C., Boothby, W. M.: The Syndrome of Hyperventilation. Proc. of Staff Meets of Mayo Clinic. Vol. 16, pages 211-213. April 2, 1941.
11. Barach, A. L., Steiner, A.: The Physiologic Action of Oxygen and Carbon Dioxide on the Coronary Circulation, as shown by Blood Gas and Electrocardiographic Studies. Amer. Ht. Jour., Vol. 22, pages 13-34. July, 1941.

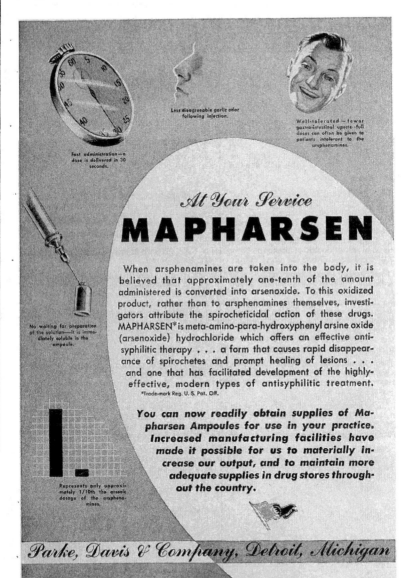

· THE PRESIDENT'S PAGE ·

"WHAT THEY THINK"

"Somewhere in the Southwest Pacific a poll-minded Army Officer whiled away his free hours making a public opinion survey among U. S. Troops. He used the interview method, took plenty of time, quizzed more than 700 enlisted men . . . His results:

Do you favor socialization of medicine?
Yes—72.2 per cent. No—27.8 per cent."

Time. Page 73-74, February 7, 1944.

The great need is for a gigantic educational effort to enlighten the public and this puts a duty squarely on the shoulders of each of us. Too long we have relied on elected officials for our organizations, or salaried employees, to do all our work for us, all our speaking for us, and some of our thinking for us. Some say they are busy practicing medicine and that they have no time to do other things, but if a pistol was put to their heads, these men could forget practicing medicine temporarily. Well, a pistol is at the head of every doctor of medicine right now—The Wagner-Murray-Dingell Bill. Are we still too busy to heed the gun! Shall we just let it go off.

Each doctor should constitute himself a committee of one to discuss this bill with his patients. Every County Society should choose its best speakers to address civic clubs, school groups, labor groups and the like. The common man esteems doctors, but he also knows it costs money to break a leg, or to have appendicitis. He is the man we must reach in this campaign. He can be shown that facilities are now available to care for his medical catastrophes—through industrial medical plans; industry cooperation with employees to provide group insurance: private companies providing health insurance policies; prepayment plans under physician sponsorship. He also can be shown what another 6 per cent out of his pay check will do to him.

Our campaign should center largely on the employed groups, farmers and small business men. The bankers, the insurance men, the attorneys, the men of big business are already on our side. They know that if the medical profession is socialized—they are next!

Three hundred and fifty of our members are fighting the Japs and Germans. We, at home are soldiers too—the medical profession is in the front line of battle against bureaucracy—we should be proud to be the first to be attacked. Can we forget for a time our professional dignity, take our heads out of the sand, and go to war!

Your officers have been doing everything in their power to combat this Bill, and your State Journal has spared no effort to inform you about it. But only YOU—each individual doctor—can reach the common man. It is your war! WHAT ARE YOU DOING ABOUT IT!

James Stevenson

President.

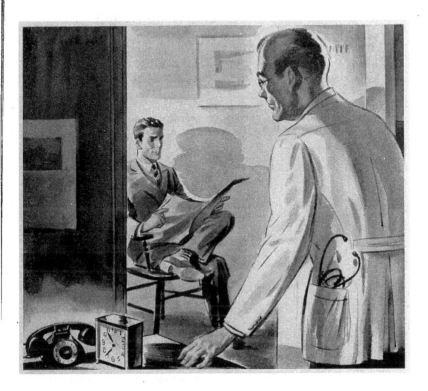

THE LAST PATIENT . . .

When day is done, and the last patient is in sight, the physician puts behind him a day of strenuous activity. On the home front, he is now doing far more than his share and is daily faced with an increasing number of patients.

Warren-Teed commends these war-time physicians . . . for their constant patience and unending sacrifice.

Well aware that "every minute counts," our courteous, professional representatives are ever mindful of the physician's time.

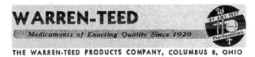

The JOURNAL Of The
OKLAHOMA STATE MEDICAL ASSOCIATION

EDITORIAL BOARD
L. J. MOORMAN, Oklahoma City, Editor-in-Chief

E. EUGENE RICE, Shawnee　　　　　　　　　　　　　　　　　NED R. SMITH, Tulsa

MR. R. H. GRAHAM, Oklahoma City, Business Manager
(Serving in the Armed Forces)

CONTRIBUTIONS: Articles accepted by this Journal for publication including those read at the annual meetings of the State Association are the sole property of this Journal.

The Editorial Department is not responsible for the opinions expressed in the original articles of contributors.

Manuscripts may be withdrawn by authors for publication elsewhere only upon the approval of the Editorial Board.

MANUSCRIPTS: Manuscripts should be typewritten, double-spaced, on white paper 8½ x 11 inches. The original copy, not the carbon copy, should be submitted.

Footnotes, bibliographies and legends for cuts should be typed on separate sheets in double space. Bibliography listing should follow this order: Name of author, title of article, name of periodical with volume, page and date of publication.

Manuscripts are accepted subject to the usual editorial revisions and with the understanding that they have not been published elsewhere.

NEWS: Local news of interest to the medical profession, changes of address, births, deaths and weddings will be gratefully received.

ADVERTISING: Advertising of articles, drugs or compounds unapproved by the Council on Pharmacy of the A.M.A. will not be accepted. Advertising rates will be supplied on application.

It is suggested that members of the State Association patronize our advertisers in preference to others.

SUBSCRIPTIONS: Failure to receive The Journal should call for immediate notification.

REPRINTS: Reprints of original articles will be supplied at actual cost provided request for them is attached to manuscripts or made in sufficient time before publication. Checks for reprints should be made payable to Industrial Printing Company, Oklahoma City.

Address all communications to THE JOURNAL OF THE OKLAHOMA STATE MEDICAL ASSOCIATION, 210 Plaza Court, Oklahoma City. (3)

OFFICIAL PUBLICATION OF THE OKLAHOMA STATE MEDICAL ASSOCIATION
Copyrighted February, 1944

EDITORIALS

THE CHEMISTRY OF THE TUBERCLE BACILLUS

At Yale University on February 3, 1944, The National Tuberculosis Association presented to President Semour more than 300 chemical products of the tubercle bacillus and other acid-fast bacilli. This work was directed by The Committee of Medical Research representing one of the activities of The National Tuberculosis Association and the costs were covered by successive grants from this organization. The work was done by Dr. R. J. Anderson, Professor of Chemistry at Yale, and his colleagues, covering a period of 17 years. The collection represents a great scientific adventure and stands as a monument to one of the world's outstanding chemists. The total cost, including time and effort, plus Yale's contribution in personnel, equipment and other facilities, is estimated at one half a million dollars. Since chemotherapy has not revealed a cure for tuberculosis, Dr. Anderson's remarkable studies may become very valuable in that the biological investigations of the various chemical fractions of the tubercle bacillus may open the way to diagnostic, preventive or curative advances.

The following informative paragraphs are quoted from the presentation statement made by the President of The National Tuberculosis Association.

"When this committee, with the approval of the National Tuberculosis Association, undertook to sponsor research in this field, its first major grant was made to Esmond R. Long at the University of Chicago. In those days, Dr. Long's thesis was that since the tubercle bacillus would grow on a synthetic medium, all the complex constituents contained in the bacillus must have been synthesized by the living cells from very simple chemical compounds of known constitution. Dr. Long thought that these substances could be isolated and that their biological action should be studied.

"Shortly after he began his work, he asked that part of his grant be given to Professor Treat B. Johnson of the Sterling Chemistry Laboratory, so that he might obtain from Dr. Johnson pyrimidine bases which are present in the tubercle bacillus, in order to determine their influence on the growth of the tubercle bacillus. Dr. Johnson, in accepting the grant, felt that he should know which pyrimidines were predominant in the bacillus. This required large quantities of bacilli for analysis, and these were provided by the Mulford Company, Sharp & Dohme, and Parke, Davis & Co. Very soon it developed that research should be devoted to the fat fractions of the bacillus, since a phosphorous-containing fat formed so large a part of the bacillary body.. Johnson suggested that the best man in the United States to undertake this study was R. J. Anderson of Cornell University, Geneva Agriculture Experiment Station. After a number of conferences and some correspondence, Anderson was presuaded to come to Yale for a sabbatical year. Thus began the long successful cooperation between Yale University and the National Tuberculosis Association. In the words of Dr. Anderson, *'It is seldom that such a long-term program has received the continuous support by any Association. It is more than likely that the results obtained could not have been achieved except by the long-term support. Short-term grants, such as are often given for a year or two, would probably have produced only meager results. Thanks to the wisdom and far-sighted outlook of the Medical Research Committee of the National Tuberculosis Association, there is now available a new chapter, not only in the chemistry of the tubercle bacillus and other acid-fast bacteria, but also in organic chemistry.'*

"A review of the vast amount of work that has been accomplished appeared in the beautiful Willard Burr Soper Memorial number of the Yale Journal of Biology and Medicine, January, 1943. Many of the chemical substances produced by Professor Anderson and his associates have opened up a whole new field in the knowledge of chemistry, and many of them are to be found only in the tubercle bacillus in minute quantities. All of them have been produced at great expense.

"With rare foresight these substances have been preserved in this exhibit, and they have been described and catalogued and their method of preparation noted, so that future scientists may have them for reference and use. This exhibit represents an enduring testimony to the fruitful colaboration between the Yale authorities and those of the National Tuberculosis Association. In pursuit of the original plan, many of these substances have been tested in the animal body to determine their biological activity, possibly leading to a cure for tuberculosis. The biological study of these fractions was pursued at the Rockefeller Institute by Dr. Florence R. Sabin and her colleagues, and they represent a tremendous effort and a great contribution to medical science.

"In furtherance of this original idea, using these fractional studies of the enzymes in their relation to resistance to tuberculosis have been undertaken by Dr. Winternitz and Dr. Gerstl in the Yale Laboratory of Pathology. In addition, efforts to find a prognostic test of value in tuberculosis have been made in the Department of Preventive Medicine by Dr. John R. Paul and Mr. Riordan. That these efforts have not yet met with complete success need not discourage us. Many of the compounds have not yet been studied and many of them are already in the hands of investigators in many parts of the world. Who can tell what these studies may divulge?

"Today we idealize a great chemist, whose untiring efforts have given us this tangible store of knowledge and material to serve as an important nucleus from which significant avenues of chemical and biological investigation may radiate with ultimate blessings to humanity."

UNFORTUNATE EXTREMES

When we were planted at Plymouth our forefathers imagined the hand of God in the plague that decimated the savages on the rocky shores of Massachusetts Bay, thereby rendering their own occupation of the land more secure. This providential viewpoint comes from the pious pen of Nathaniel Morton:

"The Lord also disposed, as aforesaid, much to waste them (the aborigines) by a great mortality . . . so as the twentieth person was scarce left alive when these people (the pilgrims) arrived, there remained sad spectacles of that mortality in the place where they seated, by many bones and skulls of the dead lying above ground; whereby it appeared that the living of them were not able to bury their dead . . . Thus God made way for his people, by removing the heathen, and planting them in the land."

While it is impossible to identify the disease, it may have been a frightful visitation of bubonic plague upon our aborigines. It could have been smallpox but the colonist should have readily recognized this condition. No doubt most of them exhibited the scars on their faces. The English people also experienced epidemics of bubonic plague in the 16th and 17th centuries but to them its manifestations might have been less familiar than smallpox which branded nearly every native British subject with the flight of adolescence. The cause of this unidentified calamity to the American Indian may have been carried by the Pilgrims or transmitted by the skirting of New England's shores by previous European vessels such as Captain John Smith's or by the escape and return of Indians who had been prisoners on European vessels.

Since that eventful period when our people blindly looked to God for health protection, American medicine has made phenominal progress in the recognition and control of disease. Apparently, the omnipotent Father of us all, saw fit to leave the care of the sick and the control of infectious diseases in the hands of those whose business it is through the grace of God to know how. It was natural for our Pilgrim fathers to think that God saved the day at Massachusetts Bay, but it seems presumptious for the law makers and the bureaucrats to think they can do the supernatural in the field of medicine. In Dante's "Purgatorio," Virgil says: "Virtue descends from on high." We suggest that each individual consider the source of his knowledge and skill and that he stick to his own job and thus avoid the danger of assuming authority on the strength of wild presumptions.

OUR DAY

Many generations ago Horace said:

"Happy the man—and happy he alone,

Who can call today his own,

He who secure within can say,

Tomorrow, do thy worst — for I have lived today."

One summer afternoon in Camden, New Jersey, Walt Whitman, after greeting a group of friendly workmen, turned to his physician, William Osler, and said; "Ah, the glory of the day's work, whether with hand or brain! I have tried 'To exalt the present and the real, to teach the average man the glory of his daily work or trade'."

Great poets and great physicians have much in common, their highest services to humanity are equally dependent upon absolute freedom of thought and freedom of action. Can you imagine Walt Whitman or William Osler reading a bureaucratic bulletin for daily guidance. Certainly not in Walt Whitman's America!

Observation and Experimentation

By simply noting facts, we can never succeed in establishing a science. Pile up facts or observations as we may, we shall be none the wiser. To learn, we must necessarily reason about what we have observed, compare the facts and judge them by other facts used as controls. But one observation may serve as control for another observation, so that a science of observation is simply about facts observed in their natural state, as we have already defined them. An experimental science, or science of experimentation, is a science made up of experiments, i. e., one in which we reason on experimental facts found in conditions created and determined by the experimenter himself.—Experimental Medicine. Claude Bernard. Page 16. The MacMillan Company. 1927.

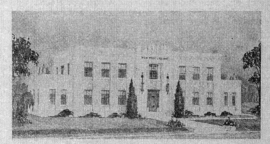

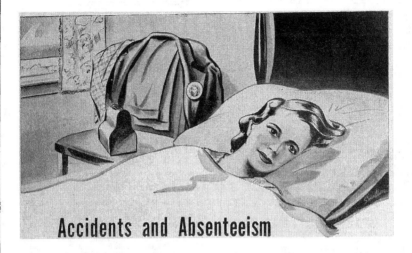

Accidents and Absenteeism

ACCIDENTS contribute to absenteeism. In women — particularly the conscientious middle-aged who try to stay on the job—the nervous symptoms associated with the menopause may directly affect their efficiency, and contribute to accidents of one kind or another.

For women in the menopause who require estrogenic therapy, the Squibb Laboratories supply *natural* estrogenic substance, Amniotin in Oil, and the *synthetic* estrogen, Diethylstilbestrol.

Physicians who prefer natural estrogens will find the vial packages of Amniotin in Oil very practical and economical. The three potencies which are available (20,000, 10,000 and 2,000 I.U. per cc.) offer a range suited to various patients. The vaccine-type cap permits the withdrawal of a dose of just the size to meet the patient's needs.

The lower cost and convenience of Squibb Diethylstilbestrol Tablets appeal to many busy physicians who are realizing more and more

that the side effects of the synthetic estrogen are generally merely temporary, and that after a few days many patients gain tolerance to the drug so that they can take the tablets without discomfort and obtain the benefits afforded by oral administration.

Amniotin and Diethylstilbestrol Squibb are supplied in a variety of dosage forms for oral and hypodermic administration. Also in pessaries (vaginal suppositories).

For literature address the Professional Service Dept., 745 Fifth Avenue, New York 22, N. Y.

E·R·SQUIBB & SONS
Manufacturing Chemists to the Medical Profession Since 1858

KEEP ON BUYING MORE WAR BONDS OF THE
COLLEGE OF PHYSICI

ASSOCIATION ACTIVITIES

POTTAWATOMIE COUNTY MEDICAL SOCIETY HOLDS ANNUAL SPRING MEETING

The Annual Spring Meeting of the Pottawatomie County Medical Society will be held on Tuesday, March 7, at the Aldridge Hotel, Shawnee, Oklahoma. Guest speakers for the Meeting include Dr. P. S. Pelouze, Philadelphia; Dr. Grady F. Mathews, Commissioner of Public Health, State of Oklahoma; Dr. James Stevenson, President of the Oklahoma State Medical Association. Chairman will be Dr. Charles W. Haygood, Shawnee, Oklahoma.

The afternoon meeting will be held at 3:00 P.M. and invitations will be sent to the doctors, nurses, public health workers, medical education committee and all others who may be interested in the discussion. Dr. Grady F. Mathews will introduce Dr. P. S. Pelouze who has chosen as his subject "Control of Gonorrhea from a Public Health Standpoint." Dr. Alfred R. Sugg, Ada, will discuss the subject. Dr. Mathews will then discuss Public Health Problems. Dr. James Stevenson will address the group on "Medical Problems During the War and Post-War."

The regular meeting which will be restricted to medical doctors only, begins at 7:00 P.M. with a buffet supper at the Aldridge Hotel. Dr. Pelouze will discuss "Treatment of Ghonorrhea," and Dr. Stevenson will then address the physicians.

This meeting is being held as a District Meeting especially for the physicians in the 7th Councilor District which includes Garvin, Hughes, Lincoln, McClain, Okfuskee, Pontotoc, Pottawatomie and Seminole counties.

DR. W. W. RUCKS, STATE CHAIRMAN OF PROCUREMENT AND ASSIGNMENT SERVICE, ILL

Dr. W. W. Rucks, Sr., Oklahoma City, State Chairman of the Procurement and Assignment Service, suffered a coronary on Sunday, January 16 and is at present in Wesley Hospital in Oklahoma City. Dr. Ruck's condition is improving.

Dr. C. R. Rountree, Assistant Chairman, has temporarily taken over Dr. Ruck's duties. Dr. Rountree is appointed by Paul V. McNutt of the War Manpower Commission in Washington, D. C.

UROLOGY AWARD

"The American Urological Association offers an annual award 'not to exceed, $500.00' for an essay (or essays) on the result of some specific clinical or laboratory research in Urology. The amount of the prize is based on the merits of the work presented, and if the Committee on Scientific Research deem none of the offerings worthy, no award will be made. Competitors shall be limited to residents in urology in recognized hospitals and to urologists who have been in such specific practice for not more than five years. All interested should write the Secretary, for full particulars.

"The selected essay (or essays) will appear on the program of the forthcoming meeting of the American Urological Association, June 19-22, 1944, Hotel Jefferson, St. Louis, Missouri.

"Essays must be in the hands of the Secretary, Dr. Thomas D. Moore, 899 Madison Avenue, Memphis, Tennessee, on or before March 15, 1944."

WASHINGTON BIRTHDAY CLINIC

The Washington Day Birthday Clinic will be held at the University Hospital on February 22, 1944, under the auspices of the Oklahoma City Internist Association. All members of the State Medical Association are cordially invited. Classes will be held from 10 A.M. to 4 P.M. and luncheon will be served in the dining room of the University Hospital.

FORTIETH ANNUAL CONGRESS ON MEDICAL EDUCATION AND LICENSURE, FEBRUARY 14 AND 15

The Fortieth Annual Congress on Medical Education Licensure was held February 14 and 15, 1944 in the Red Laequer Room of the Palmer House in Chicago. The Council on Medical Education and Hospitals of the American Medical Association conducted the Monday morning and afternoon meetings. The Chairman of the Council, Ray Lyman Wilbur, M.D., Stanford University, California, opened the meeting with the Introduction to the Fortieth Annual Congress. Other speakers and subjects of the morning session included: The Medical School Program, Harold S. Diehl, M.D., Minneapolis; Hospital Training of Medical Graduates, Samuel Soskin, M.D., Chicago; Readjustments of Returning Medical Officers, Wilbert C. Davison, M.D., Durham, N. C.; Financing of Higher Education, Fred J. Kelley, Ph. D., Washington, D. C.; Distribution of Medical Care, Samuel Proger, M.D., Boston.

Wartime Problems in Medicine and Medical Education was the theme of the afternoon session. Subjects and speakers included: The Army Medical Officer in Action, Major George F. Lull, M.D.; Medicine in the Navy, Rear Admiral Ross T. McIntire, M.D.; The Expanding Field of Public Health, Thomas Parran, M.D., Washington; Medical Manpower for Civilians, Harvey B. Stone, M.D., Baltimore; Wartime Graduate Training, Commander Edward L. Bortz, M.D., Philadelphia.

The Federation of State Medical Boards conducted the evening session, beginning with the Federation Dinner. Licensure Trends and Medicine were discussed by Alphonse M. Schwitalla, S. J., Ph. D., of St. Louis, and the Annual Report was given by Frank M. Fuller, M.D., Keokuk, Iowa. A round table discussion followed concerning State Board problems.

The Tuesday meeting was built on the Accelerated Medical Training and Related Licensure Implications. The following were subjects and speakers: Premedical Training, Victor Johnson, M.D., Chicago; Basic and Clinical Medical Sciences, E. M. MacEwen, M.D., Iowa City; Hospital Internship, Jean A. Curran, M.D., Brooklyn; Medical Licensure Aspects, J. E. McIntyre, M.D., Lansing, James D. Osborn, M.D., Frederick, Oklahoma, Robert R. Hannon, M.D., Albany.

On Tuesday, a luncheon was held for the Lay Boards of Hospitals and Public Health Nursing Organizations and the Address was given by Miss Lucile Petry, Washington, D.C., Director, Division of Nurse Education of the United States Public Health Service.

The Meetings concluded Tuesday afternoon with the following program: The Amended Nebraska Medical Practice Act, George W. Covey, M.D., Lincoln, Neb., Medical Legislation, J. W. Holloway, Jr., Chicago. A General Discussion followed and an Executive Session ended the meeting.

Dr. James Stevenson, Tulsa, Dr. C. R. Rountree and Dr. Tom Lowry, Oklahoma City, attended the Congress.

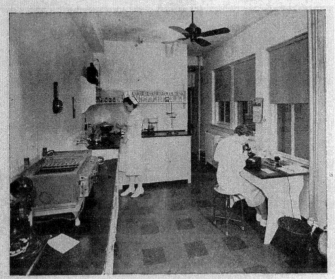

Accepted

An advance in diabetic control

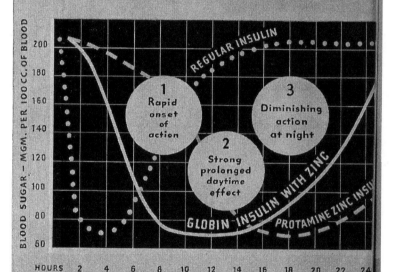

Insulin action conforming to patients' needs

The above diagram shows the effects of comparable doses of various insulins on the blood sugar level of a *fasting* diabetic patient. Note the *intermediate type of action* of globin insulin as compared with regular insulin and protamine zinc insulin.

Special Article[*]

The Physician's Federal Income and Victory Tax

Prepared by the Bureau of Legal Medicine and Legislation

Federal income and victory taxpayers, last September, filed a declaration of estimated tax covering the calendar year 1943. This was the second step to put taxpayers on a current payment basis, the first step having been taken when the withholding provisions of the current tax payment act became operative on July 1, 1943. In this declaration, estimates of income and deductible expenses were made and taxes were computed on these estimates. The tax estimated to be due was either paid in full at the time the declaration was filed or one half then and the remainder on or before December 15. Persons in the armed forces on September 15 were excused from then filing the declaration.

Final Return for 1943

On or before March 15, a final return for 1943 must be filed. This return, in effect, will be in substantiation of the declaration that was filed in September. It will be based on the provisions of the revenue act of 1942 and of the current tax payment act of 1943. The new revenue bill now pending in Congress need not be given any consideration in filing the return. The purpose of the final return is to place the taxpayer on an actual tax basis instead of an estimated tax basis and to permit readjustments. If the taxpayer has already paid more during 1943 than his final return to be filed on or before March 15 indicates he should have paid, he will be entitled to a refund or credit. If he paid less, then he will be required to pay the difference.

Tax Forgiveness

In connection with this return, consideration must be given to the tax forgiveness provisions of the current tax payment act of last year. That act provided for an abatement of 75 per cent of one year's tax or the first $50 thereof, whichever amount is the greater. The abatement is based on the lower tax of the two years 1942 and 1943 except in the case of taxpayers in service. If the 1943 tax is lower, 75 per cent of it is abated. If the 1942 tax is lower as shown on the return that was filed last March, 75 per cent of it is abated. The unabated portion will become a liability on March 15 of this year. The taxpayer may either pay the unabated portion in full at that time or he may pay one half of it at that time and the remainder on or before March 15, 1945.

If a taxpayer was in the armed forces at any time during the taxable year of 1942 or 1943, and his tax for 1942 was greater than the tax for 1943, the forgiveness will be increased to the extent that the excess of the 1942 tax over the 1943 tax is attributable to the inclusion of net income. A detailed explanation of this special provision in favor of persons in the service was included in THE JOURNAL, Aug. 14, 1943, page 1134. Physicians in service should review that explanation.

The Victory Tax

The method of computing the victory tax was explained in THE JOURNAL, Aug. 14, 1943. There has been one modification of the method of computation made effective since that time. Initially the revenue act conditioned the option that was accorded a taxpayer to take credit currently for the postwar credit on his having paid premiums on life insurance, purchased obligations of the United States or reduced indebtedness in an amount equal to the credit allowed. By Public Law No. 178, Seventy-Eighth Congress

[*]Reprint from the Jour. A. M. A., January 29, 1944

approved Oct. 28, 1943, the postwar credit provisions of the revenue act were repealed and the taxpayer allowed an unconditional current credit against the victory tax as follows:

1. SINGLE PERSONS.—In the case of a single person, a married person not living with husband or wife, or an estate or trust, an amount equal to 25 per cent of the victory tax or $500, whichever is the lesser.

2. HEADS OF FAMILIES.—In the case of the head of a family, an amount equal to 40 per cent of the victory tax or $1,000, whichever is the lesser.

3. MARRIED PERSONS.—In the case of a married person living with husband or wife—

(a) if separate returns are filed by each spouse an amount equal to 40 per cent of the victory tax or $500, whichever is the lesser, or

(b) if a separate return is filed by one spouse and no return is filed by the other spouse, or if a joint return is filed, only one credit not exceeding 40 per cent of the victory tax or $1,000, whichever is the lesser.

4. DEPENDENTS.—For each dependent, excluding as a dependent in the case of the head of a family one who would be excluded for income tax purposes, an amount equal to 2 per cent of the victory tax or $100, whichever is the lesser.

If the status of the taxpayer changed during the year with respect to his marital relationship or with respect to his dependents, other than a taxpayer who uses the simplified return form, the amount of the credit will be apportioned, under rules and regulations prescribed by the Commissioner of Internal Revenue with the approval of the Secretary of the Treasury, in accordance with the number of months before and after such change. For the purpose of such apportionment, a fractional part of a month will be disregarded unless it amounts to more than half a month, in which case it will be considered as a month.

Exemptions

The revenue act of 1942 under which the final return will be filed reduced the personal exemption of single persons from $750 to $500 and of married persons or heads of families from $1,500 to $1,200. It also reduced the credits for dependents from $400 to $350. The current tax payment act of 1943 provides a special exemption for members of the armed forces, in addition to the personal exemption. The first $1,500 of the service pay of members of the armed forces, including commissioned officers, is nontaxable.

Tax Rates

The basic rate of taxation remains at 6 per cent. The surtax rate begins at 13 per cent on the first $2,000 of surtax net income and increases in rate for incomes in the higher brackets. The earned income credit of 10 per cent remains as heretofore, claimable in connection with the normal tax but not with the surtax. The pending tax bill proposes to eliminate this credit, applicable to 1944 income.

Simplified Tax Schedule

The provision for a simplified tax schedule for use by taxpayers having gross incomes of $3,000 or less, derived wholly from salaries, wages or other forms of compensation for personal services, dividends, interest, rents, annuities or royalties is continued. The use of the simplified form is optional. Generally speaking, if a taxpayer has no deductions it will be to his advantage to use this form.

Who Must File Returns

1. IN GENERAL—Returns must be filed by every unmarried person and by every married person not

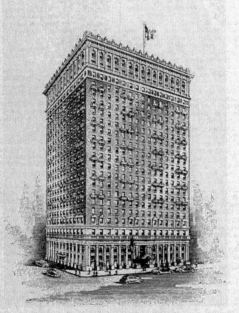

living with spouse, if gross income during 1943 was $500 or more.

2. Returns must be filed by every married person who lived with spouse, if gross income during 1943 was $1,200 or over. If both husband and wife had income and their combined gross income was $1,200 or over, they must either file separate returns or, if both are citizens or residents of the United States and if they were living together at the end of the taxable year, they may file a joint return. If a person was married and lived with spouse for only part of 1943, special rules apply with respect to the filing of returns and physicians who come within this classification should read carefully the instructions given on the tax return blanks.

If the status of a taxpayer, so far as it affects the personal exemption or credit for dependents, changed during the year, the personal exemption and credit must be apportioned, under rules and regulations prescribed by the Commissioner of Internal Revenue with the approval of the Secretary of the Treasury, in accordance with the number of months before and after such change. For the purpose of such apportionment a fractional part of a month should be disregarded unless it amounts to more than half a month, in which case it is to be considered as a month.

PHYSICIANS IN MILITARY AND NAVAL SERVICE.—While a physician in the armed forces was not required to file a declaration of estimated income last September, the fact of service does not of itself excuse a failure to file the return next March. It is understood that if because of the inaccessibility of necessary records a physician in service is unable to file a complete return, he may file a tentative return on which he must estimate his income, deductions and tax as best he can and indicate on the return his reasons for following this procedure. At a later date, if that procedure is followed, a completed return must be filed and necessary adjustments in tax will be made. What has just been said relates to physicians in service who are stationed in this country.

If a physician in service is on duty outside the United States, no income tax return or payment of income tax will become due, generally speaking, until the 15th day of the 4th month following the month in which the physician ceases, except by reason of death or incompetency, to be a member of the military forces on sea duty or in service outside the continental United States, or the 15th day of the third month following the month in which the present war is terminated, whichever may be the earlier.

Gross and Net Incomes: What They Are

GROSS INCOME—A physician's gross income is the total amount of money received by him during the year for professional services, regardless of the time when the services were rendered for which the money was paid, assuming that the return is made on a cash receipts and disbursements basis, plus such money as he has received as profits from investments and speculation and as compensation and profits from other sources.

If a physician receives a salary as compensation for services rendered and in addition thereto living quarters or meals, the value to the physician of the quarters and meals so furnished ordinarily constitutes income subject to tax. If, however, living quarters or meals are furnished for the convenience of the employer, the value thereof need not be computed and added to the compensation otherwise received by the physician. As a general rule, the test of "convenience of the employer" is satisfied if living quarters or meals are furnished to a physician who is required to accept such quarters and meals in order to perform properly his duties. For example, if a physician employed by a hospital is subject to immediate service at any time during the twenty-four hours of the day and therefore cannot obtain quarters or meals elsewhere without material interference with his duties and on that account is required by the hospital to accept the quarters or meals

furnished by it, the value thereof need not be included in the gross income of the physician.

NET INCOME.—Certain professional expenses and the expenses of carrying on any enterprise in which the physician may be engaged for gain may be subtracted as "deductions" from the gross income, to determine the net income on which the tax is to be paid. An "exemption" is allowed, the amount depending on the taxpayer's marital status during the tax year as stated before. These matters are fully covered in the instructions on the tax return blanks.

EARNED INCOME.—In computing the normal tax, but not the surtax, there may be subtracted from net income from all sources an amount equal to 10 per cent of the earned net income, except that the amount so subtracted shall in no case exceed 10 per cent of the net income from all sources. Earned income means professional fees, salaries and wages received as compensation for personal services, as distinguished from receipts from other sources.

The first $3,000 of a physician's net income from all sources may be regarded under the law as earned net income, whether it was or was not in fact earned within the meaning set forth in the preceding paragraph. Net income in excess of $3,000 may not be claimed as earned unless it in fact comes within that category. No physician may claim as earned net income any income in excess of $14,000.

Physicians in Military or Naval Service

Physicians in service are as much subject to the income tax law as are physicians engaged in civilian practice, except when expressly excluded from a requirement. The service pay of such physicians must be reported as income. Commutation of quarters and rental value of quarters occupied by medical officers, however, are not taxable income.

If the ability of physicians in service to pay income taxes is materially affected by such service, payment of the tax falling due before or during the service may be deferred for a period extending not more than six months after termination of service. This deferment is authorized by section 513 of the Soldiers' and Sailors' Civil Relief Act of 1940 and applies to all members of the Army, Navy, Marine Corps and Coast Guard, and to all officers of the United States Public Health Service detailed by proper authority for duty either with the Army or Navy, on active duty or undergoing training or education under the supervision of the United States preliminary to induction into service. This does not apply to the tax imposed on employers by section 1400 of the Federal Insurance Contributions Act. This deferment is not automatic. The taxpayer must present evidence to show that his ability to pay the tax is materially impaired by reason of military service. Proof of that impairment should be submitted at the time the tax is due, on a form procurable from the offices of the collectors of internal revenue. A copy of the form was reproduced in the Feb. 28, 1942 issue of THE JOURNAL on page 737.

Any tax liability owed by a member of the military or naval forces who dies in service will be canceled, this relief being retroactive to Dec. 7, 1941. If a tax has already been assessed at the time of the death of a person in service it will be abated. If the tax has already been collected, it will be refunded as an overpayment. This tax forgiveness applies only to income taxes and not to the estate tax.

Deductions for Professional Expenses

A physician is entitled to deduct all current expenses necessary in carrying on his practice. The taxpayer should make no claim for the deduction of expenses unless he is prepared to prove the expenditure by competent evidence. So far as practicable, accurate itemized records should be kept of expenses and substantiating evidence should be carefully preserved. The following statement shows what such deductible expenses are and how they are to be computed:

OFFICE RENT.—Office rent is deductible. If a physician rents an office for professional purposes alone, the entire rent may be deducted. If he rents a building or apartment for use as a residence as well as for office purposes, he may deduct a part of the rental fairly proportionate to the amount of space used for professional purposes. If the physician occasionally sees a patient in such dwelling houses or apartment, he may not, however, deduct any part of the rent of such house or apartment as professional expense; to entitle him to such a deduction he must have an office there, with regular office hours. If a physician owns the building in which his office is located, he cannot charge himself with ''rent'' and deduct the amount so charged.

OFFICE MAINTENANCE.—Expenditures for office maintenance, as for heating, lighting, telephone service and the services of attendants are deductible.

SUPPLIES.—Payments for supplies for professional use are deductible. Supplies may be fairly described as articles consumed in the using; for instance, dressings, clinical thermometers, drugs and chemicals. Professional journals may be classified as supplies and the subscription price deducted. Amounts currently expended for books, furniture and professional instruments and equipment, ''The useful life of which is short,'' generally less than one year, may be deducted, but if such articles have a more or less permanent value, their purchase price is a capital expenditure and is not deductible.

EQUIPMENT.—Equipment comprises property of a more or less permanent nature. It may ultimately wear out, deteriorate or become obsolete, but it is not in the ordinary sense of the word ''consumed in the using.''

The cost of equipment such as has been described, for professional use, cannot be deducted as expense in the year acquired. Examples of this class of property are automobiles, office furniture, medical, surgical and laboratory equipment of more or less permanent nature,

and instruments and appliances constituting a part of the physician's professional outfit, to be used over a considerable period of time, generally over one year. Books of more or less permanent nature are regarded as equipment and the purchase price is therefore not deductible.

Although the cost of such equipment is not deductible in the year acquired, nevertheless it may be recovered through depreciation deductions taken year by year over its useful life, as described later.

No hard and fast rule can be laid down as to what part of the cost of equipment is deductible each year as depreciation. The amount depends to some extent on the nature of the property and on the extent and character of its use. The length of its useful life should be the primary consideration. The most that can be done is to suggest certain average or normal rates of depreciation for each of several classes of articles and to leave to the taxpayer the modification of the suggested rates as the circumstances of his particular case may dictate. As fair, normal or average rates of depreciation, the following have been suggested: automobiles, 25 per cent a year; ordinary medical libraries, x-ray equipment, physical therapy equipment, electrical sterilizers, surgical instruments and diagnostic apparatus, 10 per cent a year; office furniture, 5 per cent a year.

The principle governing the determination of all rates of depreciation is that the total amount claimed by the taxpayer as depreciation during the life of the article, plus the salvage value of the article at the end of its useful life, shall not be greater than its purchase price or, if purchased before March 1913, either its fair market value as of that date or its original cost, whichever may be greater. The physician must in good faith use his best judgment and claim only such allowance for depreciation as the facts justify. The

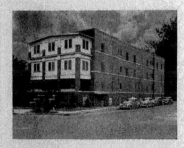
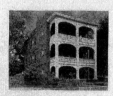

estimate of useful life, on which the rate of depreciation is based, should be carefully considered in his individual case.

MEDICAL DUES.—Dues paid to societies of a strictly professional character are deductible. Dues paid to social organizations, even though their membership is limited to physicians, are personal expenses and not deductible.

POSTGRADUATE STUDY.—The Commissioner of Internal Revenue holds that the expense of postgraduate study is not deductible.

TRAVELING EXPENSES.—Traveling expenses, including amounts paid for transportation, meals and lodging, necessarily incurred in professional visits to patients and in attending medical meetings for a professional purpose, are deductible.

AUTOMOBILES.—Payment for an automobile is a payment for permanent equipment and is not deductible. The cost of operation and repair, and loss through depreciation, are deductible. The cost of operation and repair includes the cost of gasoline, oil, tires, insurance, repairs, garage rental (when the garage is not owned by the physician), chauffeur's wages, and the like.

Deductible loss through depreciation of an automobile is the actual diminution in value resulting from absolescence and use and from accidental injury against which the physician is not insured. If depreciation is computed on the basis of the average loss during a series of years, the series must extend over the entire estimated life of the car, not merely over the period in which the car is possessed by the present taxpayer.

If an automobile is used for professional and also for personal purposes—as when used by the physician partly for recreation, or so used by his family—only so much of the expense as arises out of the use for professional purposes may be deducted. A physician doing an exclusive office practice and using his car merely to go to and from his office cannot deduct depreciation or operating expenses; he is regarded as using his car for his personal convenience and not as a means of gaining a livelihood. What has been said in respect to automobiles applies with equal force to horses and vehicles and the equipment incident to their use.

Miscellaneous

CONTRIBUTIONS TO CHARITABLE ORGANIZATIONS.—For detailed information with respect to the deductibility of charitable contributions generally, physicians should consult the official return blank or obtain information from the collectors of internal revenue or from other reliable sources. A physician may not, however, deduct as a charitable contribution the value of services rendered an organization operated for charitable purposes.

BAD DEBTS.—Physicians who make their returns on a cash receipts and disbursements basis, as most physicians do, cannot claim deductions for bad debts.

TAXES.—Taxes generally, either federal or state, are deductible by the person on whom they are imposed by law. Both real and personal property taxes are deductible; but so-called taxes, more properly assessments, paid for local benefits, such as street, sidewalk, and other like improvements, imposed because of and measured by some benefit inuring directly to the property against which the assessment is levied, do not constitute an allowable deduction from gross income. Physicians may deduct state gasoline taxes and state sales taxes. In some states sales taxes are imposed on the seller, but, if they are passed on to the buyer, the latter may deduct them.

State income and use taxes are deductible; federal income taxes are not. Among the federal taxes that a physician may deduct are those on admissions, dues, initiation fees, safety deposit boxes, tax on telegraph, telephone, cable and radio messages, and the federal use tax on automobiles. State automobile license fees

are deductible. If a state or local fee is imposed for regulatory purposes, and not to raise revenue, the fee may not ordinarily be deducted as a tax. If such fees, however, are classifiable as a business expense, they are deductible as such. Annual registration fees imposed on physicians probably come within the category of regulatory fees and should be deducted as a business expense rather than as taxes. Local and state occupational taxes imposed on physicians are deductible either as taxes or as a business expense, depending on the purpose for which the tax is imposed.

The excise taxes imposed on employers by section 804, title VIII, and section 901, title IX, of the Social Security Act, commonly referred to as old age and unemployment benefit taxes, are deductible annually by employers in computing net income for federal income tax purposes. If the taxpayer's return is made on a cash basis, as are the returns of practically all physicians, the taxes are deductible for the year in which they are actually paid. If the return is made on an accrual basis, the taxes are deductible for the year in which they accrue, irrespective of when they are actually paid. Employees, including physicians whose employment brings them within that category, may not deduct the tax imposed on them by section 801, title VIII, of the Social Security Act, generally referred to as the old age benefits tax. If, however, the employer assumes payment of the employee's tax and does not withhold the amount of the tax from the employee's wages, the amount of the tax so assumed may be deducted by the employer, not as a tax paid but as an ordinary business expense.

MEDICAL EXPENSE.—A taxpayer may deduct amounts expended for medical, dental and hospital care, not compensated for by insurance or otherwise, including amounts paid for accident and health insurance, according to a prescribed formula. Deductions will be permitted to the extent that such expenses exceed 5 per cent of the net income of the taxpayer but not in excess of $2,500 in case of the head of a family, or $1,250 in case of other individual taxpayers.

EQUIPMENT NECESSITATED BY MILITARY SERVICE.—The cost of equipment of an Army officer to the extent only that it is especially required for his profession and does not merely take the place of articles required in civilian life is deductible. The cost of a uniform is considered a personal expense and hence not deductible.

LABORATORY EXPENSES.—The deductibility of the expenses of establishing and maintaining laboratories is determined by the same principles that determine the deductibility of corresponding professional expenses. Laboratory rental and the expenses of laboratory equipment and supplies and of laboratory assistants are deductible when under corresponding circumstances they would be deductible if they related to a physician's office.

LOSSES BY FIRE OR OTHER CAUSES.—Loss of and damage to a physician's equipment by fire, theft or other cause, not compensated by insurance or otherwise recoverable, may be computed as a business expense and is deductible, provided evidence of such loss or damage can be produced. Such loss or damage is deductible, however only to the extent to which it has not been made good by repairs and the cost of repair claimed as a deduction.

INSURANCE PREMIUMS.—Premiums paid for insurance against professional losses are deductible. This includes insurance against damages for alleged malpractice, against liability for injuries by a physician's automobile while in use for professional purposes, and against loss from theft of professional equipment and damage to or loss of professional equipment by fire or otherwise. Under professional equipment is to be included any automobile belonging to the physician and used for strictly professional purposes.

EXPENSE IN DEFENDING MALPRACTICE SUITS.—Expense incurred in the defense of a suit for malpractice is deductible as a business expense.

SALE OF SPECTACLES.—Oculists who furnish spectacles etc., may charge as income money received from such sales and deduct as an expense the cost of the article sold. Entries on the physician's account books should in such cases show charges for services separate and apart from charges for spectacles, etc.

Nontrade or Nonbusiness Expenses

A new provision in the Revenue Act of 1942 permits, in the case of an individual, the deduction of all the ordinary, necessary expenses paid or incurred during the taxable year for the production or collection of income, or for the management, conservation or maintenance of property held for the production of income. While the phraseology of this provision is very broad, the Commissioner of Internal Revenue has by regulation ruled that the following expenses, among others, are not deductible under it: Commuters' expenses; expenses of taking special course of training; expenses in seeking employment or in placing one's self in a position to begin rendering personal services for compensation; bar examination fees and other expenses incurred in securing admission to the bar, and corresponding fees and expenses incurred by physicians, dentists, accountants and other taxpayers for securing the right to practice their respective professions.

Declaration of Estimated Tax for 1944

In addition to filing the final return for 1943, individual taxpayers above the income levels described in THE JOURNAL, Aug. 14, 1943, must file another declaration of estimated tax on or before March 15, covering the anticipated tax for the calendar year 1944. This declaration, it is assumed, will be similar in form to the declaration filed last September. Forms on which it is to be filed have not as yet been distributd. They have been withheld, no doubt, because of the pendency of tax legislation in Congress that will apply to 1944 taxes.

In completing this declaration, taxpayers will follow the same procedure utilized in completing the September declaration. They must estimate their income for the year, their exemptions and deductions, and compute the tax on the basis of such estimates. One fourth of the estimated tax must be paid when the declaration is filed, except in the case of taxpayers subject to the withholding provisions of the current tax payment act. Ample provision is made for the filing of amended declarations periodically in case the original estimates are too far out of line.

When Congressional action has been completed on the pending legislation, a statement will be prepared for publication in THE JOURNAL to aid physicians in complying with its requirements.

Hidden Phenomena

Only within very narrow boundaries can man observe the phenomena which surround him; most of them naturally escape his senses, and mere observation is not enough. To extend his knowledge, he has had to increase the power of his organs by means of special appliances; at the same time he has equipped himself with various instruments enabling him to penetrate inside of bodies, to dissociate them and to study their hidden parts. A necessary order may thus be established among the different processes of investigation or research, whether simple or complex; the first apply to those objects easiest to examine for which our senses suffice; the second bring within our observation, by various means, objects and phenomena which would otherwise remain unknown by us forever, because in their natural state they are beyond our range. Investigation, now simple, again equipped and perfected, is therefore destined to make us discover and note the more or less hidden phenomena which surround us.—Experimental Medicine. Page 5. The MacMillan Company. 1927.

A new semester started on January 5 with 76 students in the Freshman Class, 72 in the Sophomore Class, 72 in the Junior Class, and 56 in the Senior Class. The majority of the students are attending school under the Specialized Training Programs of the Army and Navy.

Previous to the inauguration of the accelerated program,.all students in the School of Medicine were required to purchase their own microscope. As a result of the limitation of critical materials it was not possible for each student to have his own microscope. The School of Medicine consequently was able to purchase 132 new microscopes to be rented to medical students.

Dr. H. A. Shoemaker, Assistant Dean, and Dr. Arthur A. Hellbaum, Professor of Pharmacology, attended a conference of the Board of Medical and Dental Interviewers of the Eighth Service Command, Dallas, Texas, on January 12.

Dr. Tom Lowry, Dean, and Mr. Howard R. Dickey, Chief Clerk of the University Hospitals, had a conference with officials of the F.W.A. in Fort Worth, Texas, Monday, January 10, regarding the addition to the University Hospital.

Dr. Ernest Lachman, Associate Professor of Anatomy, read a paper before the Tulsa Cancer Society on January 4. The title of the paper was ''The Anatomical Pathways for the Spread of Cancer of the Breast.''

Dr. Anderson Nettleship has been appointed Associate Professor of Pathology, assuming his duties on January 1. Dr. Nettleship received the B.S. degree from the University of Arkansas in 1931 and the M.D. degree from Johns Hopkins University School of Medicine in 1935. Dr. Nettleship has held appointments in Cornell Medical School, New York Hospital, Duke University Hospital, Vanderbilt University Hospital, and Union University, Albany, New York. He has also served as Director of Laboratories, Montgomery County, New York. He comes to the medical school from Bethesda, Maryland, where he has been serving as Passed Assistant Surgeon, R, U.S.P.H., National Cancer Institute.

Dr. Nettleship is a Diplomate of the American Board of Pathology in Anatomy and Clinical Pathology, a member of the American Association of Pathologists and Bacteriologists, American Society for Experimental Pathology, American Association for Cancer Research, the Society for Experimental Biology in Medicine, and the International Association of Medical Museums.

He is the author or co-author of 17 scientific publications.

Dr. E. R. Kellersberger, General Secretary of the American Mission to Lepers, gave an illustrated lecture in the auditorium of the Medical School on Friday afternoon, January 14, and spoke on his experience in tropical medicine. Dr. Kellersberger served as a medical missionary in the Belgian Congo for 24 years.

Dr. John F. Hackler and Dr. Donald B. McMullen, Professor and Associate Professor respectively in the Department of Public Health and Preventive Medicine, participated in the Kay County Medical Society held at the City Hospital in Tonkawa on the evening of January 13. Dr. McMullen was the principal speaker, giving an account of his recent work in Tropical Medicine in Central America. Dr. Hackler discussed his presentation.

★ FIGHTIN' TALK ★

LT. RUFUS C. GOODWIN, Oklahoma City, has been ordered to active duty. He was sent to Camp Barkley, Texas, after completing his internship at the Presbyterian Hospital in Philadelphia.

The following have received recent promotions: from Lieutenant to Captain; SAM R. FRYER, Oklahoma City; HAROLD B. WITTEN, Harrah; R. L. ALEXANDER, Okmulgee; from Major to Lt. Colonel; F. S. ETTER, Bartlesville.

The following three Oklahomans graduated, on December 16, from the Medical Field Service School, Carlisle Barracks, Pa., LT. LAWRENCE S. SELL, LT. RICHARD H. GRAHAM of Oklahoma City; LT. WILBUR F. BOHLMAN of Watonga.

LT COL. W. T. DUNNINGTON, Cherokee, has recently returned to the United States after having spent two years overseas.

CAPT. WILLIAM CAMPBELL, Fairland, graduate of the University of Oklahoma School of Medicine in 1939, entered service immediately upon completion of residency. He has recently returned from overseas duty and just reported to the School of Aviation Medicine, Randolph Field, Texas. He was a recent dinner guest of Dr. Tom Lowry, Dean of the Medical School.

CAPT. ROGER REID, Ardmore, is now in Atlantic City, New Jersey, where he is on duty at the England General Hospital.

MAJOR FREDERICK R. HOOD, Oklahoma City, has recently been promoted to Lt. Colonel. He is stationed at La Garde General Hospital in New Orleans where he is assistant chief of medical service and chief of cardio-vascular section. Lt. Colonel Hood was Assistant Professor of Medicine at the University of Oklahoma School of Medicine.

MAJOR PAT NAGLE, Oklahoma City, who spent the past twelve months in the Southwest Pacific Area, is at home for a fifteen-day leave. He is visiting his wife and three children at 121 N. E. 15th St., Oklahoma City.

Major Nagle was Chief of Surgery for an army field hospital in the fighting zone and is high in his praise of the army's medical service in the maintaining of morale of the fighting men. Major Nagle says in part:

"The knowledge that they have readily available very good medical facilities, including adequate supplies of blood plasma, is an important morale factor among our men. Blood plasma was the bulwark in the treatment of burns. It may be repetitious, but public support in maintenance of adequate supplies of blood plasma is no little contribution to the war in the Pacific. We never at any time had a lack of plasma."

Major Nagle will go from Oklahoma City to Hot Springs, Arkansas for reassignment.

CAPT. J. O. AKINS, Tulsa, who was wounded at Salerno, recently arrived in the United States aboard the Hospital Ship Acadia. From the port, Capt. Akins was taken to a hospital.

LT. COL. S. F. WILDMAN, landed in the United States on Christmas Day to spend a 30-day leave after nearly a year in North Africa, having recently been released from a hospital where he had been convalescing with his second siege of malaria. It is the opinion of Colonel Wildman that malaria is one of America's greatest post-war problems.

Colonel Wildman spent two years of World War No. I in the ambulance division of the Rainbow Division during its occupation of Germany. In 1942 he reached Casablanca in January and traveled overland 1,800 miles to Gafso, in Tunisia. There, he helped direct the supplying of medical equipment and medicines to the hastily constructed hospitals.

Colonel Wildman states; "The doctors and nurses are doing a fine job at the front. Most of the hospitals are hastily erected tents, offering problems of cleanliness and sanitation not found where structures can be permanent—and I never heard a single complaint, no matter how hard they worked."

COMDR. C. C. FULTON, Oklahoma City, has spent nineteen months in his present overseas area, and is getting a little anxious to return to the U.S.A. Comdr. Fulton reports that he has recently seen DRS. DICK FORD, Tulsa, JOHN CUNNINGHAM, Oklahoma City and ROY L. SMITH, Tulsa, and that they are all in good health.

CAPT. FRED T. PERRY, Healdton, sends his regards from 'somewhere in Italy' to Drs. Tom Lowry, Wann Langston, Gregory Stanbro, Joe Kelso, "Charlie" Bondurant and many others on the home front. Capt. Perry says in regard to the Post-War Planning "Please know that whatever your efforts do produce, however great or small, it will be very greatly appreciated by those of us who have been away, have lost a golden opportunity at times, seems quite discouraging."

The following anonymous reply to one of the Post-War Planning questionnaires was received from overseas: "I would like to have an opportunity to practice honest surgery without governmental interference. Those of us who have been away, have lost a golden opportunity of laying away a 'nest egg' for the future, not only monetarily but in the establishment of a local surgical reputation. It is my earnest hope that I shall be physically qualified and governmentally free to do all of the work that comes my way so that I may become economically independent as are other professionally trained individuals."

MAJOR HERVEY A. FOERSTER, Oklahoma City, has recently been transferred to Camp Reynolds, Greenville, Pennsylvania, from Camp Maxey, Texas. Also Major Foerster, was certified on November 5, 1943, by the American Board of Dermatology and Syphilology.

MAJOR CHARLES J. ROBERTS, Enid, has been in the Hawaiian Islands since March, 1942 and states that is a long time to be away from home. He is Chief of the Medical Service at the location and CAPT. DWIGHT PIERSON, Buffalo, is in the same organization, where he is Chief of the Surgical Service. Here's hoping they get their wish to come home before too much longer.

The Executive Office has received a long and most interesting letter from COLONEL REX BOLEND who is overseas with an Evacuation Hospital (Editors Note: *We beg forgiveness for calling the Hospital an Evacuation Unit. We have thoroughly enjoyed Colonel Bolend's* letter and wish that it were possible to print all of it in the Journal). The letter, in part, is as follows:

"Our Evacuation Hospital is comparable to the Army Jeep. The Jeep, as you know, is capable of going anywhere, any time, under all conditions of roads and terrain, with heavy or light load. It will surely get you there but with few refinements. There is no soft spring or cushion, it is neither warm nor air-cooled. We are completely equipped and self-contained and operate as an independent unit. We can go into the open field and in the matter of a very few hours be ready to receive and care for completely a great number of patients. We have all departments of a well organized hospital. Our x-ray is perhaps as modern and complete as any. Our Pharmacy and Medical Supplies are as complete as any modern hospital. The Laboratory is capable of considerable more than routine work. Our Operating Room is quite as modern and well equipped as any first class civilian hospital. This same thing applies to Orthopedic Department, Urological Department and General medicine.

"Now with this more or less elaborate set-up we could still be called the Jeep because we do not have, and you can readily see, could not carry the refinements. For example, our hospital is set up entirely in tents, with cots for hospital beds, mostly lanterns for light, no iceboxes, refrigeration system, rocking chairs or desks, etc., that go to make for comfort and convenience of either doctors or patients. In other words, I would say that we are set up to take care of a large number of any type cases quickly and make a rapid turn-over when necessary.

"I rather surmise the censor would not permit an exact recital of our operations at present. However, I feel safe in saying to you that you could and would have considerable glow of pride to see how this unit has taken their primary duties and with what thoroughness and carefulness they are attending to patients in this hospital. I can tell you truthfully that they have already made themselves felt and are looked upon as one of the strong and dependable organizations in the South Pacific. This is not our own opinion, it has been told to us from all echelons of command and from the mission and objectives they have set for us, it seems to be quite true. While I am telling you these things, I would be an ungrateful commander if I did not mention the enlisted men and the work they did in building, establishing and finally assuming their normal duties in this hospital. I realize this is not so important from the doctors' standpoint, but as you well know, a hospital cannot run without the necessary and efficient manpower."

Classified Advertisements

Experience

In French the word experience in the singular means, in general and in the abstract, the knowledge gained in the practice of life. When we apply to a physician the word experience in the singular, it means the information which he has gained in the practice of medicine. It is the same with the other professions; and it is in this sense that we say that a man has gained experiences, or that he has experience. Subsequently the word experience (experiment) in the concrete was extended to cover the facts which give us experimental information about things.—Experimental Medicine. Claude Bernard. The MacMillan Company. 1927. Page 11.

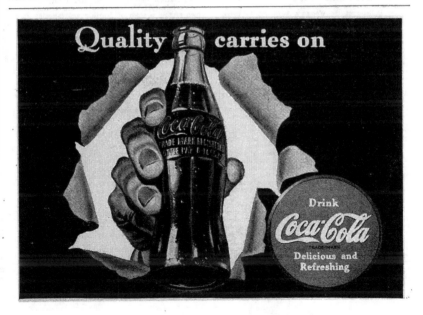

WOMAN'S AUXILIARY NEWS

A Message From Our President

"The private practice of medicine is being challenged by legislative measures. Because of the limited amount of time at the disposal of each doctor, because of the added duties in practice, the Auxiliary must necessarily undertake the serious task of informing the public concerning these legislations. The Wagner-Murray-Dingell Bill, Senate Bill 1161, is vicious in its socialization of medicine. Each Auxiliary member should be fully informed on this Bill before she endeavors to explain or refute it to her neighbor or the laity. The purpose is lost if she attempts to defeat the Bill without definite knowledge and support for her arguments.

"It is not necessary to remind you of the critical times and conditions under which we are living. Each of us has a feeling that we and our patients are being tried just a bit more now than previously and perhaps we are justified in our convictions. We, as Auxiliary members and helpmates to our husbands, who are members of the Medical Profession, are intensely conscious of the pressing tasks of service. Tasks, not in the sense that they are something that must be done, but with the inert feeling that we want to do everything that is humanly possible and we will take a real delight in doing, because they are for the real benefits of our country and for the grand profession of our life's partner, our husband, the Doctor of Medicine."

Mrs. F. Maxey Cooper, *President*

The following excerpt is from the article "The Woman's Auxiliary in This Great Crisis" written by Ernest D. Hitchcock, M.D., 1943 President of the Montana State Medical Association. The article appeared in the Bulletin of the Woman's Auxiliary, February, 1944.

"The women of America are contributing their all to the war effort, not only are they sending their sons over the seven seas but their daughters are taking their places in the front ranks. The young women of this country are working in the factories and ferrying the great bombers through the skies. Women are taking their place in war and must take their place in the making of a just peace.

"The Woman's Auxiliary to the American Medical Association has now come of age, being twenty-one years old this year. You are organized in 40 states and the District of Columbia so I am told. It has been repeatedly said that 'women have no place in politics,' that they belong in the home and should not concern themselves with national affairs. I do not know of any group who is more vitally concerned in just and proper laws or in a just and lasting peace than woman.

"We need a Woman's Auxiliary of a medical association of one-hundred-thousand strong. In numbers there is strength when united in a common purpose. I am satisfied that the time will come when the physicians of this nation will need the Woman's Auxiliary to help save those fundamental principals of free practice that have made American medicine great.

"Recently President Roosevelt sent to Congress the proposals of the National Planning Board and recommended its passage. This is the so-called 'American Beveridge Plan' or as the newspapers put it, 'The Cradle to the Grave Security Plan.' Part of this plan American medicine can endorse wholeheartedly. We all want better coordination of medical and health facilities. American medicine recognizes its obligation to the American people. We have always taken care of the poor; in fact, it is a truism that the rich and the poor get the best and fullest treatment while the middle classes suffer. In order to adequately provide medical care for all the people in this country the Public Health Service must be extended, for in many of our countries the population will not support a physician. This is especially true in the deep South.

"The health of America depends to a great measure on the health of the whole world. An epidemic of yellow fever in Africa today is a direct threat to our own states in the South. The men and women of America have made this country great not only through their industry and initiative but they have 'dreamed dreams' of a better land and a better world. We want to save all that was good in pre-war America. We want above all the principle of freedom of choice and freedom of opportunity. We want free choice of the school one attends, the church one worships in, the physician, the dentist or lawyer one consults. We want freedom of want not only for ourselves but for all people. Do the boys in Africa and Guadalcanal want to come back to the America that they knew so well, or do they want a new world to result from this conflict? An advertisement which has caught the public fancy says in part: '*Back home to the same town—to the same job you like so much—to the same America we have always known and loved, where you can work and plan and build; where there are no limits to any man's, and woman's or any child's opportunity. That is the America I want when I come back. Don't change that ever. Don't let anyone tamper with the way of living that works so well*'."

Tulsa County

The Tulsa County Medical Auxiliary's regular monthly luncheon was held January 2 at 12:30 P.M. in the Oklahoma Natural Gas club rooms. Mrs. C. H. Haralson gave a talk, "If We Must Cook". Mrs. Haralson has been making a study of Wartime and rationing food recipes and had formulated several new ideas which help conserve food and aid the War effort. The War Aid Committee report that they are sending out a questionnaire to each member to fill out on War work and hope to have a full report very soon. Red Cross workers are busy at present on surgical dressings.

Pittsburg County

The Pittsburg County Medical Auxiliary has had no formal meeting this year. The first event planned is a tea the first week in February at the home of Mrs. L. S. Willour, President, with Mrs. J. F. Park assisting. The Tea is planned in honor of the wives of the Medical Officers stationed at the Prisoner of War Camp and the Naval Ammunition Depot here.

War work has been the chief concern of most of the Auxiliary members; some do knitting, surgical dressings and Nurses' Aide Work.

Mrs. Willour, as Chairman of the Pittsburg County Tuberculosis Seal Sales, has just succeeded in raising $1,489.11 for the current campaign.

Mrs. W. H. Kæiser assists regularly in the offices of Dr. Kæiser and Dr. T. H. McCarley. Her work is along the Doctors' Aide line, but even more strenuous in that she makes post-partem visits to their patients.

Mrs. J. F. Park is continuing her duties this year at Red Cross Headquarters as instructor in Home Nursing and Nurses' Aide Classes.

Mrs. W. J. Dell has joined her husband who is stationed in Camp Abbott, Oregon.

Dr. Floyd Bartheld is in service, but Mrs. Bartheld is living in McAlester.

Dr. and Mrs. Mills are stationed in Utica, New York. Mrs. F. L. Watson's death has not been reported, although she died last year.

Pontotoc County

The members of the Auxiliary were guests of the Pontotoc Medical Society at a dinner given at the Al-

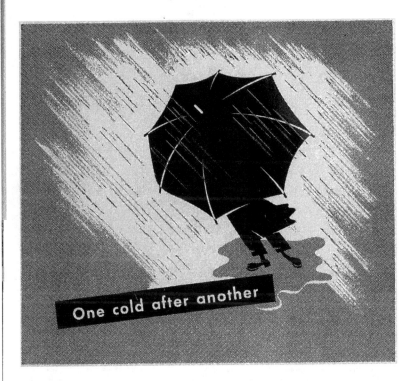

dridge Hotel on the night of January 12, 1944. Dr. and Mrs. Clinton Gallaher from Shawnee were guests. Dr. Gallaher, as councilor, was speaker for the evening and the new officers took office.

Mrs. E. M. Gullatt is teaching a class of volunteer Nurses' Aides for the Red Cross.

Cleveland County

Officers of the Cleveland County Auxiliary

President ....Mrs. Warren T. Mayfield
Vice-President ....Mrs. Charles Brake
Secretary ....Mrs. Curtis Berry
Treasurer ....Mrs. Tom Atkins

Oklahoma County

The January meeting of the Oklahoma County Auxiliary was held in the Y.W.C.A. on January 26. Mrs. Wolf, Public Relations Chairman, gave a report on the Wagner Bill. Mrs. Joseph W. Kelso gave a brief report of the Woman's Auxiliary Meeting at the Southern Medical Association held in Cincinnati in November. A more detailed report will be presented at the February meeting by the other representative, Mrs. Ray M. Balyeat.

Members of the Auxiliary worked on surgical dressings of various kinds for the University Hospital, also making glove wrappers, glove cases and students gowns.

Report of finances—Three $100.00 Bonds and three $25.00 Bonds have been purchased by the Auxiliary with money from their Emergency Fund. A $10.00 donation was made to the Hospital Piano Fund of Will Rogers Field.

PROPOSED HEALTH BILL IGNORES THE QUALITY OF MEDICAL CARE

Journal Says Wagner- Murray-Dingell Bill Focuses Attention On The Political Machinery To Distribute Service

The Wagner-Murray-Dingell focuses attention on the political machinery that will distribute medical service and ignores the quality of service itself, The Journal of the American Medical Association for October 30 points out in the last three editorials analyzing the measure:

"Revolutions often produce dictators who rise by force of personality or leadership but usually only after the revolution has run much of its course. The Wagner-Murray-Dingell Bill proposes to supply the dictator for American medicine even before the revolution begins. Compulsory sickness insurance produces the least evils when control of the actual practice of medicine is placed under the democratic management of medical associations. The quality of the medical service under such systems deteriorates least in proportion to the extent to which the establishment and maintenance of standards and quality of medical practice are confided to medical organizations. The authors of S. 1161 have overlooked this lesson as they have many others in the field of medical practice. But they had little apparent medical aid in formulating their blueprint for American medicine.

"In the Netherlands and Norway the medical profession resisted the attempts of Naziism to break down the autonomy of the medical profession in spite of severe persecution. In so doing, these physicians followed age-long professional tradition. The whole body of physicians acting autonomously and democratically is the only institution that has ever succeeded in creating and enforcing standards of conduct not only in practice but in medical education and the operation of medical institutions.

"S. 1161 makes a shallow pretense of recognizing this fact by proposing to create a committee containing representatives of the organizations concerned with medical practice. This committee is to be purely 'advisory,' without powers and with indefinite functions. It is to be appointed by the dictator whom it is supposed to advise. Provisions are not suggested whereby state or local professional bodies may exercise judgment and supervision at the only point where such judgment and supervision can be effective.

"While the Surgeon General of the United States Public Health Service is proposed as the dictator, it must be assumed that he will follow the pattern of administrative organizations and appoint subordinates responsible to him alone. Does any one believe he can avoid political considerations in making such appointments? He is to have the power to determine who will be specialists, what specialities they will follow and who will remain general practitioners. In fact, the fate of all phases of medical practice is vested in this dictator.

"The framers of the proposed law apparently neglected any consideration of the quality of the medical service to be distributed. More than fifty pages of the bill are given to the details of administration and financial arrangements; not one word is printed as to how the standards of medical practice shall be kept at their present high stage. Mention is not made of measures that might maintain the steady upward progress of those standards that has had characteristic of the period during which their establishment and maintenance have been entrusted to the medical profession.

"In the familiar pattern of advocates of compulsory sickness insurance, attention is focused on the political machinery that will distribute medical service; the quality of the service itself receives no notice. Medical care is a service given by physicians; the ability to diagnose and treat disease and protect the health of the public depends on the qualifications of the physician—on his education and training, his integrity, skill and initiative. The Wagner-Murry-Dingell plan is a blueprint for medical revolution, dealing with the sick and with the physicians who care for them as inanimate units to be moved at a dictator's will."

OFFICIAL WARNS DOCTORS TO BE ON GUARD AGAINST DRUG ADDICTS

Commissioner Of Narcotics Says Physicians Are Being Imposed On With Increasing Frequency Due To Drug Shortage

To the Editor:—Because of the shortage of narcotic drugs in the illicit traffic, drug addicts are calling on members of the medical profession looking for a "soft touch." This is the addict's term for a doctor who will write a narcotic prescription after listening to a plausible tale. Hundreds of such cases are coming to our attention.

A drug addict goes into a doctor's office and simulates a bad cough. He tells the doctor that the only thing that will help him is a drug, the name of which he has on a slip of paper. He shows the doctor this slip of paper, on which the word Dilaudid is written. He takes a chance that the doctor is unaware of the fact that this drug is a derivative of morphine. It is surprising how many doctors follow the addict's suggestion and write a prescription for Dilaudid.

When addicts find a notice of a doctor's death in an obituary column they sometimes call on the bereaved widow on the day following the death alleging that they are narcotic inspectors and have come to take charge of the doctor's morphine stock.

Pharmacists are being deluded with forged narcotic prescriptions. Blank pads are stolen from doctors' desks by addicts. Several times we have referred to numerous thefts of physicians' bags containing narcotics. A doctor's bag left in a parked automobile near a hospital is invariably stolen by a drug addict.

Physicians are being imposed on with increased frequency. I know they are extremely busy during this emergency. They should be warned to be on guard when a stranger tries to induce them to write a narcotic prescription. Many of the drug addicts today tell us they are obtaining narcotics to satisfy their various craving by going to various physicians and simulating some serious physical ailment.

H. J. Anslinger, Washington, D.C.
Commissioner of Narcotics.

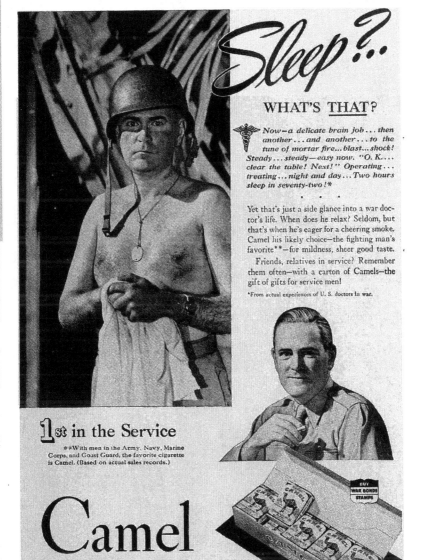

Sleep?...

WHAT'S THAT?

Now—a delicate brain job... then another... and another... to the tune of mortar fire... blast... shock! Steady... steady—easy now. "O. K.... clear the table! Next!" Operating... treating... night and day... Two hours sleep in seventy-two!*

. . .

Yet that's just a side glance into a war doctor's life. When does he relax? Seldom, but that's when he's eager for a cheering smoke. Camel his likely choice—the fighting man's favorite**—for mildness, sheer good taste.

Friends, relatives in service? Remember them often—with a carton of Camels—the gift of gifts for service men!

*From actual experiences of U. S. doctors in war.

1st in the Service

**With men in the Army, Navy, Marine Corps, and Coast Guard, the favorite cigarette is Camel. (Based on actual sales records.)

BUY
WAR BONDS
STAMPS

Camel
costlier tobaccos——

New reprint available on cigarette research—Archives of Otolaryngology, March, 1943, pp. 404-410. Camel Cigarettes, Medical Relations Division, One Pershing Square, New York 17, N. Y.

BOOK REVIEWS

"The chief glory of every people arises from its authors."—Dr. Samuel Johnson.

BRUCELLOSIS IN MAN AND ANIMALS. I. Forest Huddleson, D.V.M., M.S., Ph.D., Research Professor in Bacteriology, Michigan State College. Contributing authors: A. V. Hardy, M.S., M.D., Dr. P. H., Associate Professor of Epidemiology, DeLamar Institute of Public Health, Columbia University Medical School, Consultant, U. S. Public Health Service. J. E. Debono, M.D., M.R.C.P., Professor of Pharmacology and Therapeutics, Royal University of Malta. Ward Giltner, D.V.M., M.S., Dr. P.H., Dean of Veterinary Division and Professor of Bacteriology, Michigan State College. Revised Edition. Published, 1943, in New York by The Commonwealth Fund. 379 pages. Price $3.50.

This book contains a compilation of material never before presented in medicine. It is such as anyone interested in the subject, either a veterinarian, public health doctor, or practicing physician, could not afford to be without.

It is a treatise which is strictly scientific and apparently not proposed, altogether, as a direct clinical aid. The description of the organisms "the genus brucella," the methods of its isolation, and the differentiation of the various species are accurately described. One chapter on brucellosis in human beings gives an interesting historical survey and covers (by A. V. Hardy, M.S., M.D., Dr. P.H.) the epidemiology, incubation period, pathology, clinical types, clinical analysis of symptoms, sequelae, and duration of physical findings in connection with the cases in the United States.

A separate chapter (by Dr. J. E. Debono, M.D., M.-R.C.P., Royal University of Malta) gives a description of brucellosis in Malta.

Brucellosis in Animals is an extremely interesting chapter and one which seems to set forth many fundamental principles which establish sound basic study for the human form.

The laboratory diagnosis, including the serological methods, the agglutination test for human beings and for cattle are itemized and tabulated and their values and interpretations set forth in a very interesting manner.

The allergic tests, or skin tests, are given in a separate chapter and the opsonocytophagic test thoroughly described and evaluated.

Finally, there is a chapter by Ward Giltner on the irradication, or control, on sources of brucellosis infection.

The entire book is adequately and very nicely illustrated in both black and white and color. Important data from several investigators have been included. Twenty-four case reports are to be found in the appendix. These are all interesting and instructive.

I believe the book may be considered indispensable to any person seriously interested in any phase of the disease, and the authors deserve praise for their contribution.—Hugh Jeter, M.D.

DISEASES AND INJURIES OF THE LARYNX. Chevalier Jackson and Chevalier L. Jackson. Second Edition. The MacMillan Company. New York. 1943. $8.00.

This comprehensive textbook is the latest book published by these two authors. Every known laryngeal malady is discussed. Definition, etiology, pathology, symptoms, clinical findings, diagnosis, differential diagnosis, association with systemic diseases, treatment, prognosis and sequelae are considered. Practically all the material from "Diseases of the Larynx" and "Cancer of the Larynx" by these same authors is included. There are meticulously detailed descriptions of various techniques employed in diagnosis and treatment of laryngeal conditions. The text, as in all of Jackson's works, is easily readable. It gives the author's personal opinions regarding all subjects but does not neglect to consider the contributions of other laryngologists. There are eleven color plates, over 100 halftones and 221 pen and ink drawings.

The chapter on war surgery of the larynx is entirely new and will be of great value to military and naval surgeons.

The book is recommended to anyone interested in the diagnosis and care of diseases of the larynx.—L. Chester McHenry, M.D.

CLINICAL SIGNIFICANCE OF THE BLOOD IN TUBERCULOSIS. Gulli Lindh Muller, M.D. The Commonwealth Fund. New York City. 516 pages, price $3.50.

In Part One, the author gives a concise review of the physiology of the blood and discusses the cellular response in the tissues to the tubercle bacillus in experimental and in human tuberculosis. In Part Two, the author takes up changes in the circulating blood in tuberculosis and first discusses the neutrophil shift, pointing out that in active lesions there is a shift to the left which becomes more marked as the lesion becomes more advanced, and that a shift to the right suggests greater resistance or improvement in the state of the patient. Dr. Muller thinks that, while the "shift" may be of some value in diagnosis, it is of more value in differentiating active from inactive forms and that it is of considerable use in prognosis.

There usually is a monocytosis which increases with increasing activity of the process. Lymphocytic changes correspond to the activity of the lesion, the lymphocytes increasing with improvement. Several chapters are devoted to other leucocytes, leucocytic formulæ, etc. Several anemia is not frequently found, but all types, macrocytic, normocytic and microcytic, have been observed. The importance of the sedimentation rate is indicated by the fact of five chapters of the book being devoted to it.

The book seems to me to be of considerable interest to the hematologist and to the specialist in the tuberculosis, but is too voluminous to be of great use to the general practitioner.—Wann Langston, M.D.

METHODS OF TREATMENT. Eighth Edition. Logan Clendening and Edward H. Hashinger. C. V. Mosby Company. St. Louis. 1943. 1008 pages. Price $10.00.

This is a book written both for medical students and practitioners of the profession. The book is not devoted exclusively to drugs, but practically all of the therapeutic procedures are brought together in this one volume and discussed in the usual Clendening style.

Realizing the rapid change and progress which has recently been made in therapeutic procedures, it was necessary that many chapters of the book be entirely rewritten and some new chapters included. This has been adequately done by the authors and their collaborators. Such new chapters include the chapters on Chemotherapy for Coccal Diseases; Back Ache; Peripheral Vascular Diseases; Deficiency Diseases; Anesthetics; and Gout. Completely rewritten chapters include those in Intestinal Parasites; Syphilis; Vitamins; and Ductless Glands.

The first part of the book describes each procedure under the heading of drugs, diets, hydrotherapy, etc. The second considers the application and the results to be expected under the heading of the various diseases.

It is both interesting and encouraging to see the first

chapter devoted to a discussion of the therapeutic value of nature's best remedy, "Rest," and to read: "Rest in bed will do more for more diseases than any other single procedure"; and further, !"Immature faddists are continuously proclaiming the value of exercise; four people out of five are more in need of rest than exercise." How difficult it is for us to convince, sometimes ourselves, but more often our patients of this fact.

To one who has found Dr. Clendening's practical psychology and philosophy always interesting, his chapter devoted to psychotherapy is another stimulus. He describes it as "Intrinsically, treatment of the soul." In addition, "The profession as a whole is more indifferent to, and neglectful of, psychotherapy than any other form of therapeutics."

The details and technique of mechanical therapeutic procedures such as lumbar puncture, blood transfusions, duodenal drainage and paracentesis abdominalis are explained so thoroughly and simply that it might tempt a freshman medical student to action. In fact, the subjects so ably covered in this book make it a first-class textbook of medicine.—Tom Lowry, M.D.

THE NATURE AND TREATMENT OF MENTAL DISORDERS. Dom Thomas Verner Moore, O.S.B., Ph. D., M.D. Grune & Stratton, Inc. New York. 1943.

This book is not large but the author has given an outline and concept of mental disorders along with his experience in treating them without burdening the text with high-sounding and technical phrases. In Part I he outlines what he terms psychopathology and speaks of the advantages and disadvantages of Freud's conception that all mental disorders are due to sex maladjustment in early life. He discusses the theory of Jung with respect to the introvert and the extrovert, also of Adler's idea of the superiority and inferiority complexes. He comes to the conclusion that some mental disorders at least must be looked upon as truly psychic in nature and do not have a specific organic cerebral pathology. He recognizes of course that some forms of mental abnormality have their foundation in the accidental localizations of certain types of cerebral lesions but states that this is not sufficient to explain all forms that the psychobiological constitution of the patient must be considered.

This establishes the foundation for his methods of treatment. He emphasizes the necessity for chemotherapy in organic disorders and of psychotherapy in functional disorders. He takes up individual cases, discusses their probable cause and follows them through to a conclusion whether the result is favorable or not.

This book can be read and easily understood by the average practitioner and in it he would find illustrations of many of the problems which he faces in his daily contact with patients. It also gives the specialists many constructive ideas. The author does not stress the importance of placing each patient in a certain category, although in the Appendix he has listed the classification and definition of mental disorders as approved by the American Psychiatric Association.—John L. Day, M.D.

ALLERGY. Erick Urbach & Phillip M. Gottlieb. Grune & Stratton, Inc. New York. 1014 pages. Price $12.00.

From an infant who was still in the diaper stage a little more than two decades ago, allergy has grown to be one of the lustiest among specialists in medicine. This is evidenced by the voluminous literature on the subject, nearly twenty-five hundred authors being cited in the work.

Dr. Urbach is a teacher and writer of prominence. In this book he shows that much time, thought and research have combined to produce a work rarely excelled for thoroughness. He analyzes previous and contemporary studies in allergy and enables his readers to make practical application of the accumulated facts.

For convenience and practical use the book is divided into three parts, "Fundamentals of Allergy", "Etiologic Agents" and "Symptomatology and Therapy".

Unlike many works on the various specialities, this book is of great value to the general practitioner and should be very helpful to him in adding to his knowledge of etiology and treatment of many allergic diseases.

The large number of clear, vivid illustrations, the many tables and charts as well as the exhaustive description of testing methods and the graphic pollination calendars, should all be valuable aids in differential diagnosis.

Typographically, the book comes up to the best standard of medical publications.

The author is to be congratulated on the production of a work which is so easily read and which is a valuable addition to the medical library and is of great help to the general practitioner in his diagnosis and treatment of allergic conditions and diseases.—J. V. Athey, M.D.

A Surgeon's Prayer in Wartime

"God of Battle, grant that the wounded may swiftly arrive at their hospital haven, so that the safeguards of modern surgery may surround them, to the end that their pain is assuaged and their broken bodies are mended.

"Grant me as a surgeon, gentle skill and intelligent foresight to bar the path to such sordid enemies as shock, hemorrhage and infection.

"Give me plentifully the blood of their non-combatant fellowman, so that their vital fluid may be replaced and thus make all the donor people realize that they, too, have given their life's blood in a noble cause.

"Give me the instruments of my calling so that my work may be swift and accurate; but provide me with resourceful ingenuity so that I may do without bounteous supplies

"Strengthen my hand, endow me with valiant energy to go through day and night; and keep my heart and brain attuned to duty and great opportunity.

"Let me never forget that a life or a limb is in my keeping and do not let my judgment falter.

"Enable me to give renewed courage and hope to the living and comfort to the dying.

"Let me never forget that in the battles to be won, I too must play my part, to the glory of a great calling and as a follower of the Great Physician. Amen."

John J. Moorhead, Colonel M. C.
Trippler General Hospital,
Honolulu, T. H.

Christmas Night, 1941.
William R. Warner & Co., Inc.

The Discoverer

The discoverer of natural knowledge stands apart in the modern world, an obscure and slightly mysterious figure. By the abstract character of his researchs his individuality is obliterated; by the rational form of his method is concealed; and at best he can be known only through an effort of the imagination. This is perhaps inevitable. But the unfortunate effects are enhanced by convention which today prescribes a formal, rigorous and impersonal style in the composition of scientific literature. Thus while it is no more difficult to know Galileo and Harvey than Cervantes and Milton through their writings, or to perceive their habits and methods of work, psychological criticism will often seek in vain the personality and the behavior of the person behind the modern scientific printed page. Yet, whoever fails to understand the great investigator can never know what science really is.—Experimental Medicine. Claude Bernard. Page 5. The MacMillan Co. 1927.

Are you finding more Tuberculosis
in your practice?

TUBERCULIN PATCH TEST
(Vollmer)
Lederle

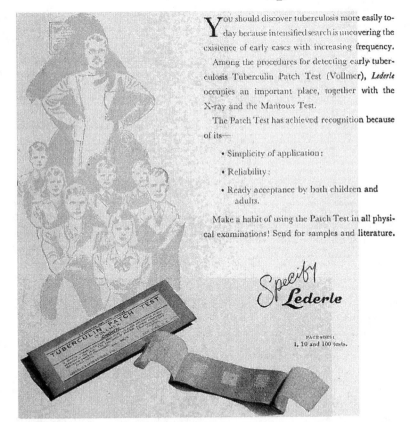

You should discover tuberculosis more easily to-day because intensified search is uncovering the existence of early cases with increasing frequency.

Among the procedures for detecting early tuberculosis Tuberculin Patch Test (Vollmer), *Lederle* occupies an important place, together with the X-ray and the Mantoux Test.

The Patch Test has achieved recognition because of its—

- Simplicity of application;
- Reliability;
- Ready acceptance by both children and adults.

Make a habit of using the Patch Test in all physical examinations! Send for samples and literature.

Specify Lederle

PACKAGES:
1, 10 and 100 tests.

MEDICAL ABSTRACTS

"THE PRACTICAL MANAGEMENT OF HEADACHE."
Arthur W. Proetz. Annals of Otology, Rhinology and Laryngology. Vol. 52, No. 2, pages 409-418. June, 1943.

There is no generally accepted classification of headache, although various ones to be found in recent publications fairly parallel one another. While the local mechanisms which produce headache are of only two or three types, many remote conditions provoke them by activating these mechanisms. In general it may be said that all headaches must be the result of disturbances transmitted through the sensory cranial nerves. The sensitive structures may be designated as: the dural arteries, the cerebral arteries at the base of the brain, arteries outside the cranium, the great venous sinuses and the basal portions of the dura itself.

In a case of headache the first and most important step is to project the case into one of the following classes: having (a) definite demonstrable causes, (b) semi-demonstrable causes, and (c) undemonstrable or only remotely suggestive causes. Under Class A are included local conditions which include demonstrable eye, ear, nose, brain and dental lesions; specific nerve affections such as trigeminal nerve pains and nasal ganglion syndromes; injuries; tumors and infections; remote conditions such as constipation and other digestive disturbances; organic disease whose characteristic toxic mechanical aberrations produce referred pains in the head; allergic conditions definitely traceable to known antigents; anemias; histamine poisoning.

Under Class B are grouped migraine, psychoneurotic disturbances, fatigue and kindred relatively definite processes. Under the C group come headaches which might once have been described as idiopathic. They appear to be due to vascular changes occasioned by all manner of influences, arise probably from acute distentions and more particularly rapid collapses and spasm of blood vessels, alterations in blood pressure, in fact any change in local vasomotor tone. These merge into the neuralogic and the toxic pains. The three are often related to such demonstrable lesions as arthritis and arteriosclerosis.

To find the proper place for a case of headache, the most reliable method is a standardized headache history, recording upon special forms. Such a record serves to segregate the findings pertaining specially to headache and throws them into juxtaposition so that their relationships become more apparent. The patient also records foods and drugs ingested during a specific period, usually extending several weeks, also some of his more important contacts. Such a record of the personal life of the patient will demonstrate the patient's eating habits, idiosyncrasis of diet, intake of alcohol, smoking propensities, and exposure to industrial dusts and fumes.

A complete physical and laboratory examination follows. After such examination the Class A cases take care of themselves. The remedy is obviously the removal of the cause when that is possible. As mentioned before, such cases may be caused by a sinus infection, a hyperphoria, a brain tumor, or any of a great number of disturbances by the examination.

Patients classified under B will be apt to require readjustment in their occupations or some other dominant factor in their daily lives. Their problem is often for the sociologist. For the person whose headache turns out to be hereditary there is no help.

Class C comprises the most perplexing but at the same time the most satisfactory cases. For the treatment of such cases, the author considers various experimental measures. He begins with alteration of the vascular tone. Unless there is hypertension, the patient is given ephedrine orally (together with seconal or some other barbiturate to minimize the unpleasant effect). Many headaches disappear promptly and many are controlled by this means alone. The ephedrine is given in doses of three-eighths grain twice daily and, if effective, is continued for a week. If, after the drug is withdrawn, the headache returns, it may be resumed, but a long continued course of ephedrine is not to be recommended. Some persistent headaches can be controlled with occasional courses of ephedrine. If they are affected at all, the suspicion of their vascular origin is confirmed.

If this is unsuccessful, and especially if the patient complains of lassitude and fatigue, thyroid extracts take the place of ephedrine. Of course, the thyroid administration should be very cautious. If it succeeds, then the dosage is subsequently determined by the symptomatology rather than the metabolic rate. These patients are apt to complain of deep boring or bursting headache and there may be sensitivity of the anterior deep temporal artery.

The third experimental measure consists in evacuating the lower bowel, preferably with enema, at the very onset of the attack, regardless of the patient's statement that his habits are regular. Headache, usually basilar or occipital, may result from obvious constipation, but similar headaches may be produced by some local retention or possibly by the absorption of toxic products without demonstrable stasis. Abdominal discomfort often announces or is coincident with headache and has been described as of allergic origin.

Minor episodes of starvation, especially by a long period between breakfast and lunch, can produce typically basilar and occipital headaches. Although these headaches may be prevented by the taking of food before they begin, once they occur, the ingestion of food will not diminish them; in fact, they may persist for several hours in spite of it. The remedy lies in a bite to eat between meals, with an eye to the choice of food.

In regard to the ingestion of alcoholic drinks it is important to determine not only the amount ingested but the time in relation to eating, sleeping and exercise, and the type of drink, also the time relation between drink and pain. Smoking habits must be also determined. Local irritations from tar deposits are especially common in patients with septal spurs or other constrictions, deviations and obstructions, and headaches from such irritations are not uncommon.

Headache may result from sleeping overlong, especially if ventilation is faulty. Lack of humidification in heated houses causes a parched membrane and produces a characteristic boring type of pain, usually referred to the forehaad and the bridge of the nose. Faulty posture in typists, pianists and technical workers produce pain in the occiput and shoulders which is sometimes persistent for a time after the condition is corrected.—M.D.H., M.D.

"EQUALIZING THE LOWER EXTREMITIES: A CLINICAL CONSIDERATION OF LEG LENGTHENING VERSUS LEG SHORTENING." George S. Phalen and C. C. Chatterton. Surgery. Vol. XII, page 769. 1942.

The authors refer to the psychological and physical difficulties developing from a shortened lower extremity, and discuss the advantages, disadvantages, and techniques of various methods of leg-lengthening and leg-shortening operations, and the indications and contra-indications for their use.

Before the operation for leg lengthening is performed, the patient should wear an elevated shoe not only to correct secondary conditions such as scoliosis and poor posture, but also to determine the amount of lengthening which will give the optimal improvement in function. In some instances, a leg-lengthening operation may so change the leverage of weakened muscles that the gait will be worse rather than better after the operation.

The article is based on the authors' experience with forty-five patients, twenty-six of whom had leg-lengthening, and nineteen, leg-shortening operations. The authors prefer leg-shortening operations and believe that the leg-lengthening procedures should be limited to a small, carefully chosen group of patients who are either unwilling or ill able to sacrifice any fraction of their height.—E.D.M., M.D.

"NONSURGICAL ASPECT OF OCULAR WAR INJURIES. Frederick C. Cordes. American Journal of Ophthalmology. Vol. 26, pages 1062-1071. October, 1943.

There are certain basic causative agents that produce eye injuries in warfare. These are: 1. Artillery fire, 2. High-explosive bombs, 3. Incendiaries, 4. Flame burns, 5. Contact burns, and 6. War gas burns. One basic principle underlying the treatment of ocular war injuries is the avoidance of too early and too much interference.. Some of these cases, exclusive of gas injuries, may be let alone for 24 or more hours. Patients who exhibit considerable shock and restlessness are treated for shock and allowed to recover from it before the eye is treated. Patients exposed to affects of demolition bombs are wisely treated so that the conjunctival sac is irrigated gently a number of times at hourly intervals with very mild antiseptics before surgery or repair is attempted. The only urgent operation is excision of prolapsed irides and coverage of wound with a flap.

Lid injuries, conjunctival tears, corneal wounds, various types of penetrating injuries of the globe, prolapsed irides, are all surgical problems that require immediate care. Immediate repair of lid wound is important in order to avoid notching and to protect the eye. If facilities are not available the wound is cleaned up gently and moist compresses applied over the eye; the patient is sent to a base hospital where proper repair can be made.

Single foreign bodies of the cornea are handled as in the civilian practice. If there is a circle of rust that cannot be removed easily it is well to keep the eye bandaged for 24 hours, at the end of which time enough infiltrate will have formed around the foreign body to facilitate its removal. The use of dental burr often aids greatly in this procedure. Multiple foreign bodies are frequent. They should not be attempted to be removed at once; the eye should be washed and cleaned out, bandaged, and further removal attempted after 24 or 48 hours.

The cornea has a tendency to extrude foreign bodies. After 24 or 48 hours many of the minute foreign bodies are found in the conjunctival sac. Inert foreign bodies deeply imbedded may be left alone, if their removal would cause much more damage; but limestone must be removed always.

In case of intraocular foreign bodies detailed examination of the fundus and x-ray study are indicated even for the apparently well eye. In war injuries of the eye, 90 per cent of the intraocular foreign bodies are principally sand, stone, debries, and glass; even the rest of, foreign body cases, though metallic, is nonmagnetic. Considering the good tolerance of the eye to such foreign bodies, and the possibility of spontaneous extrusion,

one should be patient with removal. Copper and its alloys are well tolerated, but if it remains in the eye, chalcosis may develop. In this condition the lens has a disciform opacity in its central area, of greenish gray color; the iris may be also discolored. If the copper particle is absorbed or removed, the chalcosis may also disappear.

Iron may spontaneously disappear, but the resulting siderosis is so disastrous that removal of iron or steel particles is a necessity. Removal should be made, however, only under favorable circumstances. Glass is well tolerated, but usually the eye itself is severely damaged and little can be done for saving it from enucleation.

Contusions of the eyeball usually are complicated with rupture of the chorid, retinal hemorrhage and detachment. Eye contusions are common and very destructive in the present war. The care of contusions from without is the same as in the civilian practice. Orbital contusions are caused by missiles passing into or through the orbits above the level of the zygoma. Very severe damage can be seen, and usually the optic nerve is also injured. All orbital injuries above the level of the zygoma should be considered as brain cases until proved otherwise. The optic nerve may receive direct injuries. Windage, or remote effect of explosive bombs together with sudden atmospheric expansion, may cause some queer and rather severe ocular injuries; proptosis, rupture of the eyeball, and rupture of the choroid.

In case of burns of the eyelids, the burned area is not to be treated with tannic acid; the area should be gently cleansed with warm saline and the surrounding area with soap. Blisters should be opened and loose epidermis removed. After this a dressing is applied that will keep the burned area clean and that upon removal will not be damaging to the new epithelium. Scorching burns resulting from explosions sometimes may be rather severe; searing of the cornea will be seen, but the corneal epithelium will, as a rule, regenerate in 24 to 48 hours. Contact burns with molten metal, wood, etc., are more serious than scorching from flames. Treatment is similar to that used in civil life. Anesthetics should not be applied to eye; if pain is present, it should be controlled by oral or hypodermic administration.

War-gas burns of the eyes or exposure to war gas requires immediate attention. The most effective universal treatment, irrespective of the type of gas, or in the event of a mixture of gases, would appear to be that based on alkaline hydrolysis by the use of approximately 2 per cent sodium bicarbonate. This can be simply made by dissolving a teasponful of baking soda in a glass of water. In any case of war-gas burn the patient should be reassured that he is not blind. Dark glasses should be used, but no bandages on gassed eyes, and the dark glass should be removed as early as possible to prevent neurasthenic symptoms.—M. D. H., M.D.

E. D. M. ....Earl D. McBride, M. D.
H. J. ....Hugh Jeter, M. D.
M. D. H. ....Marvin D. Henley, M. D.

For the General Practitioner

For the general practitioner a well-used library is one of the few correctives of the premature senility which is so ape to overtake him. Self-centered, self-taught, he leads a solitary life, and unless his every-day experience is controlled by careful or by attrition of a medical society it soon ceases to be of the slightest value and becomes a mere accretion of isolated facts, without correlation. It is astonishing with how little reading a doctor can practice medicine, but it is not astonishing how badly he may do it.—Aecquanimitas and other Addresses. Sir William Osler. 3rd Edition.

OFFICERS OF COUNTY SOCIETIES, 1944

★

COUNTY	PRESIDENT	SECRETARY	MEETING TIME
Alfalfa	H. E. Huston, Cherokee	L. T. Lancaster, Cherokee	Last Tues. each Second Month
Atoka-Coal	R. C. Henry, Coalgate	J. S. Fulton, Atoka	
Beckham	G. H. Stagner, Erick	O. C. Standifer, Elk City	Second Tuesday
Blaine	L. R. Kirby, Okeene	W. F. Griffin, Watonga	
Bryan	John T. Wharton, Durant	W. K. Haynie, Durant	Second Tuesday
Caddo	E. L. Patterson, Carnegie	C. B. Sullivan, Carnegie	
Canadian	P. F. Herod, El Reno	A. L. Johnson, El Reno	Subject to call
Carter	J. R. Pollock, Ardmore	H. A. Higgins, Ardmore	
Cherokee	P. H. Medearis, Tahlequah	*James K. Gray, Tahlequah	First Tuesday
Choctaw	C. H. Hale, Boswell	E. A. Johnson, Hugo	
Cleveland	F. T. Gastineau, Norman	Iva S. Merritt, Norman	Thursday nights
Comanche	George L. Berry, Lawton	Howard Angus, Lawton	
Cotton	A. B. Holstead, Temple	Mollie F. Scism, Walters	Third Friday
Craig	Lloyd H. McPike, Vinita	Paul G. Sanger, Vinita	
Creek	J. E. Hollis, Bristow	W. G. Bisbee, Bristow	
Custer	F. R. Vieregg, Clinton	C. J. Alexander, Clinton	Third Thursday
Garfield	Julian Feild, Enid	John R. Walker, Enid	Fourth Thursday
Garvin	T. F. Gross, Lindsay	John R. Callaway, Pauls Valley	Wednesday before Third Thursday
Grady	Walter J. Baze, Chickasha	Roy E. Emanuel, Chickasha	Third Thursday
Grant	I. V. Hardy, Medford		
Greer	R. W. Lewis, Granite	J. B. Hollis, Mangum	
Harmon	W. G. Husband, Hollis	R. H. Lynch, Hollis	First Wednesday
Haskell	William Carson, Keota	N. K. Williams, McCurtain	
Hughes	Wm. L. Taylor, Holdenville	Imogene Mayfield, Holdenville	First Friday
Jackson	C. G. Spears, Altus	E. A. Abernethy, Altus	Last Monday
Jefferson	F. M. Edwards, Ringling	L. I. Wade, Ryan	Second Monday
Kay	J. Holland Howe, Ponca City	G. H. Yeary, Newkirk	Second Thursday
Kingfisher	A. O. Meredith, Kingfisher	H. Violet Sturgeon, Hennessey	
Kiowa	J. William Finch, Hobart	William Bernell, Hobart	
LeFlore	Neeson Rolle, Poteau	Rush L. Wright, Poteau	
Lincoln	W. B. Davis, Stroud	Carl H. Bailey, Stroud	First Wednesday
Logan	William C. Miller, Guthrie	J. L. LeHew, Jr., Guthrie	Last Tuesday
Marshall	O. A. Cook, Madill		
Mayes	Ralph V. Smith, Pryor	Paul B. Cameron, Pryor	
McClain	W. C. McCurdy, Sr., Purcell	W. C. McCurdy, Jr., Purcell	
McCurtain	A. W. Clarkson, Valliant	N. L. Barker, Broken Bow	Fourth Tuesday
McIntosh	Luster I. Jacobs, Hanna	Wm. A. Tolleson, Eufaula	First Thursday
Murray	P. V. Annadown, Sulphur		Second Tuesday
Muskogee-Sequoyah Wagoner	H. A. Scott, Muskogee	D. Evelyn Miller, Muskogee	First Monday
Noble	C. H. Cooke, Perry	J. W. Francis, Jerry	
Okfuskee	C. M. Cochran, Okemah	M. L. Whitney, Okemah	Second Monday
Oklahoma	Walker Morledge, Oklahoma City	E. R. Musick, Oklahoma City	Fourth Tuesday
Okmulgee	S. B. Leslie, Okmulgee	J. C. Matheney, Okmulgee	Second Monday
Osage	C. R. Weirich, Pawhuska	George K. Hemphill, Pawhuska	Second Monday
Ottawa	Walter Kerr, Picher	B. W. Shelton, Miami	Third Thursday
Pawnee	E. T. Robinson, Cleveland	R. L. Browning, Pawnee	
Payne	H. C. Manning, Cushing	J. W. Martin, Cushing	Third Thursday
Pittsburg	P. T. Powell, McAlester	W. H. Kaeiser, McAlester	Third Friday
Pontotoc	A. R. Sugg, Ada	R. H. Mayes, Ada	First Wednesday
Pottawatomie	E. Eugene Rice, Shawnee	Clinton Gallaher, Shawnee	First and Third Saturday
Pushmataha	John S. Lawson, Clayton	B. M. Huckabay, Antlers	
Rogers	R. C. Meloy, Claremore	Chas. L. Caldwell, Chelsea	First Monday
Seminole	J. T. Price, Seminole	Mack I. Shanholtz, Wewoka	Third Wednesday
Stephens	W. K. Walker, Marlow	Wallis S. Ivy, Duncan	
Texas	T. G. Obermiller, Texhoma	Morris Smith, Guymon	
Tillman		O. G. Bacon, Frederick	
Tulsa	Ralph A. McGill, Tulsa	E. O. Johnson, Tulsa	Second and Fourth Monday
Washington-Nowata	K. D. Davis, Nowata	J. V. Athey, Bartlesville	Second Wednesday
Washita	A. S. Neal, Cordell	James F. McMurry, Sentinel	
Woods	Ishmael F. Stephenson, Alva	Oscar E. Templin, Alva	Last Tuesday Odd Months
Woodward	H. Walker, Buffalo	C. W. Tedrowe, Woodward	Second Thursday

*(Serving in Armed Forces)

THE JOURNAL

OF THE

OKLAHOMA STATE MEDICAL ASSOCIATION

| VOLUME XXXVII | OKLAHOMA CITY, OKLAHOMA, MARCH, 1944 | NUMBER 3 |

Surgical Indications In Glaucoma[*]

DONALD V. CRANE, M.D.

TULSA, OKLAHOMA

The subject of glaucoma occupies a position of enormous diagnostic and therapeutic importance in the field of Ophthalmology. In fact, it is a disease of vital interest and significance in the whole domain of medicine. Occurring in the unwholesome proportion of one-2 per cent of all diseases the eye is subject to, and acting as the cause of blindness in 9 per cent of all cases, its seriousness in this age, demanding good vision, cannot be overlooked. It is unfortunate that a condition known since the era of Hippocrates should today be so prevalent, so insidiously sinister in producing blindness, and also so resistant to the investigation of its etiology, pathogenesis and hence accurate treatment.

The term glaucoma to the ophthalmologist does not indicate a disease entity, but rather a group of pathological processes, the clinical manifestations of which are dependent upon, and dominated by, an elevation of the intra-ocular pressure and the clinicopathological sequelae of this event. It has been generally regarded that the intra-ocular hypertension is the disease itself. However, instead of this, it would be better to consider the increased tension more as a symptom or sign of a complex pathological change involving not only the eye, but also the entire systemic physiology. In this new light, the elevated pressure could well be compared to the symptom of jaundice which has an extremely varied etiology and pathology as we well know.

Because of the relative scientific ignorance pertaining to glaucoma, it has been neces-sary to divide the etiology of this disease into two major portions designed arbitrarily as primary and secondary. In the former, no discoverable cause for the elevated tension can be found clinically. In reality however, the hypertension is secondary to various physiological disturbances which are at present unknown. In the secondary type a disturbance of intra-ocular circulation, to which is added an obstruction to the drainage of the intra-ocular fluids, is caused by an obvious pre-existing lesion. Unfortunately, the variability of this lesion is manifold in type and character. Among such conditions may be included acute or chronic intra-ocular inflammations, trauma, intra-ocular tumors, congenital anomalies, changes in the crystalline lens, obstruction of the central retinal vein, etc. As will be noted, these lesions either reduce the volume of the globe, disturb the intra-ocular circulation, or interfere mechanically or osmotically with the drainage of the intra-ocular humors. The treatment of the secondary type of glaucoma is directed at the pre-existing lesion or condition and surgical intervention is considered as a secondary factor in the usual case. One of the most commonly used procedures is a paracentesis to temporarily relieve the increased tension and this may be repeated at indicated intervals or the wound may be kept open. Except for the glaucoma secondary to congenital anomalies, the usual surgical measures are not followed by successful end results.

It is the so-called glaucoma in which we are especially interested for the purpose of our present discussion. Primary glaucoma

[*]Read before the Annual Meeting held in Oklahoma City, May 11-12, 1943.

can be arbitrarily divided into two major clinical groups; non-congestive, perhaps better known as chronic simple glaucoma, and congestive glaucoma. The latter type has an acute and chronic phase and when seen in the acute form often presents the picture of one of the calamities seen in medicine. In the final stages of disease, the terms of absolute glaucoma and degenerative glaucoma graphically describe the condition of the eye.

To discuss the treatment of primary glaucoma is difficult because of the limitation of our knowledge of the etiology of this disease. Since the rationale of successful treatment is directed primarily against the cause of a disease, and secondarily against the manifestations of its symptoms, we are at present confined to a very limited scope from a therapeutic point of view. Etiologically we know that this disease is the result of factors causing disturbances in the venous-capillary circulation, in capillary permeability, in the central mechanism regulating the physiological tonus of the eye and finally in the drainage of the intra-ocular fluids. In most instances the impairment of drainage is only a contributory or precipitating factor. However, surgical treatment has been confined to its correction alone, because of its relative ease of study and because of the extreme complexity of the other etiological factors. The various surgical approaches therefore, attempt to increase the amount of drainage of fluids from the eye and thereby reduce the hypertension. Procedures have been designed to accomplish this by either re-opening normal pathways of drainage, by establishing additional intra-ocular pathways or by the development of extra-ocular drainage.

Before continuing in more detail with the surgical approaches to this problem, it would be well to mention the other therapeutic measures used in the treatment of primary glaucoma. These include; medical methods to reduce the elevated tension i.e. miotics; physical procedures i.e. massage, osmotic drugs, etc.; and finally systemic measures designed to improve the general health and hygiene of the patient. In glaucoma these therapeutic adjuncts are analogous to the use of dietary regulation in the control of a well established case of diabetes mellitus. They act as measures to ameliorate the disease processes. In this analogy, the use of surgical measures added to the above adjuncts resembles the addition of insulin therapy in the severe diabetic. Just as the severe diabetic will not do well without insulin neither will the established primary glaucoma patient do as well without surgery as with it. The role of operative intervention is thus easily realized.

With regard to the various technical procedures in common use today each has a fairly definite indication, depending upon the various stages in which the disease is encountered. There is no argument but that the acute congestive attacks which fails to respond to thorough medical measures in 24 hours, should be treated by the classical Graefe basal iridectomy. If the attack has been successfully controlled by medical treatment, the indications for surgery are still imperative, and the most widely accepted procedure is to establish extra-ocular drainage by the use of a corneo-scleral trephining operation. If the problem at hand is an instance of the chronic congestive phase, extra-ocular drainage can be obtained by the use of the corneo-scleral trephine, the La Grange irido-scerectomy, or one of the various iris-inclusion operations such as iridencleisis or irido-tasis. In my personal use the procedures are listed according to preference with the Elliot corneo-scleral trephine the method of choice.

The question of chronic simple (non-congestive) glaucoma is one of great interest, and of course the problem of early diagnosis is all important. For those patients seen in the early stages, carefully controlled medical treatment alone is sufficient, providing the tension is within the limits of a high normal and only slight evidences of impaired function exist. However, at the very earliest indication of any deterioration in the central visual fields examined with the 1-2000 isopter or in the stability or level of the tension, surgical interference should be contemplated immediately. The procrastination of operating in these cases has been responsible for more failures in end results than any other factor. The choice of procedure is determined by the clinical evidence at hand. If the tension is relatively low and visual field studies reveal that slow deterioration is occurring in the face of adequate medical care, a cyclediałysis has the definite advantages of few complications, not disturbing the integrity of the globe, and ease of repetition and performance. A geniotomy may also be considered. If the disease were of a more serious nature or if these procedures were not successful, a filtering operation should be done. A corneo-scleral trephine, La Grange irido-sclerectomy, or iridencleisis in the order named would then be the procedures of choice. Aside from the occurrence of late infection through the bleb, the trephine operation has been found to be the most advantageous with regards to results.

To mention absolute glaucoma and degenerative glaucoma, it has been found that constructive surgical methods are usually of no avail in the treatment of these conditions. As soon as the associated pain becomes of

sufficient intensity to be intolerable, enucleation should be done if possible. The various
procedures to abolish pain alone are not
without criticism because of the presence of
neoplasms within the globes of about 10 per
cent of the eyes diagnosed as absolute glaucoma.

In conclusion, therefore, we may consider
the present day treatment of primary glaucoma to be resolved into an attempt to correct the more fundamental etiological factors, insofar as they can be determined, by
regulating the patients hygiene, counteract-
ing any constitutional diathesis, and by using
medicinal methods to try to maintain the
tension of the eye within normal limits. If
these are not successful and the tension remains elevated or fluctuates undesirably, or
if a deterioration of function continues, operative measures as outlined above must
be undertaken. With no treatment of any
kind the disease will progress to complete
bilateral blindness. With adequate treatment the majority of patients retain useful
vision until death. The two essential features
in obtaining successful results are early diagnosis and continuous adequate treatment.
When we consider that glaucoma causes 27
per cent of all blindness before 45 years of
age, and that it is the ranking cause of blindness after this age has been reached and that
it causes 60 per cent of all blindness present
in individuals over 60 years of age, its importance becomes vivid to us and should
stimulate each one of us to be on the look-
out for its occurrence so that early diagnosis
and the proper treatment may be instituted.

DISCUSSION

C. GALLAHER, M. D.
SHAWNEE, OKLAHOMA

I do not deserve the privilege of being
asked to open the discussion of Dr. Crane's
paper on the subject "Surgical Indications
in Glaucoma." But I do appreciate the opportunity of a review and I hope that each
of you will find enough time to read and consider it carefully when it is made available
in the Journal of the Oklahoma State Medical Association. Dr. Crane is not only well
informed on the subject of which he has

written, but the material which he presents
is well organized and accurate.

It is particularly satisfactory to note Dr.
Crane's careful attention to the definition of
glaucoma, to see that he is sharply aware of
the fact that this is a group of pathological
processes, that it embraces a composite of
pathological conditions which have the common feature that their clinical manifestations are to a greater or lesser extent dominated by an increase in the
intra-ocular pressure and its consequences.
Glaucoma is as definitely a symptom complex as asthma and a failure to bear in
mind this basic concept would be incompatible with intelligent discussion of the subject.

It does not appear that I have anything
to add to the technical considerations which
he has so ably discussed. I should like however to ask you to consider for a few moments, the patient's view-point of this matter, as I believe it should be interpreted to
him by his physician. The patient who is
in need of surgical treatment for glaucoma,
may often have difficulty in realizing the
degree of necessity. And unless he can become sincerely convinced that this is the
best possible course, he may resist or refuse
until it is impossible to give any where near
as good results as might earlier have been
expected. In our attempts therefore to preserve vision, to prevent loss of vision, and
in some cases to improve vision it is important that we be able to explain the situation clearly to our patients. Few can fail
to make correct decisions when they truly
appreciate the nature of the problem, the
consequences of neglect or improper treatment and the hope which is justified with
adequate management. When the physician
in charge has determined that a surgical procedure must be included in the treatment
of choice in a given case and has made up
his own mind what shall be done, he should
adapt his language to the patients limits
of understanding of technical terms and proceed to explain.

The prime objective is to secure a lowered
tension, with minimal danger of hemorrhage
or infection, either immediate or late, and
thus preserve both the central vision and the
field of vision for the patient. It is true
that when the process has advanced to a

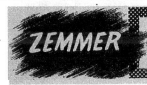

stage where the central vision is greatly re-
.duced, and the field of vision diminished to
20 degrees or less, the progressive optic atrophy may continue. It is entirely reasonable
however to assume that the relief of the etiological factor may arrest or at least decrease the rate of opic nerve atrophy. It
is more reasonable to assume that when the
intra-ocular pressure is reduced, thus
releasing the pressure on the blood vessels
which supply the retina, there should be
more of a tendency to improve this vision
than otherwise.

The objection is frequently raised that
surgical treatment in glaucoma has a tendency to produce cataract formation, or to increase the opacity of an already cloudy lens.
Although this is true in a limited number of
cases, it is equally true that much greater
danger to vision is sustained by permitting
the pressure to continue, and a cataract, if
it should develop, can be dealt with at a later
date. Moreover, the glaucoma per se has a
tendency to produce cataract formation
whether the patient has surgical treatment
or not.

A patient should usually be informed that
however effective the medical management
is at a given date, it is only a matter of time
when all non-surgical treatment is apt to become of little or no avail. Many patients
too, will develop a sensitiveness to pilocar-
pine or eserine and become unable to continue the use of either.

Even though an operation may not improve vision it will usually preserve such
vision as the patient has, or at least afford
him the best possible chances for preserving
it.

Patients should be informed that the operation is not without danger, that the eye
could be lost by the accidents of hemorrhage,
acute infection, or the development and cin-
tinuation of a chronic ureitis.

The Clinical Importance of Refractive Errors[*]

A. C. McFARLING, M.D.

SHAWNEE, OKLAHOMA

In view of the intensely interesting neurologic aspect of this case, I herewith outline
very briefly the clinical history as follows:

T. M., a white child, 10 years of age, was
presented for the examination of his eyes
which were entirely normal as to appearance
of external tissues.

During a retinoscopic examination which
lasted no more than two or three minutes,
the patient became greatly agitated, was exceedingly pale, and twitching of the facial
muscles was observed. Also there was inco-
ordinated movements of the lower limbs and
arms which were spasmodic in character and
of sufficient severity to interfere with loco-
motion though the patient walked with some
difficutly when supported by an attendant.
He was moaning, not so much as if in pain,
but the character of moaning that one might
hear in a convulsive seizure. There was no
frothing at the mouth and no change in the
size or shape of the pupils.

*Read before the Annual Meeting held in Oklahoma City,
May 11-12, 1943.

The examination was interrupted at this
point—the patient vomited two or three
minutes later and the symptoms disappeared after a short lapse of time. A cyclo-
plegic was found and the patient was told
to return in 72 hours, which he did, at which
time the examination was completed without
further difficulty.

The refractive error found was as follows:

Right Eye: Plus 7.75, plus 2.00, Axis
90, Vision equals 20/40;

Left Eye; Plus 7.75, plus 1.00, Axis
90, Vision equals 20/40.

Thus it will be seen that the total hyperopia existing for each eye was almost 10 di-
optres which is approximately the total refractive power of the normal crystalline lens.
This patient, in order to see his way, was
obliged to drive the accomodative mechanism
of his eyes to its maximum effort during all
his waking hours.

In discussing the important role of eye
strain in the causation of a symptom com-

plex such as that so briefly outlined in the foregoing case history, I shall consider the diagnostic methods employed and the corrective measure advised as routine and, therefore, unimportant, but shall attempt to discover the manner in which eye strain may operate through the medium of the brain to bring about such a state of incoordination of the physiological functions of the body as that described in the foregoing history.

Since the brain, the great central station of the nervous system whose complex function serves not only to generate and control the working forces of the body but spans the chasm would otherwise separate the spiritual from the physical aspect of the mind, is the clearing house through which every organ of the body must receive its impulses, I shall, therefore, review briefly the anatomical and physiological characteristics of the nervous and mental processes by which we perceive those of the forces and the forms of energy in the world with which we are cognizant, to-wit: Sensation, perception, association, concentration and inhibition.

The fundamental element or unit of the nervous tissue is the neuron—a cell with many processes projecting from it—some short and branching; one or sometimes two of which often extend a long way and usually become the axon of a medullated nerve fiber and in some cases gives off a few collateral branches. Both axons and dendrons are composed of delicate fibrillae which pass directly without interruption through the cell body. Of these neurons varying in form and size and supported by the delicate framework of the neuroglia, the entire nervous system is composed.

The fundamental physiological characteristics of the nervous tissues are excitabilty and transmission—the power of receiving an excitation and not only transmitting it from one end of the neuron to the other but also of transmitting it to other neurons with which the first is in anatomical and physiological relationship. By its dendrons the nerve cell receives nervous impulses and by its axons sends out its own impulses. There is experimental evidence which tends to prove the activity of a nerve cell is the result of chemical reactions while the conduction along nerve fibers is mainly a physiological process. The transmission of energy from one neuron to another in contrast with it seems to depend upon differences in the tension of this energy in the two neurons. The cellular activity is, therefore, easily exhausted while the activity of the nerve fiber is not easily exhausted. Thus it will be seen that a nerve fiber may continue to transmit impulses received from other cells long after its own cellular exhaustion would have precluded the possibility of modification of such impulses by inhibition or promotion.

When the various impulses have passed along the various tracts and have traversed and been interrupted by several masses of gray matter, they reach the sensory area of the cerebral cortex and there give rise to a new form of energy called sensation, that is, to say, a physical force is converted in a terminal organ into nervous energy and as such, having traversed the sensory tracts, reaches the cerebral cortex. It is there transmitted into a new form of energy as, for instance, the sensation of light which takes place in the brain—not the eye—and has no similarity to the undulations of either from which it orginates and it may be caused not only by this but also may originate in perfect darkness from mechanical irritation of the eye or from the optic nerve. The same is true of other nerves, thus; if we mechanically irritate the auditory nerve, the impulse will be interpreted in the brain as sound or if the impulse be given to a motor nerve, we may likewise expect a muscular contraction.

Sensation is the simplest manifestation of consciousness or cognition and like electricity requires for its production a certain degree of intensity of the nervous impulses. Below this point of intensity the cortex may be in activity but sensation will not result, the activity will be sub-conscious. A series of these slight impulses may by summation cause sensation. There is, therefore, a minimum of intensity necessary for sensation just as electricity passing through a wire must have a certain intensity before the wire glows and light is produced. There is also a maximum beyond which, no matter how great the irritation, there is no increase in sensation but rather a diminution from exhaustion of the nerve cells. Between this minimum and maximum point, sensibility increases or diminishes by little steps in definite ratio to the stimulus.

Sensation is thus a special individual force produced in the cerebral cortex and has its special individual characteristics. A complex manifestation of this force constitutes consciousness and personality. Sensation and all other forms of mental activity are absolutely dependent upon a fairly healthy cerebral cortex and a fairly abundant blood supply. If the cortex be destroyed in large part or the blood supply be cut off, then sensation, preception, memory,thought, ethics, association of ideas, etc., are all partially or entirely suspended until such time as the normal blood supply be re-established.

This brings us to the consideration of perceptions and concepts which for the purpose of this paper it will suffice to say that a perception consists of a combination of sensations which are received from various sensory nerves and organs but all of which proceed, usually simultaneously, from the same external object.

Passing to a study of association we recall the essential physiological characteristics of nervous tissue which are:

1. Its excitability, its reaction to stimulation by the discharge of nervous energy stored within it.

2. Its transmissibility.

This energy when produced does not long remain localized but tends to pass along nerve fibers throughout its own neuron and to other neurons. The channels along which it will pass depend upon the anatomical arrangement of the fibers. In consequence of heredity and evolution, certain channels are easier for the passing of this nervous impulse than others. This is especially true of certain reflexes which are present at birth such as breathing, etc.

When a perception occurs, impulses radiate out along the association fibers from which it is produced. If at the same time another perception takes place in another portion of the cortex, the association fibers connecting these two portions of the cortex, being acted upon at the same time, will convey impulses more readily than the other association fibers. The longer and more frequently the association fibers are traversed by these impulses, the better conductors they become and these two perceptions become more and more excited, the one by the other. The activity in the cortex does not long persist and when the associated idea is in consciousness, the orginal perception which awoke it is already, or soon will be, subconscious yet they are so firmly associated that in the future when one enters into activity it may excite the other.

At this juncture, let us review the more salient features of the process known as concentration. It seems to be a general law in the physiology of the nervous system that when there is a strong activity in one part, the activity of the rest of the nervous system is inhibited, thus reflex activity can be inhibited by strong pain and the reflex activity of the spinal cord is more or less inhibited when the brain is in activity. In the brain itself, when a portion of the cortex or a group of nerve cells is in activity, the activity of the other cortical areas as well as that of the lower centers is inhibited. The stronger the local activity, the greater and more this active portion will have a free and uninterrupted field. Naturally, consciousness remains limited to this strong activity for a long time. When an unusual or very vivid perception is in consciousness it occupies the center of the stage. Consciousness is limited to this one vivid perception or idea and its associations so that milder activities occurring in the cortex at the time which should ordinarily produce perceptions and associations, remain sub-conscious. This phenomenon is called concentration and is a very important function in nervous physiology since the laws governing the same are applicable not only consciousness but to the sub-conscious process as well, many of which have to do with the regulation of those important physiological processes and functions whose sum total constitute the physical aspect of the phenomenon we call life.

Before pursuing further, and in connection with our study of inhibition, it will be remembered that our study of sensation discloses the fact that when a perception or sensation at a given point in the cortex, the energy or impulse does not long remain localized but travels along the fibers of its own neuron and by the association fibers to other neurons. It will be seen that when a nerve cell, or cell unit, in sending out impulses to an organ of the body, a muscle, or group of muscles over whose function it is its duty to preside, does not possess the ability to limit such impulse to that particular muscle or organ for which it was normally intended but, on the other hand, unavoidably transmits a portion of such impulse to those nerve cells or cell units which are in anatomical and physiological relationship with it. This law of the transmission of impulses is an invariable one which fact does not preclude the possibility of an impulse radiation from a given point in the cerebral cortex to a contiguous cell or cell unit. This impulse, if elaborated and promoted by the synergic action of the contiguous cell, would be antagonistic or detrimental or the normal function of that muscle or organ over which such contiguous cell unit presides. It does not necessarily follow, however, that such association impulse would be promoted by the contiguous cell but instead would in the normal physiological course of events be neutralized according to this same law of the transmission of impulses by other impulses generated and sent out by the contiguous cell in the regular performance of its duty. This constitutes what we call inhibition and may in some degree be likened unto the rights of citizenship under the laws of a democracy whose constitution accords to every citizen the right to follow the bend of his own mind in the pursuit of happiness and the acquisition of wealth, so long as such pursuits do not interfere with the rights of others. Thus it may be seen that if two cell units in the cortex in anatomical relationship with each other be in simultaneous activity, their respective association impulses will, if they be of the same degree of intensity, exactly neutralize each other but, if the impulse originating in one cell unit be abnormally strong, then that portion of energy which travels by the association fibers will be proportionately stronger and will override the weaker associational impulse which it may meet and will, therefore, succeed in reaching the other cell unit and there register itself as a distinct impulse.

Now let us assume that the cell unit from which this stronger impulse originates is the organization of cells which control the physiological functions of the eyes. Let us assume further the existence of a muscular inbalance or a refractive error, or both, in a degree approaching the maximum amount which can be corrected by the ocular muscles. It is well known that the brain will not tolerate anything in such a case except perfect, single, binocular vision. It is self-evident that the exaggerated muscular contractions necessary to correct this visual defect must necessarily be actuated and maintained by corresponding exaggerated impulses from the brain centers which control the musculature of the eyes.

It is also evident that by reason of this greater activity more blood will be attracted to these occulomotor centers than would be demanded for normal work. In consequence there will be a diminution of the normal blood supply of the adjacent tissues and a proportionate reduction in the inhibitive influence which these adjacent centers would normally exercise toward the excited oculomotor centers. It is equally obvious that these exaggerated motor impulses radiating in rapid succession from the oculo-motor centers will, by association, reach and register themselves upon all the adjacent cells with which they are in anatomical and physiological relationship.

Since the gray matter possesses the inherent faculty of summation it necessarily follows that when these impulses have been repeated a sufficient number of times sensation will result—the nature of which will be determined in each instance by the normal function of the cell so affected. In case a motor nerve cell were so influenced the result would be an involuntary contraction of the muscle which it supplies; if a sensory cell, pain may be excited; if a cell unit controlling a gland or organ, we may expect some alteration in the nature or amount of the secretion of the gland or a perversion of the function of the organ so supplied.

In view of the fact that the intensity of a sensation occurring at a given point is in a direct ratio to the stimulus, we may safely assume the existence of a ratio between the intensity of the sensation and the impulses which may go out from the central cell receiving the sensation.

If the exaggerated impulses radiating from the oculo-motor centers in their exaggerated effort at correcting the visual defects assumed in our hypothetical case, be capable of transmission by association to all the adjacent cells with which they are in relationship thus confusing and causing them to send out impulses at variance with their normal functions, we may likewise expect their confusion and excitement to spread to still other cells.

Since the incentive to perfect vision is absolutely constant in the brain and since this state of confusion and excitement does not depend upon the intensity of one impulse or sensation but rather upon their frequent repetition over a long period of time, we may safely assume the possibility and probability of this excitement spreading from cell to cell until the entire working forces of the brain would be thrown into a functional discord. In consequence of the incoordination of the working forces of the brain which control and regulate the vital functions incident to life, will necessarily follow the incoordination of the functions themselves.

By way of condensing and summing up the foregoing arguments, we may conclude: (a) the nerve centers which control the normal functions of the body exercise a normal inhibitive influence toward each other which eventuates in the proper coordination of these functions and (b) any form of irritation, either central or peripheral in orgin, whose intensity is of a degree above the minimum required for sensation in the particular cell involved, if sufficiently prolonged will derange the normal inhibition of the cells as a result of which the impulses radiating from a cell subjected to such irritation, being of a much higher degree of intensity than normally required, will be super-imposed upon all the cells with which that cell is in anatomical and physiological relationship.

If at this point we recall the fact that the ocular muscles derive their nerve supply from the third, fourth, and sixth cranial nerves while the stomach, for example, is supplied by the pneumogastric nerve, all of which have their origin from nuclei situated beneath the aquaduct of sylvius in the floor of the fourth ventricle ,we may, in the light of the foregoing deductions reasonably conclude that in this manner eye strain, when present, may be instrumental in producing not only the gastric symptoms noted in the foregoing case history but in like manner spread the existing stimulus by association to other parts of the brain until the resultant nervous incoordination may reach the proportions of a conclusive crisis.

DISCUSSION

F. MAXEY COOPER, M.D.

OKLAHOMA CITY, OKLAHOMA

Dr. McFarling is to be complimented on his paper. I was struck by the unusual clarty and scholarly choice of English and composition, the talent for which is rare in physicians.

This paper effectually reminds us that eye strain does not manifest itself in local eye symptoms alone but frequently causes disturbances of more distant functions, and logically explains the mechanism by which such disturbances are caused.

To emphasize his point a case history is given in which a child was so upset by a very high hyperpia with astigmatism that he was thrown into convulsions of the clonic type by a short retinoscopic examination. Perhaps in this case that is true. On the other hand it is hard to say that epilepsy of the sub-clinical type could have been present.

To give a really good discussion of this paper, one should be a neurologist or psychiatrist. I am neither, so my observations must be drawn from what experience I have had in dealing with patients. It has seemed to me that patients with errors of refraction —both of hyperopia and astigmatism, complain less of all symptoms than those with moderate errors. Usually the child with high hyperopia comes in saying his only trouble is that he can't see well and his teacher suggested he have his eyes examined. When this patient tells you that he does not see well it means that he has given up the struggle to maintain enough accommodation to obtain acute vision. He has surrendered to a superior foe and his nervous system has given up the battle. With more moderate errors he can maintain the acute vision he has, an instinctive desire for and throughout his waking hours expends much nervous energy. If this is too great a drain he is warned by the various signs that he is straining.

In my opinion the symptoms of eyestrain are usually moderate. Headaches which cannot be relieved by aspirin or a good nights sleep are probably not due to strain. Acute abdominal pain cannot be blamed on the eyes, but spastic, colitis, chronic indigestion, or gastric ulcer may be due to eyestrain.

On the other hand we should not forget that this experience may be reversed. All of the symptoms of eyestrain may be experienced by normal eyes. If a person is under par due to systemic disease so that he lacks the normal nervous energy to run his pair of eyes, that lack of energy produces the same headache, burning, and watering. Normal eyes show typical signs of strain in gastrointestinal troubles. From the patients history it is impossible to tell which comes first, the eyestrain or the stomach trouble, until a refraction is done. Either one may affect the other. One of our best gastro-interologists is very insistent that his patients wear constantly small astigmatism corrections where they are present and has found its effective over a long period of practice. It is the strain that is tolerable that we carry for long periods. If it is too great our protective mechanism forces us to give up the struggle by submitting to lowered visual acuity.

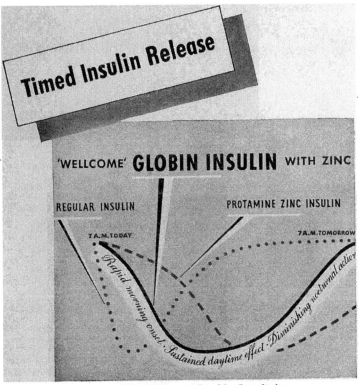

Timed Insulin Release

'WELLCOME' GLOBIN INSULIN WITH ZINC

REGULAR INSULIN   PROTAMINE ZINC INSULIN

7 A.M. TODAY   7 A.M. TOMORROW

Rapid morning onset · *Sustained daytime effect* · *Diminishing nocturnal action*

A schematic representation of the effects of various
insulins on the blood sugar of a fasting diabetic.

● 'Wellcome' Globin Insulin with Zinc, a new type of insulin, provides more efficient timing of action. Its rate of insulin release is such that its prompt effect meets the morning requirements; strong prolonged daytime action coincides with the period of peak need; and diminishing action during the night minimizes the possibility of nocturnal insulin reactions.

'Wellcome' Globin Insulin with Zinc conforms to the needs of the patient. *A single injection* daily has been found to control satisfactorily many moderately severe and severe cases of diabetes. 'Wellcome' Globin Insulin with Zinc, a clear solution, is comparable to regular insulin in its freedom from allergenic skin reactions.

'Wellcome' Globin Insulin with Zinc was developed in the Wellcome Research Laboratories, Tuckahoe, New York. Registered U. S. Patent Office, 2,161,198. Available in vials of 10 cc., 80 units in 1 cc.   'Wellcome' Trademark Registered

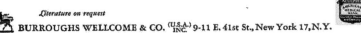

Literature on request

BURROUGHS WELLCOME & CO. (U.S.A. INC.) 9-11 E. 41st St., New York 17, N.Y.

· THE PRESIDENT'S PAGE ·

Like most physicians, I feel tired, overworked and generally abused. I went to Shawnee recently to a very fine, well attended District Councilor meeting. Councilor Clinton Gallaher had worked very hard to have an attractive meeting and deserves much praise. I phoned an old friend of mine—Dr. "Johnny" Walker, who for many years was Councilor from the Seventh District. Doctor Walker is over eighty years of age. He was "out" making calls, and would not be back in his office until 6:30 P.M. Later, I saw this grand old man—he admitted that he, too, got tired at times—but that he was taking things easy, rarely getting up in the morning before 7:00 A.M.

At the recent National Conference on Medical Service (Chicago, February 13, 1944) much of the confusion of thought in medical circles was exposed. No fewer than five proposals of programs sponsored by local or regional areas that had ambitions to perform public relations for American Medicine, were advanced:

1. The Lake County, Indiana, Plan, which has recently been sent in the form of an eight-page newspaper to all of us.

2. Proposals of the six New England Medical Societies offering alternatives to the Wagner-Murray-Dingell Bill.

3. The Western Health League of six far western states, which is establishing a public relations representative in Washington.

4. The National Physicians Committee for the Extension of Medical Service. This organization has furnished each of us with an analytical pamphlet, taking the Wagner Bill apart. More recently they have conducted two polls, in the nature of "gallop" polls, to determine the public's attitude toward medicine and medical economics. Results of these polls are now beginning to appear in the Journal of the American Medical Association.

5. The newly created Council on Medical Care and Public Relations of the American Medical Association. The most recent activity of this Council is set forth on Page 714, Journal of the American Medical Association, March 11, 1944.

Out of this apparent overlapping effort, good will come, and eventually the common goal of all will be realized and one organization will survive which we can all support. It is heartening that so many physicians now realize that we must come out of our shell and tell our story to the people. Six years ago we engaged Dick Graham, and he helped immensely as a liason officer between the lay public and the profession in this State. The same thing can be done on the national level.

A member of the Council on Medical Care and Public Relations, Dr. Alfred W. Adson, Rochester, Minnesota, will discuss this problem of public relations at our State Meeting—do not miss hearing him!

James Stevenson

President.

The JOURNAL Of The
OKLAHOMA STATE MEDICAL ASSOCIATION

EDITORIAL BOARD
L. J. MOORMAN, Oklahoma City, Editor-in-Chief

E. EUGENE RICE, Shawnee

NED R. SMITH, Tulsa

MR. PAUL H. FESLER, Oklahoma City, Acting Business Manager

EDITORIALS

THE ANNUAL MEETING

It is gratifying to know that the plans for the State Meeting are well under way. The Program, already well filled, promises much for the busy doctor. Overworked doctors are entitled to a few days in a different environment with opportunities for relaxation and the acquisition of new knowledge. The doctors on the home front must remember that the men in the military service are constantly on their toes because of the stimulating environment, the anticipated responsibility and the element of emergency. Although the doctor in civilian practice may find little time for study, this handicap can be overcome in part by attending the Annual Meeting.

Date yourself for a good time including social, intellectual, gastronomic and professional opportunities. If you miss your State Meeting, you are slipping.

THE DESIRABILITY OF A STATE BOARD OF HEALTH

In Oklahoma, the State Commissioner of Health cannot properly coordinate all Public Health Agencies, State Hospitals and Sanatoria because of divided authority. A nonpartisan State Board of Health appointed by the Governor with authority over all agencies and institutions concerned with the health of our citizenry, would relieve the Governor of a heavy responsibility; serve as a guide to and check upon the State Health Commissioner; forward the interests of public health and prove a great savings to taxpayers. This method of Public Health Administration is now employed in at least 21 states.

The State Board of Health should consist of 5 or 7 members with two or three representatives from the medical profession, one or two from the dental profession and the other representatives should be chosen because of special interests or qualifications from other professions or from the business world. The original appointment should be made in such a way that the retirement of individual members will be staggered. All subsequent appointments or reappointments should be for a period of 5 or 7 years. In this way the Board will always have the services of seasoned members familiar with the established policies and practices, and thus escape the dangers of sudden changes consequent upon shifting politics and executive policies.

Under this plan, the State Health Commissioner should be chosen by the Board and should be responsible to the same for the judicious and efficient performance of the functions of his office.

The medical profession of Oklahoma should give serious consideration to this long neglected question. Giving advice, helping determine policies and devising ways and means are among the obligations the doctor owes the people of his community and the state. The approaching meeting of the State Medical Association offers an opportunity for collective consideration and discussion of this important subject.

WHAT'S THE MATTER WITH SOCIALIZED MEDICINE

According to a recent broadcast, the only picture of Hitler appearing in recent German newspapers represent "Der Fuerer" presenting a medal to his personal physician. According to our estimate of this mass murderer, any doctor from Bismark's gang would be good enough for him. But apparently the diabolical beast who delights in the wholesale destruction of other people's lives is not willing to entrust his own to the mill run from the government controlled medical service, which long ago was set up as a political sop for his unhappy subjects.

Fortunately, the law of compensation, good or bad, outstrips the doctors skill. Even though Hitler's personal physician may be a good psychiatrist, he cannot ward off a just retribution.

DRAFTING YOUR WASTEBASKET

The War Production Board has sent an appeal to medical journals under the following caption; "Hospital Waste Paper Container Re-Use Program." The worthy appeal is 7 pages long and every paragraph contains vital facts. We are not printing this in full for two reasons: First, because the State Medical Journal has been on a paper saving schedule since War was declared; second, because Oklahoma Hospital authorities need only to be apprised of a war need to bestir themselves toward its execution.

Without delay, hospital management in Oklahoma will go from basement to garrett and clean out all available paper, cardboard containers, etc. Day by day the waste paper will be accumulated for war rather than stuffed in the fire. Read the following from the War Production Board's appeal and do your duty now.

"From the day a soldier goes to war, he is dependent on paper. From his draft card to his honorable discharge, his records are kept on it.

"His records are packed in it; his cartridges are wrapped in it; his shoes are lined with it; his letters are written on it.

"His barracks are built with paper wallboard, paper roofing, paper insulation.

"He shoots at paper targets, eats from paper plates, drinks from paper cups.

"His battles are planned, his orders are issued, on paper.

"Literally, he lives, trains, travels and fights, with paper, his indispensable ally.

"And, of course, his 'honorable discharge' will be handed to him on a piece of paper—after a beaten Axis has signed the peace terms . . . on paper!"

Every member of the State Medical Association who holds an appointment on a hospital staff should clip this editorial and hand it to the superintendent of the hospital with an urgent request that all paper products be saved and turned over to the proper authorities.

THE DECLINE IN AIR-BORNE DISEASES

Dwight O'Hara in his recently published book "Air-Borne Infections," points out the fact that for several decades we have experienced a gradual decline in air-borne infections. Chief among the diseases transmitted through the air are tuberculosis, pneumonia, measles, scarlet fever and whooping cough.

There is no definite way to determine all the factors responsible for this decline or to accurately figure the relative importance of the known factors. Certainly the educational program carried on by the National Tuberculosis Association and other public health agencies over a period of 40 years has had its influence. In addition to the common methods of prevention these agencies have taught the people the importance of adequate nutrition, sleep, fresh air and above all, the danger of fatigue.

The apparent increase in resistance to air-borne infections is not as spontaneous as it seems. True, it is in part due to better living and greater prosperity but in turn, better living and, to some extent, greater prosperity is due to the program initiated by the National Tuberculosis Association and persistently pursued over a period of 40 years.

In the case of pneumonia and certain of the streptococcus infections, we must consider the influence of anti-pneumococcus serum and the sulfonamides. These therapeutic agents have cut short the period of morbidity, thus reducing the duration of contact, and no doubt their bacteriostatic and bacteriscidal effects have materially lessened the danger of contact.

It is remarkable that in the mobilization of the largest Army in the history of our country we have escaped serious epidemics of respiratory infections.

TIME AND TROUBLE
TAKE THEIR TOLL

The speed of the sand in the hourglass of life is always accelerated by troubles. Statistical studies show that in New York City there were 6,000 more deaths among elderly people in 1943 than in 1942. This increase is apparently due to the influence of strain and stress upon the degenerative diseases with the War as the chief contributing factor. Th· latter observation seems justifiable, since the increased mortality is out of all proportion to that reported in other groups.

In these columns, the growing need of a revival in the art of medicine has received repeated notice. The above figures should have careful consideration by every doctor, because they reveal an important trend which must be met by a calm, logical, hopeful approach to the mounting problems of life. While the young are holding the battle front on the firing line, those of us who have silently slipped into the realm of the degenerative diseases, should muster all possible poise in order to prolong our hold upon life and our efficiency on the home front. We owe this to those who follow on. The example of deliberate action with studied expedition and undaunted courage, will not only help defer the evil day for the doctor, but it will help keep his patients on the beam. Amiel says, "To know how to grow old is the master-work of wisdom, and one of the most difficult chapters in the great art of living." There is every reason why the doctor should know how to grow old and excel in the great art of living, thus exerting a chastening and stablizing influence upon those with whom he comes in contact. Growing old need not discourage us as wisdom and art travel with age, and according to Cicero, an honored old age has great authority. Even though we may be acquiring the Shakespearean characteristics of age, "a moist eye, a dry hand, a yellow check, a white beard, a decreasing leg," we must keep a clear head, conserve every unit of energy and work with a will for the duration, whether of life, or the War.

Many a good doctor has earned a long rest on the Riviera di Ponente, below the Maritime Alps, but remains in the harness at home in order that his young colleagues may go to the Mediterranean, and to other parts of the world to fight it out with the enemies of our way of life. For such there must be a celestial coast with palms and pomegranates and the fragrance of hyacinths.

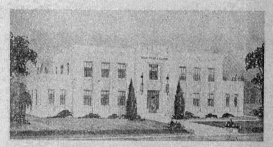

VON WEDEL CLINIC

PLASTIC and GENERAL SURGERY
Dr. Curt von Wedel

TRAUMATIC and INDUSTRIAL
SURGERY
Dr. Clarence A. Gallagher

INTERNAL MEDICINE and DIAGNOSIS
Dr. Harry A. Daniels

Special attention to cardiac and gastro
intestinal diseases

Complete laboratory and X-ray facilities.
Electrocardiograph.

610 Northwest Ninth Street
Opposite St. Anthony's Hospital
Oklahoma City

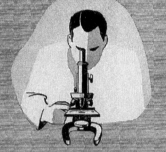
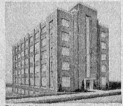

ASSOCIATION ACTIVITIES

POSTGRADUATE STUDY IN SURGICAL DIAGNOSIS

The new course in Surgical Diagnosis, by Dr. A. G. Fletcher of Philadelphia, opened in Northeastern Oklahoma the week of February 14. The enrollments at the time of the opening in the teaching centers were as follows:

Miami	21
Vinita	10
Bartlesville	21
Claremore	7
Pryor	8

Dr. Fletcher has made elaborate plans for bringing a practical course to general practitioners of the state, supplementing his didactic lectures with models, demonstrations, lantern slides and movies, both silent and talking.

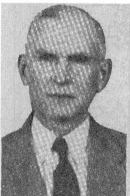

This course will recess during the week of the Oklahoma State Medical Meeting which will be held at the Mayo Hotel in Tulsa, April 24, 25, 26. Dr. Fletcher will attend the State Meeting and many physicians and County Medical Society Officers will be able to meet him on the 16th floor at the Postgraduate Booth. Mrs. Orene Ramsey, from the Postgraduate office, will be at the booth to answer all inquiries as to dates and points of information regarding this course.

The Experimental Method

The experimental method, then, cannot give new and fruitful ideas to men who have none; it can serve only to guide the ideas of men who have them, to direct their ideas and to develop them so as to get the best possible results. The idea is a seed; the method is the earth furnishing the conditions in which it may develop, flourish and give the best of fruit according to its nature. But as only what has been sown in the ground will ever grow in it, so nothing will be developed by the experimental method except the ideas submitted to it. The method itself gives birth to nothing. Certain philosophers have made the mistake of according too much power to method along these lines.—Experimental Medicine. Claude Bernard. Page 34. The MacMillan Company. 1927.

TEMPORARY EXECUTIVE SECRETARY APPOINTED

Mr. Paul H. Fesler has been employed on a temporary basis to act as Executive Secretary during the absence of Mr. Richard H. Graham.

Mr. Fesler is especially well qualified for the position having served as Superintendent of the University Hospital in Oklahoma City and as Superintendent of the Minnesota Hospital in Minneapolis. He has also been connected with the Wesley Hospital in Chicago as Superintendent and is past president of the American Hospital Association.

Mr. Fesler has a wide acquaintance among the profession of this State and his services will prove valuable to the State Association.

OKLAHOMA CITY ROENTGENOLO-GICAL CLUB ORGANIZED

On January 24, 1944, the Oklahoma City Roentgenological Club was organized, held its first meeting and presented a short program. The purpose of this group will be to present and discuss subjects relating to roentgenological diagnosis and therapy. The following men attended: Drs. J. E. Heatley, Ralph Myers, C. P. Bondurant, E. Lachman, P. E. Russo, L. Shyrock and Lt. Wilmer of Will Rogers Field. Meetings will be held on the last Monday of each month at 7:30 P.M., Classroom A, University Hospitals.

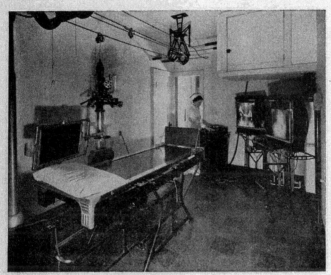

AMERICAN COLLEGE OF SURGEONS TO HOLD 22 WAR SESSIONS

Twenty-two cities distributed throughout the United States and Canada have been selected by the American College of Surgeons as headquarters for one-day War Sessions to be held in March and April, 1944. Advancements in military medicine and developments in civilian medical research and practice under the spur of the war emergency will be presented by authorities representing government agencies and by civilian physicians and surgeons.

The meetings will be open to the profession at large, including medical officers of the Army and the Navy, residents, interns, medical students, and executive personnel in hospitals. For the latter special hospital conferences, to be held simultaneously with the scientific sessions, are being arranged. Those who plan to attend the War Sessions may select the meeting which in place or time is most convenient, regardless of the states and provinces which, for the purpose of organization, are designed on the schedule as participating in a given meeting.

The United States Army, Navy, Public Health Service, Veterans Administration, Procurement and Assignment Service, and the Office of Civilian Defense, are assigning representatives to participate in the meetings. In Canada, the corresponding agencies are likewise assigning official representatives. Experiences of medical officers who have been on active duty in combat zones will be especially featured. In the hospital conferences, such agencies as the War Production Board, the War Manpower Commission, the American Red Cross, and groups interested in student nurse recruitment, will be represented.

Each meeting will open at 8:30 A.M. with the showing of official U.S. Army and U.S. Navy films on medical and surgical subjects, such as evacuation of the wounded, fractures, bomb blast, burns, and treatment of wounds. From 9:30 to 11:30 Army and Navy representatives who have been on active duty abroad will report; from 11:30 to noon representatives of the Public Health Service will report on measures for the control of endemic and epidemic diseases. Current problems of the Procurement and Assignment Service will be presented by a representative at the luncheon from 12:15 to 2:00 o'clock. Between 2:15 and 5:00 P.M., three scientific presentations by medical members of the Armed Forces and by civilian members of the medical profession will be made; a scientific presentation will be made by a representative of a medical service in industry; and the program for veterans will be presented by a representative of the Veterans' Administration. From 5:00 to 5:80 P.M. the need for protective services in time of war will be presented by a representative of the Office of Civilian Defense. The concluding session will be a dinner meeting and open forum with all participants in the day's program as the panel of experts to lead discussion of any subjects presented during the day together with other problems of interest to the medical and hospital professions. The motion picture showing, public health service session, luncheon conference, civilian defense program, and the dinner meeting and open forum will be attended by both the medical and hospital groups. The hospital representatives will discuss wartime hospital problems and how they are being solved, from 9:30 to 11:30 A.M., and will hold a round table conference on "Wartime Hospital Service" from 2:15 to 5:00 P.M.

Preliminary Schedule of 1944 War Sessions

Date	City	States and Provinces	Headquarters
February 28, Monday	Winnipeg	Manitoba, Saskatchewan	The Fort Garry
March 2, Thursday	Minneapolis	Minnesota, North Dakota, South Dakota	Hotel Nicollet
March 4, Saturday	Des Moines	Iowa, Nebraska, Missouri	Hotel Ft. Des Moines
March 6, Monday	Chicago	Illinois, Wisconsin	The Stevens
March 8, Wednesday	Cincinnati	Ohio, Kentucky, Indiana, West Virginia	The Netherland Plaza
March 10, Friday	Detroit	Michigan	Hotel Statler
March 13, Monday	Rochester	New York State	The Seneca
March 15, Wednesday	Toronto	Ontario	Royal York
March 17, Friday	Montreal	Quebec, New Brunswick, Nova Scotia, Prince Edward Island, Newfoundland	Mount Royal Hotel
March 20, Monday	Springfield	Massachusetts, Maine, New Hampshire, Vermont, Rhode Island, Connecticut	Hotel Kimball
March 22, Wednesday	Philadelphia	Pennsylvania, New Jersey, Delaware	The Bellevue-Stratford
March 24, Friday	Baltimore	Maryland, District of Columbia, Virginia	Lord Baltimore Hotel
March 27, Monday	Jacksonville	Florida, Georgia, North Carolina, Eastern Tennessee	The George Washington
March 29, Wenesday	Jackson	Mississippi, Louisiana, Western Tennessee, Alabama	Hotel Heidelberg
April 1, Saturday	San Antonio	Texas, New Mexico, Mexico	The Gunter Hotel
April 4, Tuesday	Tulsa	Oklahoma, Kansas, Arkansas	The Mayo
April 7, Friday	Denver	Colorado, Wyoming, Western Nebraska	Hotel Utah
April 11, Tuesday	Salt Lake City	Utah, Idaho	Cosmopolitan Hotel
April 14, Friday	Spokane	Washington, Northern Idaho, Oregon, Montana	The Davenport Hotel
April 18, Tuesday	Vancouver	British Columbia, Alberta	Hotel Vancouver
April 24, Monday	San Francisco	Northern California, Nevada	Mark Hopkins Hotel
April 27, Thursday	Los Angeles	Southern California, Arizona	The Biltmore Hotel

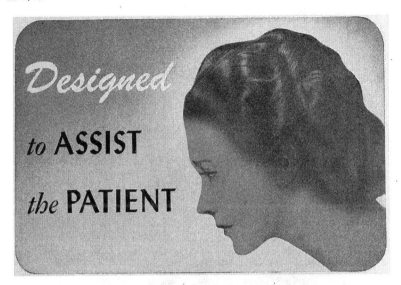

GUEST SPEAKER

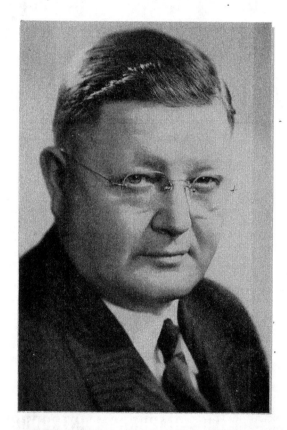

ALFRED W. ADSON. M.D., Rochester Minnesota. Member of the Council on Medical Service and Public Relations of the American Medical Association.

PROGRAM

Fifty-Second Annual Session of the Oklahoma State Medical Association Tulsa, April 24, 25 and 26, 1944

GREETINGS FROM THE TULSA COUNTY MEDICAL SOCIETY

This year it is again the privilege of the Tulsa County Medical Society to act as host at the Fifty-second Annual Convention of the Oklahoma State Medical Association in Tulsa, April 24, 25 and 26. It is always a genuine pleasure to welcome the doctors of Oklahoma to Tulsa as it provides a much-needed opportunity of returning the hospitality which is shown Tulsa doctors in other cities and towns of the state.

In the midst of the third war year, the average doctor is a busy man with the cares of a heavy practice. For that reason, any activity which takes the physician from his professional duties must be well justified. The convention program this year does justify that expenditure of time and money through the educational facilities it affords. The Tulsa County Medical Society will see that additional justification is provided through enjoyable social events which provide much-needed relaxation.

You are invited to attend a Buffet Dinner at 6:00 P.M., on the opening night, Monday, April 24, at the Mayo Hotel in the Junior Ballroom. A short program of entertainment will follow. The Dinner will be complimentary. This event will be a stag, and is presented by the Tulsa County Medical Society.

The Ladies Auxiliary of the Tulsa County Medical Society has planned an attractive program of entertainment for wives of attending doctors. Make your plans to bring your wife with you.

We believe that you will find the annual convention of 1944 a most interesting and enjoyable meeting. The members of the Tulsa County Medical Society look forward to welcoming you again to Tulsa.

Ralph A. McGill, M.D., President
Tulsa County Medical Society

General Information

HEADQUARTERS
Mayo Hotel

REGISTRATION
Sixteenth Floor

Registration will be on the Sixteenth Floor, Mayo Hotel. All physicians except those from outside the state, visiting guests, and those on military assignment, must present membership cards for 1944 before registering. Dues will not be accepted at the Registration Desk except from County Secretaries.
Registration will open at 8.00 A.M., Monday, April 24.

GUEST SPEAKERS

Walter C. Alvarez, M.D., Internist, Professor of Medicine, Graduate School, University of Minnesota, Mayo Clinic, Rochester, Minn.; Duff S. Allen, M.D., Surgeon, Assistant Professor of Clinical Surgery, Washington University School of Medicine, St. Louis, Mo.; Cecil K. Drinker, M.D., Physiologist, Professor of Physiology, Harvard Medical School and Graduate School, Boston, Mass.; Harry S. Mustard, M.D., Director, DeLamar Institute of Public Health, Columbia University, New York, N. Y.

GENERAL SESSIONS

The General Sessions will be held at 1:15 P.M., Tuesday, April 25, and 1:30 P.M., Wednesday, April 26, in the Crystal Ballroom, Sixteenth Floor, Mayo Hotel.

SECTION MEETINGS

All Section Meetings will be held on Tuesday and Wednesday mornings, April 25 and 26, on the Sixteenth Floor, Mayo Hotel.

HOUSE OF DELEGATES

The House of Delegates will meet Monday, April 24, at 8.00 P.M., immediately following the Buffet Dinner of the Tulsa County Medical Society, and at 8.30 A.M., Tuesday, April 25, in the Ivory Room, Mezzanine Floor, Mayo Hotel.

COUNCIL

The Council will convene at 1.30 P.M., Monday, April 24, in the English Room, Mezzanine Floor, Mayo Hotel, and thereafter on call of the President.

WOMAN'S AUXILIARY

Registration will be on the Mezzanine Floor of the Mayo Hotel. The complete Program may be found on page 114 of this Program.

TECHNICAL EXHIBITS

The Exhibits will be displayed on the Sixteenth Floor, Mayo Hotel.

TULSA COUNTY MEDICAL SOCIETY BUFFET DINNER

The Buffet Dinner will be Monday evening, April 24, at 6:00 P.M. in the Junior Ballroom, Mayo Hotel. All members of the Association and guests of the Association are to be Guests of the Tulsa County Medical Society. An interesting program has been arranged.

OKLAHOMA UNIVERSITY MEDICAL ALUMNI LUNCHEON

The Luncheon will be at 12.15 P.M., Tuesday, April 25, at the Tulsa Club. The complete program appears on page 119. Tickets will be on sale at the Registration Desk.

PRESIDENT'S INAUGURAL DINNER DANCE

The President's Inaugural Dinner Dance will be held in the Crystal Ballroom, Sixteenth Floor, Mayo Hotel, at 7:30 P.M., Tuesday, April 25. Dr. Alfred W. Adson, member of the Council on Medical Service and Public Relations of the American Medical Association, Rochester, Minn., will be Guest Speaker. Guests will meet on the Mezzanine Floor. Ticket reservations must be made at the time of registering due to food rationing.

GOLF TOURNAMENT

There will be no Golf Tournament at the 1944 Meeting; however, arrangements have been made for anyone to play at the Tulsa Country Club and at the Southern Hills Country Club. The player will pay the regular green fee. Cards may be obtained at the Registration Desk. Charles H. Haralson, M.D., Chairman.

RESOLUTIONS

Resolutions to be submitted should be prepared and presented at the first meeting of the House of Delegates.

Woman's Auxiliary Program

Oklahoma State Medical Association

State Auxiliary Officers

President
Mrs. F. Maxey Cooper
Oklahoma City

Secretary
Mrs. Charles R. Rountree
Oklahoma City

President-Elect
Mrs. Clarence C. Young
Shawnee

Treasurer
Mrs. C. P. Bondurant
Oklahoma City

Vice-President
Mrs. Warren T. Mayfield
Norman

Historian
Mrs. Alfred R. Sugg
Ada

Parliamentarian
Mrs. Frank L. Flack
Tulsa

CONVENTION PROGRAM

Mrs. J. W. Rogers, Tulsa, Convention Chairman
Monday, April 24, 1944

9.00 A.M.   Registration ....Mezzanine Floor, Mayo Hotel.
6.00 P.M.   Buffet Dinner and Pre-Convention Execution Executive Board Meeting in the home of Mrs. John Perry, 2928 South Columbus Place, Tulsa. **Tuesday, April 25, 1944.**
9.00 A.M.   Registration ....Mezzanine Floor, Mayo Hotel.
10.00 A.M. Annual Business Meeting ....Room. B, Mezzanine Floor, Mayo Hotel
1:00 P.M.   Luncheon—First Methodist Church, 1115 South Boulder Avenue, Tulsa. All visiting ladies invited.
3:00 P.M.   Post-Convention Board Meeting ....Methodist Church
7:30 P.M.   President's Inaugural Dinner Dance ....Crystal Ballroom, Sixteenth Floor, Mayo Hotel

OFFICERS
of
Oklahoma State Medical Association
1943-44

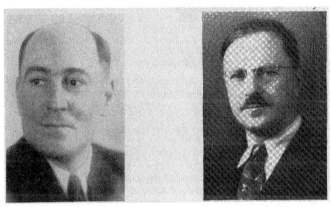

C. R. Rountree, Oklahoma City
President-Elect

James Stevenson, Tulsa
President

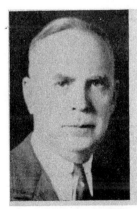

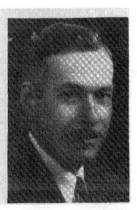

Lewis J. Moorman, Oklahoma City
Secretary-Treasurer

George H. Garrison, Oklahoma City
Speaker, House of Delegates

SCIENTIFIC PROGRAM

All Sections will meet on the Sixteenth Floor, Mayo Hotel

GENERAL SESSIONS

The General Sessions will meet in the Crystal Ballroom, Sixteenth Floor, Mayo Hotel

SECTIONS

Section on Eye, Ear, Nose and Throat—Parlor A, 9:00-10:30 A.M., Tuesday, April 25.

Section on Urology and Syphilology—Parlor B, 9:00-10:30 A.M., Tuesday, April 25.

Section on General Medicine—Crystal Ballroom, 9:00-12:00 A.M., Tuesday, April 25.

Section on Pediatrics—Parlor A, 10:30-12:00 A.M., Tuesday, April 25.

Section on Dermatology and Radiology—Parlor B, 10:30-12:00 A.M., Tuesday, April 25.

Section on Public Health—Parlor A, 9:00-12:00 A.M., Wednesday, April 26.

Section on Neurology, Psychiatry and Endocrinology — Parlor B, 9:00-10:30 A.M., Wednesday, April 26.

Section on General Surgery—Crystal Ballroom, 9:00-12:00 A.M., Wednesday, April 26.

Section on Obstetrics and Gynecology—Parlor B, 10:30-12:00 A.M., Wednesday, April 26.

Scientific Program

Oklahoma State Medical Association

April 25 and 26, 1944

Sixteenth Floor, Mayo Hotel

Tulsa

Tuesday, April, 25, 1944

General Chairman, Maurice J. Searle, M.D., Tulsa

Parlor A

Sixteenth Floor, Mayo Hotel

9:00—10:30 A.M.

SECTION ON EYE, EAR, NOSE AND THROAT

Leo F. Cailey, M.D., Oklahoma City, Chairman

Hugh J. Evans, M.D., Tulsa, Secretary

9:00   "Corneal Ulcer"—Marvin D. Henley, M. D., Tulsa.

9:20   Discussion—James R. Reed, M.D., Oklahoma City.

9:30   "Eye Conditions Among Military Men"—Major W. W. Sanger, M.C., Station Hospital, Camp Gruber. (Formerly of Oklahoma City).

9:50   Discussion—D. L. Mishler, M.D., Tulsa.

10:00   "Otitis Media—Pathology and Treatment"—O. Alton Watson, M.D., Oklahoma City.

10:20   Discussion—J. C. Macdonald, M.D., Oklahoma City.

Parlor A

Sixteenth Floor, Mayo Hotel

10:30—12:00 A.M.

SECTION ON PEDIATRICS

Luvern Hays, M.D., Tulsa, Chairman

G. R. Russell, M.D., Tulsa, Secretary

10:30   Chairman's Address—"Acute Anterior Poliomyelitis"—Luvern Hays, M.D., Tulsa.

11:00   "Rheumatic Fever in Children"—Clark H. Hall, M.D., Oklahoma City.

11:20   Discussion—Ben H. Nicholson, M.D., Oklahoma City.

11:30   "Observations in 'Thymus Disease' "—G. R. Russell, M.D., Tulsa.

11:50   "Discussion—Maurice J. Searle, M.D., Tulsa.

GUEST SPEAKERS

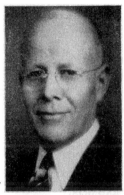

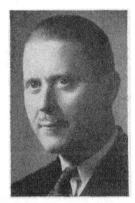

Walter C. Alvarez, M.D., F.A.C.P., Internist, Mayo Clinic, Rochester, Minn. Cooper Medical College, San Francisco, 1905. American Board of Internal Medicine, Association of American Physicians, American Gastro-Enteroligical Association, American Society for Clinical Investigation. Professor of Medicine, Graduate School, University of Minnesota.

Duff S. Allen, M.D., Surgeon, St. Louis, Mo. Washington University School of Medicine, 1919. American Board of Surgery, American Association for Thoracic Surgery. Assistant Professor Clinical Surgery, Washington University School of Medicine, St. Louis, Mo.

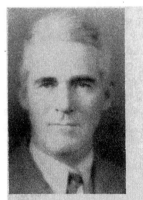

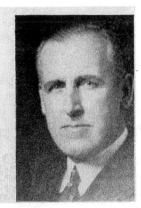

Cecil K. Drinker, M.D., Physiologist, Boston, Mass. University of Pennsylvania School of Medicine, Philadelphia, 1913. Association of American Physicians, American Society for Clinical Investigation. Professor of Physiology, Harvard Medical School and Graduate School, Boston, Mass.

Harry S. Mustard, M.D., Public Health, New York, N.Y. Medical College of the State of South Carolina, Charleston, 1911. Editor of Journal of the American Public Health Association. Director, De Lamar Institute of Public Health, Columbia University, New York N.Y.

Tuesday, April 25, 1944

General Chairman, Alfred R. Sugg, M.D., Ada

PARLOR B

Sixteenth Floor, Mayo Hotel

9:00—10:30 A.M.

SECTION ON UROLOGY AND SYPHILOLOGY

Alfred R. Sugg, M.D., Ada, Chairman

J. W. Rogers, M.D., Tulsa, Secretary

9:00   Chairman's Address—"Management of Urinary Tract Stones"—Alfred R. Sugg, M.D., Ada.
9:30   "Modern Concepts in the Treatment of Syphilis"—Charles B. Taylor, M.D., Oklahoma City.
9:50   Discussion—Major C. A. Shumate, M. C., Rush Springs. (*By Invitation*).
10:00   "Urological Pain with a Negative Urinalysis"—W. F. Lewis, M.D., Lawton.
10:20   Discussion—Joseph Fulcher, M.D., Tulsa.

Parlor B

Sixteenth Floor, Mayo Hotel

10:30—12:00 A.M.

SECTION ON DERMATOLOGY AND RADIOLOGY

Walter S. Larrabee, M.D., Tulsa, Chairman

John Heatley, M.D., Oklahoma City, Secretary

10:30   Chairman's Address—"The Science of Radiology"—Walter S. Larrabee, M.D., Tulsa.
11:00   "Para Basedowian Syndromes"—L. S. McAlister, M.D., Muskogee.
11:20   Discussion—Leon H. Stuart, M.D., Tulsa.
11:30   "Fever Treatment"—M. O. Nelson, M. D., Tulsa.
11:50   Discussion—C. P. Bondurant, M.D., Oklahoma City.

Tuesday, April 25, 1944

Crystal Ballroom

Sixteenth Floor, Mayo Hotel

9:00—12:00 A.M.

SECTION ON GENERAL MEDICINE

Mary V. S. Sheppard, M.D. Oklahoma City, Chairman

H. A. Ruprecht, M.D., Tulsa, Vice-Chairman

Philip M. Schreck, M.D., Tulsa, Secretary

9:00   Chairman's Address—"Typhoid Outbreak in Oklahoma City"—Mary V. S. Sheppard, M.D., Oklahoma City.
9:30   "Some Observations of the Clinical Use of Penicillin"—Lt. Col. E. Rankin Denny, M.C., Chief of Hospital Services, Gardiner General Hospital, Chicago, Ill. (Formerly of Tulsa).
9:50   Discussion—Ian MacKenzie, M.D., Tulsa.
10:00   "Diabetes in Pregnancy"—Paul B. Cameron, M.D., Pryor.
10:20   Discussion—C. J. Fishman, M.D., Oklahoma City.
10:30   "Clinical Diagnosis of Malignancies"—Hugh Jeter, M.D., Oklahoma City.
10:50   Discussion—Paul B. Champlin, M.D., Enid.
11:00   "Peptic Ulcer and Related Conditions"—Lt. Col. J. C. Cain, M.C., Chief of Medical Service, Station Hospital, Camp Gruber. (*By Invitation*).
11:20   Discussion—Arthur W. White, M.D., Oklahoma City.
11:30   "Some Laboratory Phases of Clinical Diagnosis"—I. H. Nelson, M.D., Tulsa.
11:50   Discussion—Elizabeth M. Chamberlin, M.D., Bartlesville.

Annual Spring Meeting of the Oklahoma University Medical School Association

Tulsa Club

12:15 P.M.

PROGRAM

J. William Finch, M.D., Hobart, Presiding

Honor Classes — 1914, 1924, 1934, 1944

Special Tables

Honoring R. M. Howard, M.D., (Professor Emeritus, Surgery, Oklahoma University School of Medicine) — F. M. Lingenfelter, M.D.,

Honoring E. S. Lain, M.D., (Professor Emeritus, Dermatology and Syphilology, Oklahoma University School of Medicine) — M. W. Wickham, M.D.

Introducing Class of 1914—Powell L. Hays, M.D., Vinita.

Introducing Class of 1924—William O. Armstrong, M.D., Ponca City.

Introducing Class of 1934—Herbert A. Masters, M.D., Tahlequah.

Representing Class of 1944—Mr. Millington Young, Valedictorian, Senior Class.

Remarks—Tom Lowry, M.D., University of Oklahoma School of Medicine.

Tuesday, April 25, 1944

GENERAL SESSION

James Stevenson, M.D., Tulsa, Presiding

Crystal Ballroom

Sixteenth Floor, Mayo Hotel

1:15   "The Restoration of Breathing in Emergencies and the Maintenance of Respiration in Non-Breathing Patients"—Cecil K. Drinker, M.D., Boston, Mass.

2:00   "Sick Headaches"—Walter C. Alvarez, M.D., Rochester, Minn.

2:45   "The Diagnosis and Treatment of Cancer of the Lung" — Duff S. Allen, M.D., St. Louis, Mo.

3:30   "Trends in Public Health"—Harry S. Mustard, M.D., New York, N. Y.

Entertainment Program

Tuesday, April 25, 1944

7:30 P.M.

PRESIDENT'S INAUGURAL DINNER DANCE

Crystal Ballroom

Sixteenth Floor, Mayo Hotel

W. A. Showman, M.D., Tulsa General Chairman, Presiding

Program

Introduction of Guests .... W. A. Showman, M.D., Tulsa

Address of Welcome—Ralph A. McGill, M.D., President, Tulsa County Medical Society.

Response and Introduction of President-Elect—James Stevenson, M.D., Tulsa, President, Oklahoma State Medical Association.

President's Response—and Introduction of President's Guest Speaker—C. R. Rountree, M.D., Oklahoma City.

Guest Speaker's Address

"The Federal Challenge to Practitioners of Medicine"

Alfred W. Adson, M.D., Member of the Council on Medical Service and Public Relations of the American Medical Association, Rochester, Minn.

(Tickets must be purchased at time of registering due to food rationing).

Wednesday, April 26, 1944

Parlor A

Sixteenth Floor, Mayo Hotel

9:00—12:00 P.M.

SECTION ON PUBLIC HEALTH

John W. Shackelford, M.D., Oklahoma City, Chairman

Carl Puckett, M.D., Oklahoma City, Vice-Chairman

Charles W. Haygood, M.D., Shawnee, Secretary

9:00   "Comparative Values in Public Health Activities" — Harry S. Mustard, M.D., New York, N. Y. *(By Invitation)*.

9:30   "Wartime Tuberculosis Control in Oklahoma"—Richard M. Burke, M.D., Oklahoma City.

9:50   Discussion—Carl Puckett, M.D., Oklahoma City.

10:00   "A Physician's View of Health Education"—Clinton Gallaher, M.D., Shawnee.

10:20   Discussion—Charles W. Haygood, Shawnee, and Helen Martikainen, M.P.H., Shawnee. *(By Invitation)*.

10:30   "The Significance of Abnormal Spinal Fluid Findings in the Diagnosis and Treatment of Neurosyphilis"—William E. Grraham, M.D., Medical Officer in Charge, U. S. Public Health Service Hospital, Hot Springs, Ark. *(By Invitation)*.

POLIOMYELITIS

11:00   "Epidemiological Observations"—Grady F. Mathews, M.D., Commissioner of Health, Oklahoma City.

11:20   "Diagnosis and Pediatric Care"—Carroll M. Pounders, M.D., Oklahoma City.

11:40   "Treatment and Orthopedic Care"—D. H. O'Donoghue, M.D., Oklahoma City.

Wednesday, April 26, 1944

General Chairman, Ben H. Nicholson, M.D., Oklahoma City.

Parlor B

Sixteenth Floor, Mayo Hotel

9:00—10:30 A.M.

SECTION ON NEUROLOGY, PSYCHIATRY AND ENDOCRINOLOGY

C. T. Steen, M.D., Norman, Chairman

Charles E. Leonard, M.D., Oklahoma City, Vice-Chairman

Coyne H. Campbell, M.D., Oklahoma City, Secretary

9:00   Chairman's Address—"Historical Aspects of Psychiatry in Oklahoma"—C. T. Steen, M.D., Norman.

9:20   Discussion—Felix M. Adams, M.D., Vinita.

9:30   "Diagnosis of Ruptured Intervertebral Disc"—Arnold H. Ungerman, M.D., Tulsa.

9:50   Discussion—Harry Wilkins, M.D., Oklahoma City.

10:00   "Treatment of Neuroses in General Practice"—Hugh M. Galbraith, M.D. Oklahoma City.

10:20   Discussion—Major Moorman Prosser, M. C., Station Hospital, Camp Gruber, (Formerly of Norman).

Parlor B

Sixteenth Floor, Mayo Hotel

10:30—12:00 A.M.

SECTION ON OBSTETRICS AND GYNECOLOGY

Edward N. Smith, M.D., Oklahoma City, Chairman

Roy E. Emanuel, M.D., Chickasha, Secretary

10:30   Chairman's Address—"Functional Uterine Bleeding"—Edward N. Smith, M.D., Oklahoma City.

11:00   "The Present Status of Pain Relief During Labor"—Major Silas H. Starr, M.C., Chief of Surgical Section—Officers and Women, Borden General Hospital, Chickasha. *(By Invitation)*.

11:20   Discussion—Harry B. Stewart, M.D., Tulsa.

11:30   "An Unusual Complication in Obstetrics"—Carl F. Simpson, M.D., Tulsa.

11:50   Discussion—J. B. Eskridge, Jr., M.D., Oklahoma City.

Wednesday, April 26, 1944

Crystall Ballroom

Sixteenth Foor, Mayo Hotel

9:00—12:00 A.M.

SECTION ON GENERAL SURGERY

Oscar White, M.D., Oklahoma City, Chairman

Gregory E. Stanbro, M.D., Oklahoma City, Vice-Chairman

John C. Perry, M.D., Tulsa

9:00   Chairman's Address—"Surgery of the Spleen"—Oscar White, M.D., Oklahoma City.

9:30   "Lessons Learned from the Use of the Roger-Anderson Apparatus"—Major T. Wiley Hodges, M.C., Chief of Orthopedic Section, Glennan General Hospital, Okmulgee. *(By Invitation)*.

9:50   Discussion—W. K. West, M.D., Oklahoma City.

10:00   "Carcinoma of the Rectum"—Neil W. Woodward, M.D., Oklahoma City.

10:20   Discussion—R. M. Howard, M.D., Oklahoma City.

10:30   "Reformed Gall Bladders"—George H. Miller, M.D., Tulsa.

10:50   Discussion—F. S. Watson, M.D., Okmulgee.

11:00   "Care of Chest Injuries"—Major William F. Hoyt, M.C., Chief of Surgical Section, Glennan General Hospital, Okmulgee. *(By Invitation)*.

11:20   Discussion—Harold M. McClure, M.D., Chickasha.

11:30   "Intestinal Obstructions in Childhood"—E. Eugene Rice, M.D., Shawnee.

11:50   Discussion—John F. Park, M.D., McAlester.

Wednesday, April 26, 1944

GENERAL SESSION

C. R. Rountree, M.D., Oklahoma City, Presiding.

Crystal Ballroom

Sixteenth Floor, Mayo Hotel

1:30   "Thyrotoxicosis in Older People"—Duff S. Allen, M.D., St. Louis, Mo.

2:15   "Implications of Tropical and Imported Diseases from a Public Health Standpoint"—Harry S. Mustard, M.D., New York, N. Y.

3:00   "Nervous Breakdowns and Their Causes"—Walter C. Alvarez, M.D., Rochester, Minn.

3:45   "An Analysis of the Modern Treatment of Severe Burns"—Cecil K. Drinker, M.D., Boston, Mass.

DELEGATES AND ALTERNATES SELECTED FOR ANNUAL MEETING

In compliance with the By-Laws of the Oklahoma State Medical Association, the following listed delegates and alternates have been certified to the Executive Office as representatives of their respective counties at the Annual Meeting.

Credential cards have been mailed to the delegates and alternates, who in turn must present their credentials to the Credentials Committee prior to the first meeting of the House of Delegates on Monday evening, April 24.

COUNTY	DELEGATE	ALTERNATE
Alfalfa	Forrest Hale, Cherokee	
Atoka-Coal	H. C. Huntley, Atoka	W. W. Cotton, Atoka
	J. B. Clark, Coalgate	R. C. Henry, Coalgate
Beckham	G. H. Stagner, Erick	O. C. Standifer, Elk City
Blaine	A. K. Cox, Watonga	
Bryan	O. J. Colwick, Durant	John A. Haynie, Durant
Caddo	F. L. Patterson, Carnegie	C. B. Sullivan, Carnegie
Canadian	J. T. Phelps, El Reno	M. E. Phelps, El Reno
Carter	F. W. Boadway, Ardmore	G. E. Johnson, Ardmore
	J. Hobson Veazey, Ardmore	T. J. Jackson, Ardmore
Cherokee	W. M. Wood, Tahlequah	H. A. Masters, Tahlequah
Choctaw	C. H. Hale, Boswell	Fred D. Switzer, Hugo
Cleveland	F. T. Gastineau, Norman	Iva S. Merritt, Norman
	M. M. Wickham, Norman	Carl T. Steen, Norman
Comanche	George S. Barber, Lawton	William C. Cole, Lawton
Cotton	George A. Tallant, Walters	George W. Baker, Walters
Craig	F. M. Adams, Vinita	W. R. Marks, Vinita
Creek	J. B. Lampton, Sapulpa	E. W. King, Bristow
Custer	Ellis Lamb, Clinton	C. Doler, Clinton
	McLain Rogers, Clinton	Ross Deputy, Clinton
Garfield	D. S. Harris, Drummond	
	V. R. Hamble, Enid	
Garvin	M. E. Robberson, Wynnewood	G. L. Johnson, Pauls Valley
Grady	H. M. McClure, Chickasha	L. E. Woods, Chickasha
Greer	J. B. Hollis, Mangum	J. T. Lowe, Mangum
Harmon	W. G. Husband, Hollis	W. M. Yeargan, Hollis
Haskell	J. C. Rumley, Stigler	William S. Carson, Keota
Hughes	W. L. Taylor, Holdenville	W. E. Floyd, Holdenville
Jackson	E. S. Crow, Olustee	E. W. Mabry, Altus
Jefferson	L. L. Wade, Ryan	
Kay	Dewey Mathews, Tonkawa	L. H. Becker, Blackwell
	Philip C. Risser, Blackwell	J. C. Wagner, Ponca City
Kingfisher	A. O. Meredith, Kingfisher	
Kiowa	J. M. Bonham, Hobart	J. William Finch, Hobart
LeFlore	S. D. Bevill, Poteau	E. M. Woodson, Poteau
Lincoln	J. W. Adams, Chandler	U. E. Nickell, Davenport
Logan	L. A. Hahn, Guthrie	
Marshall	J. F. York, Madill	J. L. Holland, Madill
Mayes	Carl Puckett, Oklahoma City	
McClain	R. L. Royster, Purcell	S. C. Davis, Blanchard
McCurtain	W. W. Williams, Idabel	R. H. Sherill, Broken Bow
McIntosh	W. A. Tolleson, Eufaula	F. R. First, Checotah
Murray	W. P. Rudell, Sulphur	
Muskogee-Sequoyah-Wagoner	C. E. White, Muskogee	L. S. McAlister, Muskogee
	E. H. Fite, Muskogee	J. R. Rafter, Muskogee
	H. K. Riddle, Coweta	J. H. Plunkett, Wagener
	J. A. Morrow, Sallisaw	
Noble	T. F. Renfrow, Billings	
Okfuskee	A. S. Melton, Okemah	L. J. Spickard, Okemah
Oklahoma	L. Chester McHenry, Oklahoma City	C. M. O'Leary, Oklahoma City
	W. F. Keller, Oklahoma City	Harper Wright, Oklahoma City
	R. Q. Goodwin, Oklahoma City	John H. Lamb, Oklahoma City

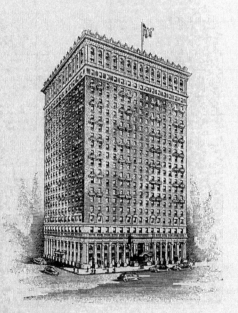

Welcome To . . . . .

THE MAYO

TULSA

Official Headquarters

Oklahoma State Medical Association

1944 Annual Convention, April 24-26

JOHN D. MAYO, Managing Director

COUNTY	DELEGATE	ALTERNATE
	Robert H. Akin, Oklahoma City	Oscar White, Oklahoma City
	C. M. Pounders, Oklahoma City	J. H. Robinson, Oklahoma City
	D. H. O'Donoghue, Oklahoma City	James R. Reed, Oklahoma City
	W. E. Eastland, Oklahoma City	F. M. Lingenfelter, Oklahoma City
	Walker Morledge, Oklahoma City	Ben H. Nicholson, Oklahoma City
	O. A. Watson, Oklahoma City	H. L. Deupree, Oklahoma City
	Neil W. Woodward, Oklahoma City	Leo J. Starry, Oklahoma City
	W. K. West, Oklahoma City	E. R. Musick, Oklahoma City
	M. F. Jacobs, Oklahoma City	Jolin F. Burton, Oklahoma City
Okmulgee	G. Y. McKinney, Henryetta	A. R. Holmes, Henryetta
	J. C. Matheney, Okmulgee	Fred Watson, Okmulgee
Osage	G. I. Walker, Hominy	Roscoe Walker, Pawhuska
Ottawa	Walter C. H. Kerr, Picher	F. L. Wormington, Miami
	B. Wright Shelton, Miami	M. M. DeArman, Miami
Pawnee	J. L. LeHew, Sr., Pawnee	
Payne	L. A. Mitchell, Stillwater	R. E. Leatherock, Cushing
Pittsburg	T. H. McCarley, McAlester	W. C. Wait, McAlester
	L. S. Willour, McAlester	F. J. Baum, McAlester
Pontotoc	Sam A. McKeel, Ada	C. F. Needham, Ada
	O. H. Miller, Ada	M. M. Webster, Ada
Pottawatomie	G. S. Baxter, Shawnee	E. Eugene Rice, Shawnee
	W. M. Gallaher, Shawnee	C. C. Young, Shawnee
Pushmataha	John S. Lawson, Clayton	E. S. Patterson, Antlers
Rogers	G. D. Waller, Claremore	C. L. Caldwell, Chelsea
Seminole	Mack I. Shanholtz, Wewoka	A. B. Stephens, Seminole
Stephens	A. J. Weedn, Duncan	W. Z. McClain, Marlow
Texas	R. B. Hayes, Guymon	D. S. Lee, Guymon
Tillman	J. D. Osborn, Frederick	T. F. Spurgeon, Frederick
Tulsa	W. Albert Cook, Tulsa	M. V. Stanley, Tulsa
	W. A. Showman, Tulsa	W. A. Walker, Tulsa
	Marvin D. Henley, Tulsa	J. J. Billington, Tulsa
	Ralph A. McGill, Tulsa	James L. Miner, Tulsa
	John C. Perry, Tulsa	Henry S. Browne, Tulsa
	L. C. Northrup, Tulsa	F. L. Underwood, Tulsa
	W. S. Larrabee, Tulsa	D. J. Underwood, Tulsa
	H. B. Stewart, Tulsa	Hugh J. Evans, Tulsa
Washington-Nowata	H. C. Weber, Bartlesville	R. E. Beechwood, Bartlesville
	J. G. Smith, Bartlesville	L. D. Hudson, Dewey
	S. A. Lang Nowata	K. D. Davis, Nowata
Washita	A. H. Bungardt, Cordell	A. S. Neal, Cordell
Woods	D. B. Ensor, Hopeton	W. F. LaFon, Waynoka
Woodward	Roy E. Newman, Shattuck	M. H. Newman, Shattuck
	John L. Day, Supply	D. W. Darwin, Woodward
	D. W. Vincent, Vici	

University of Oklahoma School of Medicine

Dr. Donald B. McMullen, Associate Professor of Preventive Medicine and Public Health, is giving a refresher course in Parasitology at Tulsa. The course is being given at the University of Tulsa with the full cooperation of that institution. More than 30 medical technologists and others interested in Parasitology are attending this course. The course consists of eight weekly lectures and laboratory periods.

Dr. McMullen is also giving a series of lectures on "Malaria Control" to the students under the Army Specialized Training Program at Norman. Approximately 1,500 students make up this group.

According to a recent release three medical students have been chosen to appear in the 1943-44 edition of Who's Who Among Students in American Colleges and Universities: Robert Edwin McCurdy, sophomore student from Purcell; Edwin Patrick Shanks, sophomore from Drumright, and Lylith Medbery, freshman from Clinton. Since enrollment, however, Miss Medbery has found it necessary to withdraw from school. McCurdy is President of the Sophomore Class, having served in the same capacity during his Freshman Year.

Dr. Donald Slaughter, Acting Dean of the Medical School of Southwestern Medical Foundation, Dallas, was a recent visitor at the School of Medicine.

The Library Staff wishes to call attention to the following books among many new one that have recently been received:

Berlinger—Biomicroscopy of the Eye

Bruner—Treatise of the Canon of Medicine of Avicenna

Lewis—Diseases of the Heart—Third Edition.

Kahn—Man in Structure and Function

Thorex—Surgical Errors and Safeguards

What is probably the world's largest and most complete collection of medical literature is now available to you at no cost. The Army Medical Library has extended its free microfilm service, furnishing films of any periodical article desired without charge to libraries or to individuals. The Library has an Argus Reader and a convenient place for viewing these films as you would read a book—or, if you prefer, projecting them and viewing them as you would a movie. All physicians are cordially invited to take advantage of this service.

Lt. (jg) Francis Randall Buchanan, MC-V(G), USNR, Class of 1942, has just completed the basic course of instruction at the Naval Medical School, National Naval Medical Center, Bethesda, Maryland.

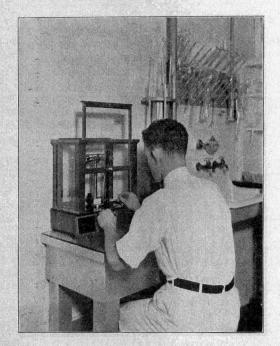

• OBITUARIES •

Roy Wilton Dunlap, M.D.
1878-1944

Dr. Roy Wilton Dunlap, 65, veteran Tulsa opthalmologist-otolaryngologist, died January 28 in a Tulsa hospital following a brief illness. His death came as a result of complications of a cerebral hemorrhage and collapse at the Armed Forces Induction Station where he was a member of the examining staff.

Born in 18.8, Dr. Dunlap attended the Fort Worth School of Medicine at Fort Worth, Texas, from which he received his medical degree in 1901. He practiced for several years in Texas. Following the first world war, during which he served as a First Lieutenant in the Medical Corps, he came to Tulsa and established his practice in 1918.

Dr. Dunlap was President of the Tulsa County Medical Society in 1923 and served for many years as Secretary of that organization and in other capacities. More recently, he was Chairman of the Welfare Committee. Dr. Dunlap was also an active member of the Oklahoma State Medical Association and the American Medical Association. He was prominent in civic and fraternal groups in Tulsa and had attained distinction as an amateur horticulturist.

He is survived by his wife, Mary Dunlap, and one son, Captain Roy W. Dunlap, Jr., now stationed in the South Pacific. Funeral services were held January 31 at the First Christain Church of Tulsa.

The following resolution was passed by the Tulsa County Medical Society at the meeting of February 14, 1944.

Resolution

WHEREAS, the members of the Tulsa County Medical Society were saddened by the death of Dr. Roy Wilton Dunlap last January 28, and

WHEREAS, Dr. Dunlap was a valued member of the Tulsa County Medical Society, serving in the capacity of President and in other official positions, and exerting his abilities and influence in the interests of organized medicine over a period of thirty years, and

WHEREAS, the loss of Dr. Dunlap will be keenly felt in the medical profession of this city and state, Now Therefore

BE IT RESOLVED, that this resolution serves to commemorate the death of Dr. Dunlap and remain as a tribute to the high respect in which this venerable physician was held by his friends and associates, and

BE IT FURTHER RESOLVED, that the Tulsa County Medical Society take this means of conveying its heartfelt sympathy to the members of Dr. Dunlap's family who survive him, and to his many friends and associates.

Approved at the meeting of the Tulsa County Medical Society, February 14, 1944.

Attest: J. Fred Bolton, M.D.
Chairman, Welfare Committee

Fred Yohn Cronk. M.D.
1884-1944

Dr. Fred Yohn Cronk, noted Tulsa surgeon, died February 13 at his home of a sudden heart attack. He was sixty years of age.

A graduate of Johns Hopkins University in 1907, Dr. Cronk was resident surgeon at Lakeside Hospital- in Cleveland and later at St. Agnes Hospital in Baltimore during the following four years. He came to Oklahoma in 1911 as chief surgeon at the Methodist Hospital of Guthrie, removing to Tulsa six years later Dr. Cronk won ready recognition as a surgeon and as a civic leader. He was most active in the Tulsa Rotary Club, the First Presbyterian Church of Tulsa, and the Southern Hills Country Club.

Dr. Cronk was a member of the Tulsa County Medical Society and the Oklahoma State Medical Association. At the time of his death, he was chief surgeon of the Mid-Continent Petroleum Company and a director of the Tulsa County Public Health Association.

He is survived by his wife, Mildred M. Cronk; and three sons, Fred Y. Cronk, Jr., a medical student at Baylor University, Dallas; and Gerald T. and Thomas N. Cronk, twin sons, both now students of medicine at Duke University, Durham.

Funeral services were held February 16 at the First Presbyterian Church of Tulsa.

The following resolution was passed by the Tulsa County Medical Society.

Resolution

WHEREAS, the membership of the Tulsa County Medical Society was greatly saddened by the sudden passing of Dr. Fred Yohn Cronk last February 13, and

WHEREAS, Dr. Cronk was held in high professional esteem as a distinguished physician and surgeon by his fraternal brothers, and

WHEREAS, Dr. Cronk contributed much to the progress of organized medicine through his unselfish efforts and contributions, and to the improvement of the civic virtues of the city and state in which he lived, and

WHEREAS, Dr. Cronk's passing will be a great loss to his many friends outside of the medical profession as well as within, Now Therefore

BE IT RESOLVED, That this resolution serve to commemorate his passing and pay tribute to the accomplishments of his knowledge, skill and effort during his lifetime.

BE IT FURTHER RESOLVED, That this resolution express to the family, friends, and associates of Dr. Cronk the deepest sympathy of the Tulsa County Medical Society.

The Tulsa County Medical Society
J. Fred Bolton, M.D., Chairman
Welfare Committee.

Pettis M. Richardson. M.D.
1879-1944

Dr. Pettis M. Richardson was killed instantly January 10, when his car was hit by a train.

Dr. Richardson was born at Owensville, Missouri, August 21, 1879. He attended Southwest Baptist College, Boliver, Missouri, the Ava Academy, Ava, Missouri, and Medical schools at Texarkana, Texas. Serving his internship at Shreveport, Louisiana, and later taking special courses in surgery at Chicago. He has been practicing medicine in Cushing since 1917.

He was a member of the Oklahoma State Medical Association and of the Payne County Medical Society. Dr. Richardson was also a member of the Masonic Lodge, Baptist Church, Rotary Club and was City Health Officer of Cushing.

He is survived by his son Major Clarence Richardson on foreign duty, one daughter, Mrs. Dale Fenton of Stillwater, four sisters, one brother and one nephew.

Doctor's Wife Has Her Own Ten Commandments
(Taken from the Illinois Medical Journal, August, 1940)

She must not know the meaning of the word "jealous".
She must never gossip.
She must run a cafeteria, serving meals at all hours for her husband.
She must be—like Caesar's wife—above reproach.
She must have self-reliance and self-control.
She must be able to think quickly and sanely in emergencies.
She must be a diplomat, see all, hear all, say a lot, yet say nothing.
She must learn to bear stoically and without complaint, disappointments in her personal plans.
She must be a good mother and father, because doctors are often too busy to discipline their own children.
She must be a good "doctor" because doctors never take time to doctor themselves.

—*Author Unknown, Wichita Medical Bulletin.*

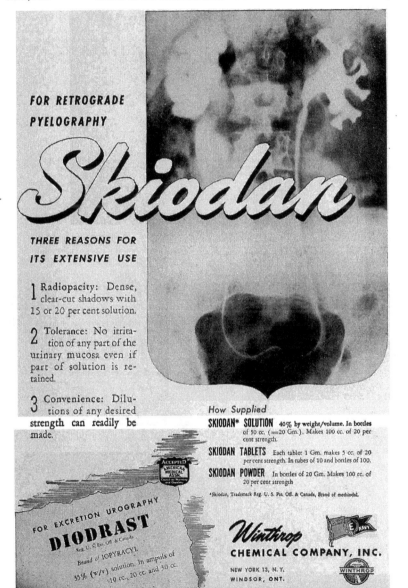

COMMITTEE REPORTS

ANNUAL REPORT OF DISTRICT NO. 1

To the President and House of Delegates
Oklahoma State Medical Association
Gentlemen:

Because of present conditions, I have not visited each County in my Distirct during the past year. There is only one doctor in Cimarron County, and it is 235 miles to the town in which he lives. I have written numerous letters to Beaver and Texas Counties. I have visited all the rest of the Counties at least once during the past year.

We have societies in Alfalfa, Woods and Woodward Counties. The Woodward County Society serves Harper, Dewey and Ellis Counties. I have attended meetings at all points where they are regularly held, having been to Shattuck and Supply each two times.

I have assisted in the collection of annual dues and cooperated with the work of the Procurement and Assignment Committee. At some trouble and numerous telephone calls, I arranged for Ross Rizley, United States Congressman from this District, to speak at Alva and hold a conference with the physicians. He also spoke at Cherokee. I gave out literature on S. B. 1161 at the Rotary and Kiwanis Clubs, and gave out literature to each doctor in Woods County. In addition to above-mentioned activities, I attended a Council Meeting in Oklahoma City on September 26, 1943; organized a Crippled Children's Clinic on November 29, 1943, and assisted in the organization of a Postgraduate course in Internal Medicine held at Alva which began in June of 1943 and extended over a period of ten weeks.

Two doctors of my District have passed away during the year: namely, Dr. E. P. Clapper of Waynoka and Dr. Issac S. Hunt of Freedom, both of whom were Honorary Members of the Oklahoma State Medical Association.

Respectfully submitted,
O. E. TEMPLIN, M.D.
Councilor, District No. 1

ANNUAL REPORT OF DISTRICT NO. 4

To the President and House of Delegates
Oklahoma State Medical Association
Gentlemen:

It has been most gratifying to me to represent the Fourth Councilor District during the past three years, and it is my desire at this time to express my deep appreciation for the hearty cooperation that has been extended in my behalf by the profession in my District. It has indeed been a pleasure to work with those who comprise the membership of the Societies.

The Fourth District is composed of six counties: namely, Blaine, Canadian, Cleveland, Kingfisher, Logan and Oklahoma, all of which have active County Medical Societies; however, it has been necessary because of present world-wide conditions to curtail activities somewhat since those on the home front are extremely busy caring for the civilian population.

As of March 1, there is a total of 385 paid members in the District, 97 of whom are Service Members. Of those now serving in one of the branches of the Armed Forces, one is from Blaine, one from Canadian, eight from Cleveland, two from Kingfisher, two from Logan and 83 from Oklahoma.

At a recent Council Meeting, it was the consensus of opinion and so moved and passed that the Councilor of each District would be most willing to act in an advisory capacity to the local County Committee with regard to information concerning malpractice insurance and approval for those who might desire to make application for participation of the Group Policy of the Association through Eberle and Company, local agents of the London and Lancashire Indemnity Company. Participation in this Policy for malpractice insurance will result in an individual saving due to reduced rates.

Your Councilor kept in touch with the activities of the members of this District, and aided and advised to the best of his ability the State Secretary in her contacts and correspondence with the members—most questions concerning Procurement and Assignment and approval for malpractice insurance. It was a pleasure for the Oklahoma County Medical Society to invite the Presidents and Secretaries of the County Societies of this District to the Annual Inaugural Banquet of the Oklahoma County Medical Society in Oklahoma City on January 29.

A Councilor District Meeting will be held in Oklahoma City during the latter part of March at which time there will be a detailed discussion concerning prepayment surgical insurance.

It is urged that the members of the profession individually support their County Medical Society to the fullest extent as it is only in this manner that fellowship which now exists can continue to prevail.

Respectfully submitted,
TOM LOWRY, M.D.
Councilor, District No. 4

ANNUAL REPORT OF DISTRICT NO. 7

To the President and House of Delegates
Oklahoma State Medical Association
Gentlemen:

In accordance with the custom established by the By-Laws and by long continued usage, the Councilor of the Seventh District herewith submits a brief report for the fiscal year beginning May, 1943.

Activities in the Seventh District have been characterized by an increasing interest in the study of medical care and in the establishment and maintenance of closer harmony and understanding among all of the physicians of the District. In spite of the increasing case load which every doctor has sustained, it is found that the meetings occur more frequently and attendance is in general better than previously. In so far as it is possible under present conditions, meetings are held in all of the Societies at intervals of one month or less and at least two of the County Medical Societies have three or more regular meetings, well attended. In addition to this, members within the Seventh District have shown no hesitancy to continue attending state and national medical meetings and assemblies of various kinds.

The Seventh District has been unusually active in their effort to tell the people of the District about the tendency toward socialized medicine and to ask their cooperation in its control. Members of the Seventh District have been unusually active in sustaining the efforts of those who are attempting to keep Senate Bill 1161 in the Committee where it belongs. Toward this effort, we have added the active assistance of the American Legion, newspapers, radio and civic clubs. Physicians have consistently shown themselves ready, willing and able to present the situation under almost any circumstances in the manner in which we feel it deserves to be understood by the people. The Representative from this District says "I am unalterably opposed to socialized medicine in any of its forms, or anything tending that way," and his action confirms the conviction of his words.

During this past year, special attention has been given to the project of merging two of our County Medical Societies. Depleted by the fact that several of its physicians have entered the Armed Forces, the Murray County Medical Society was conducting regular meetings with difficulty and the suggestion was made that a merge with the Pontotoc County Medical Society might strengthen both organizations and be beneficial to them. Upon the presentation of a petition to this effect, signed by all members of the Murray County Medical Society, the Pontotoc County Medical Society voted favorably. The Councilor from the Fifth District, Dr. J. I. Hollingsworth, expressed his favorable opinion of the merge, and the Councilor of the Seventh District, Dr. Clinton Gallaher, has lent his efforts to completing this union.

Physicians of this District are ready at all times to lend their active support to do anything which will promote peace, harmony and unity among physicians.

Respectfully submitted,
CLINTON GALLAHER, M.D.
Councilor, District No. 7

ANNUAL REPORT OF DISTRICT NO. 9

To the President and House of Delegates
Oklahoma State Medical Association
Gentlemen:

The Ninth Councilor District has not changed since the report of one year ago, except in that Pittsburg County does not have as many new people to be cared for since the completion of the construction work on the Naval Ammunition Depot. This was an extremely heavy load on our doctors while it lasted.

Each County Society is in a healthy condition and holding its meetings regularly. Reports are that the members are paying their dues very promptly.

The District has cooperated with the State Office each time a request has been made.

There is to be a District Meeting and Conference in McAlester on March 8 at which time Dr. P. S. Pelouze of the University of Pennsylvania Medical School will be our guest. It is anticipated there will be a good attendance and that much good will come from this conference. Dr. Pelouze is being brought to the State by the Oklahoma State Health Department, and we feel particularly fortunate in having him as our guest.

Due to war restrictions, I have not visited my District but will do so before the meeting in April. I have, however, kept in touch with counties in my District during the entire year.

Respectfully submitted,
L. C. KUYRKENDALL, M.D.
Councilor, District No. 9

REPORT OF THE COMMITTEE ON POSTGRADUATE MEDICAL TEACHING

The Committee on Postgraduate Medical Teaching submits the following report to the House of Delegates.

The postgraduate program in internal medicine conducted by L. W. Hunt, M.D., of Chicago, Illinois, which was completed February 4, 1944, was a success from every viewpoint. The course was offered in 46 teaching centers. Total registration numbered 1,046 with an average attendance of 85 per cent. Doctor Hunt held 1,106 private consultations with physicians and conducted clinics with a total of 556 patients. This is excellent considering the fact that many actual and potential registrants have been called to military duty.

Receipts from all sources amounted to $30,983.00. Total disbursements were $25,100.98. Balance at the close of the program was $5,882.02, which amount was prorated back to the participating agencies according to the percentage of their contributions. Bound copies of the instructor's lectures were distributed to the physicians enrolled and a total of 855 Certificates of Attendance were issued to those whose attendance averaged 70 per cent or more.

The Committee thanks The Commonwealth Fund of New York, the Oklahoma State Health Department, the United States Public Health Service, and the Oklahoma State Medical Association for their cooperation and financial assistance. It further recommends that the House of Delegates, by resolution, express its appreciation to these agencies.

We are pleased to announce that a two-year program in surgical diagnosis is now in progress. A. G. Fletcher, M.D., F.A.C.S., Philadelphia, Pennsylvania, began instruction in northeastern Oklahoma, February 14. Teaching centers for the first circuit are Miami, Vinita, Bartlesville, Claremore, and Pryor. Approximately 80 per cent of the physicians practicing in this section of the state have enrolled. The second circuit will open

May 1, in the southeastern part of the state with Ada, Sulphur, Durant, Hugo and Idabel as teaching centers.

Further information regarding this course may be obtained at the Postgraduate Booth during the State Medical Meeting at Tulsa. Physicians will have the opportunity of meeting Doctor Fletcher in person at the State Meeting.

Respectfully submitted,
Gregory E. Stanbro, M.D., Chairman
D. B. Ensor, M.D.
J. C. Matheney, M.D.
H. M. McClure, M.D.
M. J. Searle, M.D.
H. C. Weber, M.D.

REPORT OF COMMITTEE ON JUDICIAL AND PROFESSIONAL RELATIONS

The Committee on Judicial and Professional Relations submits the following report to the House of Delegates:

Your Committee on Judicial and Professional Relations desires to report that during 1943-1944 there have been no requests made for assistance from the Medical Defense Fund. Of the two cases previously filed, one has been settled by a verdict in favor of the defendant and the other case has not come to trial.

As of March 1, there was on deposit in the Medical Defense Fund $619.34 augmented by bonds as shown in the audit report of the Association.

Respectfully submitted,
S. A. Lang, M.D., Chairman
J. M. Bonham, M.D.
Claude S. Chambers, M.D.

REPORT OF MEDICAL ADVISORY COMMITTEE TO THE STATE DEPARTMENT OF PUBLIC WELFARE

The Medical Advisory Committee submits the following report to the House of Delegates:

In the early part of the year of 1941, the Department of Public Welfare became increasingly aware of the need for assistance in evaluation of claims of physical disability of parents who apply for aid to dependent children. At that time, the case histories were obtained by a process which included the report from a medical examiner. These examiners were selected at random, usually by the applicant, and they were asked to present a report without compensation. These reports were reviewed by lay members of the Department in the Oklahoma City office who encountered much difficulty in the interpretation of the degree of disability, if any.

For these and other reasons, an appeal was made to the Oklahoma State Medical Association for assistance, and it was suggested that the formation of a Medical Advisory Committee should be considered. This matter was discussed by Dr. Finis. W. Ewing, who was at that time the President of the Oklahoma State Medical Association; Mr. J. B. Harper, Director of the Department of Public Welfare; Mr. R. H. Graham, Executive Secretary of the Oklahoma State Medical Association; Miss Lorraine Ketchum, Assistant Director of the Department of Public Welfare, and Miss Olivia Hemphill, Assistant Supervisor in the Department of Public Assistance.

Dr. Ewing presented the names of five Oklahoma physicians and recommended to the Department of Welfare that these be appointed to this committee. The first meeting was held in the office of the Public Welfare Department in the State Capitol Office Building, on Sunday, July 20, 1941. Members of the Medical Advisory Committee, in addition to those previously mentioned, in attendance were Drs. C. R. Rountree, Oklahoma City; A. R. Sugg, Ada; R. M. Shepard, Tulsa; F. Redding Hood, Oklahoma City, and Clinton Gallaher, Shawnee.

The personnel of the Committee has been changed somewhat by deliberate intent and by the necessity of war. Dr. Moorman P. Prosser of Norman served on the Committee as the advisor in psychiatry. When it became necessary for him to resign, Dr. Hugh Galbraith was appointed. Dr. F. Redding Hood was obliged to resign to report for active duty in the Army. Dr. A. R.

Sugg also felt obligated to resign. Dr. Walker Morledge, Oklahoma City, was appointed to the Committee to replace Dr. Hood, and Dr. Mack I. Shanholtz, Wewoka, was appointed to fill the vacancy created by the resignation of Dr. Sugg. The consulting assistance of Dr. Tullos O. Coston, Oklahoma City, has also been secured.

It became at once apparent that the major project of this Committee would be concerned with the improvement of reports of medical examinations from physicians throughout the state and a more satisfactory interpretation of these reports through better acquaintance of the members of the Committee and the physicians making the examinations. For this reason, the state was somewhat arbitrarily divided into several districts and each district assigned to the particular interest of a certain Committee member.

Certain changes in the original methods have been made as follows: 1. The form of the physician's examination report has been changed and another change is now being contemplated. 2. Arrangement was made for payment of physicians' for examinations. 3. Arrangement has been made to provide special examining procedures as, for example, x-ray, basal metabolic rate, blood chemistry, and other laboratory procedures. 4. The internal organization of the Committe itself has been changed particularly in regard to the formation of a sub-committee consisting of the Chairman and an Assistant Director from the Department of Public Welfare.

Whereas it is freely admitted that the review of cases applying for aid does not yet permit a complete physical and psychiatric inventory, it is the opinion of most of those who are interested and aware of the nature of this work, that there has been distinct improvement in the relative accuracy of evaluating the claims. It is now possible for the Committee collectively, and for its members separately, to consider tolerably complete evidence both medical and social before arriving at any decisions as to recommendation which shall be made.

The regular procedure of an applicant now includes the following conditions. The county director assembles such evidence as appears to be needed in regard to a given case and forwards it to the Oklahoma City office. From this office, the cases are distributed to the several members of the Medical Advisory Committee for recommendation. Recommendation may include straight approval, request for further information—social or medical, or denial. Cases which are approved go on the rolls immediately and in a normal course of events will receive aid for a period of twelve months unless the member of the Committee specifically requests a re-examination at sometime prior to the expiration of the twelve-month period. Cases where further information is requested will be returned to the county director and the additional information added and returned to the Committee member. When denial is recommended however, it is the desire of the Committee that it be the unanimous consent of all members. All denials, therefore, are subject to review by the Committee before the decision is final. When the Committee, as a whole denies aid, no further action is taken by the Department. However, if the applicant is dissatisfied, he may enter what is called an appeal for a fair hearing, in which case a Committee member is asked to name a medical consultant who will act as a referee and the case is no longer in the province of the Medical Advisory Committee. Fair hearing cases are encountered rarely.

It is the opinion of the Medical Advisory Committee that the honest appraisal of a physician who examines a given case should be given strong consideration in any disposal which is made. We are convinced that the physicians are apt to be much better acquainted with the circumstances of a given applicant than any other who expresses opinions concerning his eligibility. It is true that other factors enter into the consideration of a case, but it is true also that a physician examining an applicant, who satisfies himself that the claim should be denied or approved and substantiates his reason for

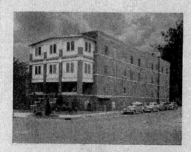
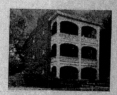

so doing, will usually find his impression is sustained by the Medical Advisory Committee.

We feel that every doctor in the State should be, and is, interested in the evaluation of these claims. We have been able to provide a certain amount of compensation for these examinations. We have been able to more properly evaluate the validity of claims because of the very fine cooperation which we have received from every doctor who has ever been asked to submit a report. The Medical Advisory Committee, in principle at least, is simply trying to interpret the impression and wish of the physicians of this State in regard to the granting or withholding of claims which are presented to the Welfare Board. We hope all physicians continue to be fair and just, and pledge our sustained cooperation in all efforts that seem proper.

Statistical Data Regarding the Activities of the Medical Advisory Committee for the Year 1943

There was a total of 1,116 cases studied by the Medical Advisory Committee for the period January 9, 1943, to January 8, 1944, inclusive. One hundred and two of these cases were carried over from the previous quarter; 667 were new applications, and 130 were presented to the committee because the county department questioned whether or not the parent continued to be incapacitated. Eight cases were re-submitted by the county department for further study by the committee, and 193 were studied because re-examinations had been made at the request of the committee. Sixteen were Fair Hearings.

Of the 1,116 cases studied, the parent was considered incapacitated in 871 cases and not incapacitated in 257 cases. Twenty-two cases were disposed of for ''other'' reasons, and 56 cases are pending.

Of the 1,038 cases in which a final opinion was given by the committee, the committee concurred with the county in 919 cases but did not concur in 119 cases.

A sample of 111 cases from 13 counties by the agency during the three months ending December, 1943, revealed the following information regarding treatment: Treatment was recommended in 95 of the 111 cases. Sixty-one of these 95 cases had been studied by the Medical Advisory Committee. Of the 95 cases where treatment had been recommended, the examining physician recommended treatment in 77 cases, the Medical Advisory Committee recommended treatment in three additional cases, and in 15 cases it was not recorded as to who recommended the treatment. Treatment was provided in 46 of the cases. Treatment was not provided in 47 of the cases, and there was no record of treatment in two of the cases.

Treatment was provided for 46 patients by:

Treatment was provided for 46 patients by: Cost included in the assistance plan, 10; University Hospitals, 9; Private physicians, 2; County Health Physician, 1; Institutional care, 14; Other, 10.

Treatment was not provided in the 47 cases for the following reasons: Treatment not available, 1; Plan initiated but not completed, (Reason for failure to complete not given), 7; Patient refused treatment, 24; No plan initiated, 13; Other, 2.

The treatments recommended and refused by the patients in the majority of cases were as follows: surgery, hospitalization, and institutional care.

Sixteen cases were studied as a result of a request for Fair Hearing. Twelve of these cases were accepted for assistance, one was rejected, one request was withdrawn because of employment and two are pending.

Approximately 2,820 families were receiving aid to dependent children as of January 1, 1944, on the basis of physical or mental incapacity of a parent.

During 1943, a total of $3,611.00 for examinations and laboratory work was paid 366 physicians. Transportation for clients in connection with examinations to determine eligibility for assistance amounted to approximately $85.00 for the calendar year.

Respectfully submitted,

Clinton Gallaher, M.D., Chairman   Walker Morledge, M.D.
C. R. Rountree, M.D.   Hugh Galbraith, M.D.
R. M. Shepard, M.D.   Mack I. Shanholtz, M.D.

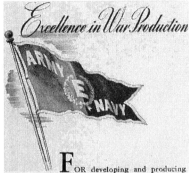
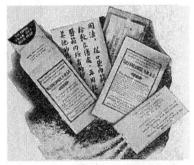

REPORT OF COMMITTEE ON PUBLIC POLICY

The Committee on Public Policy submits the following report to the House of Delegates:

Your Committee wishes to report that its principal activity during the past year has been directed toward the defeating of Senate Bill 1161 more commonly known as the Murray-Wagner-Dingell Bill which purports to create a unified national social insurance system. Because of the implications as it pertains to the medical profession, it is important that every doctor in this country should be well versed on the provisions as set forth in the Bill.

It is the opinion of the Committee that the newly created Council on Medical Service and Public Relations established by the American Medical Association at its Annual Meeting in June, 1943, will be most active in acquainting and advising the physicians of this country with regard to the provisions and import of this bill and likewise in taking suitable measures to combat its passage.

An analysis of the above-named bill with reference to details as pertain to its effect upon medicine prepared by the Bureau of Legal Medicine and Legislation of the American Medical Association appeared in a June issue of the Journal of the American Medical Association. In turn, a reprint of the above was forwarded to each member of the Oklahoma State Medical Association in August of 1943 under the direction of your Public Policy Committee, with the request that each member of the profession contact the Congressman of his District in order that our representatives at the National Capitol might be informed with reference to our attitude as physicians of Federalized Medicine. As a profession, physicians are vitally interested in this legislation for the purpose of protecting the health of the people of the United States.

Senate Bill 1161 is quite detailed and lengthy and endeavors to cover all of the social security in this country in regard to sickness and the provisions of medical and hospital care from the "cradle to the grave." With this thought foremost in our minds, the bill should be of interest to us not only from a physician's standpoint but that of a citizen as well.

Respectfully submitted,

J. D. Osborn, M.D., Chairman
J. T. Martin, M.D.
Frank W. Boadway, M.D.

REPORT OF COMMITTEE ON STUDY AND CONTROL OF TUBERCULOSIS

The Committee on the Study and Control of Tuberculosis submits the following report to the House of Delegates:

A number of conditions have arisen during the past year which have, more or less, affected tuberculous people of the State of Oklahoma.

Great numbers of people have been going to work at defense plants on the West Coast, unaware that they had tuberculosis until they worked there from three months to a year. When it is discovered they are a victim of advanced tuberculosis of the lungs and they are returned to their homes.

There is a decrease in the number of patients being hospitalized at the sanatorium, and I think this is due to the increase of income of all classes. Many are financially able to take rest treatment under the supervision of their local physicians.

The poor housing facilities in these defense areas will cause an increased incident of tuberculosis, which will show up more as time goes on.

Of course, the lack of proper personnel such as doctors, nurses and attendants, still exists at the sanatorium and, in fact, has grown more acute in the past year. This condition will not improve as long as work on the outside is so plentiful and salaries so high.

Your Committee desires to advise that the National Tuberculosis Association and the American Trudeau Society now have a Committee on Therapy to check through

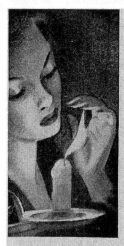

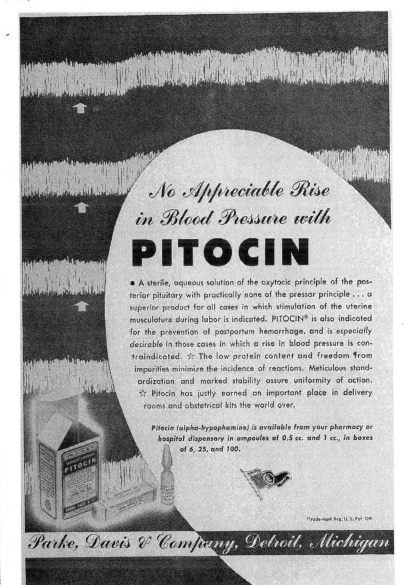

the results of treatment from the new drug diazone with the purpose of helping to keep us well informed. Thus far, there seems to be no bona fide evidence of a cure. Your Committee is advised that the National Tuberculosis Association is contemplating the appointment of an additional Committee for the purpose of inspecting the work in the 20 sanitoria selected for the therapeutic tests of this drug. Their chief purposes are to apprise results and to try to bring about standardized methods with reference to discharge and apprisal of results.

It appears that tuberculosis is going to be one of our major problems after the war; therefore, we should be planning for the future now.

Respectfully submitted,
F. P. Baker, M.D., Chairman
Floyd Moorman, M.D.
R. M. Shepard, M.D.

REPORT OF COMMITTEE ON PUBLIC HEALTH

The Committee on Public Health submits the following report to the House of Delegates:

Your Committee on Public Health during the past year was approached by the local branch of the War Food Administration with reference to the problem of special diets for those under the care of the physician and for hospitals in their care of patients requiring special diets brought forth by the inauguration of the point system of rationing foods.

The appeal for advice on the part of the War Food Administration from the Public Health Committee of the Oklahoma State Medical Association was occasioned by the fact that point rationing covers a large range of meats, fats and processed foods, therefore, making it necessary that extra points be allowed those requiring special diets.

After careful study and research, the Committee presented its recommendations to the Board at which time they were accepted. Certificates requesting extra rations are furnished by local rationing boards and are honored only when the attending physician is licensed to practice medicine and/or surgery in the State of Oklahoma.

A complete listing of the Committee's recommendations for special diets appeared in the December, 1943, issue of the Journal, therefore, will not be repeated in this report.

Respectfully submitted,
Carroll M. Pounders, M.D., Chairman
E. H. Werling, M.D.
Philip C. Risser, M.D.

REPORT OF THE COMMITTEE ON MILITARY AFFAIRS

The Committee on Military Affairs submits the following report to the House of Delegates:

Your Committee on Military Affairs desires to report that it has referred physicians with military experience to County Medical Societies at their request for the purpose of appearing before the meeting of the local Societies to discuss the topics of physical fitness for the Army and Allied subjects.

The Committee recommends that the various County Societies take advantage of the opportunity offered to secure medical personnel of the Armed Forces stationed in Oklahoma to discuss post-war rehabilitation of these men disabled at the battle front.

Since this is the first year the Committee has been appointed, and in view of the fact that some of the military hospitals will be maintained within the State, the Committee further recommends that all members of the profession familiarize themselves with the rehabilitation therapy as used in the various hospitals.

Respectfully submitted,
Louis H. Ritzhaupt, M.D., Chairman
Ralph V. Smith, M.D.
P. P. Nesbitt, M.D.

REPORT OF THE COMMITTEE ON MEDICAL ECONOMICS

The Committee on Medical Economics submits the following report to the House of Delegates:

In 1943, mention was made in the report of your Committee on Medical Economics that the problem concerning cooperation between the Farm Security Administration and the county medical societies had been discussed at various meetings with the decision that the Oklahoma Blue Cross Plan was the logical organization to carry out a hospitalization program.

At this time, your Committee desires to report that thus far enrollment has been completed in nine of the 77 counties; namely, Canadian, Creek, Garfield, Grant, Noble, Okfuskee, Okmulgee, Osage and Pontotoc. The total participants with relation to this program in the above-named counties number 300,905 at the present time.

It is the further information of the Committee from those responsible for the conducting of the hospitalization program that a number of the other counties are now enrolling, and it is anticipated that within two or three months a good percentage will be complete. All of the member hospitals of Blue Cross which total 73 are participating under the ward contract as well as semi-private care.

In last year's report reference was also made with regard to the fact that this committee through the State Association and the local County Medical Societies concern themselves with the economic rehabilitation of the physicians who will return from the present world conflict.

Your Committee desires to report in this respect that a special Committee known as the Post-War Planning Committee was appointed by your President. This Committee presented its recommendations before the Annual Secretaries Conference in October, and they were published in the November issue of the Journal. It is our understanding that a further report will be made by the Post-War Planning Committee setting forth statistics and data secured from conducting the survey among the members of our profession now serving in the Armed Forces before the House of Delegates at its Annual Meeting, April 24.

It is the further desire of your Committee at this time to state that it heartily endorses the recommendations as set out in the preliminary report of the Committee as mentioned above.

Respectfully submitted,
McLain Rogers, M.D., Chairman
H. M. McClure, M.D.
L. R. Kirby, M.D.

REPORT OF COMMITTEE ON MALPRACTICE INSURANCE

The Committee on Malpractice Insurance submits the following report to the House of Delegates:

Your Committee on Malpractice Insurance desires to report to you that on the second anniversary date of the transfer of the Group Policy from the Tulsa County Medical Society to the Oklahoma State Medical Association there was on record with the London and Lancashire Indemnity Company, represented by the local agents Eberle and Company, Oklahoma City, a total of 430 certificates spread over 47 of the 77 counties. They are as follows:

Atoka 1, Beckham 3, Blaine 6, Bryan 4, Caddo 4, Canadian 4, Carter 9, Cleveland 12, Coal 1, Comanche 7, Craig 3, Creek 6, Custer 7, Ellis 5, Garfield 13, Garvin 4, Grady 3, Greer 1, Harmon 1, Hughes 1, Kay 10, LeFlore 1, Lincoln 1, Logan 2, Major 2, Marshall 1, Mayes 2, Muskogee 11, Nowata 1, Okfuskee 3, Oklahoma 132, Okmulgee 10, Osage 6, Ottawa 5, Pawnee 1, Payne 6, Pittsburg 13, Pontotoc 10, Pottawatomie 8, Rogers 2, Seminole 1, Sequoyah 1, Stephens 3, Tulsa 87, Wagoner 1, Washington 10 and Woodward 5.

This represents an increase over 1943 of eight counties and 143 certificates.

During the past year, your Committee contacted the Presidents of the County Medical Societies and requested they appoint a local Committee to approve requests for the issuing of malpractice insurance under the Master Policy of the Association when contacted by the Executive Office. This procedure is followed since it is the opinion of your State Committee that Local Societies are more familiar with their individual members. In some counties blanket approval of the membership has been given by the local Committee, whereas in others approval is periodically requested. Many times the Committee is a blind appointment known only to the President.

At the 1943 meeting of the House of Delegates, it was the recommendation of your Committee that the period of time limit of the Master Policy be extended to cover three years in order that a three-year policy might be obtained at a ten per cent reduction. It is the privilege of the individual applicant to secure a one-year policy however, if he so elects. Statistics as secured from London and Lancashire indicates that 45 three-year certificates have been issued under the Master Policy since April, 1943. Further information reveals that five one-year certificates have been changed to three year terms during this same period.

At a meeting of the Council on October 17, 1943, it was the consensus of opinion of the individual Councilors and so moved and passed that they would be willing to act in an advisory capacity with the local committees and counties in their Districts with reference to information concerning malpractice insurance under the Master Policy should any question arise pertaining thereto.

Your Committee recommends that local county societies continue to urge their membership to secure the benefit of the Group Policy malpractice insurance coverage because of its reduced rate due to the fact that it is available only to members of the Association.

Respectfully submitted,
V. K. Allen, M.D., Chairman
John R. Walker, M.D.
L. J. Starry, M.D.
L. B. Oldman, M.D.

REPORT OF THE COMMITTEE ON INDUSTRIAL MEDICINE AND TRAUMATIC SURGERY

The Committee on Industiral Medicine and Traumatic Surgery submits the following report to the House of Delegates:

Your Committee has met twice during the past year for the purpose of discussing compensation law changes. We have surveyed the legislation of other states covering occupational diseases and providing death benefits, and wish to make the following recommendations:

That the Public Policy Committee be directed by the House of Delegates to contact the State Legislation at its next regular session to discuss amending the present compensation laws to include occupational diseases and to provide for the payment of death claims resulting from occupational injury or disease.

It is the opinion of your Committee on Industrial Medicine and Traumatic Surgery that this coverage is proper and that such revision will not add an appreciable burden to industry. We will be at the service of the Public Policy Committee at any time they may desire assistance in the assembling of any information which we have that might be of value.

Respectfully submitted,
J. S. Chalmers, M.D., Chairman
D. H. O'Donoghue, M.D.
C. E. Northcutt, M.D.

REPORT OF CRIPPLED CHILDREN'S COMMITTEE

The Crippled Children's Committee submits the following report to the House of Delegates:

As is true in all agencies and organizations, the Oklahoma Commission for Crippled Children has likewise felt the effect of the war upon its activities and work during the past year. A number on the professional staff have been called to duty with the various branches of the military. Because of the loss of trained personnel and due to the lack of replacements, work has of necessity been curtailed and a greater burden has been placed on the remaining surgeons and nurses. In addition to the shortage of trained personnel, the lack of hospital beds due to over-crowded conditions and trans-

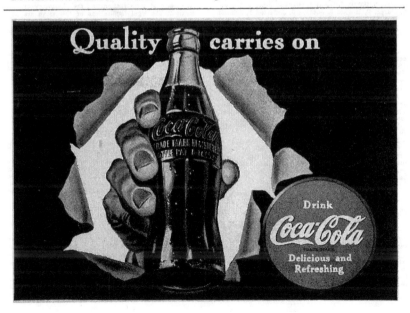

portation difficulties have likewise presented serious problems.

At the time of the outbreak of poliomyelitis in Oklahoma during the summer of 1943, your Committee in cooperation with the University Medical School, its teaching hospitals, the Oklahoma Commission for Crippled Children, the State Health Department and other interested agencies released a bulletin to all members of the Association outlining the program of treatment in effect at the Crippled Children's Hospital for the combating of polio. Likewise, every cooperation in the treatment of acute cases was extended by the State Chapter of the National Foundation for Infantile Paralysis.

With the increase of cases, it was later necessary to enroll the facilities of hospitals in other sections of the State and those points selected were Clinton and Tulsa.

Information received from Joe N. Hamilton, Secretary of the Oklahoma Commission for Crippled Children, reveals that the County Chapters of the National Foundation of Infantile Paralysis in Oklahoma contributed $24,905.76 during the 1943 epidemic for use in the concentrated points. In turn, this was distributed as follows: Western State Charity Hospital, Clinton, $3,538.35; St. John's Hospital and Junior League Home, Tulsa, $9,554.18, and Crippled Children's Hospital, Oklahoma City, $11,813.23. In addition, the National Foundation, New York, contributed a total of $9,200.00 for help in the program which was distributed in the following manner: Tulsa $5,200.00; Oklahoma City, $3,000.00, and Clinton, 1,000.00.

In statistics just released from the State Department of Health, it is indicated there was a reported total of 594 cases of poliomyelitis in Oklahoma during 1943. These are listed on a statewide scale with only four of the counties reporting no cases: namely, Adair, Cimarron, Haskell and Ottawa. Other counties and the reported number of cases are as follows:

Alfalfa 1, Atoka 1, Beaver 3, Beckham 8, Blaine 5, Bryan 6, Caddo 11, Canadian 12, Carter 11, Cherokee 5, Choctaw 7, Cleveland 18, Coal 4, Comanche 22, Cotton 1, Craig 1, Creek 8, Custer 11, Delaware 1, Dewey 5, Ellis 1, Garfield 8, Garvin 7, Grady 8, Grant 2, Greer 1, Harmon 1, Harper 2, Hughes 9, Jackson 3, Jefferson 2, Johnson 1, Kay 15, Kingfisher 1, Kiowa 4.

Latimer 2, LeFlore 12, Lincoln 7, Logan 10, Love 3, McClain 7, McCurtain 10, McIntosh 3, Major 4, Marshall 5, Mayes 8, Murray 3, Muskogee 14, Noble 4, Nowata 1, Okfuskee 3, Oklahoma 79, Okmulgee 7, Osage 7, Pawnee 4, Payne 7, Pittsburg 13, Pontotoc 13, Pottawatomie 18, Pushmataha 2, Roger Mills 5, Rogers 3, Seminole 27, Sequoyah 6, Stephens 7, Texas 19, Tillman 6, Tulsa 38, Wagoner 4, Washington 14, Washita 4, Woods 2 and Woodward 7.

It is interesting to note by color distinction that of the total number of cases, 551 were white, 24 were negro, eight were Indian and eleven unknown. Of this number, ten were military personnel.

The total number of deaths resulting was 33 reported from 19 counties and all were white.

It is the recommendation of your Committee that in order to properly carry on the Crippled Children's program, the cooperation of all interested agencies engaged in this particular type of work, including health departments, the medical profession, hospitals and nurses, be continued at all times.

Respectfully submitted,
Ian MacKenzie, M.D., Chairman
Carroll M. Pounders, M.D.
L. S. Willour, M.D.

REPORT OF COMMITTEE ON CONSERVATION OF VISION AND HEARING

The Committee on Conservation of Vision and Hearing submits the following report to the House of Delegates:

Your Committee has worked with the Crippled Children's Commission in devising and carrying on a program to provide glasses for under-privileged children. In brief, the child is checked by the social service workers, sent to a qualified Specialist as determined by the State Medical Association Committee, and is examined for a fee of $5.00.

The glasses are provided by the Crippled Children's Fund. The examiner assumes the responsibility of seeing that the prescription is filled correctly and the glasses properly adjusted. The fee of $5.00 amounts to approximately half price for the same service rendered to private patients and, of course, the patients must be in the financially dependent group.

Respectfully submitted,
F. Maxey Cooper, M.D., Chairman.
Charles H. Haralson, M.D.
J. B. Hollis, M.D.

REPORT OF COMMITTEE ON MATERNITY AND INFANCY

The Committee on Maternity and Infancy submits the following report to the House of Delegates:

A meeting of the Committee was held in Tulsa, April 1943, at which time the plans for the coming year were discussed. The Committee then appeared before the Muskogee County Medical Association and presented maternal mortality statistics before that group.

At the annual convention of Presbyterian ministers held at Enid, Oklahoma in June, 1943, the Committee appeared by invitation and discussed the problem of abortions in Oklahoma. By unanimous vote, the ministerial group voted to make this material available to the individual ministers, and a resolution was passed recommending this subject for discussion from the pulpit on the next ensuing Mother's Day.

The same subject was discussed before the Ministerial Alliance in Oklahoma City at its noon luncheon, and several individual ministers promised to use the subject for pulpit discussion.

The Committee met with Mr. A. L. Crable, State Superintendent of Schools, at which time plans were discussed for the preparation of a small booklet which would be available for high-school students explaining the physiology of menstruation and the physiology of conception. The legal implications of this move are now under consideration.

At the present time an effort is being made to contact the ministers of various denominations and to make available to them the factual material contained in the annual report of maternal mortality, with the view to the utilization of this material from the pulpit in a state wide campaign to educate the pregnant woman to avoid the abortionist, and to report early for ante partum care.

Respectfully submitted,
Edward N. Smith, M.D., Chairman
J. T. Bell, M.D.
E. O. Johnson, M.D.

REPORT OF COMMITTEE ON NECROLOGY

The Committee on Necrology submits the following report to the House of Delegates:

In the present world-wide emergency, medicine's duty to humanity finds physicians on all fronts. Their duty is to save rather than to take life. Many physicians are paying the supreme sacrifice on the battle front; likewise, other physicians are performing their service on the home front.

In honor of those members of the Association who have passed away during the past year, the Committee on Necrology submits the following resolution for adoption by the House of Delegates:

WHEREAS, 16 of our members have passed to the Great Beyond since the 1943 report of the Committee on Necrology of the Association,

THEREFORE, BE IT RESOLVED, That the House of Delegates of the Oklahoma State Medical Association recognize the demise of these fellow members and instruct the Secretary to inscribe with honor and regret the following names upon the records of the Association:

*H. P. Wilson	Wynnewood	May 1, 1943
U. S. Cordell	Macomb	May 28, 1943
F. R. Buchanan	Canton	June 30, 1943
C. E. Bradley	Tulsa	July 6, 1943
S. S. Garrett	Duncan	August 8, 1943
Charles T. Schrader	Bristow	August 27, 1943
Marion O. Brice	Okemah	September 7, 1943
John L. Fortson	Tecumseh	September 10, 1943
Sam H. Williamson	Bethany	September 14, 1943
C. C. Bombarger	Paden	September 18, 1943
*Issac S. Hunt	Freedom	October 15, 1943
John P. Rutherford	Bennington	October 31, 1943
*E. P. Clapper	Waynoka	November 28, 1943
James R. McLauchlin	Oklahoma City	December 26, 1943
Benjamin W. Slover	Blanchard	January 8, 1944
P. M. Richardson	Cushing	January 10, 1944
Roy W. Dunlap	Tulsa	January 28, 1944
Fred Y. Cronk	Tulsa	February 12, 1944

* Honorary

Respectfully submitted,
J. S. Fulton, M.D., Chairman
O. S. Somerville, M.D.
John A. Walker, M.D.

HONORARY MEMBERSHIP APPLICATIONS

In accordance with the provisions of Chapter I, Section 3, Subsection (b), of the By-Laws, the following names have been submitted to the Executive Office of the Association for election to Honorary Membership:

N. N. Simpson, Henryetta
J. M. Postelle, Oklahoma City
W. H. Livermore, Chickasha
Walker W. Beesley, Tulsa
J. E. Brookshire, Tulsa
Paul R. Brown, Tulsa
Gilbert H. Hall, Tulsa
Joel S. Hooper, Tulsa
James L. Reynolds, Tulsa
Albert W. Roth, Tulsa

ASSOCIATE MEMBERSHIP APPLICATIONS

In compliance with the provisions of Chapter I, Section 3, Subsection (d), of the By-Laws of the Association, the names of the following physicians have been submittd to the office of the Association for election to Associate Membership. The Pottawatomie County Medical Society has proposed the name of Dr. Ralph M. Alley of Shawnee, and the Council of the Association desires to offer the name of Dr. David A. Myers of San Francisco, Calif., past President of the Oklahoma State Medical Association in 1910-1911.

ANNUAL AUDIT REPORT

February 21, 1944

James Stevenson, M.D., President
Oklahoma State Medical Association
210 Plaza Court
Oklahoma City, Oklahoma

Dear Sir:

We have completed the audit of the financial records of

THE OKLAHOMA STATE MEDICAL ASSOCIATION

Oklahoma City, Oklahoma

for the period from January 1, 1943, to December 31, 1943, and submit herewith the following Exhibits:

EXHIBIT "1"—BALANCE SHEET

EXHIBIT "2"—STATEMENT OF CASH RECEIPTS AND DISBURSEMENTS

EXHIBIT "3"—OPERATING STATEMENT

EXHIBIT "4"—BANK RECONCILIATION

EXPLANATION

Since the Association operates on a Cash Receipts and Disbursements basis, the disbursements for December, which are paid in January, are included in the report for the following year.

We wish to thank you for this audit, and if we can be of further service, please feel free to call upon us.

Respectfully submitted,
H. E. COLE COMPANY

EXHIBIT "1"

OKLAHOMA STATE MEDICAL ASSOCIATION
Oklahoma City, Oklahoma

BALANCE SHEET
Dec. 31, 1943

ASSETS	Total	Membership Fund	Journal Fund	Medical Defense Fund	Annual Meeting
Petty Cash	$ 10.69	$ 10.69	$	$	$
Bank	10,316.20	7,843.55	1,260.81	606.84	605.00
U. S. Treasury Bonds	6,178.88	1,235.78		4,943.10	
U. S. Defense Bonds	3,220.00			3,220.00	
U. S. Savings Bonds	1,000.00	1,000.00			
TOTAL ASSETS	$20,725.77	$10,090.02	$ 1,260.81	$ 8,769.94	$ 605.00

LIABILITIES

Operating Reserve	$20,725.77	$10,090.02	$ 1,260.81	$ 8,769.94	$ 605.00
TOTAL LIABILITIES	$20,725.77	$10,090.02	$ 1,260.81	$ 8,769.94	$ 605.00

EXHIBIT "2"

OKLAHOMA STATE MEDICAL ASSOCIATION
Oklahoma City, Oklahoma

STATEMENT OF CASH RECEIPTS & DISBURSEMENTS
January 1, 1943 to December 31, 1943

	Total	Membership Fund	Journal Fund	Medical Defense Fund	Annual Meeting
Cash Balance—January 1, 1943	$ 6,076.43	$ 4,069.46	$ 1,321.63	$ 685.34	$
Petty Cash Balance—January 1, 1943	11.37	11.37			
Transfer from Membership Fund*	1,000.00		1,000.00		

RECEIPTS:

Membership Dues 1943	$15,257.00	$15,257.00	$	$	$
Membership Dues 1942	10.00	9.00		1.00	
Journal Advertising & Subscriptions	7,969.81		7,969.81		
Government Bond Interest	147.50	27.00		120.50	
Exhibit—1942 Meeting	55.00	55.00			
Refund—Social Security	459.17	459.17			
Annual Meeting 1943	828.00	828.00			
Annual Meeting 1944	605.00				605.00
Total Cash to be Accounted for	$32,419.28	$20,716.00	$10,291.44	$ 806.84	$ 605.00

DISBURSEMENTS:

Expenses for 1943	$20,092.39	$10,861.76	$ 9,030.63	$ 200.00	$
U. S. Savings Bonds	1,000.00	1,000.00			
Transfers	1,000.00	1,000.00			
	$22,092.39	$12,861.76	$ 9,030.63	$ 200.00	$
Bank Balance—December 31, 1943	$10,316.20	$ 7,843.55	$ 1,260.81	$ 606.84	$ 605.00
Petty Cash—December 31, 1943	10.69	10.69			
	$10,326.89	$ 7,854.24	$ 1,260.81	$ 606.84	$ 605.00

* NOTE—Transfer of $1,000.00 was made from Membership Fund to Journal Fund to take care of Publication Deficit.

OKLAHOMA STATE MEDICAL ASSOCIATION
Oklahoma City, Oklahoma

EXHIBIT "3"

OPERATING STATEMENT
1943

	Total	Membership Fund	Journal Fund	Medical Defense Fund	Annual Meeting
REVENUES:					
Membership Dues 1943	$15,257.00	$15,257.00	$	$	$
Membership Dues 1942	10.00	9.00		1.00	
Journal Advertising & Subscriptions	7,969.81		7,969.81		
U. S. Government Bonds Interest	147.50	27.00		120.50	
Exhibit 1942 Meeting	55.00	55.00			
Annual Meeting 1944	605.00				605.00
Annual Meeting 1943	828.00	828.00			
Social Security Refund	459.17	459.17			
TOTAL REVENUE	$25,331.48	$16,635.17	$ 7,969.81	$ 121.50	$ 605.00

EXPENSE:

Salaries	$ 7,998.80	$ 3,967.50	$ 4,031.30	$	$
Telephone & Telegraph	657.40	657.40			
Rent	300.00	150.00	150.00		
Stationery & Printing	565.08	483.99	81.09		
Office Supplies	272.74	272.74			
Traveling Expense	628.82	628.82			
Journal Printing & Mailing	4,343.87		4,343.87		
Journal Engraving	152.06		152.06		
Auditing & Legal	350.00	75.00	75.00	200.00	
Express	5.91	5.91			
A. M. A. Delegate Expense	275.56	275.56			
Postage	445.28	345.07	100.21		
Engraving Cards	20.91	20.91			
Social Security Refunds to employees	198.71	198.71			
Post Graduate Committee	2,000.00	2,000.00			
Repair—typewriter	15.00	15.00			
Sundry Expense	62.95	62.95			
Annual Meeting Expense	1,333.02	1,333.02			
Surety Bond	57.61	57.61			
Pictures & Framing Past Presidents	192.53	192.53			
Annual Secretaries Conference	119.04	119.04			
History of Okla. Medicine	97.10		97.10		
TOTAL EXPENSES	**$20,092.39**	**$10,861.76**	**$ 9,030.63**	**$ 200.00**	
Revenue over Expenses	$ 5,239.00	$ 5,773.41	—$ 1,060.82	—$ 78.50	$ 605.00

OKLAHOMA STATE MEDICAL ASSOCIATION
Oklahoma City, Oklahoma
EXHIBIT ''4''
BANK RECONCILIATION
December 31, 1943

Liberty National Bank

MEMBERSHIP FUND

Balance per Bank Statement	$ 7,896.85
Deposit of 12-24-43, posted to Defense Fund by Bank	25.50
	$ 7,922.35
Outstanding Checks:	
Voucher No. 1185 ....$78.80	$ 78.80
Balance Per Books	$ 7,843.55

JOURNAL FUND

Balance Per Bank Statement	$ 1,324.01
Outstanding Checks:	
Voucher No. 1183 ....$63.20	$ 63.20
Balance Per Books	$ 1,260.81

ANNUAL MEETING FUND

Balance Per Bank Statement	$ 605.00
Balance Per Books	$ 605.00

MEDICAL DEFENSE FUND

Balance Per Bank Statement	$ 606.84
Balance Per Books	$ 606.84
TOTAL MONEY ON DEPOSIT	$10,316.20

★ FIGHTIN' TALK ★

The following appointments and promotions have been reported: Ordered to Active Duty: LT. COL. HARVEY C. HARDEGREE, Muskogee; MAJOR JAMES H. PARKER, Muskogee; MAJOR GILBERT H. ALEXANDER, Muskogee; CAPT. ALBERT ROME, Muskogee; LT. JAMES C. AMSPACHER, Norman; LT. JON DEWITT ASHLEY, JR., Oklahoma City; LT. HARVEY C. ROYS and LT. ALBIN MONROE BRIXEY, JR., Norman; LT. CHARLES SHELLY GRAYBILL, Lawton; LT. MASON R. LYONS, Anadarko; LT. CLEVE BELLER, Stigler; LT. OLIVER HAROLD THOMPSON, Tulsa; LT. JOHN BENNETT JARROTT, Oklahoma City; LT. GEORGE LOGAN TRACEWELL, Okmulgee. Promoted from lieutenant to captain: CAPT. SAMUEL BREWSTER LESLIE, JR., Okmulgee; CAPT. RALPH W. MORTON, Sulphur; CAPT. WALDO B. NEWELL, JR., Enid. Promoted from captain to major: MAJOR D. L. EDWARDS, Tulsa; MAJOR WILLIAM K. ISHMAEL, Oklahoma City; MAJOR RALPH W. RUCKER, Bartlesville; MAJOR FLOYD T. BARTHELD, McAlester; MAJOR JAMES S. PETTY, Guthrie.

COLONEL REX BOLEND arrived in Oklahoma City on leave from the Pacific theater of war. Colonel Bolend has been connected with the University of Oklahoma Evacuation Hospital and is home for surgical treatment. Twenty seven of the 37 doctors and dentists serving on the Staff of the Hospital are Oklahomans. COLONEL GEORGE H. KIMBALL and COLONEL BERT MULVEY are top ranking officers. Colonel Bolend says that the Hospital and all the staff are "on the job" and are saving hundreds of lives. He will leave shortly for the West Coast where he will be reassigned.

CAPT. H. MYLES JOHNSON, Supply, has recently had a hand in saving the lives of 2,000 Chinese soldiers on the battlefields of Burma. Capt. Johnson is attached to the famous Seagrave Hospital Unit headed by Lt. Col. Gordon S. Seagrave, author of the book "Burma Surgeon." The unit is with General Stilwell's forces who are clearing the northern Burma so that American engineers can extend the Ledo road to the Burma road.

MAJOR PATRICK H. LAWSON, Marietta, in charge of a medical station on the Anzio beachhead in Italy, experienced a German bombing recently. Major Lawson says that the Germans dropped a bomb in the hospital area which landed near the hospital kitchen, wounding two men. Several hospital tents were struck but there were no other casualties.

LT. COMDR. JOHNNY A. BLUE, Guymon, commissioned in the Navy two years ago, has recently been transferred to the base hospital at Pearl Harbor. Lt. Comdr. Blue was medical officer at the navy recruiting office in Oklahoma City.

Word has been received from MAJOR PAUL B. LINGENFELTER, Clinton. Major Lingenfelter is in the Southwest Pacific and says that they are all working hard and are set up so that they can do excellent work.

CAPT. ZALE CHAFFIN, who was with the city Health Department before entering the Army two years ago, has been on Los Negros island. It is reported that the going was a bit rough with Japs, rain and mud to battle.

LT. HAROLD J. BINDER, Oklahoma City, is now stationed at Lawson General Hospital in Atlanta, Georgia, where he was sent from Carlisle Barracks. Lt. Binder has completed the course of Military Neuropsychiatry at the Mason General Hospital and feels that he is now "a full-fledged army neuropsychiatrist."

LT. LOGAN A. SPANN, Tulsa, writes to us from the South Pacific area and states that he has seen a group of the Oklahoma doctors recently. He says that they all have a nice sun-tan but that somebody made a mistake on the posters depicting the beautiful tropical South Sea Islands.

LT. (jg) LOUIS R. DEVANNEY, recently had a little difficulty with his Draft Board. A card was sent to Lt. Devanney to report for pre-induction examination. When he did not appear, inquiries were made as to his whereabouts. The Marine Corps advised that he may be found in the Marshall Islands where he is busy taking care of a little business with the Japs.

CAPT. ISADORE DYER, Talequah, has recently had a promotion. He writes us from his station at Biggs Field, Texas and encloses a very interesting caricature of himself depicting him as a Flight (?) Surgeon with dreams of the proverbial stork. Capt. Dyer is at Biggs Field training heavy bombardment crews for overseas. He states that at a high altitude on a clear day he can almost see the smoke rising from some of Ed White's barbecues.

MAJOR CHARLES A. SMITH, formerly connected with the Coyne Campbell Clinic in Oklahoma City, has been overseas in the South Pacific about six months. He was stationed at Camp Huachuca, Arizona before going across.

LT. FRANK H. SISLER, JR., Bristow, has completed the flight surgeon's course at Pensacola and has been sent to the U. S. Naval Air Station at Glenview, Illinois. We enjoyed the letter from Lt. Sisler.

A very interesting V-Mail was recently received from Capt. J. R. Ricks, Oklahoma City. His letter reads in part:

"I spent a year in Panama training in jungle warfare. I liked that command and we worked and trained hard all year long. The last of December 1942, I was given this Company to come to the Southwest Pacific. We trained in Australia and have been out of there ten months now and are on our third straight mission since then when we made our first amphibious landing unopposed. We set up the hospital with my fine officers and men and ran mostly medical cases. We then got our first combat mission and managed to do O. K. We were bombed and straffed a lot in landing, while we were there, and as we left. Spent our time living in fox holes and slit trenches when we weren't doing surgery or medicine in our improved bomb proof dugout. We were then pulled out and sent on this mission but it has been as easy as pie. We are located in a dense forest of huge hardwood trees with beautiful overhead cover for concealment. It is like living in a huge air cathedral since you look up 80 to 100 feet to see the light filtering down to us. Rains a lot and we have a problem trying to dry patient's pajamas. Doing surgery and plenty of tropical medicine."

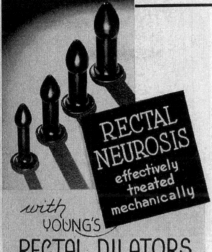

OFFICERS OF COUNTY SOCIETIES, 1944

★

COUNTY	PRESIDENT	SECRETARY	MEETING TIME
Alfalfa	H. E. Huston, Cherokee	L. T. Lancaster, Cherokee	Last Tues. each Second Month
Atoka-Coal	R. C. Henry, Coalgate	J. S. Fulton, Atoka	
Beckham	G. H. Stagner, Erick	O. C. Standifer, Elk City	Second Tuesday
Blaine	L. R. Kirby, Okeene	W. F. Griffin, Watonga	
Bryan	John T. Wharton, Durant	W. K. Haynie, Durant	Second Tuesday
Caddo	F. L. Patterson, Carnegie	C. B. Sullivan, Carnegie	
Canadian	P. F. Herod, El Reno	A. L. Johnson, El Reno	Subject to call
Carter	J. R. Pollock, Ardmore	H. A. Higgins, Ardmore	
Cherokee	P. H. Medearis, Tahlequah	W. M. Wood, Tahlequah	First Tuesday
Choctaw	C. H. Hale, Boswell	E. A. Johnson, Hugo	
Cleveland	F. T. Gastineau, Norman	Iva S. Merritt, Norman	Thursday nights
Comanche	George L. Berry, Lawton	Howard Angus, Lawton	
Cotton	A. B. Holstead, Temple	Mollie F. Seism, Walters	Third Friday
Craig	Lloyd H. McPike, Vinita	Paul G. Sauger, Vinita	
Creek	J. E. Hollis, Bristow	W. G. Bishee, Bristow	
Custer	F. R. Vieregg, Clinton	C. J. Alexander, Clinton	Third Thursday
Garfield	Julian Feild, Enid	John E. Walker, Enid	Fourth Thursday
Garvin	T. F. Gross, Lindsay	John R. Callaway, Pauls Valley	Wednesday before Third Thursday
Grady	Walter J. Baze, Chickasha	Roy E. Emanuel, Chickasha	Third Thursday
Grant	J. V. Hardy, Medford		
Greer	R. W. Lewis, Granite	J. B. Hollis, Mangum	
Harmon	W. G. Husband, Hollis	R. H. Lynch, Hollis	First Wednesday
Haskell	William Carson, Keota	N. K. Williams, McCurtain	
Hughes	Wm. L. Taylor, Holdenville	Imogene Mayfield, Holdenville	First Friday
Jackson	C. G. Spears, Altus	E. A. Abernethy, Altus	Last Monday
Jefferson	F. M. Edwards, Ringling	L. I. Wade, Ryan	Second Monday
Kay	J. Holland Howe, Ponca City	G. H. Yeary, Newkirk	Second Thursday
Kingfisher	A. O. Meredith, Kingfisher	H. Violet Sturgeon, Hennessey	
Kiowa	J. William Finch, Hobart	William Bornell, Hobart	
LeFlore	Newson Rolle, Poteau	Rush L. Wright, Poteau	
Lincoln	W. B. Davis, Stroud	Carl H. Bailey, Stroud	First Wednesday
Logan	William C. Miller, Guthrie	J. L. LeHew, Jr., Guthrie	Last Tuesday
Marshall	J. A. Holland, Madill	J. F. York, Madill	
Mayes	Ralph V. Smith, Pryor	Paul B. Cameron, Pryor	
McClain	W. C. McCurdy, Sr., Purcell	W. C. McCurdy, Jr., Purcell	
McCurtain	A. W. Clarkson, Vallinut	N. L. Barker, Broken Bow	Fourth Tuesday
McIntosh	Luster I. Jacobs, Hanna	Wm. A. Tolleson, Eufaula	First Thursday
Murray	P. V. Annadown, Sulphur	J. A. Wrenn, Sulphur	Second Tuesday
Muskogee-Sequoyah			
Wagoner	H. A. Scott, Muskogee	D. Evelyn Miller, Muskogee	First Monday
Noble	C. H. Cooke, Perry	J. W. Francis, Jerry	
Okfuskee	C. M. Cochran, Okemah	M. L. Whitney, Okemah	Second Monday
Oklahoma	W. E. Eastland, Oklahoma City	E. R. Musick, Oklahoma City	Fourth Tuesday
Okmulgee	S. B. Leslie, Okmulgee	J. C. Matheney, Okmulgee	Second Monday
Osage	C. R. Weirich, Pawhuska	George K. Hemphill, Pawhuska	Second Monday
Ottawa	Walter Kerr, Picher	B. W. Shelton, Miami	Third Thursday
Pawnee	E. T. Robinson, Cleveland	R. L. Browning, Pawnee	
Payne	H. C. Munning, Cushing	J. W. Martin, Cushing	Third Thursday
Pittsburg	P. T. Powell, McAlester	W. H. Kaeiser, McAlester	Third Friday
Pontotoc	A. R. Sugg, Ada	R. H. Mayes, Ada	First Wednesday
Pottawatomie	E. Eugene Rice, Shawnee	Clinton Gallaher, Shawnee	First and Third Saturday
Pushmataha	John S. Lawson, Clayton	B. M. Huckabay, Antlers	
Rogers	R. C. Meloy, Claremore	Chas. L. Caldwell, Chelsea	First Monday
Seminole	J. T. Price, Seminole	Mack I. Shanholtz, Wewoka	Third Wednesday
Stephens	W. K. Walker, Marlow	Wallis S. Ivy, Duncan	
Texas	R. G. Obermiller, Texhoma	Morris Smith, Guymon	
Tillman	C. C. Allen, Frederick	O. G. Bacon, Frederick	
Tulsa	Ralph A. McGill, Tulsa	E. O. Johnson, Tulsa	Second and Fourth Monday
Washington-Nowata	K. D. Davis, Nowata	J. V. Athey, Bartlesville	Second Wednesday
Washita	A. S. Neal, Cordell	James F. McMurry, Sentinel	
Woods	Ishmael F. Stephenson, Alva	Oscar E. Templin, Alva	Last Tuesday Odd Months
Woodward	H. Walker, Buffalo	C. W. Tedrowe, Woodward	Second Thursday

*(Serving in Armed Forces)

THE JOURNAL

OF THE

OKLAHOMA STATE MEDICAL ASSOCIATION

| VOLUME XXXVII | OKLAHOMA CITY, OKLAHOMA, APRIL, 1944 | NUMBER 4 |

Surgical Complications of Pregnancy and Their Complications[*]

GERALD ROGERS, M.D.

OKLAHOMA CITY, OKLAHOMA

Pregnancy does not preclude the occasional necessity for surgical procedures. These, if major, unquestionably increase both maternal and fetal morbidity and mortality. The internist who has studied various medical conditions in pregnant women is cognizant of the fact that pregnancy alters both the anatomy and physiology of not only the abdominal organs, but of the body as a whole. These changes must be understood by the obstetrician and the surgeon before they can accurately diagnose and treat non-obstetric surgical complications of pregnancy. Symptomatology is often obscure, laboratory procedures may confuse, and delay may proportionately increase both maternal and fetal morbidity and mortality. In general, it should be emphasized that the principles of recognizing and handling acute abdominal emergencies during pregnancy are the same whether the patient is pregnant or not. Furthermore, it should be remembered that a differential diagnosis is not always possible. It is of the highest importance, above all, to recognize that an acute abdominal emergency exists, and to manage the situation accordingly. It is the purpose of this discussion to enumerate and review cases seen in my private practice during the past five years which have demanded surgical intervention and management .

In general, two types of surgical complications in the abdomen may occur during pregnancy, those which involve the organs of reproduction, and those which occur in other organs but may also be found during the period of gestation. In the former group we

*Read before the Annual Meeting held in Oklahoma City, May 11-12, 1943.

find ectopic gestation with accompanying hemorrhages. I have excluded from this discussion these cases. Table No. 1 lists the major complications which were treated during this five year period.

Nine of these cases were subjected to laparotomy during pregnancy. Only one case aborted. While there are certain precautions and a few "don'ts" which were carefully observed, I would not assume credit for any unusual surgical skill. The use of progesteon in adequate dosage both pre-operatively and post-operatively, in my opinion, is the responsible factor. The big problem is to determine how much to give. We have no practical hormone assay technique. The expense, if obtainable, would cost more than a few extra doses of progestin. I am certain my cases received more than was necessary. All elective cases received five units the night before and morning of operation. The preparation was given every six to eight hours post-operatively the first three days, and then five units daily until the patient was out of bed.

The optimum time to perform an indicated elective laparotomy during pregnancy is at the twelfth to the fourteenth week. Prior to this period there is greater hazard of abortion, and afterward the mechanical difficulties attendant to adequate surgical exposure of pathology may produce unnecessary trauma.

These cases were operated under ethylene, cyclopropaine and local infiltration anesthesia. Cyclopropane is unquestionably the ideal anesthetic agent for major obstetrical procedures. Extreme Trendelenberg position minimized packing away of intestines and adjacent viscera. Use warm packs, not hot packs, and be gentle! A wider use of local anesthesia will insure the last point. Adequate post-operative fluids and narcosis is indicated. It is my observation that less nausea is seen by use of pantopon and dilaudid. Post-operative nausea and vomiting are contributory factors to exciting uterine cramps.

FIBROMYOMA UTERI COMPLICATING PREGNANCY

The presence of small uterine fibromyoma is one of the very common pathological conditions noticed during pregnancy and rarely is there occasion for alarm as to the prognosis of labor or the possibility of postpartum hemorrhage. As a general rule, there should be no fear of fibroids in pregnancy as they may be considered as one of the many things incidental to the pregnancy, and in most instances we merely treat the pregnancy and take the fibroids as they come. Certain myomas, however, may act as an obstruction to labor, become incarcerated in the cul-de-sac, produce a retention of urine and, in rare instances, undergo necrosis and necrobiosis causing severe abdominal pain and hyperpyrexia, necessitating their enucleation during pregnancy. It is my policy not to advise operation for fibromyomata during pregnancy unless the size of the tumor and location would indicate that pressure symptoms might arise late in pregnancy or pain would indicate acute degeneration or pedicle tortion. In event of the former, an operation should be performed only if one is positive that the fibroid has a pedicle. If there is a definite obstruction to the birth canal by the tumor, a cesarean section, myomectomy or hysterectomy should be performed as deemed advisable at term. In general, in treating the pregnant patient with uterine fibroid the following management is advised:

1. There should be careful observation during the course of the pregnancy without interference unless symptoms of sufficient magnitude arise.

2. Natural delivery should be allowed to go on unless the size or the location of the tumor produces obstruction to the passage of the fetus.

3. A trial of labor should be permitted in doubtful cases.

4. When operative interference prior to delivery is indicated by necrosis in the tumor, by obstruction to the birth canal or by failure of a normal uterine mechanism it should consist of Cesarean section with myomectomy, or preferably hysterectomy.

5. If operative interference becomes necessary during puerperium hysterectomy is usually the procedure of choice. This state-

ment is adequately confirmed by the literature in case reports.

6. From reported cases in the literature myomectomy with Cesarean section carries an appreciably greater mortality and therefore its employment is generally contraindicated.

7. Fibromyomatas, per se, do not necessarily indicate either hysterectomy or myomectomy. A brief summary of the cases in this series necessitating surgical intervention is given.

CASE No. 1

Mrs. T. W., age 43, Para O. Gravida I. First consulted her physician at third month.

Diagnosis: Pregancy and multiple fibroids, size of six months gestation. Elected to go to term.

I saw this patient in consultation because she had stopped labor and had been dilated several hours, 48 hours after rupture of membranes. Condition critical, temperature 101, pulse 120. Uterus ligneous. Fetal heart tones absent. Mal-odorous, purulent vaginal drainage. Labor induced — castor oil and quinine totaling 36 grains in 3 grain doses. Sterile vaginal revealed a hard spherical tumor pushing against perineum. Cervix closed and pulled up behind pubes.

Diagnosis: Intra-uterine pregnancy at term.

1. Multiple fibroids.
2. Obstructed labor.
3. Tetanic uterus.
4. Dead baby.
5. Intra-partum sepsis.

Consultants: Drs. Dick Lowry and E. F. Allen.

Operation: Poro-hysterectomy.

Post-operative Course: Stormy for first ten days, then prognosis seemed very favorable. Sudden death, apparently from pulmonary embolus on 17th post-operative night. A classical example of mal-obstetric judgment and management of labor.

CASE No. 2

Mrs. V. Y., age 30, Para O. Gravida I. This patient was first seen June 1935 because of signs of threatened abortion. A patient in Moorman Sanatorium, she had had bilateral phrenicectomy for extensive bilateral bronchiectasis. Diagnosis of complicated fibroid made. Patient responded to treatment.

Labor: Onset at 36 weeks, November 27, 1938. Six hours test of labor. Tumor in lower segment prevented engagement.

Diagnosis: Intrauterine pregnancy 36 weeks, position and presentation Sc. C. T. (confirmed by x-ray). Bilateral bronchiectasis with bilateral phrenicectomy. Fibroid obstructing labor.

Consultants: Drs. Floyd Moorman and Dick Lowry.

Operation: Laparo-trachelotomy and myomectomy, local anesthetic.

Post-operative course: Two febrile readings.

CASE No 3

Mrs. D. E., age 26, Gravida I. Last menstraul period October 23, 1940. This patient was admitted to the hospital January 2, 1941 complaining of retention of urine and amenorrhea.

Diagnosis: Pregnancy of 11 to 12 weeks. Incarcerated fibroid with retroversion. Retention of urine, acute.

Operation: January 3, myomectomy, nodule 11-12 cm in diameter beneath symphysis.

Post-operative Course: Afebrile. No uterine cramps.

Delivery: At term, July 30, 1942, low forceps, episiotomy and repair.

CASE No. 4

Mrs. H. M., age 37, Para O. Gravida I. Married 11 years. First seen December 18. This patient's chief complaint was amenorrhea since September 26. Pelvic pressure, constipation, tender breasts with slight enlargement.

Examination: Uterus boggy, size 8 to 10 weeks gestation. Displaced anteriorly by solid, somewhat irregular neoplasma filling cul-de-sac, separate from uterus.

Diagnosis: Intrauterine pregnancy complicated by fibroid and possible cancer of the ovary.

Laparotomy: January 14, 1942. Myomectomy.

Pathological Diagnosis: Dr. Keller. Degenerating pedunculated fibromyoma 12x14x 16 cm., benign.

Post-operative Course: Four febrile readings. No cramps. Delivery at term July 12, 1941, spontaneous with episiotomy and repair.

OVARIAN CYST

Four patients were seen in which removal of the tumor was necessary during the pregnancy. As a general rule if the patient is seen in the first half of pregnancy and an ovarian tumor of the diameter of six centimeters or greater is present which with a short period of observation does not regress, laparotomy is indicated. In the four patients operated in this series, two were removed because of adnexal tortion. Three continued to term. All were delivered by the vaginal route. The patient in this group which aborted had a gangrenous ovarian cyst as a result of acute tortion. Differential diagnosis at time of operation was that of acute adnexal tortion or the possibility of an ectopic pregnancy with large hemotocele. Spontaneous, complete abortion on the fourth postoperative day.

CASE No 1

Mrs. W. M., age 30, Para O. Gravida I. First seen April 23, 1940. This patient complained of amenorrhea, painful breast, left lower quadrant pain.

Examination: Uterus slightly enlarged, third degree retroverted and displaced to left side by tender, semi-fluctuant mass. Temperature 99.6, pulse 88, blood pressure 100/60. Red blood count 3,760,000, white blood count 12,000, hemoglobin 78 per cent.

Impression: Intra-uterine pregnancy with complicating ovaries cyst.

Tubal abortion with hematocele

Operated: May 2, 1940. Findings: Intra-uterine pregnancy six weeks and gangrenous twisted corpus luteum cyst 8 centimeters in diameter.

Post-operative Course: Seven febrile readings. Spontaneous, complete abortion on the fourth post-operative day.

CASE No. 2

Mrs. G. O., age 28, Gravida I. First seen 1939, six weeks post-operative removal right tube and right ovary (ovarian cyst), and resection of cystic left ovary.

Returned for sterility investigation eight months later. Lipiodol revealed tubal occlusion of fimbriated end and marked tortuosity. Repeated injection under fluorscopic and manometric control established potency.

Ovarian cyst discovered at first prenatal visit which increased rapidly in size.

Operation: April 5, 1941 Cyst-oophorectomy remaining ovary (15 cm, in. diameter, filling cul-de-sac and displacing uterus superiorly and to the right.) Dense omental adhesions.

Post-operative Course: 5 units progestin every 6 hours pre-operatively one day, postoperatively 4 days. Five febrile readings.

Delivered: At term, October 10, 1941. Episiotomy, low forceps and repair, normal uterine motility. No milk. Hot flashes began at the 6th puerperal week.

CASE No. 3

Mrs. R. T., age 24. Para O. Gravida I. First seen October 19, 1937. This patient complained of pain in right lower quadrant. Amenorrhea 6 weeks. Sore breasts.

Examination: Intrauterine pregnancy four to six weeks; uterus displaced posteriorly by tender fluctuant spherical mass filling the right lower quadrant.

Operation: October 29, 1937. Right cyst-oophorectomy for ovarian cyst, measuring 14 to 16 cm. in diameter, complete torsion two times counter clock-wise.

Post-operative Course: Uneventful. Three febrile readings.

Delivered: May 4, 1938 at term, episiotomy, low forceps and repair. Baby had bi-lateral talipes valgus.

CASE NO. 4

Mrs. M. S., age 25, Para O. Gravida 1 First seen January 10, 1941. This patien complained of amenorrhea. Frequency. Pain in left lower quadrant.

Diagnosis: Intrauterine pregnancy six weeks. Left ovarian cyst 10 cm. in diameter. Observation for six weeks, gradual enlargement of tumor with increasing pelvic pain and urinary symptoms.

Operated: March 2, 1941. Left cyst-oophorectomy.

Post-operative Course: Two febrile readings.

Delivered: At term on August 14, 1941. Episiotomy, low forceps and repair.

The second case, Mrs. G. O., presented features of unusual clinical interest:

1. Relative sterility as result of post-operative adhesions for cyst-oophorectomy.

2. Successful salpingostomy by transuterine injection of lipiodol under fluoroscopic and manometric control.

3. Successful removal of remaining neoplastic ovary at three and a half months.

4. Opportunity to observe uterine motility in labor in a castrate.

5. Opportunity to observe effect of castration on lactation.

6. Opportunity to observe onset and severity of menopause in the above individual.

HYPERTHYROIDISM AND THYROIDECTOMY

The diagnosis of hyperthyroidism in pregnancy is not always easy to make. The indications for surgical treatment of disorders of the thyroid gland during pregnancy are infrequent. Some physicians have advocated thyroidectomy for slight exacerbations or hyperthyroidism early in pregnancy, whereas others prefer medical treatment unless the hyperthyroidism is severe. The risk of complications following a thyroidectomy during the latter part of pregnancy is greater and in most instances it may be advisable to treat the patient conservatively. Should operation be indicated in the latter part of pregnancy, it is better to perform the thyroidectomy first, and then if obstetric complications develop to take care of them as may be indicated. In my opinion, a thyroidectomy should be performed if the patient has a rather marked hyperthyroidism and is seen before the 24th week. On the other hand, if she is seen in the last trimester most careful evaluation is indicated and in most instances she should be given Lugols solution and operated sometime after delivery. A thyroidectomy for a non-toxic goitre should not be done during pregnancy unless there

is a marked tracheal compression which embarrasses respiration.

CASE NO. 1

Mrs. I. H., age 30, Para O. Gravida II. L.M.P. May 3, 1936.

Complaint: Thyrotoxicosis first and second trimester. Lobectomy for respiratory embarrassment and tracheal compression. Dr. Lingenfelter on December 9, 1936. Acute fulminating pre-eclampsia, December 22, 1936.

Labor: December 23, 1936 at 34 weeks. Ruptured membranes.

Delivery: December 24, midforceps. Pudenal block and oxygen anesthetic.

Lobectomy: February 2, 1937. Dr. R. M. Howard.

Follow-up: Satisfactory.

APPENDICITIS WITH APPENDECTOMY

The incidence of appendicitis is no greater during pregnancy than at any other time, although some authors have made the statement that pregnancy tends to cause exacerbations in a chronically inflamed appendix. There is usually little difficulty in making a diagnosis of acute appendicitis during the first trimester, although the symptoms of hyperemesis and the possibility of an extra-uterine pregnancy may add difficulty to the differential diagnosis. During the second and third trimester the symptoms and clinical course may be atypical. The one reliable symptom, pain, may first appear as an epigastric discomfort or even be more or less generalized, with subsequent localization in the right lower quadrant or umbilical region. As the pregnant uterus enlarges, the appendix is displaced upward. The absence of nausea and vomiting does not rule out appendicitis. During the seventh, eighth and ninth months the incidence of appendicitis is apparently lower than during the first and second trimesters. The severity of appendicitis and the incidence of obstetric complications are much greater during the last trimester, which might be explained by several factors. The diagnosis of appendicitis during the last three months is much more difficult and the physician is therefore more reluctant to consider surgical intervention because of possible complications. It is probable that mild attacks subside undiagnosed, or, if diagnosed, as some inherent discomfort or pain of pregnancy. This would tend to lead to fewer appendectomies during this period and among the operative cases, there would be a higher incidence of neglected appendicitis with abscess or spreading peritonitis. Furthermore, when appendicitis becomes suppurative with localized or spreading peritonitis, there is a tremendously increased hazard during the last three months of pregnancy as compared with the first six months. One factor in this greater hazard is the obliteration of the cul-de-sac by the large uterus which consequently prevents localization of the inflammatory process in this favorable site. Another factor is that the uterus makes an unsatisfactory wall for localizing abscess because of contractions and its mobility which tends to break down fresh fibrinous adhesions. There is also a greater hazard to the patient during the puerperium. A parurient uters is a potential menace in that the extension of the inflammatory process to it would superimpose a puerperal sepsis on an already exceedingly serious condition. There is a difference in opinion as to the surgical management in cases of appendicitis occurring at or just before term. As to whether to intervene obstetrically immediately before or after the removal of an acute uncomplicated appendicitis or to wait for the natural onset of labor. A few surgeons and some obstetricians have favored Cesarean section in this case with removal of the appendix through the same or a separate incision. I am of the positive opinion that no obstetrical procedure should be performed at the time of appendectomy unless there is a definite obstetrical indication such as active labor, complicated by acute appendicitis with evidence of cephalo-pelvic disproportion. Such a combination with pathology would be very rare indeed. With the current use of intraperitoneal sulfonamides and the ability to retard the onset of labor by use of adequate dosage of progestin modern recommendations for management of this serious complication must be altered. If there is reasonable doubt as to a diagnosis of acute appendicitis than exploratory laparotomy is indicated in view of the serious morbidity and even mortality associated with neglected appendicitis during the pregnancy or puerperium.

CASE No. 1

Mrs. T. S., age 32, Para O. Gravida I. First seen in consultation October 2, 1939. Normal spontaneous delivery thirty-six hours before. Her chief complaint was a right lower quadrant pain and tenderness, nausea and vomiting following indefinite cramping pain in region of umbilicus. Temperature 100.5., pulse 100, white blood count 16,500. Polys 86 per cent. Diagnosis: probable acute appendicitis. Differential diagnosis. adnexal torsion or acute adnexal inflammation. Exploratory Laparotomy: right rectus incision — acute gangrenous appendix. Post-operative course uneventful. Four febrile readings.

CASE No. 2

Mrs. S. M., age 21, Para 1. Gravida 11. Admitted to the hospital May 26, 1942, with symptoms and signs of acute appendicitis with probably perforation at 24 weeks gestation. An appendectomy was performed on May 26 — acute gangrenous appendix with much free fluid. Special treatment; intraperitoneal sulfanilamide 6 grams—5 U. Progestin every 4 hours for three days. Postoperative course: three febrile readings—no uterine cramps. Delivered at term September 5, 1942, low forceps extraction.

CARCINOMA OF THE CERVIX

Carcinoma of the cervix was encountered in two cases. The first case an early clinical group 1 carcinoma which was picked up on routine speculum examination, and in which the symptom which brought the patient to the office was that of amenorrhea and nausea. The second case was that of an advanced late group IV carcinoma of the cervix seen at term on the clinical service at the hospital. Carcinoma in any part of the body offers a much more serious prognosis during pregnancy than at any other time. In considering these two patients I might quote from the English edition (1634) of Ambrose Pare's work: Hippocrates is credited with saying, "Such as have hidden and are not ulcerated cancers, had better not cure them, for healed they quickly die, not cured they live longer." Such were these cases. The incidence of carcinoma of the cervix and uterous complicating pregnancy is extremely rare. During a six year period at the Chicago Lying-In Hospital and Clinic, during the examination of over 20,000 pregnant women, Dieckmann reports only three cases were observed. Emphasis should be placed on the importance of routine inspection of the cervix of every pregnant woman when she is first examined and of the obtaining of a biopsy from any lesion suspected of being malignant. The treatment naturally depends upon the period of gestation and the extent of the malignancy. The management must be individualized to suit the conditions that exist. The following general principles may be stated: in early pregnancy the treatment should consist of extensive radiation and irradiation of the tumor itself. Later in pregnancy, as the period of viability is approached, the application of a moderate dosage of radium, 2,000 to 3,000 mg hours "will serve to inhibit the growth and extension of the cancer." At or near term the pregnancy should be terminated by cesarean or porrocesarean section in most instances, because of the possible dangers of exsanguinating hemorrhage as a result of laceration into the lower segment and large uterine vessels. It should be stressed that carcinoma of the cervix is usually infected, and that the induction of labor is very apt to be followed by a puerperal infection. If the patient is seen and delivered at term, extensive radia-

and multiple transfusions. The patient died June 29, 1942 due to infection resultant from phyometra and attributal to inadequate follow-up.

CASE No. 2

Mrs. C. L., age 39, Para III, Gravida IV, No. 115588. This patient was admitted to St. Anthony Hospital on May 10, 1938 with chief complaint of vaginal bleeding of one month and uterine pregnancy at or near term. The clinical diagnosis revealed intrauterine pregnancy approximately 40 weeks, epidermoid cancer of the cervix, clinical group IV, histologic grade III. A laparotrachelotomy was performed on May 14, 1938, under local anesthesia. The post-operative course was afebrile and the patient was given Roentgen therapy as an outpatient. The result was death.

CONCLUSIONS

Pregnancy, labor, and the puerperium do

TABLE NO. 1
MAJOR SURGICAL COMPLICATIONS

	Total No.	Surgical Treatment of Complications During: Pregnancy	Labor	Puerperium
FIBROMYOMATA	5			
Myomectomy		2	2	
Hysterectomy			1	
OVARIAN CYST	4			
Cyst-oophorectomy		4		
HYPERTHYROIDISM	1			
Thyroidectomy (two-stage)		Lobectomy		Lobectomy
APPENDICITIS	2			
Appendectomy		1		1
CANCER OF CERVIX	2	1		1

tion therapy should be instituted at the end of the puerperium.

CASE No. 1

Mrs. V. H., age 30, Para O. Gravida 1. Her chief complaints were relative sterility and nine days past time of expected menses. The examination revealed questionable early pregnancy and a peculiar hard hypertrophic lesion,, anterior lip of the cervix. Biopsy was made March 4, 1942 with discovery of epidermoid cancer, clinical group I, histologic group III. Roentgen therapy began March 7 with spontaneous abortion of tissue histologically proven placenta three weeks later. Radium applied April 2, 4500 mg. hours by in trauterine tandem and interstitial needles into nodules; Roentgen therapy as an outpatient, with rather severe reaction. The follow-up was inadequate and the patient was admitted to St. Anthony Hospital on June 4, 1942. Diagnosis was made as follows: extensive pelvic cellulitis, pelvic peritonitis, poymetra; progressive septic course despite drainage of broad ligament abscess, chemotherapy

not contraindicate the performance of necessary operations for non-obstetric complications.

The physiologic changes and altered anatomy of normal pregnancy may mask pathology and increase diagnostic problems. A knowledge of these changes is of great importance in the art of surgery and obstetrics. The use of large doses of progestin both pre-operatively and postoperatively is a valuable addition to our surgical armantarium.

DISCUSSION

JAMES F. McMURRY, M.D.

SENTINEL, OKLAHOMA

Dr. Rogers has presented an excellent paper. His case reports demonstrate well the proper handling of surgical complications of pregnancy. I certainly agree with him on his handling of fibromyomata and ovarian cysts during pregnancy.

With regard to hyperthyroidism, I am definitely of the opinion that a pregnant woman who has an enlarged thyroid and who has had two or more exacerbations of even relatively moderate hyperthyroidism, should have a thyroidectomy done during the fourth month of her pregnancy. If done under nerve block anesthesia, there is very little shock or danger of disturbing the fetus. Pregnancy greatly stimulates the thyroid and we avoid having the patient go through a period of hyperthyroidism which may not be completely controlled by iodine. One should remember, however, that following a thyroidectomy, the patient is hypothyroid and thyroid extract should be given.

Acute appendicitis is probably the most frequent surgical complication of pregnancy and demands immediate operation regardless of the stage of pregnancy. During the first four months, the diagnosis is usually relatively simple but during the third trimester, the diagnosis is more difficult due to the displacement upward and rotation of the appendix. However, if the obstetrician makes a careful check of any abdominal pain that lasts more than three hours particularly if it originates around the umbilicus or epigastrium the diagnosis is not likely to be missed. It is important to remember that there may be no vomiting. An abscessed or ruptured appendix occurring after mid term probably carries a mortality of over fifty per cent due to the changed location of the appendix and to the fact that almost all these cases go into labor and spread the infection.

Dr. Rogers reported one case of acute appendicitis following delivery. This case is interesting to me because the diagnosis might easily be missed.

There are two other surgical complications I would like to mention. One of them is carcinoma of the breast. Fortunately, this is not a common complication of pregnancy but the mortality is terrific. Some authors report only 20 per cent five year survivals in cancer of the breast occurring during pregnancy in spite of treatment. The discovery of a malignancy of the breast during pregnancy calls for a therapeutic abortion or induction of labor followed by radical mastectomy and x-ray. Cancer of the breast is one very good reason for checking the breasts every two months during the pregnancy.

The other complication of pregnancy I would like to mention is cholecystitis. Fortunately, severe attacks of cholecystitis usually do not occur until late in pergnancy and frequently not until after delivery. It is probably always better to defer operation until after delivery due to technical diffculties and to the fact that delivery usually occurs without serious risk to mother or child.

If the attacks have been severe, particularly if the patient has been jaundiced, cholecystectomy should be done within a reasonable time after delivery. In such cases there is usually considerable liver damage and if the patient is to have more babies, she is sure to have other attacks and the gall bladder had better be out.

To me a study of this subject emphasizes, as Dr. Rogers has shown in his report of cases, that good obstetrical care and judgement combined with gentle surgery practically always resolves these complications without great risk to the mother and little for the child but if badly handled can result in disaster.

Androgen Therapy In The Female[*]

J. WILLIAM FINCH, M.D.

HOBART, OKLAHOMA

Recently, in medical literature, there has been a considerable volume of material published relative to androgen therapy of females. This paper is intended neither to uphold nor condemn the use of androgens in this type of therapy, but is an effort to correlate present day knowledge of the subject so that logical conclusions may be drawn regarding such therapy.

Androgens have been credited with being

*Read before the Annual Meeting held in Oklahoma City, May 11-12, 1943.

indicated in the treatment of functional uterine bleeding, the menopausal syndrome, primary dysmenorrhea, frigidity and advocated for inhibiting lactation and for the relief from afterpains. Likewise, they have been condemned as producers of ovarian atrophy, deepening of the voice and hirsutism.

Certainly, long continued dosage of a contrasexual hormone or of the use of such hormone in contraphysiological dosage at any time is to be condemned. With almost equal certainty, however, the judicious use of androgens in certain well defined cases may be indicated.

Although the use of androgens in the female is frequently specified as "contra-sexual", I wonder if we can truthfully designate it as such. Theoretically it is possible for the ovaries to secrete androgen since this action has been demonstrated in the mouse under certain experimental conditions. Furthermore, an ovarian tumor, (Arrhenoblastoma), in women secretes androgens, as is evidenced by its masculizing effect, and in addition the hilus of the normal ovary contains cells with potentially androgenic properties. The normal ovary, as indicated by assays, probably secretes only small amounts of androgen since women who have had their ovaries re-'

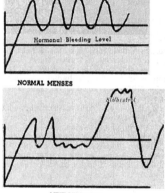

NORMAL MENSES

METRORRHAGIA
CONTROLLED BY ESTROGEN THERAPY

moved excrete abnormal amounts of androgen, probably of adrenal cortex origin. Nevertheless, there is considerable evidence that women with ovarian dysfunctions excrete abnormal amounts of androgen, frequently in quantities which approximate the amounts found in the urine of normal males[1]. The excretion of androsterone and other metabolities of testosterone is rather uniform throughout the menstrual cycle. Hamblen, Pattee and Cuyler[2] found that during the menopause the average daily amount of androgen excreted was elevated from the normal of 3.4 to 8.4 mg. In hypo-ovarianism values were 7. mg. daily and in menorrhagia about 6 mg. daily. In women whose breasts were recurrently painful with the menstrual cycle the daily androgen excretion averaged 5.1 mg., in women with functional dysmenorrhea, 6.6 mg., and in women with menstrual headaches 5.8 mg. It is interesting that

estrogen administration lowered those values somewhat.

Therapeutic effectiveness of androgens depends on their ability to (1) nullify or modify the action of estrogens on endometrium, myometrium and vaginal mucosa, (2) suppress or decrease estrogen production by the ovary and (3) inhibit gonado-tropic activity of the hypophysis.

Geist and Salmon[3] report the administration of androgen to 422 women with a number of different types of functional gynecologic disturbances. From their results they conclude that androgen therapy properly administered is rational and effective in certain types of these disorders.

They found that dosages of testosterone propionate were sufficient to cause cessation

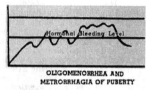

OLIGOMENORRHEA AND
METRORRHAGIA OF PUBERTY

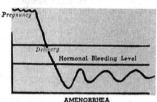

AMENORRHEA
FOLLOWING DELIVERY

of menstruation and involutional changes in the vaginal mucosa also occasionally producing acne and virilizing effects such as deepening of the voice, hypertrichosis and enlargement of the clitoris. None of these effects was noted in doses of 50 to 250 mg. per month. They conclude that androgens exert their therapeutic effect in subarrhenomimetic doses, namely, less than 300 mg. per month. Above 500 mg. per month the incidence of virilizing phenomena was 21 per cent. Satisfactory results were obtained in 91 per cent of 33 cases of functional uterine bleeding with 150-250 mg. testosterone propionate per month. They found it advisable to forestall recurrences by continuing therapy in small doses (10 mg. once or twice weekly) for several months after normal menstruation was established. In cases in which abnormal bleeding was due to submucous myomas, the drug was of little if any value.

Satisfactory results were obtained in the treatment of functional dysmenorrhea, 18 or 25 patients being relieved during treatment which consisted of testosterone propionate in doses not exceeding 250 mg. per month. Following initial treatment, oral therapy consisting of 10-20-mg. of methyl testosterone for 14 consecutive days beginning on the 12th day of the cycle was continued for two to three months. This appeared to lengthen the period between cessation of treatment and recurrence of symptoms.

Cases of premenstrual tension and premenstrual mastopathy were treated by giving 25 mg. testosterone propionate twice a week beginning on the 12th day of the cycle and continuing for 2 cycles, using supplementary therapy of 10 mg. methyl testosterone daily for several months.

These same authors report androgen therapy effective in treatment of the menopausal syndrome but that is a slower and more expensive method of obtaining the same result achieved by estrogens.

Before we can intelligently discuss the desirability of using any drug in the treatment of functional uterine bleeding we should arrive at some sort of working hypothesis as to the physiology of menstruation. Markee[4] and Bartelmez[5] have in their work indicated the effect of the fluctuating level of estrogens on the spiral arterioles of the endometrium is the true cause of menstruation. A high level causes a dilation of these arterioles with a resulting good nutrient activity on the endometrium and an absence of menstruation, whereas a low level of estrogen causes a constriction of these arterioles resulting in blood stasis and in necrosis of the endometrium, and menstruation. Karnaky[6] has advanced the theory that there is a certain estrogen level at which a woman will menstruate and that above or below this level there is no menstruation.

To prove this theory Karnaky gives enormos doses of diethystilbestrol to a bleeding patient, whether she be pregnant, threatening to abort, a case of menopausal metrorrhagis or metrorrhagia in a young girl. He claims that results are almost immediate. The exponents of androgen therapy for functional uterine bleeding claim quick cessation of bleeding after the administration of testosterne propionate in 90 per cent of their cases. I can concur in these results.

Satisfactory results have been obtained in the treatment of functional dysmenorrhea with testosterone propionate in doses not exceeding 250 mg. uer month. In the presence of chronic pelvic inflammatory disease or endometriosis, androgens are not effective in relieving dysmenorrhea. Results from androgenic therapy of menstrual cramping are in all probably due either to a lessening of uterine contractions as seems to be the case in the treatment of afterpains with androgens or due to a change in the salt-water balance of the body. Elimination of estrogens, or neutralization of estrogens may allow excretion of the sodium ion with less water retention intracellularly.

Testosterone propionate in doses of 10 to 20 mg. daily for 12 days beginning the second day postpartum or methyl testosterone in doses of 30 to 90 mg. daily has been recommended to inhibit lactation.

Although sentimental, phychologic and anatomic factors greatly influence libido nevertheless the role of the hormone has also been proved a definite influencing factor. According to Greenblat, Mortara and Torpin[7], androgens cause an increase in the sexual urge and progesterone may be administered to depress excessive libido when present. They recommend pallet implantation of 100 mg. testosterone propionate although they state they have had no virilization in doses up to 400 mg. In almost every patient who once knew libido, a resurgence has followed pellet implantation. These facts may provide a working basis for treatment. The psychotic tendencies of the nymphomaniac, the neuroses and unhappiness of the frigid female and the problems of the incompatible couple with their sociologic implications, may be amenable to hormone therapy. The mechanism of this reaction is not clear. Possible engorgement and enlargement of the clitoris may be responsible for the increase in libido. It is paradoxical that testosterone which antagonizes or neutralizes the female sex hormone should increase sex desire in the female.

I believe that anyone who had experience using both the estrogens and the androgens in female therapy will agree that many

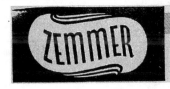

symptom complexes amenable to one are also amenable to the other. The main decision lies in which drug to use, which is most efficacious, lest harmful and most practical.

In general, let it be stated that of the two therapeutic agents, natural estrogens are expensive and effective only parentally. The synthetic estrogen, diethylstilbestrol is quite inexpensive and also quite effective orally as well as parenterally, whereas the androgens are very expensive whether given orally as methyl testosterone or parenterally as testerone propionate. Not many patients can afford an adequate dose of either form of the drug. Side effects such as nausea and vomiting are almost nil with androgens. Nausea and vomiting follows the administration of diethylstilbestrol in 20 per cent to 30 per cent of all cases unless the initial dose is quite small. All vomiters from this drug, however, are those who have had, or will have, nausea and vomiting of early pregnancy. Thus they may be predicted from their histories. If sensitive to the drug, they may be desensitized[3]. If the patient is carefully observed in her progress I feel that the carcinogenic powers of estrogen therapy are very slight. Androgens, however, are stated to be suppressive to growth of gynecological maligancies.

In the treatment of functional uterine bleeding, I think the decision lies in whether we would rather lower our estrogen level to a sub-bleeding level from suppression of the ovary and neutralization of the estrogens or whether we wish to raise it above the bleeding level with estrogens and maintain this level with moderate doses until what should be a premenstrual interval at which time the drug can be discontinued with resulting withdrawal bleeding. Frequently such treatment for two or three consequetive months, especially if progesterone is also administered in the latter half of the cycle, is followed by an apparent hormonal balance and normal menses.

This is more often true in the younger patient. I favor this therapy over androgen therapy. In the menopausal patient with functual bleeding of severity, it may often be wiser to used androgens and drop the estrogen level to a sub-bleeding zone, especially if the patient has had recurrent attacks.

Since androgen therapy of the menopausal syndrome is a much slower and more expensive method of obtaining the results achieved by estrogens I can see no excuse for the use of androgens except in the following groups: (1) patients with carcinoma; (2) patients whose symptoms are partially relieved by estrogens (and psychotherapy) ; (3) postmenopausal patients who are distressed by the uterine bleeding which may result from estrogen therapy; (4) patients who have

been castrated for the treatment of endometriosis.

I have used both androgen therapy and diethylstilbestrol in treatment of functional dysmenorrhea. Using either drug, about 80 per cent of patients are relieved to some degree during treatment and with either drug a large percentage has recurrence of their cramping on cessation of therapy. A few patients will obtain permanent relief from either form of treatment. Since estrogen therapy causes some enlargement of infantile genitalia and since there is some evidence that stilbestrol causes some definite. ovarian stimulation I feel that it should be given first choice in treatment. If no relief is obtained from it, one might be justified in the use of testosterone. With either drug, the psychic effect of a few painless menses may alone be worth the treatment.

I can see no reason to use androgens in the inhibition of lactation with the exception of the very occasional case which will have severe afterpains from the effects of estrogen administration for this purpose. Rutherford[9] states that estrogens retard postpartum involution of the myometrium and endomentrium although epithelization of mucosal surfaces proceeds at a normal rate. With androgens, in as small amount as 10 mg. daily there is no delay in involution but repair is stopped and mucosal surfaces remain denuded. The delay in involution by estrogens is of small import for it is seldom necessary to give stilbestrol more than four to six days to prevent breast engorgement. The delay of mucosal repair for that many days from androgen therapy is of much more importance.

I cannot approve androgen therapy for premenstrual tension. Here, as well as some cases of premenstrual migraine and dysmenorrhea, the actual cause of the symptoms may be a disturbance of the salt-water balance with retention of the sodium ion. A salt-free diet plus administration of potassium or ammonium chloride is so much easier, cheaper and more rational that I feel it should be used until more positive indications for androgenic therapy are uncovered.

Testosterone propionate is more effective in the relief of premenstrual nastalgia than any other therapeutic agent I have tried. Symptoms usually recur within a few months after cessation of treatment, however.

No case should be given androgen therapy without having a careful and repeated vaginal smear examinations. These may be very simply done. It is not even necessary to stain them but they should be examined. As soon as involutional changes in the vaginal mucosa are noted, dosage should be diminished or stopped.

In conclusion let us say that the use of androgens in women is not contraphysiological but that it is a very expensive type of therapy which should be used only when the patient can be very carefully supervised and after a most careful study of the case indicates its need. Doses over 250 to 300 mg. per month should never be used for fear of virilizing effects. It is of definite value in chosen cases of patients suffering from functional uterine bleeding, menopausal syndrome, functional dysmenorrhea and premenstrual mastalgia. It is inferior to diethylstilbestrol inhibiting lactation. It is a definite stimulant to libido in women.

BIBLIOGRAPHY

1. (a) Kenyon, A. T.; Gallagher, T. F.; Peterson, D. H.; Dorfman, R. I. & Koch, F. C.: Urinary Excretion of Androgenic and Estrogenic Substances in Certain Endocrine States; Studies in Hypogonadism, Gynecomastia and Virilism. Jour. Clin. Investigation, Vol. 16, page 705. September, 1937.
(b) Dingemanse, E.; Borchardt, H., & Laqueur, E.: Capon Comb Growth—Promoting Substances in Human Urine of Males and Females of Varying Ages. Biochem. Jour., Vol. 31, page 500. April, 1937.
(c) Baumann, E. J., and Metzger, N.: Colorimetric Estimation and Fractionation of Urinary Androgens. Endocrinology, Vol. 27, page 64. October, 1940.
2. Hamblen, E. C., Pattee, C. J., and Cuyler, W. K.: Alteration of Urinary Excretion of Androgens by Estrogenic Therapy. Endocrinology, Vol. 27, page 734. November, 1940.
3. Geist, Samuel H, and Salmon, Udall J.: Androgen Therapy in Gynecology. Jour. A. M. A., Vol. 117, page 2207. December 27, 1941.
4. Markee, J. E.: Analysis of Rhythmic Vascular Changes in Uterus of Rabbit. Amer. Jour. Physiol., Vol. 100, page 374. April, 1932. Contrib. Embryol., Vol. 27, page 223. 1940.
5. Bartelmez, G. W.: Contrib. Embryol., Vol. 24, page 141. 1933.
6. Karnaky, Karl John: Endocrines in Gynecology and Obstetrics with Special Reference to Stilbestrol in the Treatment of Uterine Bleeding. Jour. Texas State Med. Ass'n., Vol. 36, page 379. September, 1940.
7. Greenblatt, Robert B., Mortara, Frank, and Torpin, Richard: Sexual Libido in the Female. Amer. Jour. Obst. & Gynec., Vol. 44, page 658. October, 1942.
8. Finch, J. William: Nausea and Vomiting Following Administration of Diethylstilbestrol. Jour. A. M. A., Vol. 119, page 500. May 30, 1942.
9. Rutherford, Robert N.: Postpartum Breast Comfort Achieved by Sex Hormone Therapy. Western Jour. Surg., Vol. 50, page 283. June, 1942.

The Anatomical Pathways for the Metastatic Spread of Cancer of the Breast[*]

E. LACHMAN, M.D.
The University School of Medicine
OKLAHOMA CITY, OKLAHOMA

The facetious saying that no surgeon, irrespective of his experience, has ever seen the deep cervical fascia in the living, applies equally well to the lymphatics of the breast. But it would be erroneous to minimize the clinical importance of this subject. Anatomical texts are often rather indefinite about the topic. Yet the physician who deals with cancer of the breast, requires a precise knowledge of the lymphatic drainage of this region. Familiarity with the subject furnishes him with an understanding of the pathways of cancerous spread and brings home to him the rationale of surgical and radiotherapeutic procedures.

The lack of clearness in the presentation of this topic and the discrepancies in the literature can be explained by the great variability of the lymphatic system and by the difficulty of exploration. In common with the fascial spaces, the lymphatic system cannot be investigated by the usual method of anatomical dissection; its study requires special methods as, e.g., injection of dyes under pressure, which of course, opens the door to artifacts not in keeping with natural conditions. As a matter of fact, discrepancies have been found between the results of anatomical studies on the lymphatic system and clinical experiences in actual cancer cases. To name just one example, anatomists rarely mention the interposition of supraclavicular lymph nodes between the highest axillary nodes and their terminal drainage by way of the subclavian trunk, yet clinically, an involvement of the supraclavicular lymph nodes following axillary metastasis is a common occurrence. Blockage of the usual drainage stations seems to open up new or anatomically preformed, but otherwise not demonstrable pathways. Insufficient data are available to present the subject of lymphatic drainage of the breast in final form. For this reason it seems more appropriate to list all possible lymph channels rather than state only those that represent the average or "the typical."

It was Sampson Handley's achievement to have placed the operative treatment of breast cancer upon a rational, i.e., anatomical basis. His theory that cancer spreads centrifugally in all directions from its point of origin by permeation of the lymphatic plexuses, while somewhat dogmatic, laid the scientific foundation for the radical surgical treatment of cancer of the breast which had been elaborated before on a more or less empirical basis. It made a study of the lymphatics imperative, since surgical cure aims at eradication of all cancerous tissues from the primary

[*]Read before the Tulsa Cancer Society, January 4, 1944.

focus to the accessible lymph plexuses and nodes.

LYMPHATICS OF THE BREAST

The lymphatics from the parenchyma of the breast arise in the perilobular connective tissue; from there they follow the lactiferous ducts to terminate in the subareolar plexus of Sappey. This plexus is located around the nipple and drains essentially by way of two trunks, one from the interior lateral, the other from the superior medial part of the plexus. On their way to the axillary nodes these trunks receive some additional tributaries from the periphery of the gland. The two trunks which represent the main channel of drainage from the mammary gland, follow the interior border of the anterior axillary fold, i.e., the lower margin of the pectoralis major, or running underneath this muscle, they course with the lateral thoracic vein paralleling the inferior border of the pectoralis minor. Their termination will be discussed in connection with the lymph nodes of the axilla.

LYMPHATICS OF THE OVERLYING SKIN

In addition to the lymphatic drainage of the breast itself, the lymphatic vessels draining the integument over the breast and the fasciae and muscles of the thoracic wall underneath the gland are of importance, since the skin and the underlying structures are frequently invaded. The skin at the nipple and areola forms a dense lymphatic meshwork which drains by means of small lymph vessels into the subareolar plexus, while the more peripheral portions of the skin, being part of the integument of the anterior thoracic wall, drain toward the nearest lymph nodes, i.e., the axillary, the supraclavicular, or the retrosternal. Some cross over the midline to the breast and axillary nodes of the other side, others may communicate with cutaneous lymph vessels draining toward the inguinal region.

LYMPHATICS OF THE UNDERLYING MUSCLES

The lymphatics of the underlying fasciae and muscles are likewise of interest, since Handley has shown that the cancer frequently spreads by way of lymphatic vessels within the deep fascia and invades from there the lymphatics of the pectorales and intercostal muscles. The lymph from these muscles is received into retrosternal and posterior intercostal lymph nodes by means of vessels that run adjacent to the underlying parietal pleura. While the posterior intercostal nodes establish direct communications with the thoracic duct, the retrosternal nodes drain into the supraclavicular nodes or directly into the venous angle. Both anastomose widely with the subendothelial plexuses of the parietal pleura. It is the cancerous infiltration of the fascial and intramuscular lymphatics which makes the removal of the pectorales muscles and their fasciae an intrinsic part of radical mastectomy. On the other hand the communications with pleural lymphatics may lead to early involvement of this serous membrane and thus frustrate surgical procedure.

THE AXILLARY LYMPH NODES

Before the further drainage of the described lymph channels of the breast is discussed, it seems indicated to take up the axillary lymph nodes which receive most of the lymph from the breast. The term "axillary lymph nodes" applies to a large aggregation of lymph glands which are located within the pyramidal space of the axilla. Their separation into individual groups of lymph nodes is somewhat artificial, but facilitates the understanding of regional drainage and helps to clarify their location. Yet it should be understood that axillary glands are subject to great variations in site and number and that the individual groups have a rich system of interconnecting anastomoses. In their location the nodes follow the larger veins of the axilla. They are grouped into three outlying and two more centrally located sets or tracts.

The three peripheral groups which can be regarded as outposts are:

1. A lateral or brachial set along the upper part of the humerus in the medial bicipital groove in relation to the axillary vein.

2. A posterior or subscapular set, following the posterior axillary fold in relation to the thoraco-dorsal and subscapular veins.

3. An anterior or pectoral set underneath the anterior axillary fold in relation to the anterior thoracic vein.

The two more centrally located sets are:

1. The central nodes formed by 3-5 rather large glands in the fat of the axilla.

2. The apical or infraclavicular set in the infraclavicular triangle behind the costocoracoid membrane in relation to the axillary vein.

Pressure on the intercosto-brachial nerve by enlarged lymph nodes explains the pain radiating down the medial side of the arm in metastatic involvement of the central nodes, while oedema of the arm in metastatic cancer is due to obstruction of the axillary vein.

The axillary nodes, taken as a whole, receive two main currents of lymph, one coming from the upper extremity, the other from the adjacent thoracic wall, particularly from the breast, and the two currents meet and fuse within the apical chain. While the lymph flow from the arm is received by the outlying brachial glands, the lymph from the breast is filtered first by the anterior or pectoral nodes, in which the two previously described lymph trunks from the breast terminate. The efferents from the pectoral nodes go to the central set which drains into the apical nodes. From there the lymph passes by way of the subclavian trunk into the toracic duct on the left or the right lymphatic duct, partly being filtered by the supraclavicular or inferior cervical nodes. Thus we have the following lymph nodes interposed in the pathway of cancerous emboli from the breast before they reach the blood stream: pectoral, central, apical, (supraclavicular). Short cuts that by-pass one, two or even three of the lower way-stations may occur. Thus direct drainage from the breast into the central or the apical or even the supraclavicular set can take place. In the latter case we would have the clinical picture of enlarged supraclavicular nodes without involvement of the axilla, a condition which, in general, would be regarded as inoperable. The direct lymphatic channels from the deeper superior portions of the mammary gland to the apical nodes is well known. It passes around the inferior border or through the substance of the pectoralis major and ascends on the surface of or behind the pectoralis minor to the apical nodes. Small interpectoral nodes may be interposed in this pathway. The potential presence of this channel confirms the need for removal of both pectorales muscles in radical mastectomy. Anastomoses between the outlying pectoral, brachial, and subscapular chains are present, so that the latter two may likewise, though rarely, be affected in cancer of the breast.

A few remarks as to the technique of examination of the axillary nodes are appropriate. The pectoral nodes when enlarged are felt beneath the anterior axillary fold, with the arm in the elevated position. The subscapular set is best examined from the back, since it lies in close relation to the posterior axillary fold. The brachial nodes are felt in the medial bicipital groove. In order to palpate the central nodes, the examining hand is inserted high into the axilla, then passed down along the lateral thoracic wall, thus compressing the nodes against the thorax. They may also be palpated from

the back in the same way as the subscapular glands. The very important involvement of the apical nodes is hard to detect. Fullness or resistance in the infraclavicular region may lead one to suspect their enlargement. It has been suggested that they be palpated by pushing the fingers of one hand into the axillary space as high as possible while the other hand tries to penetrate into the supraclavicular fossa behind the clavicle.

In view of the importance of demonstrating involvement of the axillary lymph nodes for the general prognosis, the question is indicated: How accurate are our clinical methods in detecting metastatic spread to the axilla? As Taylor and Nathanson have shown, palpability of lymph nodes is dependent on a number of considerations that have no direct bearing on the presence of metastasis, such as obesity of the patient, cooperation of the patient in relaxing her muscles and skill of the examiner. In a recent study palpable axillary nodes, interpreted as metastases, proved to be free from metastasis in 13 per cent (error of commission). On the other hand, metastasis was diagnosed anatomically in 53 per cent of cases in which no nodes were demonstrable clinically (error of omission.) In another series the figures were 25 per cent and 31 per cent respectively. As the authors rightly conclude, clinical examination is not too reliable in deciding the question of presence or absence of metastasis. Yet the question of axillary metastasis is all important in determining the prognosis, since approximately two patients in three without axillary involvement are cured, while on the other hand only one patient in four with axillary metastasis has a chance of recovery.

ACCESSORY LYMPHATIC CHANNELS

So far we have described only the principal lymphatic channels of the breast. Accessory pathways do occur and have practical importance in the spread of cancer. The communication with lymph-vessels of the other breast, particularly from the inner half of the gland, has been mentioned, likewise drainage to the opposite axilla. Important are the lymph vessels that connect the medial half of the breast with the retrosternal or internal mammary nodes. These vessels traverse the pectoralis major and internal intercostal muscle and follow in their course the perforating branches of the internal mammary vessels. They terminate in nodes located in the upper intercostal spaces in relation to the internal mammary vein close to the lateral margin of the sternum. Their involvement in cancer of the breast precludes surgical cure. Fortunately they atrophy in older age, thus eliminating this node of cancer spread.

Handley has called attention to the close proximity of the medial inferior quadrant of the breast and the epigastric triangle. According to this investigator the region adjacent to the xiphoid process represents the most common port of entry for cancer cells to the peritoneal cavity. Lymph vessels from the previously mentioned segment of the breast pass downward and medially and anastomose through the linea alba with the subperitoneal lymph plexus. Thus cancer of the breast may spread to the peritoneal cavity or to the liver, in the latter case by way of the lymphatics of the falciform ligament.

Several authors have tried to evaluate the prognosis of breast cancer based on its location in different segments of the mammary gland. In view of the fact that cancer of the lower inner quadrant may spread to the peritoneal cavity and liver and that involvement of either of the inner segments may lead to early metastasis in the mediastinum or the other breast and axilla, location in the two inner quadrants is regarded as unfavorable. The most favorable location is the upper outer quadrant, in which fortunately more than 40 per cent of all breast cancers occur (Garland). But it should be realized that the site of the tumor is only one of the factors determining prognosis. Other factors, e. g., the histological type, the size of the tumor, the age of the patient,

While the mammary cancer spreads by continuity within the lymphatics of the gland itself, the skin over it and the thoracic wall deep to the gland, cancerous emboli are transported to the lymph glands in the neighborhood and involve more and more of the lymphatic chains. Obstructions to the normal lymph current by metastatic growth may lead to reversal of the flow and to involvement of lymph glands in atypical locations, e. g., the inguinal region.

HEMATOGENOUS SPREAD

Invasion of the venous circulation may take place at any time either within the breast, the axilla, the mediastinum, or by anatomical route through the thoracic or right lymphatic duct. This seems to be more common than the pathologists used to believe. The absence of lymph vessels in brain and skeleton makes their involvement by hematogenous emboli most probable. Other organs, as the liver, the heart, the lung and the pleura, may be affected either by the lymphatic or the venous route. Handley's theory of the almost exclusive dissemination of breast cancer by way of the lymphatics is too narrow and not applicable to affection of peripheral foci such as the brain or the skeletal system. Yet the non-involvement of the lungs in remote metastasis seems hard to explain even on the basis of a breakthrough into the venous circulation. Metastatic emboli would have to travel from the breast or the axillary nodes to the right heart and from there to and through the lungs to the left heart, in order to reach the peripheral locations previously mentioned. Here a hypothesis, recently propounded in a convincing manner by Batson, is very helpful. This author has shown by injection experiments on human cadavers and living monkeys, that the vertebral plexus forms a valveless system of veins which acts as a reservoir for blood forced out of the caval system by changes in pressure conditions such as take place in straining or coughing. Ample anastomoses exist between the veins of the thoracic wall including the breast and the vertebral plexus, particularly via the intercostal veins, providing a by-pass for blood around the caval, the pulmonary, and the portal system. Batson demonstrated that injected material may be transported from the veins of the breast to the vertebral plexus and from there up and down the spine, to the brain, and into parts of the skeleton. This would explain the spread of metastasis of breast cancer to distant points of the periphery without involvement of the lungs. According to this author, cancer en cuirasse may be due not so much to permeation of the cutaneous lymphatics, but rather to cancerous emboli into the venous plexuses of the mammary skin. On the whole, it seems that the venous system equals in importance the lymphatic circulation for the spread of cancer of the breast.

BIBLIOGRAPHY

1. Batson, O. V.: The Function of the Vertebral Veins and their Role in the Spread of Metastases. Annals of Surgery, Vol. 112, No. 1, page 138. July, 1940.

2. Batson, O. V.: The Role of the Vertebral Veins in Metastatic Processes. Annals of Internal Medicine, Vol. 16, No. 1, page 38. January, 1942.

3. Deaver, J. B. and McFarland, J.: The Breast, its Anomalies, Its Diseases and their Treatment. Philadelphia, 1917.

4. Delamere, G., Poirier, P., and Cuneo B.: The Lymphatics. Chicago, 1904.

5. Garland, J. G.: Common Diseases of the Breast. The Marquette Medical Review, Vol. 8, No. 4, page 189. October, 1943.

6. Geschicketer, C. F.: Diseases of the Breast. Philadelphia, 1943.

7. Handley, W. S.: Cancer of the Breast. Philadelphia, 1943.

8. Rouviere, H.: Anatomy of the Human Lymphatic System. Ann Arbor, 1938.

9. Taylor, G. W. and Nathanson, I. T.: Lymphnode Metastasis. Oxford University Press, 1942.

10. Willis, R. A.: The Spread of Tumors in the Human Body. London, 1934.

Caudal Anesthesia Catheter Method

L. C. NORTHRUP, M.D. & HERBERT ORR, M.D.

Department of Obstetrics
Hillcrest Memorial Hospital

TULSA, OKLAHOMA

This paper is based on eight months personal experience with caudal anesthesia in a small private hospital. The object of the paper is to point out the advantages of the catheter method, and give the technique in detail.

Caudal anesthesia was attempted by us in 74 cases, during a period of eight months. In 54 cases, the results were perfect, in that no other anesthetic was needed; 17 were complete failures; 3 were only partially successful, as it was necessary to supplement the caudal with other anesthesia in order to do some operative procedure. Most of the failures were due to technical difficulties, and occurred during the first six weeks, when we were experimenting with various methods of procedure. Four failures occurred when we were sure the drug was introduced properly into the canal. There was apparently no effect. Failures were more common in obese patients. This suggested the possibility that there may be deposits of fat in the canal which might keep the anesthetic agent from coming in contact with the nerves.

There were 64 primiparae in this series. All cases were delivered by outlet forceps. Episiotomy was done on all primiparae. There were no serious maternal difficulties. There was one mild localized infection. There were no injured babies and no deaths. Respiratory difficulties were conspicuous by their absence. The dura was punctured once, and the method was abandoned. This was classified as a failure. In three cases, the method was abandoned, due to hemorrhage. In two of these cases, we were attempting to use a needle instead of a catheter. These were also classified as failures. Two patients developed severe pain in the right leg. The pain started about the time the cervix became fully di-

lated and in both cases the position was R.O.P. Six patients vomited. The vomiting usually occurred when the head was passing through the cervix. Two patients developed pain in the shoulder; one case was so severe that we abandoned the caudal and used general anesthetic.

After trying the various needles and apparatus described in the literature we are convinced that the catheter method has distinct advantages, which we will point out after first giving in detail the technique of the catheter method.

The use of a catheter for caudal anesthetic was described by S. A. Manalan[1] in October, 1942. The technique, modified by us, is as follows:

With the patient on side, or knee chest, whichever you prefer, first locate the caudal notch. The skin over the caudal notch is cleansed with full strength Zephiran. A small skin bleb is made with a 25 guage needle, using 2 per cent Metycaine; then with a 23 guage needle, anesthetize a large area around the caudal notch. The next step is the introduction of a 15 guage, 3 inch needle. For this purpose, we use a Becton-Dickson stainless steel needle, without stylette, (B-D 461-LNRC). This is a special needle designed to use with a No. 4 catheter. This needle is pushed through the skin with the bevel up at an angle of about 45 degrees. The needle is then pushed through the ligament, which covers the opening, into the canal. The needle is pushed on until it strikes bone at the back of the canal. Now the needle is turned over with the bevel down and at the same time the butt end is pushed down almost parallel with the skin surface and then gently pushed about one-half inch up into the canal. No attempt is made to force the needle farther than one-half inch. The next step is the introduction of the catheter. We use a No. 4 ureteral catheter with round tip. These catheters are graduated and come with a wire through the lumen. The catheter, with the wire in place, is pushed through the needle so that the tip extends two inches beyond the tip of the needle. You can tell by the marks on the catheter when this point has been reached. Now, while holding the catheter in place, the needle is pulled out over the catheter, the wire then being pulled out of the catheter. Sulfathiozole powder is dusted around the puncture in the skin and the catheter is fastened in place by adhesive, the first piece directly over the place where the catheter enters the skin. The catheter is brought around up over the crest of ilium to the front of the abdomen; then a piece of one inch adhesive is placed, running the full length of the catheter, the end being left exposed. Thirty cc of 2 per cent Metycaine, warmed to body temperature, is now injected into the catheter with a 20 cc syringe, using a 23 guage needle which just fits the opening in the catheter. The opening in the catheter can be plugged with an ordinary pin. Repeated injections can be made when desired.

The catheter method offers some distinct advantages over the spinal or flexible needles. It is impossible to push the soft catheter through the dura, therefore, you push the catheter up as high as you wish. It is not necessary to use a small trial dose of anesthetic and wait to see if you are in the spinal canal as the easy passage of the catheter beyond the point of the needle is usually assurance that it is in the canal. There is danger of the flexible needles working up too high when the patient moves about in bed. The needles are more traumatizing than the soft catheter and too, the catheter does away with the long rubber tubing and the accessories that are kept on the table beside the bed, therefore, the patient is allowed more freedom of movement in bed. We have found it much easier to insert the rigid 15 guage needle into the canal as the flexible needles bend so easily that it is difficult to guide the point where you want it to go. The large needle is no more painful.

The catheter is inexpensive and will outlast a flexible needle. They can be autoclaved repeatedly. The catheter we use is made especially for this purpose and sold by C. R. Bard, Incorporated, 79 Madison Avenue, New York City, Catalog No. 328, size 4 fr.

BIBLIOGRAPHY

1. Manalan, S. A.: Caudal Block Anesthesia in Obstetrics. Jour. Indiana State Med. Ass'n., Vol. 35, page 564. October, 1942.

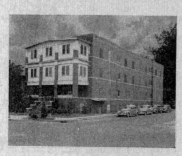
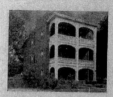

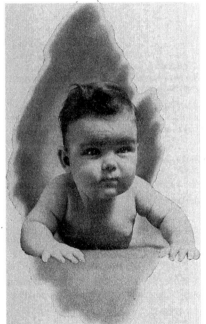
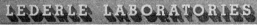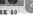

· THE PRESIDENT'S PAGE ·

It has been a pleasure to have been your servant for the past year. Without the loyalty and devotion to duty of the office force it would have been an unhappy year. There are so many routine matters in an organization as large as ours, that no practicing physician could possibly attend to. To Miss Anne Betche, Assistant Secretary, and to Mrs. Jane Firrell Tucker, Journal Assistant—my sincere thanks.

Your Councilors have been most cooperative—they have scrupulously carried out the mandates of the House of Delegates and they have been as economical in spending your money as was consistent with carrying on society affairs on a high level. They have also been charitable with my errors.

The Committees have functioned admirably and some of them have spent many, many hours over the complex problems which face American Medicine today. Their reports will be published in your Journal and should be read with great care.

Your Journal is the equal of any in the Country—Dr. Lewis J. Moorman and his Editorial Board deserve much praise.

Your Association has cooperated whole-heartedly with the war effort. The Procurement and Assignment Committee has done an outstanding patriotic duty. The Chairman, Dr. W. W. Rucks, Sr., injured his own health in his effort to be of service to his country, and others of our members have died, due to overwork on draft boards, induction centers and the like.

I know that you will give Doctor Rountree, who succeeds me in office, the same fine cooperation you have given me.

James Stevenson

President.

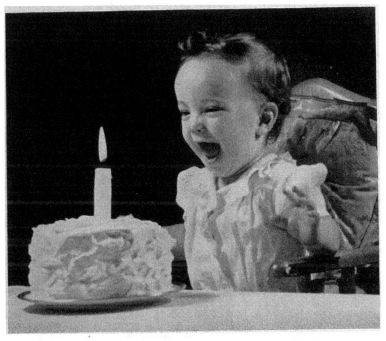

WORTH HIS WEIGHT IN RESEARCH

A generation ago more than 113 out of every thousand babies born never experienced the joy of seeing their first birthday cake.

Due to the advancement of medical science and modern hospitalization as enjoyed in our country, only 37 babies in every thousand born today fail to survive their first year.

Furthermore, babies born today have an average life expectancy 14 years longer than babies born in 1920.

Lengthening the lifeline of these healthy, growing Americans, through research, is an essential industry. We, at Warren-Teed, are proud of our contribution.

WARREN-TEED

Medicaments of Exacting Quality Since 1920

THE WARREN-TEED PRODUCTS COMPANY, COLUMBUS 8, OHIO

Visit Our Booth — No. 80 — At The American Medical Association Convention

The JOURNAL Of The
OKLAHOMA STATE MEDICAL ASSOCIATION

EDITORIAL BOARD
L. J. MOORMAN, Oklahoma City, Editor-in-Chief
E. EUGENE RICE, Shawnee
NED R. SMITH, Tulsa
MR. PAUL H. FESLER, Oklahoma City, Acting Business Manager

CONTRIBUTIONS: Articles accepted by this Journal for publication including those read at the annual meetings of the State Association are the sole property of this Journal.

The Editorial Department is not responsible for the opinions expressed in the original articles of contributors.

Manuscripts may be withdrawn by authors for publication elsewhere only upon the approval of the Editorial Board.

MANUSCRIPTS: Manuscripts should be typewritten, double-spaced, on white paper 8½ x 11 inches. The original copy, not the carbon copy, should be submitted.

Footnotes, bibliographies and legends for cuts should be typed on separate sheets in double space. Bibliography listing should follow this order: Name of author, title of article, name of periodical with volume, page and date of publication.

Manuscripts are accepted subject to the usual editorial revisions and with the understanding that they have not been published elsewhere.

NEWS: Local news of interest to the medical profession, changes of address, births, deaths and weddings will be gratefully received.

ADVERTISING: Advertising of articles, drugs or compounds unapproved by the Council on Pharmacy of the A.M.A. will not be accepted. Advertising rates will be supplied on application.

It is suggested that members of the State Association patronize our advertisers in preference to others.

SUBSCRIPTIONS: Failure to receive The Journal should call for immediate notification.

REPRINTS: Reprints of original articles will be supplied at actual cost provided request for them is attached to manuscripts or made in sufficient time before publication. Checks for reprints should be made payable to Industrial Printing Company, Oklahoma City.

Address all communications to THE JOURNAL OF THE OKLAHOMA STATE MEDICAL ASSOCIATION, 210 Plaza Court, Oklahoma City. (3)

OFFICIAL PUBLICATION OF THE OKLAHOMA STATE MEDICAL ASSOCIATION
Copyrighted April, 1944

EDITORIALS

FAILURE ON THE HOME FRONT IN TIME OF PEACE

Under the title of "The Psychoneuroses of War," Henderson and Moore[1] report 200 neuropsychiatric cases admitted for hospital care somewhere in the South Pacific. After a careful analytical study of each case, the authors conclude that broken or distorted homes constituted the most important of all the predisposing factors. In this picture, the nervous mother stands forth as the motivating influence. Though the father seems to be in the background, it was found that he drank to excess in about 50 per cent of the cases. The unstable mother sees only a hostile world and in search of comfort and sympathy she engages the children in the thought that they must stand together as a helpless unit in this hostile atmosphere. In some instances the father's alcoholism may serve as an escape from the unwholesome atmosphere, thus accentuating the childs psychological dilemma. The same influence was noted in those coming from homes broken by separation, divorce or death. In addition, it was observed that 65 of the patients had bitten their fingernails when young and the habit had been continued by the majority of them.

In the March 16 issue of the New England Medical Journal, there is an editorial "Religion and Psychology" which is indirectly related to the above mentioned trouble on the home front. Henry C. Linck, in his book The Return to Religion, shows that under the strain and stress of poverty and unemployment those who possess a belief in God often have the guts to take the gaff whereas those who have no anchor outside themselves, are cast adrift. In this connection we quote from the editorial:

"The question of the relation, if any, between psychiatry and religion is now and again propounded by someone of speculative mind. The proposal of such a question might be considered a compliment to the "Mental sciences" or it might be looked on as an attack on the body of knowledge that professes to have insight into the deepest, basic motives of human activity.

"Religious belief of some kind or other is as old as human nature and antedates the earliest beginnings of scientific inquiry. Psychiatry is a fairly young member of the scientific family. Does this child, psychiatry, dare or insist on classifying the tendency toward religious belief as founded in phantasy, delusion, wishful thinking? Is religion what Karl Marx called it, "the opium of the people"? . . .

"It may be assumed that they who do have a firm belief in the reality of an infinite being think that such faith is good. They do not berate themselves for having it and they are inclined to think that others would benefit in having the same conviction. They also would say that such trust is not selfish; that, on the contrary, it tends to make them more mindful of others. It is not compatible with religious belief for a person to be thankful that he, anyway, has his salvation whatever happens to the hindmost. The really religious person is concerned about and wants to help others.

"Anyone knows, to use that surprisingly inclusive phrase, being primarily interested in getting the biggest piece of cake for oneself is not good, farsighted or wise. Psychiatry has found and has taught for years that insofar as the patients troubles or maladjustments are not due to innate or organic abnormalities, they are dependent on the formative experiences of the early years of life. How a person meets this or that crisis or strain has a direct relation to what he has learned about self-control: to what extent he has gained the perspective which enables him to understand that his egotistic desires and needs may be of minimal importance in a vast universe of time and space.

"Psychiatry has always known and taught that having and acting on the knowledge that there is something more important than the self makes for mental health. Geniuses, in various degrees, may be exceptions, in that their egotistic desires may, in the long run, benefit others enough and more than enough to compensate for the headaches given their immediate associates by their personal idosyncrasies and selfishnesses . . .

Sigerist[2] says "Faith undoubtedly is an important therapeutic factor, whether it be faith in science, religion or in both. It is safer, however, to have mental clinics operated by medicine than by the church . . . " "As long as medicine has not reached its goal of eradicating disease there will always be patients who, hoping for a miracle, will seek help in religion or even in magic."

"Psychiatry, in therapy, does not want to take away from people their trust in God. It would prefer that they have it or that they achieve it if it can help them."

If religion can help to stabilize our reaction to environment and hold our homes unbroken, it may help directly or indirectly to hold our men on the battle line.

1. Henderson, J. L., Commander, U.S.N.R.: Moore, Merrill,
Major, M.C., A.U.S. The New England Journal of Medicine, Vol. 230, No. 10. March 9, 1944.
2. Sigerist, Henry E.: Civilization and Disease. Cornell University Press. 1943.

THE USURPATION OF FREEDOM AND THE CONFISCATION OF CAPITAL

Socialized medicine not only exacts a heavy tax from the people for its administration, but it confiscates the physician's working capital as soon as it makes it necessary for him to participate or lose his private patronage.

The physician's capital is in his head and in his acquired skills. These have come through education and experience, both of which are costly. Pressing the doctor into service is like talking over the factory, the store or the shop and saying to the owner regardless of his investments, "you are entitled to so much a month—you manage your business and we will manage you. After you are paid and those who tell you what to do are paid, the prices for your products will be scaled up or down to meet the costs of operation and the people will share the profits or pay the extra costs as the case may be.

AMERICAN MEDICINE

The remarkable accomplishments of the American Medical Association have had repeated mention in these columns and they deserve continued consideration. But it should be noted that lay publicity in connection with the alleged need of so-called better medical service is directed at the American Medical Association and occasionally, unjustly personal, as the following from one of the soundest of columnists will show:

"The American Medical Association, headed by snow-crested Dr. Olin West and the ubiquitous Dr. Morris Fishbein, have stirred a dizzy dither about it, among the already overburdened and harassed doctors of the country.

"They have circulated ominous articles, from their medical journals. National conferences have been called. Messrs. Wagner and Murray have been labelled the pre-eminent public enemies of medical science in the United States.

"The whole thing is unfortunate and somewhat tragic.

"The truth is that neither Senator Wagner nor Senator Murray commands sufficient influence in the present congress to be a competent enemy of medical science or anything else. The Wagner bill hasn't a stepchild's chance of being passed. The present congress has no stomach for such stuff, and both Wagner and Murray probably know that as well as any one."

We also call attention to the following unjust criticism of the American Medical Association by a member of the profession in a recent popular magazine.

"From all that you read in the newspapers it sounds as though all doctors were absolutely opposed to this bill. This is not true. Many of them, younger doctors in particular, understand the situation and favor such government action. It is the American Medical Association that is loudest in its criticism of the bill. The leaders of the American Medical Association and of its branches are older doctors who have been successful in establishing good practices under the present free for all system of medical care. Naturally, they resent any change which might affect their practices or their power."

Again we urge doctors to remember that the salvation of American Medicine is dependent upon the education of the public and that the members of the profession must become militant educators not with selfish motives but in behalf of the people. This is something that the American Medical Association cannot do for us; we must see that our friends and patrons understand that they have a right to the free choice of a physician and individual medical service without the annulling stroke of bureaucracy. They should know that medical care anywhere in the United States under present plans is to be had through free initiative of the individual doctor with no mandates, rules or regulations from the American Medical Association. Even our recently developed plans to meet changing social and economic conditions are stale and local, retaining in large degree free initiative in keeping with Hippocratic principles.

When American medicine loses its freedom the people will pay a frightful price and the nation will rue the day it gave professional liberty away. American doctors crave only the privilege to serve with free initiative because it is the only way they can live up to their treasured traditions through which they are giving the best medical service humanity has ever received. That people "have eyes and see not" is an old observation, consequently they are ready to consider socialized medicine. Perhaps a little clay on the lids of our law makers may save us from the threat of this nasty, Nazi situation.

It is unfortunate that those who look upon medicine as selfish and mercenary do not possess the dual conception expressed by Voltaire: "Medicine, having then become a mercenary profession in the world, as the administration of justice is in many places, has become liable to strange abuses. But nothing is more estimable than a physician who having studied nature from his youth, knows the properties of the human body, the diseases which assail it, the remedies which will benefit it, exercises his art with caution, and pays equal attention to the rich and poor." In this connection it is only fair to repeat Voltaire's famous tribute to physicians: "Men who are occupied in the restoration of health to other men by the joint exertion of skill and humanity are above all the great of the earth. They even partake of divinity since to preserve and renew is almost as noble as to create."

Rest assured that bureaucratic control would close all vistas which might otherwise open toward divinity. In this connection we are reminded of what Vasari said about the republic city of Florence four hundred years ago: "The desire for glory and honour is powerfully generated by the air of that place, in the men of every profession; whereby all who possess talent are impelled to struggle that they may not remain in the same grade with those whom they perceive to be only men like themselves, even though they may acknowledge such indeed to be masters; but all labour by every means to be formost."

Is there not much merit in leaving the men, who have to deal seriously with life and death, free to do their best with at least a chance to stand among the foremost? Doctors are seeking truth, not practicing pretension. It is our belief that two to four years in college plus the long hard discipline of a medical education should vouchsafe to the American doctor Cicero's privilege of making "his own genius the guide of his life."

Cushing's Account of Osler's Death

'The days of our age are threescore years and ten . . . so soon passeth it away, and we are gone.' The end came at 4:30 on the afternoon of December 29th, 1919, after a haemorrhage from his wound, just as the end had come to many soldiers after wounds in the war —quietly and without pain. Dr. Francis writes: 'The night before, I read to him for quite a long time, things he asked for out of the "Spirit of Man", and we finished with the last verses of "The Ancient Mariner". I thought at the time how well it fitted him, and afterwards, what an appropiate valedictory for this lover of men and books:

He prayeth best who loveth best
All things, both great and small . . .

'When I took leave of him, he said to me, as though I were still a child: "Nighty-night, a-darling!"'—The Life of Sir William Osler. Harvey Cushing. Oxford at The Clarendon Press.

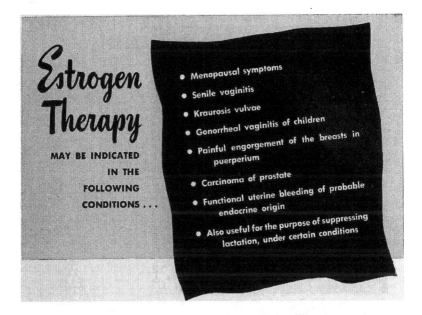

Estrogen Therapy

MAY BE INDICATED IN THE FOLLOWING CONDITIONS . . .

- Menopausal symptoms
- Senile vaginitis
- Kraurosis vulvae
- Gonorrheal vaginitis of children
- Painful engorgement of the breasts in puerperium
- Carcinoma of prostate
- Functional uterine bleeding of probable endocrine origin
- Also useful for the purpose of suppressing lactation, under certain conditions

DUPLICATING practically all the known actions of natural estrogens, having the advantage of being relatively more active upon oral administration than its natural counterparts, and being appreciably more economical, the utility of Diethylstilbestrol is gaining ever wider appreciation among clinicians.

DIETHYLSTILBESTROL SQUIBB

is available in a variety of dosage forms:

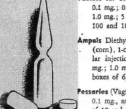

Tablets for oral administration: 0.1 mg.; 0.25 mg.; 0.5 mg.; 1.0 mg.; 5 mg.; in bottles of 100 and 1000.

Ampuls Diethylstilbestrol in Oil (corn), 1-cc., for intramuscular injection: 0.2 mg.; 0.5 mg.; 1.0 mg. and 5.0 mg. in boxes of 6, 25, 50 and 100.

Pessaries (Vaginal Suppositories) 0.1 mg., and 0.5 mg., boxes of 12 and 50.

A preparation of natural estrogens, Amniotin is also available. It is obtained from urine of pregnant mares—is a highly concentrated, non-crystalline preparation of estrone together with small varying amounts of other estrogenic ketones. It is supplied in corn oil solution for intramuscular use and in capsules for oral administration. Also in pessaries.

Particularly economical is Amniotin in Oil, in 10-cc. vials—10,000 I.U. per cc.; and 20,000 I.U. per cc.—and in 20-cc. vials containing 2000 I.U. per cc. These forms also permit utmost flexibility in adjusting dosage to meet the varying needs of patients.

For literature write the Professional Service Dept., 745 Fifth Ave., New York 22, N. Y.

E·R·SQUIBB & SONS

Manufacturing Chemists to the Medical Profession Since 1858

For Victory . . . Keep on Buying War Bonds

Special Article*

Medicine Versus Socialized Medicine

BY

LEWIS J. MOORMAN, M.D.

During the past few years there has been much agitation about the cost and distribution of adequate medical care. This is a natural outgrowth of the changing pattern of life under altered social, economic, educational, industrial, and political conditions as influenced by a period of unprecedented scientific and mechanistic progress. However, physicians and patients calmly surveying the problem in the light of experience are convinced that the people of the United States will not want any form of socialized medicine if they will first take time to carefully study our present system of medical care, and then compare the relative costs and the results achieved under this system with those reported in various European countries where medical service is largely under government control through some form of compulsory health insurance.

Unfortunately the American people have the reputation of being "down on what they are not up on." In this everchanging, fast-going, restless, highly technical, mechanistic age, it behooves us to move slowly when we are dealing with the vital agencies which have to do with "life, liberty, and the pursuit of happiness." We should be cautious in our response to the high sounding call of "social and economic security" lest we lose our priceless heritage, personal liberty.

Your attention is called, first to medicine as practiced in this country today. Medicine is a school of thought sustained and vitalized by the continued acquisition of knowledge and the application of scientific facts. In the 5th Century, B.C., Hippocrates, the recognized father of scientific medicine, broke away from magic philosophy and religious dogma and placed medicine under the rule of reason.

The practice of medicine is an art which finds its origin in "the primal sympathy of man for man." Though Hippocrates freed medicine from religious dogma, he was careful to preserve the spirit of service, which is religion's most vital contribution. The art of medicine antedated the science of medicine, however, the broad foundation laid by Hippocrates and the impartial spirit of services opened the way for science. Today the art and science of medicine go hand in hand, and the highest interests of humanity demand that they remain inseparable.

Medicine accepts everything useful in the prevention and cure of disease and the alleviation of suffering. It is interesting to note that Prof. Theodor Gomperz, in his four volume work on The Greek Philosophers of the fifth Century, B.C., refers to the oath of Hippocrates as "a monument of the highest rank in the history of civilization." Gomperz also recognizes the thoughtful and logical sources of medicine when he devotes a chapter entitled "The Age of Enlightenment" to a discussion of "The Physicians;" thus according them first place in the advance of civilization. The Hippocratic oath dealt with medical ethics, placing emphasis upon the interests of the patient. Throughout the ages, the principles laid down in this remarkable document have served as a guide to physicians and a protection to patients. Four hundred years after these principles were propounded, they were found to be in harmony with the teaching of Jesus Christ, the great physician. Today they sustain the moral integrity of the medical profession and help to maintain the intimate personal relationship between physician and patient.

Medicine successfully weathered the Dark Ages and

*Delivered to the Town Club, Oklahoma City on Thursday, January 27, 1944.

emerged with its accumulated treasures. It has been said that "Greece arose from the dead with the New Testament in one hand and the words of Aristotle in the other." It might be added that Aristotle, Hippocrates and Galen furnished the foundation for medical teaching and that the medical teachers during the Renaissance were steeped in a knowledge of the humanities and were largely instrumental in restoring interest, not only in the art and science of medicine, but in all other cultural influences.

Rapid strides in the art and science of medicine have ever safeguarded and guided the progress of civilization. Through the heroic and sacrificial pursuit of science, and the conscientious application of its revealed truths, medicine and sanitary engineering have adequately matched the needs of a restless mechanistic age. Unfortunately only physicians fully realize how well the challenge has been met. With the rapid progress of transportation and the consequent intermingling of all nations, with their various diseases and their racial susceptibilities, we would have been wiped from the face of the earth if we had not been protected by modern methods of prevention and control.

Without sanitary engineering and other preventive measures, the great cities of the world would succumb to disease within the short period of a few weeks. These achievements have come through accumulation of knowledge and skill, as a result of careful observation, scientific deduction and experimental methods.

For the benefit of the antivivisectionists, attention is called to the fact that not only have animals been mercifully sacrificed for human welfare, but members of the medical profession have voluntarily submitted to experimental methods at the risk of life, and some have made the supreme sacrifice in order that we might live.

Medicine has to its credit a long list of discoveries and inventions which have to do with the most vital interests of humanity. With few exceptions, these discoveries and inventions have come through individual effort. If they had been protected by patents, capitalized, commercialized, and paid for in proportion to their relative value, physicians and their families would now be in possession of much of the world's wealth. The members of the medical profession have preferred to say, "This will prevent or cure diseases; this will relieve suffering; this will save life; this is good for humanity and must be made available for all."

In this extravagant, swiftly-moving, luxury-loving, high-powered age, the cost of medical care has necessarily increased. However, two things are worthy of note: the physician has more than shared the cost and he had given much more than medicine could have offered in any previous age. Mechanistic, scientific, and highly technical diagnostic and therapeutic methods have not only taxed the physician's skill and ingenuity, but they have touched his purse with a heavy hand. It is difficult for the public to realize that the increased longevity, safety, and comfort now available through modern medicine is out of all proportion to the increase in cost to the patient. Since physicians throughout the history of medicine have refused to profit in a large way by their discoveries and inventions, their opportunities for the acquisition of wealth are self-limited.

Humanity carries a heavy spiritual burden which only the wise family physician can lift. Even the minister can never guess what the family doctor knows. Often a knowledge of physical phenomina serves as a clue to mental aberations. The more profound the secret, the

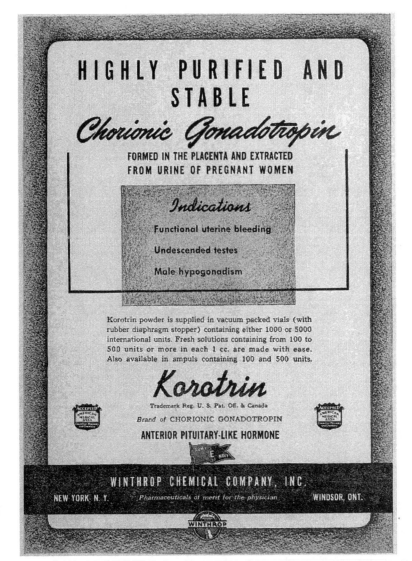

more galling the spiritual burden. The family physician, endowed with free initiative, is not a reformer, he is a mender. He takes broken bodies and lagging spirits and gently repairs damaged parts. He seeks to bring about the best possible spiritual and physical adjustments without reference to social, moral, or financial position. Medicine as now practiced in the United States is fundamental; it attends birth; it sustains life; it prevents and cures diseases; it relieves suffering; it inspires confidence, it dissipates fear; finally it contends with death; and if need be, it witnesses the separation of soul and body; often it lingers to comfort those stricken and bewildered by this last great mystery of life's incomprehensible cycle.

For twenty-five centuries physicians have known what the public seems to have suddenly discovered. I refer to the fact that poor people are in need of medical care. Physicians, more than anyone else, have realized the truth of Christ's admonition "The poor ye have always with you." They have accepted the implication and they have freely and uncomplainingly cared for the poor. Naturally they wonder why the public should suddenly become so aroused.

A few years ago the author had occasion to estimate in dollars and cents the value of free medical services given by the physicians of Oklahoma City. A conservative estimate based upon a very low fee scale indicated a total of approximately one and one-half million dollars annually. Available records indicated that members of the medical school faculty alone poured through the channels of The University and Crippled Childrens Hospitals, free services amounting to nearly one million dollars. At that time the Oklahoma City physicians were giving in free medical services five times the total budget of the Community Fund; approximately ten times the budget of the Chamber of Commerce; and more than one-half the total cost of the City Government, including the public health program.

I submit certain questions for your consideration: Would there be any economy in replacing the present plan with a regimented, tax supported form of socialized medicine, under an expensive bureaucratic control? Would it not be unfair to both physician and patient to disturb the intimate personal relationship which is possible under the present plan and often so essential in the solution of serious problems? Are the people of the United States ready to accept the cold impersonal services of an assigned government medical employee, or do they prefer to retain the right of choice with the hope of intimate, confidential, sympathetic bedside care?

Before deciding to advocate any change which will threaten the integrity of the medical profession and rob the patient of what medicine has to offer, every individual should carefully consider his own personal interests. Remember that in spite of social, religious, political, and economic upheavals, the science of medicine has steadfastly followed the pursuit of truth. With undaunted probity, it has faithfully pierced the zigzag courses of civilization and now stands efficient, ready, and willing to serve, if spared the withering hand of bureautic control.

Repeatedly, it has been said that American medicine is on trial and that the United States is facing some form of socialized or state medicine. In this free country, the people should be the judge. Next to religious freedom, comes medical freedom. There should be no lack of interest, No blind yielding to political and socialistic coercion, no passive washing of hands with the hope of shifting responsibility. After all, medicine is individual, you must make your own decision.

The above brief discussion indicates what medicine is, what it has done, and what it may do in the future if kept free and unhampered. Let us now look socialized medicine squarely in the face and exact an honest admission of its purposes and its possibilities.

Socialized medicine may be brought about in several different ways. But in the last analysis, it means medical care supported and administered by the government. It usually takes the form of so-called compulsory health insurance and the costs are paid out of a fund which is commonly composed of taxes exacted from the wages of employees, matched by the employer from income or capital.

There is no such thing as an adequate, regimented, red-taped, push-buttoned gadgeted, medical care. If you make a trade of medicine, you may expect the cold, impersonal methods of a tradesman. If you add government control you may expect political domination.

Leaving out of consideration the annulling influence of political patronage, would you like for your physician, at the bedside, to spend his time filling out reports and requisitions in triplicate to be filed for public scrutiny in the local headquarters; in the office of your State Board, and finally in Washington; when you are about to succumb to a consuming disease, an excruciating pain or a mortal fear?

Under the orders of his lay board and the pressure of other assignments, would you like for your physician to hastily review your case and record the superficial facts to meet stereotyped requirements while burning with suppressed profanity because of the gross injustice of an unnatural relationship which threatens his self-respect, destroys his initiative, and robs you of his best efforts? Would you not prefer to have your family advisor, your physician of choice, sit leisurely at your bedside, willing and ready to give your story an intelligent and sympathetic hearing; first of all for guidance in the deliberate application of the art and science of medicine to your physical and spiritual demands, and second to make private, confidential records of your mental and physical condition and your professional needs, to be placed in his own personal files which are kept inviolate against all demands unless accompanied by your written authorization or a court order.

Reputable, reasonable, conscientious, and intelligent members of the medical profession are opposed to all forms of socialized or state medicine because there is no such thing as "security against sickness" and because there can be no "economic security" in any program which immediately doubles the cost of medical care. Physicians have sought in vain for justification of the claim that socialized medicine will reduce the cost and bring about a state of economic security. A recent report from one of the departments of the Federal Government indicates that according to statistical studies, the best medicine in the world today, costs the people of the United States approximately one and one quarter billion dollars annually. If the provisions for socialized medicine proposed in the Wagner-Murray-Dingell Bill calling for a witholding tax of more than three billion dollars were to be approved by Congress, the Government would face the embarrassing paradox of promising better medicine at less cost, while actually lowering the quality at more than double the present cost.

Not only has the cost of medical care increased under socialized medicine in other countries, but the deterioration in the quality of service is confirmed by the increase in malingering, in morbidity, and mortality rates. This is not speculation, but a matter of record based upon statistical studies. The morbidity and mortality rates in the United States are lower than in the European countries now under compulsory health insurance. This is doubly significant when we take into account the fact that we are handicapped by having the American Indians and the colored race with marked susceptibility to, and high mortality from, certain diseases. Also a relatively large population in outlying, sparsely settled sections of the United States where medical care is now inadequate, and where adequate care under any plan would be next to impossible.

Worthy of note is the fact that physicians and dentists must negotiate the longest and most difficult educational program known. Physicians must spend eight to twelve years, after highschool, in preparation for practice. The cost is approximately $2,000.00 annually. Medicine, under any form of governmental control, will lose much of its present appeal, ambitious young men and women will seek professions and vocations with greater opportunities for independent self-expression and economic security. This will soon result in lower standards for medical education.

Under the plan proposed in the Wagner-Murray-Dingell Bill, each person in the designated bracket is compelled to participate. He is forced to pay into the fund according to his income and not according to established need for medical services. Would it not be better for the individual employee and better for his country if he would insist upon retaining his self-respect through independent initiative and attempt to budget for medical care and pay what he can when care is needed? The good family physician is always ready to meet the worthy patient half-way; money is not all the physician gets out of medical services; he is grateful for being called. According to the beloved Dr. John Brown, "He makes capital, makes knowledge, and therefor power, out of every case he has." Though he is entitled to an honest living, he would rather tighten his belt and go hungry than sell his freedom for a mess of porridge mixed by a bureaucratic board.

Do not these pertinent facts cause you to ask the question; who wants compulsory health insurance? Certainly not the physicians who know so well what it would mean; obviously not the employees and employers when fully informed. Apparently the movement may be traced to uninformed or possibly designing politicians, to sociologists, to some public health workers, and to agencies and foundations manned by socially minded individuals who with incomplete knowledge and limited vision think in terms of the masses and forget that the finer things of life are individual, personal, sacred, and beyond the influence of common currency.

SAYS WALKING IS NO SISSY EXERCISE; TELLS HOW TO DO IT

Walking is no sissy exercise—for men and women of 35 to 40 years of age and over it is the perfect exercise, George Weinstein, Newark, N. J., advises in the May issue of *Hygeia, The Health Magazine*. It not only will improve one's physical condition but it also can be a good cosmetic and the answer to the problem of falling asleep nights, he explains.

Boxers, football players and track athletes consider walking an important part of their training routine, Mr. Weinstein says, explaining that "It can be quite strenuous! enough so to give you almost as stiff a workout as a set of tennis or a game of handball. If you don't believe it, try a 4-mile an hour pace for the full hour. You'll know that you've been through something —but with this big difference: You will not have subjected your body to those unpredictable, helter-skelter movements that tax your vital organs to the utmost.

"Doctors and physical fitness experts rate walking as an ideal exercise for all ages. For men and women of 35 to 40 and over it rates as *the* perfect exercise.

WASHINGTON OFFICE OPENED

An Office of Information in Washington, D. C., was opened on April 3 by the Council on Medical Service and Public Relations of the American Medical Association, *The Journal* of the Association reports in its April 8 issue. It is located in suite 900, Columbia Medical Building, 1835 I Street, Northwest. A large number of booklets, pamphlets and other published material are being sent to Washington, where they will be readily available to those desiring information concerning the various fields of medicine and the activities of the Association.

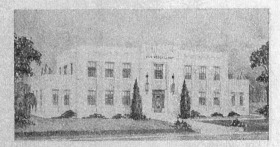

VON WEDEL CLINIC

PLASTIC and GENERAL SURGERY
Dr. Curt von Wedel

TRAUMATIC and INDUSTRIAL SURGERY
Dr. Clarence A. Gallagher

INTERNAL MEDICINE and DIAGNOSIS
Dr. Harry A. Daniels

Special attention to cardiac and gastro intestinal diseases

Complete laboratory and X-ray facilities. Electrocardiograph.

610 Northwest Ninth Street
Opposite St. Anthony's Hospital
Oklahoma City

PENICILLIN-C.S.C.

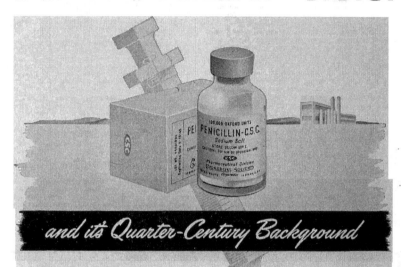

and its Quarter-Century Background

Ehrlich's prophetic vision of the "magic bullet" which would combine deadly efficacy against pathogenic bacteria with perfect compatibility in the human organism, approaches fulfillment in penicillin. Contrary to Ehrlich's expectation, this magic bullet is not a synthetic drug developed by a chemist—it results from the metabolism of a mold. Biologic production of a chemotherapeutic agent thus is now applied in the pharmaceutical field, a new approach.

Instead of the pure rationale of chemical formulas, the life habits of a microorganism are the controlling factor in the manufacture of penicillin; the chemist's important function here consists of guarding his microbian "workmen" and leading them to maximal production.

It is this type of work in which Commercial Solvents Corporation has been engaged since its beginning. For a quarter century, the life habits of bacteria and molds have been the study to which an ever increasing number of scientists in the C. S. C. Research Laboratories are devoting their lives. From their studies have come valuable products, such as butanol, acetone, vitamins, etc., achieved by exacting standards of sterility, an extremely important factor in the working of the highly sensitive microorganisms. What other manufactruer of any kind in the United States has had comparable experience in the application of microbiologic methods to mass production?

With the confidence born of this experience Commercial Solvents Corporation built, with its own funds, what now may well be the largest penicillin plant in the United States. It incorporates not only the fruits of 25 years of experience, but also the latest developments in the testing, handling, and packaging of a

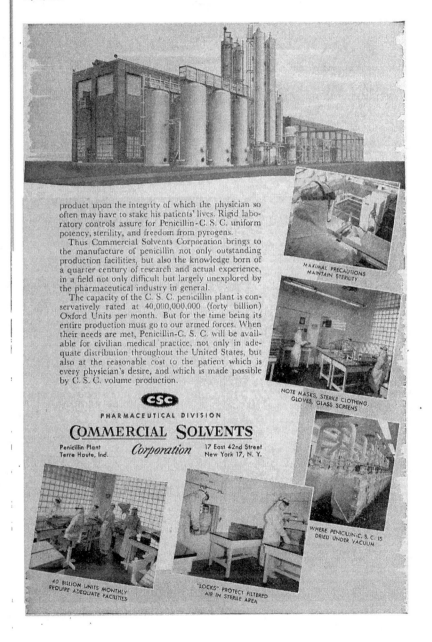

ASSOCIATION ACTIVITIES

PHYSICIANS AND HOSPITAL PERSON-NEL MEETING HELD IN TULSA

An all-day War Session for physicians, surgeons, medical students and hospital representatives of Oklahoma, Kansas and Arkansas was held under the auspices of the American College of Surgeons on Tuesday, April 4 in Tulsa.

Dr. A. W. Pigford, Tulsa, Chairman, Committee on Local Arrangements presided at the morning sessions which opened at 8:30 with the showing of military motion pictures produced for the War Department. From 9:30 to 11:30 experiences in the theaters of war were discussed by Major Clinton L. Compere, Medical Corps, United States Army, Temple, Texas, and McCloskey General Hospital, and Commander Herman A. Gross, Medical Corps, United States Navy, New Orleans, and United States Naval Hospital. From 11:30 to 12:00 "Wartime Problems in Communicable Disease Control" was discussed by Dr. Thomas B. McKneely, Surgeon, United States Public Health Service, Washington, and Chief of Emergency Medical Section.

The hospital personnel held a separate conference from 9:30 to 11:30 with Mr. E. U. Benson, Cushing, President, Oklahoma State Hospital Association, and Superintendent, Masonic Hospital Association, presiding. Wartime hospital problems were discussed by the following: Mr. R. L. Loy, Oklahoma City, Administrator, Oklahoma City General Hospital; Mr. John G. Dudley, Little Rock, Administrator, Baptist State Hospital; Sister M. Gratiana, R.N., Tulsa, Director of Nurses, School of Nursing, St. John's Hospital; Dr. Hester B. Curtis, Kansas City, Missouri, Regional Medical Consultant, Children's Bureau, United States Department of Labor; and Dr. Malcolm T. MacEachern, Chicago, Associate Director, American College of Surgeons.

At the luncheon meeting for both groups Dr. William M. Mills, Topeka, Governor, American College of Surgeons presided. Chauncey D. Leake, Ph. D., Galveston, Dean, University of Texas Medical Branch, discussed "Current Problems in Relation to the Accelerated Program for Pre-Medical and Medical Education," and Dr. C. R. Rountree, Oklahoma City, Medical Chairman for the State of Oklahoma, Eighth Service Command, Procurement and Assignment Service, War Manpower Commission discussed "Current Problems in Medical Manpower for the Armed Forces, Hospitals, and the Civilian Population."

Presiding at the afternoon meeting of the medical group was Dr. Clifford C. Nesselrode, Kansas City, Kansas, Governor, American College of Surgeons. The speakers included Colonel Bradley L. Coley, Medical Corps, United States Army, Dallas, and Surgical Consultant, Eighth Service Command, Captain Karl D. Dietrich, Medical Corps, United States Army, Chickasha, and Penicillin Officer, Borden General Hospital; Dr. Thomas J. Lynch, Tulsa; Lieutenant Colonel H. C. Hardegree, Muskogee, Chief Medical Officer, Veterans Administration Facility; and Commander Gross, Dr. McKneely, and Dr. MacEachern.

The afternoon round table conference for hospital personnel, on the relation of government agencies and voluntary organizations to hospitals in the solution of their wartime problems, was conducted by Mr. Bryce L. Twitty, Tulsa, Administrator, Hillcrest Memorial Hospital, and the participants included Mrs. Mozelle Ewing, Muskogee, Chairman, Oklahoma State Council for War Service; Alice Hyde, Oklahoma City, Chairman, Volunteer Special Services, Oklahoma City Chapter, American Red Cross; Mr. Webb Roberts, Dallas, Regional Representative Government Division, War Production Board; Mr. J. O. Bush, Jr., Oklahoma City, President Elect, Oklahoma State Hospital Association, Mr. N. D. Helland, Tulsa, Executive Director, Group Hospital Service; and Dr. Rountree, Dr. McKneely, Dr. Curtis, and Dr. MacEachern.

The War Session closed with a dinner-forum session starting at 6:15 for physicians, surgeons, and hospital representatives, with Dr. Robert M. Howard, Oklahoma City, Governor, American College of Surgeons acting as moderator. All speakers on the programs for the medical profession and the hospital conference constituted a panel of experts to lead discussion of subjects presented during the day.

HENRY H. TURNER LECTURES IN MEXICO CITY

Dr. Henry H. Turner, Oklahoma City, left on March 30 to spend the first two weeks of April in Mexico City where he was invited to lecture on Endocrinology before the Medical School and the National Academy.

JOSEPH W. KELSO APPOINTED TO MEDICAL ADVISORY COMMITTEE

Dr. Joseph W. Kelso of Oklahoma City has been appointed by Mr. J. B. Harper, Director of Public Welfare, to serve as a member of the Medical Advisory Committee to the Department of Public Welfare. Dr. Kelso's appointment was occasioned by the resignation of Dr. C. R. Rountree, Oklahoma City.

The Committee is composed of the following physicians: Clinton Gallaher, Shawnee, Chairman; Walker Morledge, Oklahoma City; R. M. Sheppard, Tulsa; Mack I. Shanholtz, Wewoka and Hugh M. Galbraith, Oklahoma City. Dr. Shanholtz was appointed in January to replace Dr. Alfred R. Sugg of Ada, who resigned.

The members of the Committee act in an advisory capacity to the Department of Public Welfare in those cases involving physical and mental incapacity.

DR. CLAUDE S. CHAMBERS ELECTED TO BOARD OF REGENTS

Dr. Claude S. Chambers, Seminole, was elected President of the University of Oklahoma Board of Regents when the board met to consider university faculty recommendations for changes in the University College Program.

"WAR CONFERENCE" ON INDUSTRIAL MEDICINE, HYGIENE AND NURSING ST. LOUIS, MAY 8-14, 1944

The Second "War Conference" of industrial physicians, industrial hygienists and industrial nurses will be held in St. Louis, Missouri, May 8-14 at the Hotel Jefferson. The participating organizations are the American Association of Industrial Physicians and Surgeons, American Industrial Hygiene Association, National Conference of Governmental Industrial Hygienists, and the American Association of Industrial Nurses.

The medical subjects to be presented include welding, in relation to clinical aspects and control of hazards; noise, as to medical phases and means of prevention; better health in small plants; the industrial physician's opportunity to advance medical knowledge; maladjustment and job environment; women in industry; and panel discussions on "Who Can Work?" and other timely questions.

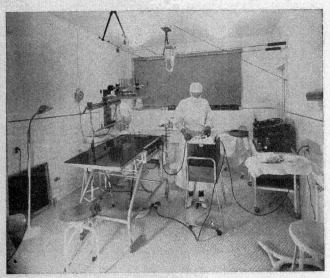

The industrial hygienists will examine the health hazards presented by the new synthetic rubber industry; radium; solvents; the toxicology of TNT; the possibilities of an excessive silica dust hazard from the extensive quartz crystal industry which has recently sprung up in many areas of the country; techniques of air sampling in specific reference to the collection of cutting oil mists and of lead fumes, the latter encountered in soldering operations where the hazard is increasing with lack of adequate tin; and hazards of exposure to cadmium, which is known to be more poisonous than lead, and has begun to cause a number of cases of poisoning.

The industrial nurses will consider postwar planning for nurses and medical services in industry; nursing ethics in industrial work; problems in industrial health and its promotion; the young nurse in the industrial environment; the industrial nurse's part in the rehabilitation of psychiatric problems; wartime industrial health; and industrial nursing and leadership.

This "War Conference" will present an unequalled opportunity for every one interested to any degree in industrial health problems—especially those of present wartime exigencies—to hear them discussed by the recognized experts in all departments of this important and growing field.

WARTIME GRADUATE MEDICAL MEETING TO BE HELD IN DENVER, JUNE 21-24

The Wartime Graduate Medical Meeting of Clinics, demonstrations and lectures under the auspices of the American Medical Association, the American College of Physicians and the American College of Surgeons will be held in Denver from June 21-24th inclusive. Officially June 24 will be the date of the regional meeting of the College of Physicians. Distinguished men of national repute are invited to attend and take part in the program.

RESOLUTION

Dr. J. T. Frizzell moved to Custer County in 1900 to engage in the practice of general medicine. In 1903 he was co-organizer of the Custer County Medical Society, and became a charter member of that group and has continuously been a member of the Custer County Medical Society since that time. He engaged in the active practice of medicine until 1942 when has was forced to retire because of ill health.

THEREFORE, BE IT RESOLVED: That in recognition of forty-two years' service to the people of Custer County, to his colleagues in the practice of medicine, and to his profession, that the Custer County Medical Society grant to Dr. Frizzell an honorary life-time membership in that society.

BE IT FURTHER RESOLVED: That the Custer County Medical Society request of the Oklahoma State Medical Association that they grant Dr. J. T. Frizzell, Clinton, Oklahoma, an honorary lifetime membership in the Oklahoma State Medical Association and that a copy of this resolution be sent to the said Oklahoma State Medical Association for their appropriate action.

F. R. VIEREGG, M.D.
President, Custer County Medical Society
C. J. ALEXANDER, M.D.
Secretary, Custer County Medical Society

Woman's Auxiliary

PRESIDENT'S REPORT TO NATIONAL ASSOCIATION

The year brought a three-fold challenge to our six groups. First, we must meet immediate war needs. Second, we must carry on as normally as the time will permit. Third, we must plan for peace and a better world of the future . . . We met these challenges as follows:

War Needs

Every county worked in all or some of the following fields: surgical dressings, nurses aides, motor corp, Gray Ladies, canteen, first aid, home nursing, nutrition, knitting, block mothers, rationing, nurses recruitment, doctors' aides, Bond booths, recruitment, Bond and Red Cross drives, speakers, bureaus, meeting Troop trains, making garments for hospitals, providing layettes for homes, helping buy equipment for recreation centers. One group took over the Tuberculosis Seal Sale in their city. The placing of Hygeia in public places in the hope of saving time of our over-worked doctors was stressed. County groups have purchased War Bonds with their savings funds. The State Treasurer was authorized to buy Bonds with our Student Loan Fund which was not needed at this time. Each County group reports on the number of hours spent in war work for the year and the total is amazing.

To Carry on Normally

We stressed the need for keeping organized, even though membership was depleted. We started the year with six groups and still have six groups. In some cases, we streamlined our meetings to fit working members. We kept in touch with "War Wives" so as to keep them interested. We entertained for new coming wives to interest them in Auxiliary Work and to make them feel at home. We tried to keep up every phase of our Auxiliary work except that of organizing new groups, striving to carry out the program of the National Auxiliary.

To Plan for Peace

Groups studied present legislative measures. A paper on "Socialized Medicine" was prepared by our State Legislative Chairman covering all phases of that subject. This paper is available for use at Auxiliary meetings and Lay meetings. Pamphlets and cartoons on the Wagner-Murray Bill were distributed. One group is studying Pan-American Relations. Groups have been asked to discuss "Peace Plans."

Our Annual meeting will be held April twenty-four and twenty-five at Tulsa, at which time our silver tray achievement award will be made to the County that carried out the National and local program to the fullest extent.

Respectfully submitted,
Mrs. F. Maxey Cooper, President

State Membership Report

Tulsa, 113 members; Oklahoma City, 114 members; Ada, 14 members; Shawnee, 16 members; Norman, 18 members.

Tulsa County

The meeting was held at the home of Mrs. Morris Lhevine with 46 members present. Mrs. Carl Hots gave a talk on "Let's Eat Victory Gardening" and the subject of home canning was discussed.

The Public Relations Committee met on March 7 with Dr. Tuzary speaking on "Pan-American Relations". Dr. Mable Hart discussed the Wagner-Murray-Dingell Bill.

URGE BLOOD STUDY FOR ALL WHO RETURN FROM MALARIOUS AREAS

Two Army Officers Find Malaria Organisms In Blood Of Italian War Prisoners Who Said They Had Never Had The Disease

The blood of all persons who have returned from areas where malaria is prevalent should be carefully examined and all those found to have in their blood the organisms that cause the disease should be treated, even though they have no symptoms. Captain Stanis P. Carney, Sanitary Corps, and Captain Noah B. Levin, Medical Corps, Army of the United States, advise in *The Journal of the American Medical Association* for April 8. In an examination of 2,723 Italian prisoners of war who had seen service for varying periods in malarious regions, the two army officers found the organisms causing malaria still in the blood of some of the prisoners months after evacuation from a region where malaria was prevalent. They found parasites in the blood of men who had maintained they never had had the disease, and also that malaria may be contracted with no symptoms of active disease until months after infection.

It is emphasized by the authors that "No expectation of the residual malarial rate of United States troops can be predicated from these [findings]. A great many of the Italians grew up in malarious regions and were exposed and infected long before their period of military service, while only a relatively small percentage of American soldiers come from areas where malaria is present in any degree at all. The antimalaria precautions taken for United States troops in the field also serve to keep the incidence of malaria down. An advice from the office of the Surgeon General of the United States Army indicates that the incidence of parasitemia [parasites in the blood] in the absence of clinical symptoms for our returned troops is much lower than the figures reported here for the prisoner group. In spite of these differential factors, we feel that this study emphasizes the necessity for careful examination of blood smears for all personnel who have returned from areas where malaria is prevalent and the need for treatment to sterilize the blood in all cases of parasitemia. This will serve the double purpose of protecting the person from further attacks and of eliminating him as a carrier."

Of the 2,723 prisoners examined, 257 or 9.7 per cent had a positive blood smear; 56 or 2.1 per cent had active malaria; 188 or 6.5 per cent had a history of malaria; 55 or 59 percent of those with active malaria had no history of malaria and 212 or 83 per cent of those with positive smears had no history of the disease.

The authors explain that it soon became apparent that malaria was going to be a problem of some concern in the prison camp "since immediately after arrival of the prisoners cases of malaria began to appear. The first question which arose was the problem of transmission of the disease to the uninfected prisoners, to the army personnel attached to the camp and to the nearby civilian population. This was satisfactorily answered by the results of two mosquito surveys made in the area in which the camp is located, one made by the state university and the other under the direction of the Seventh Service Command, in both of which no anopheline mosquitoes were found. [This is the type of mosquito that transmits malaria.] As an added precaution, however, all men hospitalized for malaria were screened by mosquito bars after dusk.

"The proposal to send some of the prisoners to work on farms in the region of the camp raised another question. Since, in many cases, side camps were to be set up, sometimes many miles away from army hospital facilities, it was decided to make an attempt to locate all men with parasitemia."

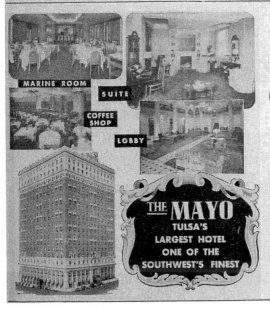

• OBITUARIES •

J. E. Crawford, M.D.
1870-1944

Dr. J. E. Crawford, member of the Washington-Nowata County Medical Society, died at his home in Bartlesville on March 19, three weeks after a coronary attack.

Dr. Crawford graduated from the medical school of the University of Nashville and served his internship in the Charity Hospital of Tulane University in New Orleans, La. For the past fifteen years he has been practicing in Bartlesville. Dr. Crawford was active in the civic affairs of Bartlesville and was a member of the Oklahoma State Medical Association, the American Medical Association, the Bartlesville Masonic Lodge and the First Methodist Church of Bartlesville.

He is survived by his widow, Mrs. Gertrude Crawford; four daughters, Mrs. J. A. Burran of Clovis, N. M., Mrs. J. R. Denison of McLean, Texas, Mrs. J. Lee Hillard of Seguin, Texas, and Mrs. H. F. Knight of Tylor, Texas; a brother, Dr. H. G. Crawford, Bartlesville, and six grandchildren, several nieces and nephews.

W. G. Bisbee, M.D.
1876-1944

Dr. Walter G. Bisbee, born August 1, 1876, in Dexter, Iowa, died March 17 at Bristow, Oklahoma. Graduate of Dartmouth Medical College, Hanover, New Hampshire, he served a years' internship at the New York Lying-In Hospital, New York. After practicing for a short time in Philadelphia, Pennsylvania, he came to Chandler, Oklahoma in 1902. He practiced in Oklahoma City for a short while, but moved to Bristow in 1922 where he practiced until the time of his death.

During the last War, Dr. Bisbee served with the United States Medical Corps, holding the rank of Captain. He was a member of the Rotary Club, Masonic Lodge, American Legion, Oklahoma State Medical Association and Secretary of the Creek County Medical Society.

Surviving Dr. Bisbee are his widow, one son, Wallace, and three grandchildren.

L. L. Wade, M.D.
1880-1944

Dr. L. L. Wade, Ryan, pioneer Jefferson County physician, died April 1, at Waurika, after an illness of several months. At the time of his death, he was Secretary of the Jefferson County Medical Society.

Dr. Wade came to Ryan before statehood as a school teacher and was the first County Superintendent of schools of Jefferson County. He laid out all of the school districts on the east side of the county. He was active not only in educational matters but all movements that had to do with the building of a good community and state. He made his influence felt in all public matters. Dr. Wade was a successful physician and will be missed in this sphere as well as others. A good citizen, a great physician and a real friend.

Surviving are his widow, Mrs. L. L. Wade of Ryan; his mother, Mrs. Peyton L. Wade, Decatur, Texas; three sons, James Peyton of Healdton; Roy Marvin and Lisby Lucius, Jr., of Ryan, at present a student in the University of Oklahoma; one grandson, two granddaughters, one brother and two sisters.

University of Oklahoma School of Medicine

While enroute to the Letterman General Hospital, San Francisco, Colonel Rex Bolend made a very interesting address to the Army and Navy Trainees in the School of Medicine. Colonel Bolend, until recently, was in command of Evacuation Hospital Number 21 in the Southwest Pacific. He has been returned for medical treatment. As well known, Evacuation Hospital No. 21 is composed chiefly of former members of the faculty of the School of Medicine and staff of the University of Oklahoma Hospitals.

Dr. P. S. Pelouze, Associate Professor of Urology, University of Pennsylvania School of Medicine and Consultant, U. S. Public Health Service, on Monday, February 28, at 2 P.M., lectured in the Auditorium of the Medical School Building on the subject "Diagnosis, Treatment, and Control of Gonococcal Infections."

The Library has just received a large number of new books and has them on display in the Browsing Corner. The following should be of interest to many, but they are only a sample. The Library staff will be glad to have you come in and see them.

Adolph—Physiological Regulations. 1943.
Bercovitz—Clinical Tropical Medicine. 1943.
Borckus—Gastro-enterology. 1943-44.
Brown—Skin Grafting of burns; primary care, treatment, repair. 1943.
Forbus—Reaction to Injury. 1943.
Goldberg—Clinical Tuberculosis. 1942.
Lewis—Introduction to Medical Mycology. 1943.
Livingston—Pain Mechanism. 1943.
Regan—Medical Malpractice. 1943.
Seagrave—Burma Surgeon. 1943.
Thorek—Plastic Surgery of the Breast and Abdominal Wall. 1942.
Trueta—Principles and Practice of War Surgery. 1943.
Wampler—Principles and Practice of Industrial Medicine. 1943.
Wolf—Human Gastric Function. 1943.

The Faculty of the Medical School entertained at Luncheon at the University Hospital the physicians who attended the Tri-State Polio Conference on February 23.

Thirty-five physicians of Oklahoma, Kansas and Texas were present, representing the pediatricians and orthopedists who took care of 90 per cent of the polio cases during the recent epidemic in the three states named.

Claude Bernard

"Nothing in his pure and harmonious life was turned aside from its chief aim. Enamored of literature, art and philosophy, Claude Bernard as a physiologist lost nothing by these noble passions; on the contrary, they all helped in developing the science with which he identified himself, and of which he is the highest and most complete embodiment. He was a physiologist such as no man had been before him. 'Claude Bernard,' said a foreign scientist, 'is not merely a physiologist, he is physiology.'

"His very death seems to make a new era in science. For the first time in our country, a man of science will receive those public honors hitherto reserved for political and military celebrities. The cabinet honored itself yesterday in asking parliment, which unanimously agreed to celebrate at state expense the solemn obsequies of the master who is no more. And one phrase of Gambetta, speaking in the name of the Budget Commission, sums up all that we have said: 'The light, which has just been extinguished, cannot be replaced'."—Paul Bert, Paris, February, 12, 1878. Experimental Medicine. Claude Bernard. Page xix. The MacMillan Co. 1927.

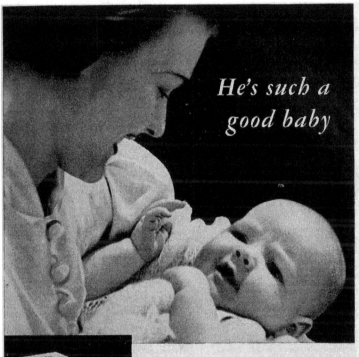

He's such a good baby

Takes his 'Dexin' formulas avidly, plays cheerfully, sleeps well. And with all this comes mother's thorough satisfaction in a smooth routine, a happy baby, and her greater enjoyment of motherhood.

'Dexin' helps assure uncomplicated infant feeding. Its high dextrin content (1) diminishes intestinal fermentation and the tendency to colic and diarrhea and (2) promotes the formation of soft, flocculent, easily digested curds.

'Dexin' promotes good feeding habits. Palatable 'Dexin' formulas are not excessively sweet, and do not dull the appetite. Babies take other bland supplementary foods with less coaxing. 'Dexin' is readily soluble in hot or cold milk.

'Dexin' reg. U. S. Patent Office

'Dexin' does make a difference

COMPOSITION

Dextrins	75%	Mineral Ash	0.25%
Maltose	24%	Moisture	0.75%

Available carbohydrate 99%
115 calories per ounce
6 level packed tablespoonfuls equal 1 ounce

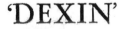

'DEXIN'

HIGH DEXTRIN CARBOHYDRATE

Literature on request

DURROUGHS WELLCOME & CO. (U.S.A.) 9-11 E. 41st St., New York 17, N. Y.

★ FIGHTIN' TALK ★

The following have been appointed to the rank of first lieutenant: JACK WENDELL MYERS, El Reno; JOHN DANIEL INGLE, Oklahoma City, now a resident at Wesley Hospital; JAMES R. McLAUCHLIN, JR., Oklahoma City, now serving as resident at St. Anthony Hospital; WILLIAM MILTON PRIER, Oklahoma City, now a resident at Hillcrest Hospital in Tulsa; JAMES ROBERT WALKER, Enid; RICHARD ALLEN CLAY, Durant; JOHN BERRY GILBERT, Oklahoma City.

The following have been called to active duty: LT. HERBERT ORR, Tulsa; CAPTAIN JAMES L. NICHOLSON, Guymon.

Some recent promotions are as follows: From lieutenant to captain; ROY MAXWELL WADSWORTH, Sand Springs; CHARLES B. OVERBEY, JR., Mangum; From captain to major: HARRY C. FORD, Oklahoma City; LEE B. WORD, Bartlesville; HILLIARD E. DENYER, Chandler; From major to lieutenant colonel; COLE D. PITTMAN, Tulsa.

CAPTAIN VAYLE HARRISON, Oklahoma City, has been killed in action in the South Pacific. Captain Harrison was graduated from the University of Oklahoma Medical School in 1937 and served his internship at Los Angeles General Hospital in Los Angeles, California. In November, before Pearl Harbor, Captain Harrison enlisted in the Army and was first stationed at Ft. MacArthur, San Pedro, California. Later he was stationed in New Guinea but recently was moved to a new base.

Captain Harrison's mother lives in Oklahoma City, and his wife and two children live in Los Angeles.

CAPTAIN E. D. PADBERG, Ada, has recently been promoted. He is now Assistant Flight Surgeon of the San Antonio aviation Cadet Center in San Antonio, Texas. Captain Padberg states that he sees and hears of a good many Oklahoma doctors and that they are all doing a ''bang-up'' job for Uncle Sam.

From somewhere in the Pacific Area comes word from CAPTAIN MYRON C. ENGLAND who says that he is receiving the Journal and letters.

CAPTAIN PHIL SALKELD, Vinita, is now stationed at Austin, Texas. After receiving our news letter, Captain Salkeld writes: ''My only other method of keeping up on the latest news is by checking dog-tags of innumerable examinees until I find an 'Okie'. Then the whole production line bogs down while we bat the breeze.'' The Air Corps stands high with Captain Salkeld and he is quite enthusiastic about flying.

From Camp Hood, Texas, comes word from MAJOR J. HOYLE CARLOCK, Ardmore. Major Carlock has been in the service almost three years and has been doing command and staff work.

MAJOR HERVEY A. FOERSTER, Oklahoma City, is now stationed in 'jolly old England'. He states that he has met quite a few Oklahoma doctors there and that everything in general is quite comfortable. Major Foerster praises the work being done by the Red Cross Canteens.

CAPTAIN LESTER P. SMITH, Marlow, is now doing hospital work in Italy. He has recently been transferred to a new unit from the Division he has been with since 1940. He is enjoying his work but is anxious for news from Oklahoma.

From the Italian Front comes a V-Mail from CAPTAIN' CLIFTON FELTS, Seminole. The following paragraph expresses well the feeling of a great many of our men who are overseas:

''Am very much interested in the socialistic trends that are being vigorously pushed by the New Dealers. Hope such measures are not allowed to become law. We in the service feel we deserve some freedom from Government supervision when we finish this stretch. I am hoping public opinion will not allow socialized medicine.''

CAPTAIN A. V. MURRY, Picher, is at Carlisle Barracks, Pa., where he will stay for six weeks, then go to Stark General Hospital at Charleston, S. C.

CAPTAIN CHARLES H. EADS, Tulsa, is stationed at the army and Navy General Hospital, Hot Springs, Arkansas. Before going to Hot Springs, Captain Eads spent several months at March Field, California and some time at Camp Robinson, Arkansas.

CAPTAIN GEORGE L. BORECKY, Oklahoma City, is now doing Venereal Disease Control Work in England. We enjoyed Captain Borecky's interesting V-Mail.

From somewhere in China, Burma or India, we received an interesting V-Mail from MAJOR RAYMOND L. MURDOCH, Oklahoma City. Major Murdoch writes as follows: ''Have seen many interesting things in Hospitals and otherwise from one end to the other of the India-Burma-China Theater. Had a nice visit with DR. W. N. DAVIDSON of Cushing in his hospital. Have come the long way around and seen and heard of numerous Oklahomans.''

Promotion of MAJOR L. H. RITZHAUPT, Guthrie, to Lieutenant Colonel, has recently been announced by the War Department of Washington. COLONEL RITZHAUPT served with the 45th Division in the Louisiana maneuvers in August, 1940 as a member of the State Staff. He was designated as State Medical Officer in October, 1940 and will remain on active duty in this capacity.

LT. NEIL T. PRICE, Oklahoma City, recent graduate of the University of Oklahoma School of Medicine, is now serving with the armed forces in Italy. Lt. Price is the father of a new son, Neil T, Price, Jr., but has not, as yet, met the new addition to the family.

LT. & MRS ROBERT MENCH, Oklahoma City, have been recent Oklahoma City visitors. Lt. Mench has been in active service with the Navy in the Pacific for the past twenty months, and is now awaiting further assignment.

LT. A. C. LISLE, JR., McLoud, graduate of the University of Oklahoma School of Medicine in May, 1943, was married on April 9 to Miss Madge Troup of Holdenville. Lt. Lisle will report for duty at Carlisle Barracks.

LT. COMDR. JAMES H. ABERNETHY, graduate of the University of Oklahoma School of Medicine in 1939, was married on April 8 to Miss Sara Wallace of Oklahoma City. Lt. Comdr. Abernethy is the nephew of Dr. E. A. Abernethy of Altus. He is stationed at the Naval Air Station, Norman.

Recently in Hawaii there has been organized the University of Oklahoma Club. The club is composed of graduates and former students from OU and consists of permanent residents of Hawaii, war workers and service personnel. It has been granted a charter by the executive board of the University of Oklahoma Association. Many interesting dinners and meetings are planned where classmates can be brought together again for the first time since their college days. The following Oklahoma physicians are charter members: COMDR. R. B. FORD, Tulsa; COMDR. C. C. FULTON, Atoka; LT. JOHN A. CUNNINGHAM, Miami.

COLONEL KENNETH A. BREWER, Oklahoma City, is commanding officer of an evacuation hospital and is now stationed in England. Colonel Brewer says that many of the officers and nurses have taken to British cycling but that he is still depending upon his feet for transit.

MAJOR HOWARD SHORBE, Oklahoma City, is now a member of a surgical team working immediately behind the front in Italy where he has been on duty for many months. Major Shorbe sees many Oklahomans who are now on active duty in that theater of operation. Recently, he received a pleasant surprise when, upon opening a box of surgical dressings, found a card on top saying "wrapped by the Oklahoma County Red Cross". This, he states, was like receiving a letter from home.

Recently Major Shorbe has seen DR. FRED PERRY,

Healdton, and MISS ERNESTINE DUFF, formerly supervisor of nurses at the Crippled Children's hospital.

Close-to-the-front surgery is relatively new and Major Shorbe has had some interesting professional sessions with the British and Italian physicians.

Medicine At War

MEDICAL ORGANIZATIONS IN THIS WAR ARE MIRACLES OF MOBILE MANAGEMENT*

Marcia Winn

The assistant surgeon general of the army sighed. "There are so many types of warfare this time." Then, with a mental glance back toward 1917-18, "we had the stable type . . . we could predict. Now we just keep moving . . . "

In that confession lies the care of American medical achievement in this war: mobility.

Medical care in this war is a far cry from the civil war, when Major Jonathan Letterman set up America's first field hospital and ambulance crops at the battle of Antietam to care for 10,000 wounded men. Major Letterman moved in after the battle. The field hospitals today move in with it. Doctors and surgeons follow the army and go with it to every front line to tend the wounded. Then they literally fly them away for immediate surgical care.

The time between injury and first aid has been cut to an average of less than one hour; the time between injury and emergency surgery is less than 10 hours; death among the wounded is the lowest in the history of warfare.

Evacuation to a base hospital by plane is only one of the various methods used. In new Guinea, the

*Oklahoma City Times, April 13, 1944.

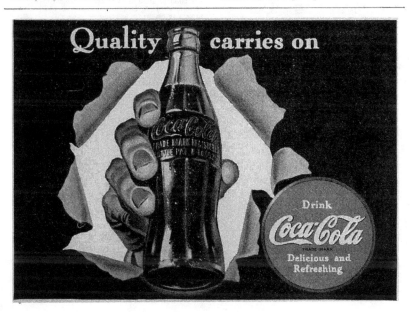

wounded were flown from the front to a field hospital back of the hills in an hour; the trip would take three weeks by pack animals. At Gaudalcanal, all the wounded eventually were evacuated by air.

In the army the procedure goes like this:

A soldier, wounded, falls. A medical man, or corpsman, examines his wound and gives him first aid—sulfa, morphine, water, if indicated, a tourniquet if necessary, a battle dressing. On a tag, he writes, with indelible pencil, what he has done and fastens it to the wounded man.

The corpsman then goes on with the advancing troops, and the litter bearers come up, often under direct fire, take him to the battalion aid station.

It may be 50 yards away, or 1,000. Here the man is given resuscitative treatment such as blood plasma, morphine, dressings, sulfa, or splints.

He then is moved back to the nearby collecting station. Here his injury is classified. From here, the man goes to a clearing station four or five miles back. If he needs an immediate operation, he gets it. A surgical team works here in a double tented operation room brought up with all its equipment by truck. Each truck-operating room can care for from 80 to 100 men in 24 hours.

From the clearing station, the man goes by jeep, bus, or plane, depending on the priority of his wound (head, chest, and abdominal wounds move first) to an evacuation hospital.

This is a conveyance line rather than an assembly line, and only emergency surgery is done, but at each stop the man is given necessary additional care. The line and its plan changes with the terrain and military strategy, but it permits life saving surgical measures and reduces serious complications.

Hand in hand with medicine is science, seen in such extraordinary aids to battle surgery as the portable X-Ray, a complete unit carried in three small foot lockers, which are borne in, set up, and taking pictures in 15 minutes. In 20 minutes the surgeon probing for bullets or shell fragments has in his hand an X-Ray of their exact location.

The army uses three types of hospitals at the front. One is the 25 bed portable surgical hospital, which can be carried into the area on canvas packboards by a crew of four doctors and 33 men. Tents and reserve supplies come up later, but the crew carries all essential equipment. One medical crew hiked from Port Moresby to Buna, bearing such a hospital, in 40 days.

Next is the semi-mobile evacuation hospital, which has to have trails or roads. It does a complete line of definitive surgery and works in tents, with wards for surgery, medical preoperative, shock, and orthopedic cases.

The navy's field hospitals, developed especially for amphibious landings, are miracles of compressed packing. Everything that goes in goes in through the water and is carried in by men, even the refrigerator, the only really bulky piece of equipment. This is estimated by weight and need down to the last bottle of soap, safety razor, and tablespoon—the latter necessary for sterilizing water for a hypodermic.

Developed under the stress of war are canvas blankets that can be carried right to the front for wounded men; a portable generator that is carried in by hand, set down, fed a pint of gasoline, and starts to generate electricity sufficient to light a field hospital; a chest pharmacy so that doctors can compound their own drugs; a portable kerosene incubator for the incubation of cultures; and an air borne surgical unit, three 16 x 16 operating rooms complete with screens, floors, and roof, that can be flown in and set up in 20 minutes.

The navy's (marine) field operation is similar, but covers less ground.

Initial beachhead casualties are evacuated to ships before the field hospitals are set up. Once the air field is established, evacuation by air begins, 20 patients at a time being flown in Douglas transports.

Doctors who go in with troops making a beachhead carry one of the neatest little packages in the history of medicine: A pocket surgical kit, battle dressings, sulfa, bandages, field splints, morphine, plasma, iodine, safety pins, a clinical thermometer, diagnosis tablets, and an indelible pencil. The corpsman substitutes a scalpel, forceps shears, and flashlight for the surgical kit, but carries everything else.

"With those, you cope with almost anything at the front," commented Capt. Warwick T. Brown, who developed many of the newer portable aids after seeing their need at Guadalcanal.

MEASLES

Reminding parents that this is the time of year when measles begins to increase, the Bureau of Publicity of the Indiana State Medical Association today issued a bulletin which pointed out that usually there is a marked rise in the number of cases through the spring, with the high point in April or May.

"The usual symptoms of measles are inflammation of the eyes and nose, and fever," the bulletin points out. "The eyes are swollen, and are irritated by light. There is usually discharge from the nose and eyes, the temperature rises and the patient complains of chilliness, cough, loss of appetite and lassitude.

"The symptoms are often not recognized as measles, so it is during this period that the infection is most likely to spread to other children. The fact that measles is transferred from person to person in the early stage before the characteristic rash appears makes it difficult to limit the spread of infection.

"The child with measles should be kept in bed in a room whose air has adequate humidity. Serum from the blood of some one who has recovered from the disease is now being used in some cases to ward off serious attacks in children who have been exposed.

"After an attack, children should be protected against possible exposure to other contagious diseases, for measles lowers the resistance to other infections, such as laryngitis, bronchitis, pneumonia and middle ear diseases.

"Parents should take every precaution to protect their children from measles. An attack, however, protects the victim from further attacks in about 95 per cent of the cases."

The Mind's Unchangeable Tripod

The human mind has at different periods of its evolution passed successively through *feeling, reason* and *experiment*. First, feeling alone, imposing itself on reason, created the truths of faith or theology. Reason or philosophy, the mind's next mistress, brought to birth scholasticism. At last, experiment, or study of natural phenomena, taught man that the truths of the outer world are to be found ready formulated neither in feeling nor in reason. These are indispensable as guides; but to attain external truths we must of necessity go down into the objective reality of things where they lie hidden in their phenominal form.

Thus, in the natural progress of things, appeared the experimental method which includes everything and which, as we shall soon see, leans successively on the three divisions of that unchangeable tripod; sentiment, reason and experiment. In the search for truth by means of this method, feeling always takes the lead, it begets the *a priori* idea or intuition; reason or reasoning develops the idea and deduces its logical consequences. But if feeling must be clarified by the light of reason, reason in turn must be guided by experiment.—Experimental Medicine. Claude Bernard. Page 28. The MacMillan Company. 1927.

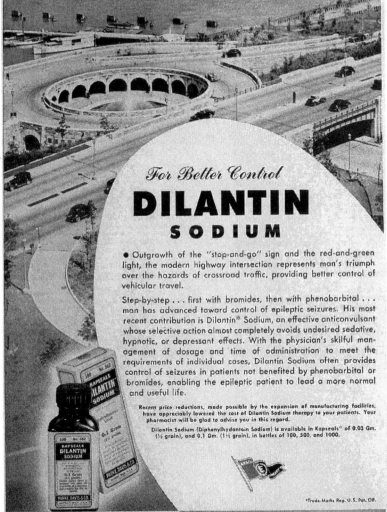

BOOK REVIEWS

"The chief glory of every people arises from its authors."—Dr. Samuel Johnson.

HUBER THE TUBER. Harry A. Wilmer, M.D. Second Edition. National Tuberculosis Association. 1942.

Harry A. Wilmer's story of tuberculosis under the above title, presents a serious drama with compelling humor. The clever illustrations with the accompanying brief descriptive paragraphs amount to easy effective lessons in anatomy and pathology and the behavior and varied manifestations of the tubercle bacillus in the broncho-pulmonary system.

The book is at once easy to read, entertaining and instructive, Not only should it be placed in the hands of every tuberculosis patient but a wide reading should be encouraged because of its public health values.

The exciting adventures of Huber the Tuber and his associates make hilarious comedy for all who read. Every doctor should have a copy on his reception room table.—Lewis J. Moorman, M.D.

ACUTE INFECTIONS OF THE MEDIASTINUM. Harold Neuhof, M.D., D.S., F.A.C.S., and Edward E. Jemerin, M.D., D.S., F.A.C.S. The Williams & Wilkins Company. 1943. 407 pages. Price $6.00.

In this important treatise, the authors have attempted to assemble all available knowledge concerning this most difficult problem. That they speak with relative authority is implied by the fact that their detailed discussions and well considered conclusions are supplemented by 100 carefully tabulated case reports, revealing exhaustive diagnostic and therapeutic considerations.

PART I. The authors devote 24 pages to the Introduction and Review of Literature.

PART II. Presentation of Cases covers 263 pages, classified as follows:

  Group A: Acute Infections of the Mediastinum Secondary to Trauma to the Esophagus.

  Group B: Acute Mediastinitis Secondary to Upper Respiratory Infection.

  Group C: Acute Mediastinitis Secondary to Infection of the Lung or Pleura.

  Group D: Acute Mediastinitis of Miscellaneous Etiology.

PART III. Fundamental Considerations.
  Surgical Anatomy.
  Classification.
  Etiology.
  Pathology and Topography.
  Bacteriology.
  Pathogenesis.

PART IV. Clinical Considerations.
  History, Symptoms, and Signs.
  Diagnostic Aspects.

PART V. Treatment and Results.
  Indications for Operation.
  Treatment.
  Results.
  Concluding Remarks.

The above outline is sufficient to show the meticulous comprehensive consideration accorded the acute infections of this small complicated anatomical area, potentially full of pathological possibilities leading to a high mortality. The anatomic considerations as presented by the authors are of vital importance to the clinician as well as the surgeon. The clinical manifestations and diagnostic features are of vital importance to every doctor seriously interested in the practice of medicine. Finally, the radiographic features, so well presented, make up the most important part of this valuable book

and definitely places the x-ray in the position of prime importance in the diagnosis of mediastinal infections.—Lewis J. Moorman, M.D.

TRAUMATIC INJURIES OF FACIAL BONES. An Atlas of Treatment. John B. Erich, M.S., D.D.S., M.D.; Louie T. Austin, D.D.S., F.A.C.D. In Collaboration with Bureau of Medicine and Surgery, U.S. Navy. W. B. Saunders Company. Philadelphia and London.

This unusual book is well worth any physician's consideration, who is called upon to treat traumatic injuries. It presents in outline form the acceptable form of treatment for every type of fracture and defect involving the mandible, maxilla, malar bones and nasal bones. It explains in detail diagnosis, emergency treatment, pre-operative preparations, operative procedures, splints, braces and various retentive appliances, as well as post-operative care and permanent prostheses.

The usual feature is the unique manner in which it is illustrated. By means of moulage models of both soft structures and the bony framework, each type of injury or fracture is reproduced. This model is then photographed and the result is a very clear-cut photograph, giving the observer detail in three dimensions. Likewise, the surgical correction, the appliance of wires, splints or appliances is shown.

The authors stress the fact that most any physician may be called upon to render first aid to these conditions, but that the best results are to be obtained by teamwork and cooperation of various branches of medicine, especially those of dentistry, otolaryngology and plastic surgery.—John F. Burton, M.D.

MINOR SURGERY. Fifth Edition. Frederick Christopher. W. B. Saunders Company. Philadelphia, 1943. 1006 pages. Price $10.00.

Sometime in the distant past all surgery was divided into major and minor surgery. That such was an unfortunate division has been held by many surgeons and physicians as well. This opinion is supported and emphasized by the Fifth Edition of Minor Surgery. The author at least implies in the Preface that there is no surgery which can rightfully be looked upon as minor.

It can well be said that this new Edition has added to and strengthened an already complete and strong text. That it is timely and distinctly up to date is emphasized by the inclusion in the contents of the treatment to increase the Ph of urine during sulfonamide administration, sternal infusions and "paratrooper fracture." The new chapter on pre-operative and post-operative care is one which appeals not only to the young surgeon but has many facts and discussions which would be of distinct benefit to the patients of the more experienced. In brief, no young graduate in or out of the armed forces, in or out of the hospital can well afford to be without this book. The general practitioner or the surgeon who is acquainted with the previous editions will be elated that Dr. Christopher has had the time to bring out this new edition.

Despite war-time restrictions, the paper, the printing, the illustrations, charts and diagrams as well as the binding adhere to the usual general excellence of a Saunders publication.—L. J. Starry, M.D.

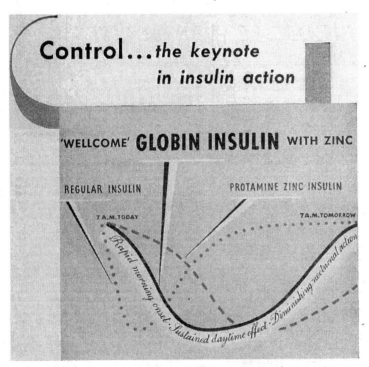

A schematic representation of the effects of various
insulins on the blood sugar of a fasting diabetic patient.

• 'Wellcome' Globin Insulin with Zinc, a new type of insulin, offers an advance in diabetic control. It provides a rapid onset of action; strong prolonged effect during the day when most needed; and diminishing action at night. Nocturnal insulin reactions are rarely encountered.

'Wellcome' Globin Insulin with Zinc conforms to the needs of the patient. *A single injection* daily has been found to control satisfactorily many moderately severe and severe cases of diabetes. 'Wellcome' Globin Insulin with Zinc, a clear solution, is comparable to regular insulin in its freedom from allergenic skin reactions.

'Wellcome' Globin Insulin with Zinc is accepted by the Council on Pharmacy and Chemistry, American Medical Association, and was developed in the Wellcome Research Laboratories, Tuckahoe, New York. Registered U. S. Patent Office No. 2,161,198. Available in vials of 10 cc., 80 units in 1 cc.   'Wellcome' Trademark Registered

Literature on request

.BURROUGHS WELLCOME & CO. (U.S.A. INC.) 9-11 E. 41st St., New York 17, N. Y.

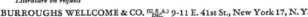

MEDICAL ABSTRACTS

"MYCOTIC ULCER OF THE CORNEA." Flavio L. Nino. Buenos Aires. Las Prensa Medica Argentina. Vol. 30. pages 797-806. May, 1943.

Corneal ulcerations caused by fungi are not as frequent in the United States as e.g. in South American countries. Even in Argentina, where such ulcers are met in the daily practice, an etiological diagnosis may be difficult. The author describes the case of a 62 year old Italian laborer whose eye disease progressed within 15 days to a status with blepharospasm, photophobia, lacrimation, pericorneal congestion, central ulceration of the cornea, iritis with posterior synechiae and precipitates in Descemet's membrane. Vision was reduced to finger counting. Intensive treatment with iodies per os, and eye washes, and excision of the lacrimal sac resulted in complete cure.

Mycological examination of the ulcer revealed the presence of a fungus, which was identified as Sporotrichum fonsecai, a fungus often found in Brazil. Various fungi have been described in connection with diseases of the anterior segment of the eye, such as the Candida albicans or the Rhinocladium schenckii. Sporotrichosis of the eye is rather rare, and it may be either primary or secondary. Almeida, of Brazil, collected 268 cases of general sporotrichosis, but only in one case did he find primary localization of this fungus on the bulbar conjunctiva.

In most cases of mycotic ulcerations of the cornea the fungus cannot be found in the necrotic tissue of the ulcer; cultivation on specially prepared media and animal inoculation is necessary to establish the correct diagnosis.—M.D.H., M.D.

"PENICILLIN." A statement released by the Committee on Medical Research. A. N. Richards, Chairman. Jour. A. M. A., Vol. 122, page 235. May 22, 1943.

A survey of the present production possibilities of penicillin is presented. At least 16 companies are now engaged in, or intend to become engaged in, the production of penicillin. In no instance is production advanced beyond the pilot plant stage; in the majority it is still in the laboratory stage. Some of the difficulties of production are mentioned.

Plans are in progress for undertaking extensive studies of the use of penicillin in wounds in 10 general Army hospitals and in venereal disease in six. The navy is planning similar studies. To date, the results in the treatment of some 300 patients have completely upheld the early promise in the reports of Florey, Chain, and other. Penicillin appears to be far superior to the sulfonamides in staphylococcus aureus infections with and without bacteremia; it is extremely effective in hemolytic streptococcus, pneumococcus and gonococcus infections resistant to the sulfonamides. It has not been found effective in sub-acute bacterial endocarditis. Studies of its local application are still inadequate.—H.J., M.D.

"OTOSCLEROSIS." Hans Brunner. The Laryngoscope. vol. 53. pages 736-742. November, 1943.

The article presents of the author's views and experiences gained over a period of more than 20 years. His observations show that, contrary to the general belief, otosclerosis is more frequent in men than in women. It is not the disease per se which is sex-linked, but the clinical progress of the disease. The chief symptoms are bilateral deafness and tinnitus.

The deafness may be due to an ankylosis of the stapes,

to a partial obliteration of the holes of the tractus foraminosus by otosclerotic bone, and to a congenital malformation of the cochlea, including and underdevelopment of the spiral nerves and ganglia. In the author's series of 17 cases there was deafness or diminished hearing in 12 cases (8 women and 4 men). Among these 12 cases, eight showed chronic diseases at autopsy, such as syphilis of the blood vessels, chronic otitis media, brain tumors, severe arteriosclerosis. Any of these diseases might impair hearing without an intercurrent otosclerosis. In the remaining four cases ankylosis of the stapes was present, also one had a congenital malformation of the cochlea, and one a simple atrophy of the cochlea.

Usually, otosclerosis is caused by stapes ankylosis. This can be diagnosed microscopically only, but it is easily overlooked. The disease as a rule is a bilateral disease, though it develops first in one ear. The conditioning may be present without causing clinical symptoms. This is usually the case in unilateral affections.

Tinnitus was present in the majority of cases, but only in one was it a predominant symptom. Very frequently, such patients forgot about their tinnitus, and do not mention it as a complaint when they seek cure of their deafness. What may be the anatomical basis of tinnitus cannot be ascertained from autopsy material.

It is known that pregnancy frequently impairs hearing, and a number of otologists strictly advise against pregnancy in otosclerosis. The author mentions a woman who had four successive pregnancies, without her hearing being impaired during otosclerosis. In another case the patient became very deaf without interfering pregnancy. A great number of clinical observations also prove the uncertainty of the relation of pregnancy to otosclerosis. The term "pregnancy" includes so many features which eventually can damage the ear that it must be stated, at first, which symptoms of pregnancy do or do not affect the hearing. It is better to avoid general statements concerning the relation of pregnancy and otosclerosis and to handle each case individually.

Frequently the findings of otosclerosis will be of less importance than other factors, such as heredity which concerns not only the ear but also mental and endocrine diseases. Furthermore, the question whether or not a woman has children may depend upon her age, general health, social circumstances and other factors. —M.D.H., M.D.

"STUDY OF THE HISTOPATHOLOGICAL CHANGES IN THE RETINA AND LATE CHANGES IN THE VISUAL FIELD IN ACUTE METHYL ALCOHOL POISONING." The British Journal of Ophthalmology. vol. 27, pages 523-543. December, 1943.

A mass poisoning by methyl alcohol in Glasgow gave opportunity to study the eyes of four victims. Methyl alcohol or methanol is rarely used as a drink; it regularly occurs in varnishes and shellacs, the fumes of which may be absorbed by the lungs. The Glasgow mass poisoning in April, 1942, was caused by drinking. Woodspirit or methanol drinking in sporadic cases may often be ignored as a cause of death. Jackson believes it to be one of the commonest causes of toxic blindness in America. Where the history of drinking is not obtained, the picture of the patient's clinical condition may be puzzling.

In case of methanol poisoning, the gravely ill are comatose, pale or cyanotic, perspiring and profoundly shocked. The pupils are widely dilated and immobile. As death approaches, the cyanosis increases and the pulse

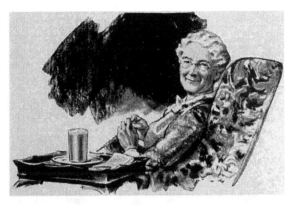

THE SUNSET YEARS AND
Adequate Nutrition

As the degenerative processes gain the upper hand during the last decade or two of life, profound changes occur in many metabolic mechanisms. The gastrointestinal tract for example becomes less tolerant of abuses, and difficulty is experienced in digesting some foods which formerly did not prove troublesome. The loss of vigor characteristic of senescence can easily be aggravated to a point of incapacitation if self-chosen eating habits are not altered to prevent nutritional deficiencies. For only by properly satisfying the nutritional requirements can adequate strength be maintained. Ovaltine is well tolerated by elderly persons. It supplies a wealth of nutrients which are readily metabolized and which are frequently lacking in the diets chosen during advanced years: biologically adequate protein, B complex vitamins, minerals, and vitamins A and D. Ovaltine is digested with ease, and its high content of diastatic enzyme makes it a valuable aid in the digestion of starchy foods. This delicious food-drink appeals to older persons, hence it can be included in their diet three times daily without meeting with resistance.

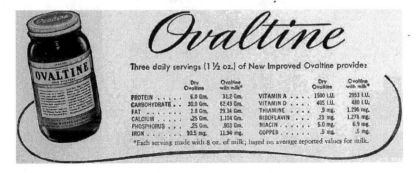

Ovaltine

Three daily servings (1 ½ oz.) of New Improved Ovaltine provide:

	Dry Ovaltine	Ovaltine with milk*		Dry Ovaltine	Ovaltine with milk*
PROTEIN	6.0 Gm.	31.2 Gm.	VITAMIN A	1500 I.U.	2953 I.U.
CARBOHYDRATE	30.0 Gm.	62.43 Gm.	VITAMIN D	405 I.U.	480 I.U.
FAT	2.8 Gm.	29.34 Gm.	THIAMINE	.9 mg.	1.296 mg.
CALCIUM	.26 Gm.	1.104 Gm.	RIBOFLAVIN	.25 mg.	1.278 mg.
PHOSPHORUS	.25 Gm.	.903 Gm.	NIACIN	5.0 mg.	6.9 mg.
IRON	10.5 mg.	11.94 mg.	COPPER	.5 mg.	.5 mg.

*Each serving made with 8 oz. of milk; based on average reported values for milk.

becomes less and less perceptible. Sometimes convulsions precede death. In the less severe type of poisoning, the patient is confused, perspiring, pale, with the cramps and abdominal pains of acute irritant poisoning. Vision may deteriorate to the perception of hand movements, but, even then, vision may be recovered. A common symptom is yellow vision. The patient may be comatose and recover, and he may be blind and recover vision, at least in large part. The milder cases have gastro-intestinal symptoms with transient dimness of vision.

Ophthalmoscopic signs are usually present in severe cases. Indistinctness of the disc edges and congestion of the veins may suggest edema of the nerve head. Edema of the retina around the disc is apparent in some cases. Gross visual loss does not necessarily accompany a degree of poisoning sufficient to produce coma. The principles of treatment employed are elimination by maintained gastric lavage and the promotion of diuresis by intravenous glucose salines, lumbar puncture, cardiac and respiratory stimulants. The elimination of methanol from the human body' is very slow.

The communications dealing with the pathological changes in the retina in methanol poisoning are few. The articles became numerous in describing an outbreak of acute methanol poisoning in 1911 in Berlin. In America during the years of prohibition there was also a great increase in the number of articles as well as addicts to denatured or dehorn alcohol. The Berlin outbreak resulted from the drinking of cheap schnapps. There were 130 cases, and 58 died. In America the first reports of poisoning appear as early as 1879. By the end of the century there were many reports of blindness from this cause, but it was not until 1906 that Congress passed the Denatured Alcohol Bill. Between that time and the advent of prohibition in 1918 there were few cases reported. Cases of poisoning from inhalation and external application were reported about this time. Some people showed a special sensitiveness to the poison. In some, 10 cc was enough to cause blindness, and 100 cc had been known to cause death. A concentration of as little as 0.2 per cent in the air had been known to cause poisoning.

The tendency to recover vision was generally considered poor. De Schweinitz reckoned that 90 per cent of cases of poisoning went on to blindness. The symptomatology is divided into general and ocular manifestations in acute cases. Headache, dizziness, nausea and vomiting, abdominal pains, cardiac weakness, slow pulse, sighing respiration, marked prostration, weakness of the extremities, delirium, convulsions, stupor, and death are the general features. The visual symptoms are loss of vision, photophobia, pain on moving the eyes, and hemeraolpia. The signs in the eye are lowered tension sometimes, dilated and fixed or sluggish pupils, normal or congested discs and central scotomas. The signs in chronic poisoning are the central scotoma with an atrophic nerve head, either complete atrophy or limited to the temporal side, with pallor.

The general pathological findings are acidosis with increased acid content of the aqueous; blood shows a reduced coagulation time, but increased viscosity with increase of erythrocytes and leukocytes and hemo-concentration. The lymphocytes, however, are decreased. There is a high output of ammonia in the urine in consequence of acidosis. The gastrointestinal tract shows mucosal hemorrhages. The blood pressure of those in whom it was recorded was systolic 110 to 140, and diastolic 78 to 90. All the patients have irregular, often labored spasmodic respiration. The rate varied, and nearing the time of death was two or three per minute. Cyanosis was marked in the late stages. Death was from respiratory failure.

The changes found post-mortem in the central nervous system were subpial and moderate cortical and subcortical interstitial edema. Only occasional focal hemorrhages were seen. On the whole the cellular changes were not marked. The author's study of the retina in methanol poisoning showed that fundal changes are not always present in the early stages of intoxication but they are of a consistent nature. Haziness of the disc margins, engorgement of the veins, and in more marked cases, edema of the retina spreading from the disc, is the picture. The fundal changes, if present, center round the nerve head. No changes in the retinal ganglion cells which could be attributed indubitably to acute methyl alcohol poisoning were found, either in the lipoid changes in the ganglion cells, or in the size and shape of the ganglion cells or the nuclear content. The optic nerves showed no abnormality. But the fact that the ganglion cells of the retina looked normal is no proof that their physiology was not impaired and that the impairment might later lead to death of the cell, with an atrophy in continuity of the neurone in the nerve.
—M.D.H., M.D.

"NASAL ALLERGY (EXCLUDING HAY FEVER)." Myles L. Formby. The Journal of Laryngology and Otology. vol. 58, pages 238-242. June, 1943.

The predominant symptom or sign of allergy varies greatly from case to case and in a few it is possible to determine the principal etiological factor from a clinical examination. If one excludes the clear cut cases of hay fever, asthma, migraine, urticaria, suppurative sinusitis or bronchiectasis there remains an enormous group whose nasal symptoms are similar to those but where underlying condition is less evident. These are the cases of allergic rhinitis, or at least each should be regarded as such until proved beyond doubt to be otherwise.

The precise etiology remains undiscovered. Age and sex throw no light on the problem. The author believes that a large number of cases of sinusitis are in the first instance uncomplicated cases of allergic rhinitis, but through unavoidable misfortune, neglect, or misguided surgical intervention, infection is superimposed.

A typical case may show a long history, with exacerbations and remissions of symptom, the influence of environment (centrally heated atmosphere and a seaside holiday both materially affecting the symptoms), the close association of nasal symptoms with physical and mental stress, the influence of normal physiological changes (pregnancy, menopause, etc.), and the association of intercurrent infection. At the onset, the picture may be that of a patient, with a susceptible nasal mucosa, who developed in the course of an influenzal epidemic an acute nasopharyngeal infection. Later, he may be seen with clinically a pansinusitis and polypi. That this is not the true sequence of events is proved by the complete absence of demonstrable organisms in the sinuses several months after the acute infection. This is no local disease of the nose but a general systemic disorder. As far as the nasal manifestations are concerned the author believes that local infection plays no important part until it has been grafted into the upper respiratory mucosa by a surgical interference. It is then a secondary infection and a complication and not a primary etiological factor.

Until we are able to either exclude or neutralize the effects of allergens, or to render susceptible individuals insensitive, we cannot hope to effect cures. The nearest approach to success has been achieved by desensitization in suitable cases. Much can, however, be done for the patients by preventive and palliative measures. Yet, in assessing treatment it is difficult to avoid self-deception and sometimes criticism is levelled at the doctor who reports success. The author's practice has been in recent years with cases where no obvious preventive measure suggested itself to prescribe full doses of colloidal calcium and vitamin D. Those whose symptoms were more severe were also given ephedrine hydrochloride, gr. one half, twice daily, by mouth, and one per cent ephedrine in normal saline as a nasal spray to relieve obstruction.

There are various palliative surgical measures. As to the value of turbinestomy, one should remember that any operation may produce apparent improvement tem-

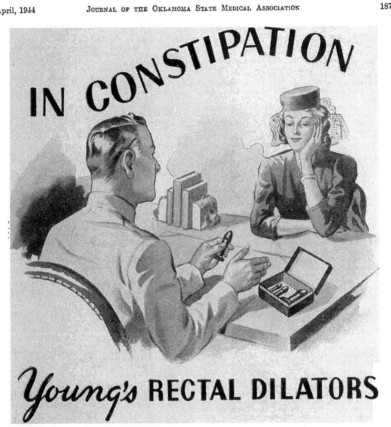
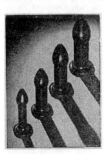

porarily. Many surgical procedures have been advocated to relieve polypoid degeneration of the nasal mucosa with complete obstruction. The author found a technic for the application of radium very successful in cases of recurrent polyps. With one exception, all patients in a series of 30 had immediate relief, all had undergone previous operation, many had multiple operations and in most secondary, sinus infection was already present.

After spraying the nose with five per cent cocaine, each side is packed for half an hour with half inch ribbon gauze soaked in equal parts of ten per cent cocaine and 1:1000 adrenalin. Under general anesthesia a submucous resection of the septum is performed if its irregularity prevents easy access to either ethmoidal region. A bilateral intranasal ethmoidectomy and bilateral intranasal antrostomy is then carried out. Two pieces of dental stent, each shaped like a lake's rubber splint, are next moulded to fit high up in the right and left ethmoidal regions. Into each piece of stent six 6.5 mgr. radium needles are inserted vertically, the stent placed in position against the roof of the nose and held in position by filling the lower part of the cavity with one inch ribbon gauze soaked in liquid paraffin. The needles are left in position for seven hours (546 mgr. hours) and then removed by withdrawing the ribbon gauze and the stent with angular forceps, morphine having been given half an hour previously if necessary.

Careful supervision for three to four days after operation is important if adhesions are to be avoided. A dense coagulum forms in the nose and must be removed daily. Regular spraying with liquid paraffin is advisable and if crusting and discharge are excessive daily douching with an alkaline lotion. Patients are generally fit to leave the hospital a week after operation but should be inspected weekly for a month and then less frequently for three to four months.—M.D.H., M.D.

"DISCUSSION ON BURNS OF THE EYELID AND CONJUNCTIVA." Cecil Wakely (et al). Proceedings of the Royal Society of Medicine. vol. 37. pages 29-33. November, 1943.

The problem of burns of the face and eyelids has been a very important one during this war and the last. Soon after the beginning of this war there was an undue number of facial burns which were the result of the man having the face completely unprotected. There was such a state of cases that at the end of 1939 an extra protection was devised. It consists of cellulose acetate goggles and eartex heat-resisting material for the nose and mouth. It can be stowed away in the soldier's helmet. By far the greatest proportion of the cases are produced by exploding bombs. The bombs may not have touched the patient at all, but the effect of the blast is to split the skin, and to produce a superficial burn of the hair and face. There are usually other lesions as well. Patients treated with triple dye jelly have done extremely well.

In a bomb-flash burn the blast may also cause the skin to split. Even though these little lesions may be deep, there is no permanent disability. An analysis of 120 cases of burns received at an R.A.F. hospital showed that 80 percent affected the face, and of this 80 per cent, 20 per cent had ectropion and 5 per cent only had the globe affected. The cause of this type of burn may be gasoline flames, incendiary and flash bombs, caustic acid and alkalis and gaseous chemicals. In facial burns, owing to the very loose supporting tissues, a tremendous amount of edema develops even in cases of moderate burn. The edema begins to make its appearance a few minutes after the accident and increases up to twelve hours. It remains at the maximum from 12 to 36 hours and then begins to subside. This has a bearing on the management of these cases, particularly of the eyes, as at this early stage it is difficult to open the eyes and therefore these patients are sent to the hospital as soon as possible. Flash burns are due to the instantaneous combustion of a magnesium used in

flash bombs. In these the exposure is a matter of a fraction of a second, whereas in the flame burn it is anything from 10 to 60 seconds, and that gives a chance for closing of the eyelids, which tends to save the globe at the expense of the lid. In the flash burn, though there is conjunctival involvement, the exposure is so brief that the burn is largely superficial. The globe in these cases is somewhat protected by the constant film of moisture which bathes the cornea and the conjunctiva. In magnesium flash burns tattooing of the globe sometimes occurs, owing to the minute particles being driven home by the force of the explosion. They are too small and too numerous to be removed surgically. Even in very bad eyelid burns, the trasal plates used to remain intact.

The present day treatment of such burns rest on simple principles, namely, to prevent infection and to do as little harm as possible to the healing tissues. If infection develops, it should be treated specifically. Early healing should be the aim, and if the case does not heal on its own, it should be assisted by skin grafting. Cetyl trimethyl ammonium bromide, in 0.75 per cent water solution, is a good antiseptic. It is applied with a swab of cotton-wool. Any loose hanging threads of epithelium are then removed. Cleansing is followed by an application of sulfonamide either as powder of three per cent cream. The face is covered by course mesh vaseline gauze, and this makes a very soft, gentle non-irritating dressing, which can be easily removed.

Penicillin has been used as a local application. Made to a strength of 100 units per gramme it was consistently effective in eliminating streptococci and staphylococci from granulating surfaces. It is applied every 24 hours, and the cases as a rule responded within four days. No coagulants should be used in the treatment of eyelids.

Grafting of the lids should be undertaken as soon as lid retraction develops. Healing is promoted and such grafts do better than expected. Burnt areas remote from the lids contribute much to the retraction and should be grafted as soon as possible. Exposed corneas may be protected by contact lenses. Early cases with loss of lid tissue may be saved by sliding down a frontal skin flap and suturing over the exposed eye. —M.D.H., M.D.

"SOME RECENT WORK ON MENIERE'S DISEASE: TREATMENT." T. E. Cawthorne. Proceedings of the Royal Society of Medicine, London. Volume 36. pages 541-546. August, 1943.

Although Meniere's Disease does not cause any obvious pathological changes in the body apart from the labyrinth it can, by the very violence of its symptoms, reduce the sufferer to a state of chronic invalidism. Thus it requires a person of robust temperament to bear with equanimity the disturbance both mental and physical that forms part of the recurrent attacks. Those who are unable to stand up to the ordeal will exhibit symptoms of nervous strain in varying degree. Such patients do not always respond easily to treatment because even if they are relieved of their severe attacks they may find difficulty in regaining self-confidence. The require constant encouragement and careful rehabilitation, particularly if they have been submitted to operation. Another factor to be considered is the natural tendency of the disease towards spontaneous remissions, and it is important to guard against attributing such a remission to a successful response to treatment.

Sedatives have long been in use and of these phenobarbital has established itself as the most popular, and rightly so, for regular doses of this drug seem to discourage the spread of the disturbance caused by an attack to other parts of the central nervous system. A regime that favors excretion of the fluid-finding sodium, has been employed often with good results. Recently much good has been observed from the adequate use of histamine, also from the use of nicotinic acid. It may also happen that eradication of

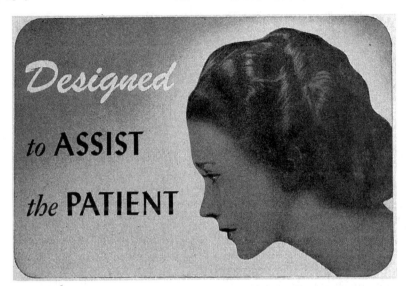
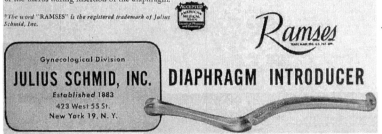

a focus of infection will lessen or stop the attacks. Causes due to focal infection are, however, very rare.

Of the operative measures employed the most rational would seem to be drainage of the saccus endolymphaticus as advocated by Portmann. Section of all or part of the eighth nerve has long been in favor, especially in America and in France. Recently all these workers have contented themselves with section of the vestibular division of the eighth nerve only, leaving the cochlear division intact so that what remains of the hearing will not be disturbed. Wright injects alcohol into the perilymph space through the tympanic membrane and stapes footplate. This gives the same result as the other forms of alcohol injection and it has the great merit of being surgically simple.

The author found in order to abolish function in the labyrinth all that is necessary is to open the endolymphatic space. The injection of alcohol is not essential as the same results can be produced by merely opening the membranous labyrinth. In order to ensure that the endolymphatic space is properly opened, the author now removes a portion of the membranous labyrinth from the external canal, this part of the labyrinth being chosen as being the most accessible. He uses a binocular dissecting microscope to magnify the field of work, and approaches the labyrinth via the mastoid, sufficient bone being removed to ensure a good view of the external semicircular canal. The bony canal is removed by means of a dental burr; then, the membranous semicircular canal is seized with a forceps, and removed.

So far 52 cases have been operated on, of which 20 occur within the series under review. All have healed by first intention and there have been no complications. The immediate postoperative effect was the same as in other cases of labyrinth destruction. Vertigo improved in most cases; tinnitus disappeared in about half of the cases. In some patients even the hearing became better.—M.D.H., M.D.

"USE OF SULFONAMIDE IN OPHTHALMOLOGY." Walther Loehlein. Berlin. Deutsche medizinische Wochenschrift. Volume No. 69. pages 420-422. May 28, 1943.

From its beginning, chemotherapy has been of special interest to the ophthalmologist, since there are many eye diseases of infectious origin, especially affecting the anterior segment of the eyeball, which is easily approachable for antibacterial medication. The superficial location of the anterior eye tissues also permits an immediate observation of the infectious process day after day, and a good checkup on any therapeutic result. No wonder that chemotherapy has frequently turned to the eye as a test object in evaluating the various newly manufactured remedies. Long before the era of sulfanilamides, a number of chemotherapeutic agents have been successfully tried out in cases of eye infections, such as optochin, and the many aniline dyes.

Sulfonamides have been tried in various eye infections, administered either perorally, or intramuscularly and intravenously, applied even locally in form of eyedrops, salves, powders, subconjunctival and intrahyaloid injections. It is very fundamental to know that the local application proved to be the least effective, which further showed that the body as a whole is indispensable for the therapeutic effect of sulfonamides. The opinions are different as to the value of sulfonamides in individual infections of the eye. Certainly, the new drugs did not show any evidence of being the long sought for therapia sterilisans magna, at least not for eye infections.

Thus, in gono-blennorrhea of the newborn many good results are reported, yet the eventual negative results caution us from abandoning the old-fashion and well-proved method of foreign protein therapy in the form of milk injections. Koch-Weeks conjunctivitis, and Morax-Axonfeld infections are, however, easily cured by sulfonamides. Similar good results are obtained in pneu-mococcic infections of the eye, as in ulcus serpens of the cornea; the ulcus will heal with much finer cicatrization than without the sulfonamides, which in itself is a great achievement. Even non-infectious inflammatory changes may become milder under sulfonamide medication, which is probably due to a special antiphlogistic effect of these drugs.

More difficult is to evaluate the action of sulfonamides in intra-ocular infections, such as seen after perforating injuries. Experiments showed that, slowly though, the intravenously injected sulfonamide will appear in the intraocular tissues. It is therefore logical to use sulfonamide as preoperative medication in eye surgery; however, it is hard to say whether there is any real prophylactic value in such a preoperative medication, since operative infections tend to become less and less frequent, even without chemotherapy.

Of special importance seems to be the behavior of trachoma under sulfonamide therapy. Repatriation of Germans from Eastern Europe gave an excellent opportunity to mass observations. There were many thousands of repatriated Germans infected with trachoma, but the use of sulfonamide made the infection much milder; the acute symptoms disappeared very soon, and there were practically no complications. The role of sulfonamides in trachoma treatment is such that the drugs will make less important to have an energetic mechanical treatment. Thus the eye is much better protected than with the older methods. · It is generally assumed by German ophthalmologists that the objective and subjective improvements is due to a direct action of sulfonamide upon the trachoma virus.—M.D.H., M.D.

KEY TO ABSTRACTORS

M.D.H., M.D. ....Marvin D. Henley, Tulsa
H.J., M.D. ....Hugh Jeter, Oklahoma City

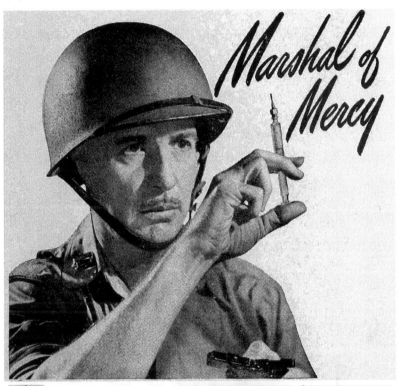

Marshal of Mercy

In war, even more than in peace... dispenser of blessed relief... his the precious power over pain.

Long hours the medical officer toils... routinely yet heroically... without thought of citation... grateful for brief moments of relaxation ... for the cheer of an occasional smoke. And likely as not, his cigarette is Camel, the favorite brand in the armed forces*... first choice for smooth mildness and for pleasing flavor. It's what every fighting man deserves... that extra measure of Camel's smoking pleasure.

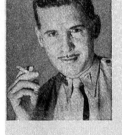

1st in the Service

*With men in the Army, Navy, Marine Corps, and Coast Guard, the favorite cigarette is Camel. (Based on actual sales records.)

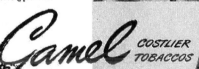

Camel   COSTLIER TOBACCOS

CAMEL
TURKISH & DOMESTIC BLEND CIGARETTES

OFFICERS OF COUNTY SOCIETIES, 1944

★

COUNTY	PRESIDENT	SECRETARY	MEETING TIME
Alfalfa	H. E. Huston, Cherokee	L. T. Lancaster, Cherokee	Last Tues. each Second Month
Atoka-Coal	R. C. Henry, Coalgate	J. S. Fulton, Atoka	
Beckham	G. H. Stagner, Erick	O. C. Standifer, Elk City	Second Tuesday
Blaine	L. R. Kirby, Okeene	W. F. Griffin, Watonga	
Bryan	John T. Wharton, Durant	W. K. Haynie, Durant	Second Tuesday
Caddo	F. L. Patterson, Carnegie	C. B. Sullivan, Carnegie	
Canadian	P. F. Herod, El Reno	A. L. Johnson, El Reno	Subject to call
Carter	J. R. Pollock, Ardmore	H. A. Higgins, Ardmore	
Cherokee	P. H. Medearis, Tahlequah	W. M. Wood, Tahlequah	First Tuesday
Choctaw	C. H. Hale, Boswell	E. A. Johnson, Hugo	
Cleveland	F. T. Gastineau, Norman	Iva S. Merritt, Norman	Thursday nights
Comanche	George L. Berry, Lawton	Howard Angus, Lawton	
Cotton	A. B. Holstead, Temple	Mollie F. Scism, Walters	Third Friday
Craig	Lloyd H. McPike, Vinita	Paul G. Sanger, Vinita	
Creek	J. E. Hollis, Bristow		
Custer	F. R. Vieregg, Clinton	C. J. Alexander, Clinton	Third Thursday
Garfield	Julian Feild, Enid	John R. Walker, Enid	Fourth Thursday
Garvin	T. F. Gross, Lindsay	John R. Callaway, Pauls Valley	Wednesday before Third Thursday
Grady	Walter J. Baze, Chickasha	Roy E. Emanuel, Chickasha	Third Thursday
Grant	I. V. Hardy, Medford		
Greer	R. W. Lewis, Granite	J. B. Hollis, Mangum	
Harmon	W. G. Husband, Hollis	R. H. Lynch, Hollis	First Wednesday
Haskell	William Carson, Keota	N. K. Williams, McCurtain	
Hughes	Wm. L. Taylor, Holdenville	Imogene Mayfield, Holdenville	First Friday
Jackson	C. G. Spears, Altus	E. A. Abernethy, Altus	Last Monday
Jefferson	F. M. Edwards, Ringling		Second Monday
Kay	J. Holland Howe, Ponca City	G. H. Yeary, Newkirk	Second Thursday
Kingfisher	A. O. Meredith, Kingfisher	H. Violet Sturgeon, Hennessey	
Kiowa	J. William Finch, Hobart	William Bernell, Hobart	
LeFlore	Neeson Rolle, Poteau	Rush L. Wright, Poteau	
Lincoln	W. B. Davis, Stroud	Carl H. Bailey, Stroud	First Wednesday
Logan	William C. Miller, Guthrie	J. L. LeHew, Jr., Guthrie	Last Tuesday
Marshall	J. L. Holland, Madill	J. F. York, Madill	
Mayes	Ralph V. Smith, Pryor	Paul B. Cameron, Pryor	
McClain	W. C. McCurdy, Sr., Purcell	W. C. McCurdy, Jr., Purcell	
McCurtain	A. W. Clarkson, Valliant	N. L. Barker, Broken Bow	Fourth Tuesday
McIntosh	Luster I. Jacobs, Hanna	Wm. A. Tolleson, Eufaula	First Thursday
Murray	P. V. Annsdown, Sulphur	J. A. Wrenn, Sulphur	Second Tuesday
Muskogee-Sequoyah			
Wagoner	H. A. Scott, Muskogee	D. Evelyn Miller, Muskogee	First Monday
Noble	C. H. Cooke, Perry	J. W. Francis, Perry	
Okfuskee	C. M. Cochran, Okemah	M. L. Whitney, Okemah	Second Monday
Oklahoma	W. E. Eastland, Oklahoma City	E. R. Musick, Oklahoma City	Fourth Tuesday
Okmulgee	S. B. Leslie, Okmulgee	J. C. Matheney, Okmulgee	Second Monday
Osage	C. R. Weirich, Pawhuska	George K. Hemphill, Pawhuska	Second Monday
Ottawa	Walter Kerr, Picher	B. W. Shelton, Miami	Third Thursday
Pawnee	E. T. Robinson, Cleveland	R. L. Browning, Pawnee	
Payne	H. C. Manning, Cushing	J. W. Martin, Cushing	Third Thursday
Pittsburg	P. T. Powell, McAlester	W. H. Kaeiser, McAlester	Third Friday
Pontotoc	A. R. Sagg, Ada	R. H. Mayes, Ada	First Wednesday
Pottawatomie	E. Eugene Rice, Shawnee	Clinton Gallaher, Shawnee	First and Third Saturday
Pushmataha	John S. Lawson, Clayton	B. M. Huckabay, Antlers	
Rogers	R. C. Meloy, Claremore	Chas. L. Caldwell, Chelsea	First Monday
Seminole	J. T. Price, Seminole	Mack I. Shanholtz, Wewoka	Third Wednesday
Stephens	W. K. Walker, Marlow	Wallis S. Ivy, Duncan	
Texas	E. G. Obermiller, Texhoma	Morris Smith, Guymon	
Tillman	C. C. Allen, Frederick	O. G. Bacon, Frederick	
Tulsa	Ralph A. McGill, Tulsa	E. O. Johnson, Tulsa	Second and Fourth Monday
Washington-Nowata	K. D. Davis, Nowata	J. V. Athey, Bartlesville	Second Wednesday
Washita	A. S. Neal, Cordell	James F. McMurry, Sentinel	
Woods	Ishmael F. Stephenson, Alva	Oscar E. Templin, Alva	Last Tuesday Odd Months
Woodward	H. Walker, Buffalo	C. W. Tedrowe, Woodward	Second Thursday

(Serving in Armed Forces)

THE JOURNAL

OF THE

OKLAHOMA STATE MEDICAL ASSOCIATION

VOLUME XXXVII	OKLAHOMA CITY, OKLAHOMA, MAY, 1944	NUMBER 5

Clinical Observations in the Use of Penicillin*

LT. COLONEL E. RANKIN DENNY
formerly of Tulsa
MEDICAL CORPS, ARMY OF THE UNITED STATES
MAJOR PAUL L. SHALLENBERGER
MEDICAL CORPS, ARMY OF THE UNITED STATES
MAJOR HAROLD D. PYLE
MEDICAL CORPS, ARMY OF THE UNITED STATES

The therapeutic value of penicillin in certain bacterial diseases is established. With each succeeding month new organisms are added to the list of those which have proven to be susceptible to penicillin. Most of the gram-positive cocci, and in addition, the meningococcus, the gonococcus, the anthrax baccillus, the organisms of gas gangrene, the Treponema pallidum, the organisms of Vincent's angina, and some strains of the actinomyces comprise this list.[1] By contrast, infections caused by the gram-negative bacilli have been found to be penicillin resistant.

Penicillin appears to have a primary inhibitory effect upon the reproduction of susceptible organisms.[2] Multiplication of the organisms is impeded by inhibition of fission. There is bacteriostasis rather than lysis. Thus its action differs from that of the sulfonamides in that the latter causes only a reduction in the rate of bacterial growth. Nor is the action of penicillin impaired by the presence of serum, pus, blood, or the products of tissue autolysis. However, the inhibitory properties of penicillin are neutralized by substances contained in certain organisms, notably the colon bacillus group.[3] This fact introduces a special therapeutic problem in the treatment of diseases caused by or associated with the colon bacillus group.

Penicillin is extremely hygroscopic and is highly soluble in water. No serious toxic effects have been reported following its clinical use. The sodium salt of penicillin is a yellow powder, furnished in sealed glass ampules. Most of the ampules contain 100,000 Oxford units. As Bloomfield[4] has said, "The clumsy Florrey (Oxford) unit—the amount of penicillin compared with an arbitrary standard which completely inhibits the growth of a test strain of Staphylococcus aureus—is still used and probably will hold its place until a chemically standard product is available."

We have found it most practicable to treat the majority of patients in a special penicillin ward. The drug is kept on the ward in refrigerators, the temperatures of which are maintained at approximately 4 degrees C. Fresh solutions are made up each day by using pyrogren-free physiological sodium chloride as the solvent. Twenty cc. syringes, sterilized by dry heat, are used in introducing salt solution into the ampules.

Following the suggestion of the Surgeon General's Office[5], a board of medical officers, consisting of officers from the Medical, Surgical, and Orthopedic Services, and the hospital bacteriologist, was appointed for the purpose of selecting patients for treatment with penicillin and for evaluating its effect. Unless the case is one of emergency, our plan consists of isolating and identifying the bacterial agent responsible for the infection, determining its penicillin susceptibility in vitro, and planning the therapeutic regime for each patient. The bacteriological study was

*Read before the Section on General Medicine. Annual Meeting, April 25, 1944 in Tulsa.

originally carried out by inoculating three blood agar plates, containing respectively 0.05 units, 0.5 units, and 5 units penicillin. Growth inhibition could thus be determined. Simultaneous studies were made upon the organism in some instances by inoculating blood agar plates impregnated with 0.25 gm per cent and 0.5 gm per cent sulfathiazole and sulfadiazine. Sulfonamide susceptibility was thus also recorded.

At least two or more members of the board planned the dosage, the route of administration, the changes in dosage, and determined when to discontinue treatment. The clinical courses of the cases being studied was noted daily and frequent bacteriological studies were made.

METHOD OF ADMINISTRATION

Intravenous administration. Penicillin is so rapidly excreted following its intravenous injection that it must be administered continuously if a constant level is to be attained. This method seems the one of choice in the treatment of the septicemias. However, it creates certain difficulties. There is a tendency for venous thrombosis to occur and this requires changing the needle position frequently. To prevent edema from the excessive use of sodium chloride, we use 5 per cent dextrose in distilled water and physiological sodium chloride as a solvent for penicillin alternately. A total of 300,000 units may be administered intravenously in 24 hours if 100,000 units are added to 1,000 cc of fluid and given at the rate approximating 40 drops per minute.

Intramuscular administration. The studies of Rammelkamp and Keefer[6] and Dawson and Hobby[7] show that following the intramuscular injection of penicillin there is a rapid rise in the blood within 15 to 30 minutes. The level attained remains stationary for about 30 minutes and then gradually falls. Small amounts are still detectable in the blood at the end of three to four hours. We feel that the intramuscular administration is the method of choice in most cases because of its simplicity. A technician can be trained to give the treatments, less supervision is required, and the majority of infections respond satisfactorily. For several months we have prepared penicillin for intramuscular injection by adding 20 cc of physiological sodium chloride to each vial containing 100,000 units, thus making a concentration of 5,000 units per cc. Recently the concentration of the drug in the solution has been doubled by using only 10 cc of solvent.

Local application. A solution containing 100 to 250 units of penicillin per cc is prepared by using physiological sodium chloride as a solvent. Where practicable, wet dressings are applied to the wound being overlayed by an impervious material. The dressings are kept moist but are changed only at 24 hour intervals. Occasionally deep seated areas of infection are treated by the introduction of penicillin via rubber tubes.

Intrathecal administration. We have had no experience with the intraspinal injection of penicillin, but the work of Rammelkamp and Keefer[8] has clearly demonstrated that penicillin does not enter the spinal fluid following the intravenous administration of the drug. Therefore, it seems necessary to introduce the drug intrathecally when dealing with infections involving the meninges. The method suggested by Rammelkamp and Keefer is as follows: Physiological sodium chloride containing 1,000 units of the sodium salt penicillin per cc is prepared. Following the removal of 10 cc of spinal fluid, from 5,-000 to 10,000 units are introduced. The injections may be repeated every 12 to 24 hours until three negative spinal fliud cultures are obtained. In patients in whom the intrathecal administration of penicillin is indicated, it seems warranted to supplement the intrathecal administration of the drug with intramuscular or intravenous treatments.

DOSAGE

The question of dosage is discretionary. In the early report of Herrell, several Staphylococcus infections associated with bacteremia were successfully treated with as little as 40,000 to 60,000 units per 24 hours. However, later reports including the War Department Technical Bulletin Med[9] indicate the need for 24 hour dosage of 400,000 units in seriously ill patients with bacteremia and especially in severe staphylococcus infections. At the onset of a severe infection, the intravenous method of administration of 100,000 units during each eight hour period is indicated. Subsequently, as improvement takes place, the plan of therapy as outlined in the above paragraph describing intramuscular administration of the drug may be followed. In the treatment of alpha and beta hemolytic streptococcus and pneumococcus infections, we have successfully used 100,000 to 150,000 units per 24 hour period, administered for the most part intramuscularly in divided doses at three hour intervals. The dosage for the treatment of uncomplicated gonorrhea is 100,000 units given in divided doses over a period of 12 hours.

ANALYSIS OF CASES

Gonorrhea

Penicillin has been found to be extremely effective in the treatment of gonorrhea which has resisted sulfonamide therapy. The patients who were considered sulfonamide resistant had received two or more courses of sulfadiazine and-or sulfathiazole, each course consisting of 30 grams administered over a period of five days. Prior to the institution of penicillin therapy, all cases showed intracellular and extracellular gram-negative diplococci in stained smears, and as will be subsequently shown, 100 of the 243 cases had cultures positive for Neisseria gonococcus. The treatment consisted of 10,-000 units of penicillin injected intramuscularly every three hours for five injections if a total dosage of 50,000 units was planned. When the total dosage planned was 100,000 units, 20,000 units of the penicillin were injected intramuscularly every three hours.

TABLE I
Results of Penicillin Therapy in
Gonococcal Infections

Groups	Total Dosage Units	No. Cases	No. Cured	No. Failures	Per Cent Cured
A	50,000	193	181	12	93.8
B	50,000	35	8	27	22.8
C	100,000	39	36	3	92.3
(Retreats)					
D	100,000	15	15	0	100.0
E	325,000 to 350,000	3	2	1	66.6
A, B, C, & D	50,000 and/or 100,000	243	240	3	98.7

Table 1 shows the incidence of cures with variable doses of penicillin. Group A consisted of 193 cases treated with 50,000 units, of which 181 (93.8 per cent) were cured. Group B consisted of 35 patients treated with 50,000 units; only 8 (22.8 per cent) were cured. We feel the low incidence of favorable results in this group may be attributed to a lot of penicillin, the potency of which was substandard. Group C consisted of the 39 failures encountered in Groups A and B, and following the use of 100,000 units, 36 (92.3 per cent) were cured. In accordance with a recent War Department directive, we started using 100,000 units in five equal doses given at three hour intervals. Group D represents 15 cases treated in this manner. All of these cases were cured. Of the three cases in Group C which failed to respond to 100,000 units, two were cured by using 325,000 and 350,000 units of penicillin respectively. The one failure was a case of gonorrheal urethritis complicated by gonorrheal ophthalmia, the clinical course of which is illustrated in Chart 1. Male, white, age 22, Case No. 188, was admitted to the Gardiner General Hospital November 30, 1943 complaining of urethral discharge of seven days' duration. The urethral smear was positive for intracellular and extracellular gram-negative diplococci. He was given tent a course of sulfadiazine therapy between December 1 and December 6. The discharge persisted and on December 8 the smear was

still positive for intracellular and extracellular gram-negative diplococci. On December 9 a second course of sulfadiazine thera-

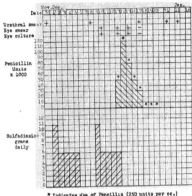

GONORRHEAL OPHTHALMIA
GONORRHEAL URETHRITIS

* Indicates use of Penicillin (250 units per cc.)
locally to the eye, applied every two hours.

CHART 1, Case No. 188: Showing the results of Sulfadiazine and Penicillin therapy and the results of bacteriological examinations of the urethral and ocular exudates chronologically.

py was initiated. He complained of pain in the right eye and the bulbar and palpebral conjunctiva was found to be injected. There was a yellowish discharge at the inner canthus. Bacteriological examination on the tenth day showed gram-negative intracellular and extracellular diplococci and the culture was positive for Neisseria gonococcus. For three days he was given hot compresses and 25 per cent argyrol instillations locally in addition to the sulfadiazine therapy by mouth. Since there was no improvement and because of the seriousness of the disease, penicillin therapy was begun as indicated in the chart on December 13. At this time the smear and culture were both positive. He received 50,000 units penicillin intramuscularly in divided doses at three hour intervals and locally every two hours, using a solution containing 250 units per cc. As indicated in the chart, the smear and culture were still positive on December 15, the third day of penicillin therapy. However, the smear and culture were negative on the fifth day of penicillin treatment. Local therapy was continued until December 20, at which time the disease appeared to be cured. However, recurrence of the urethal discharge developed throughout the subsequent four weeks and the urethal smear was positive for intracellular and extracellular gram-negative diplococci on December 31 and January 11.

Thus, of the 243 cases treated with 50,000 and-or 100,000 units, 240 (98.7 per cent) were cured. One hundred cases with positive cultures became negative after treatment with penicillin, as illustrated in Table II.

TABLE II

Incidence of Positive Cultures Before and After Penicillin Therapy in 136 Cases of Sulfonamide Resistant Gonorrhea

Number of Cases	Positive cultures before treatment Number	Per cent	Negative cultures after treatment Number	Per cent
136	100	73.6	195*	100

* 95 patients received two culture studies after treatment.

Gonococci obtained from cultures of 65 patients, whose disease was sulfonamide resistant, were subjected to sulfathiazole and sulfadiazine sensitivity tests. Chololate agar plates containing 0.25 per cent and 0.5 per cent of sulfathiazole and sulfadiazine were

and laboratory data in nine patients suffering from staphylococcus aureus infections. In three of the patients the infections were acute and localized. Although blood cultures were not obtained, it seems highly probable that there was no associated bacteremia. Among this group of acute and localized infections, the results were satisfactory and the response was particularly striking in the patient suffering from acute cellulitis of the face.

The patient (Case No. 629) with purulent conjunctivitis and punctate keratitis is of special interest. For approximately eight months he had been treated with vaccines; sulfadiazine and sulfathiazole; intra-muscular liver extract; bichloride of mercury, and boric acid. He developed drug sensitivity to mercuric chloride, boric acid and sulfadiazine. The organism isolated from the conjunctival pus was subjected to sulfadiazine and sulfathiazole sensitivity tests in vitro and was shown to be resistant to both these drugs. A rapid improvement ensued following the administration of penicillin, the cultures becoming negative on the sixth day of treatment.

TABLE III

In vito sulfathiazole and sulfadiazine sensitivity tests in 65 cases of sulfonamide resistant gonorrhea

Number of cases	Sulfathiazole Sensitive 0.25 gm. %	0.5 gm. %	Sulfathiazole Resistant 0.25 gm. %	0.5 gm. %	Per cent sensitive	Sulfadiazine Sensitive 0.25 gm.. %	0.5 gm. %	Sulfadiazine Resistant 0.25 gm. %	0.5 gm. %	Per cent sensitive
61	30	30	31	31	47	30	30	31	31	47
1	+	+	0	0		0	0	+	+	
1	0	0	+	+		+	+	0	0	
1	+	+	0	0		0	+	+	+	
1	0	+	+	0		0	0	+	+	
65 (Total)					50.7					49.3

inoculated with the organisms. Table III shows the results of this study. Although 61 patients of this group were clinically sulfathiazole and-or sulfadiazine resistant to their infection, the organism in 31 instances (50 per cent) proved to be sulfathiazole and sulfadiazine sensitive in vitro. Of the remaining four cases studied, there were variable reactions to the various concentrations of sulfathiazole and sulfadiazine. From these observations, it would seem that no close correlation exists between clinical resistance and in vitro resistance to sulfathiazole or sulfadiazine.

In only four instances were penicillin sensitivity determinations carried out in vitro using 0.05 units, 0.5 units, and 5.0 units per cc of media. The organisms were penicillin sensitive in all dilutions.

Staphylococcus aureus infections

Table IV shows the clinical, therapeutic,

Among the cases of osteomyelitis and infections complicating comminuted fractures, the results have been equivocal. In one case of osteomyelitis, there was a history of the disease of approximately eight years' duration. This patient had been subjected to repeated operative procedures, and some few weeks prior to the use of penicillin had had a saucerization performed. There remained a draining sinus. The organism cultured from the sinus was sulfadiazine and sulfathiazole resistant in vitro. The sinus drainage stopped approximately three days after the initiation of penicillin therapy and did not recur during the subsequent six weeks observation. It seems highly probable in this instance that a thorough sequestractomy had been effected. In a second patient in whom osteomyelitis co-existed with an ununited fracture of the tibia, the response to relatively large doses of penicillin was satisfactory. However, the infection involved the areas adjacent to screws fixing a vitallium plate and it was the opinion of the orthopedic surgeon that the infection and infecting organism would not be eradicated until adequate surgery was instituted. It seems reasonable to state in this connection that sequestreoctomies, the removal of foreign bodies and the institution of proper

seemed highly probable that the etiologic organism was the hemolytic staphylococcus aureus, since after the administration of relatively large doses of penicillin intramuscularly and by frequent application of the drug locally, this organism could no longer be cultured from the wound. In this instance, the wound apparently healed more rapidly than

TABLE IV
STAPHYLOCOCCUS AUREUS INFECTIONS

No.	Clinical Diagnosis	Source of Culture	How Treated, Units	Penicillin Total Dosage, Units	Results	Comment
373	Cellulitis, face	Abscess in scar	15,000 q. 3h I. M.		Satisfactory	Remarkable response; rapid localization.
531	Osteomyelitis, chronic single sinus tract	Sinus tract	15,000 q. 3h I. M.	1,235,000	Satisfactory	Organism S.T. and S.D.* resistant in vitro; Sinus drainage stopped in three days.
907	Ureteritis, cystitis, prostatitis	Ureter, Prostate	17,500 to 20,000 q. 4h I. M.	1,010,000	Satisfactory	Urine culture negative on 4th day of treatment. Cured.
653	Furuncle, posterior, cervical region	Furuncle	10,000 q. 3h I. M.	410,000	Satisfactory	Furuncle developed while convalescing from erysipelas. Cured.
950	Cyst, congenital, recurrent drainage, multiple communicating sinus tracts.	Sinus tract	12,500 q. 3h I. M.	462,500	Unsatisfactory	Three previous attempts by incision and drainage ineffective; drainage recurred; radical surgery indicated.
909	Fracture, tibia, fibula, internal fixation with plates; infected	Sinus tract	12,000 to 20,000 q. 3h to 5th I. M.; 1,000 q. 6h local	2,045,000	Unsatisfactory	Infection about steel plates; subsequent proteous bacillus infection. Improved later following removal of steel plates.
064	Osteomyelitis, nonunion fracture of tibia	Sinus tract	10,000 to 20,000 q. 2h to 4h I. M. Local irrigation 500 q. 8h	1,930,000	Unsatisfactory	Previous debridement, internal fixation with vitallion plate; bone absorption about screws; sinus drainage persisted following treatment.
629	Conjunctivitis, purulent, chronic; keratitis, punctate, chronic, left	Pus from Cul-de-sac	12,560 q. 3h I. M.; 17 q. 3h locally	1,435,000	Satisfactory	Eight months duration, treated with vaccine, sulfa drugs, I.M. liver extract; Drug sensitization to HgCl2, boric acid, sulfadiazine. Organism resistant to S.T. and S.D. in vitro. Conjunctivitis cured.
522	Fracture, compound, comminuted, tibia and fibula; infected wound	Leg wound	12,500 q. 3h 15,000 q. 3h. I. M.; local dressings	1,125,000	Satisfactory	Wound clean on 12th treatment day; fracture site firm 1 month after accident.

*S.T.—sulfathiazole; S.D.—sulfadiazine

drainage are procedures without which penicillin therapy will not avail. In addition to the cases cited in Table IV, the orthopedic department has used penicillin both locally and intramuscularly as a prophylactic measure in bone surgery with gratifying results.

Mixed infections and infections of uncertain etiology

In the group of diseases caused by or associated with mixed infections, it is at times difficult to ascertain the specific causative organism. Table V lists the data derived from nine cases of this type.

In Case No. 639, a compound comminuted fracture of the tibia and fibula infected with gram-positive spore forming organisms and hemolytic staphylococcus aureus, it

would be expected had penicillin not been used.

In Case No. 040, one of chronic osteomyelitis, the response to penicillin was unsatisfactory. This may well be attributed to our inability to improve the nutrition of the patient to a satisfactory level, and perhaps because extensive surgery did not seem practicable. The patient (Case No. 389) with acute suppurative synovitis which followed an arthrotomy recovered very rapidly following the use of relatively small doses of penicillin. The organism isolated in this case was sulfathiazole and sulfadiazine resistant, but very susceptible to penicillin in vitro.

Many students of acute rheumatic fever

feel that the disease is caused by or associated with hemolytic streptococcus of the beta type. Since this organism is highly susceptible to penicillin, it seemed worthwhile to observe the effects of penicillin in the treatment of this disease. Only four cases have been treated with penicillin. Two of the patients were suffering from a mild form of the disease. In one of these patients the disease was of the mild recurrent type manifested by a slight fever, fleeting joint pain with stiffness, erythema nodosum, increased sedimentation velocity and leukocytosis. There was a striking response within the first 48 hours following the institution of penicillin therapy as evidenced by the rapid subsidence of the symptoms and disappearance of the skin lesions, and a rapid fall in both the sedimentation velocity and white blood count. Likewise, there was a satisfactory response in the second case which was treated with penicillin from the 10th to the

22nd day of the disease. An involved phalangeal joint rapidly lost its tenderness, pain on motion, and redness of the skin overlying the joint. Furthermore, the pain, redness and tenderness of the right ankle joint, and approximately 85 per cent of the swelling, had disappeared by the fourth day of treatment. The blood sedimentation velocity in this case was 55 mm. per hour the day before penicillin therapy was started, 56 mm. on the fourth day and 15 mm. on the 12th day of treatment. The response to penicillin was considered satisfactory. However, two other cases of acute rheumatic fever were treated with penicillin and the response in these was distinctly unsatisfactory. The clinical course of one of these patients is illustrated in Chart 5. Male, white, age 21, Case No. 610, was admitted to the Gardiner General Hospital February 22, 1944 complaining of migratory joint pains involving the knees, ankles and left great toe, and the

TABLE V
MIXED INFECTION AND INFECTION OF UNCERTAIN ETIOLOGY
Penicillin

No.	Clinical Diagnosis	Source of Culture	How treated, Units	Total Dosage Units	Results	
040	Osteomyelitis, chronic suppurative, metatarsal	Draining sinuses	12,500 q. 3h I.M., 15,000 q. 4h I.M. locally	1,454,500 I.M. 41,000 locally	Unsatisfactory	Complicated case associated with Staph. albus and haem. Staph. aureus, the latter very resistant; disease of 3 yr's duration
520	Fracture, compound, comminuted, femur and patella	Wound, infected	7,500 q. 3h I.M. to 20,000 q. 4h I.M., 500 q. 4h to 1,000 q. 6h locally	2,287,500 60,500 locally	Satisfactory	Wound healed slowly; infected with Staph. citreus aureus and albus; treated 26 days; favorable response.
639	Fracture, compound, comminuted, tibia, fibula	Wound, infected	7,500 q. 3h to 20,000 q. 4h I.M. 500 q. 6h to 1,000 q. 4h locally	2,239,000 59,500 locally	Satisfactory	Infected with gram positive spore forming organism and haemolytic Staph. aureus; later eliminated from wound with relatively rapid healing.
389	Synovitis, acute, suppurative, knee joint following operation (arthrotomy)	Fluid aspirated knee joint	12,500 q. 4h I.M. 250 q. 12h locally	585,000	Satisfactory	Acute onset, rapid swelling of joint; aspirated 50 cc haemorrhagic purulent fluid containing S.T. and S.D. resistant, penicillin susceptible Staph. albus; gratifying response.
160	Rheumatic fever, acute	Pharynx Neg. for Beta haem. strep.	12,500 q. 3h I.M.	637,500	Unsatisfactory	Acutely ill patient with carditis; poor response to penicillin but rapid to salicylate therapy.
140	Rheumatic fever, acute	Pharynx blood neg.	12,500 q. 3h I. M.	1,120,000	Satisfactory	Mild case treated with penicillin from 20th to 22nd day of disease; improvement rapid.
022	Rheumatic fever, acute	Pharynx negative	12,500 q. 3h I.M.	890,000	Satisfactory	Mild case, recurrent type with erythema nodosum; gratifying response.
476	Rheumatic fever, acute	Pharynx negative	12,500 q. 3h I.M.	900,000	Unsatisfactory	Acutely ill, slight febrile response to penicillin but no symptomatic improvement; leucocyte count and sed. velocity remained markedly elevated.
453	Pneumonia, unresolved; markedly thickened pleura	Sputum beta strep. alpha strep. haem. staph. aureus	15,000 q. 3h	1,782,500	Satisfactory	Gradual recovery followed penicillin; resistant to sulfonamide.

following day the ankles were swollen and painful to the extent that he could not walk. On admission the ankles were red, hot, tender, and swollen and the knees were swollen and painful. There was tachycardia with electrocardiographic evidence of myocarditis, temperature 101 degrees. On the second hospital day the sedimentation rate was 110 mm. per hour; penicillin therapy was started

few days of treatment, but the clinical course of the disease continued unabated as evidenced by pain, persistence of polyarthritis, a persistent elevation of the white blood count and a relatively rapid sedimentation rate. In both cases there was marked improvement when they were subsequently placed on adequate salicylate therapy. Bacteriological cultures of material obtained

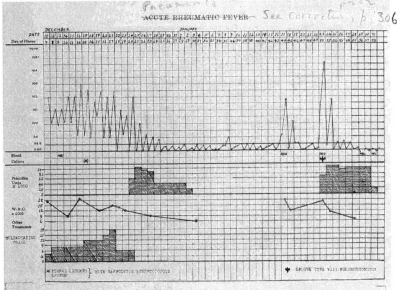

CHART 5, Case 610: Showing the dosage of penicillin and salicylate therapy, the duration and severity of the infection, the leukocyte count and sedimentation rate charted chronologically.

using 12,500 units every three hours intramuscularly. By the third day of treatment there was involvement of the left second and third metatarsal and right elbow joint. The fever persisted and a moderate tachycardia continued. The sedimentation rate had risen to 180 mm. per hour. On the seventh treatment day the heart rate was 116 per minute, there was moderate cyanosis, persistent elevation of temperature and the sedimentation rate was 160 mm. per hour; there was a moderatae degree of muscle aching and penicillin was stopped. As noted in the chart, subsequent salicylate therapy resulted in a favorable response.

Both of these patients were treated with approximately 12,500 units every three hours for 7 and 10 days respectively. There was a favorable febrile response during the last

from the tonsils, pharynx and nasopharynx of these four cases were negative for beta hemolytic streptococcus. One may not draw final conclusions relative to the use of penicillin in the treatment of acute rheumatic fever until a larger group of cases has been studied and much higher doses of penicillin have been administered. These inconclusive observations indicate the need for further study in this disabling and crippling disease.

The patient (Case No. 453) with unresolved pneumonia from whose sputum we cultured streptococci of both the beta (predominating) and alpha types, and also hemolytic staphylococcus albus, responded favorably to penicillin following a period of sulfonamide therapy. Following a transient period of improvement with sulfonamide, there gradually developed an ascending temperature curve. There was no demonstrable extension of the pneumonia by x-ray.

An interesting case of lung abcess due to bacteria not clearly differentiated is illustrated in Chart 2. Male, white, age 21, Case No. 976, was admitted to the Gardiner General Hospital January 23, 1944 complaining of cough and fever of two days' duration. Examination of the lungs revealed a few course crepitant rales over the lower lobe of the right lung. This was not associated with other positive physical findings. His

LUNG ABSCESS

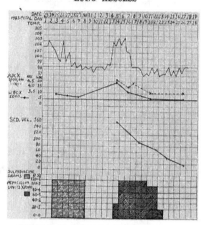

CHART 2, Case No. 976: Showing the temperature curve, the white and red cell count and the sedimentation rate of the blood, and the daily dose of sulfadiazine and penicillin charted chronologically.

temperature was 102 degrees, pulse 104, respirations 20. The white blood cells, 9,900. A smear of the pharynx showed fusiform bacilli and spirilla. There was no sputum. The blood culture was negative. An x-ray of his lungs showed an area of consolidation about 7 cm. in diameter involving the middle lobe of the right lung. This was not associated with other positive physical findings. His temperature was 102 degrees, pulse 104, respirations 20. The white blood cells, 9,900. A smear of the pharynx showed fusiform bacilli and spirilla. There was no sputum. The blood culture was negative. An x-ray of his lungs showed an area of consolidation about 7 cm. in diameter involving the middle lobe of the right lung. Following sulfadiazine therapy, the temperature fell by lysis. His clinic improvement was gradual. A second x-ray obtained on January 31 revealed an abcess cavity approximately 3 cm. in diame-

ter within the zone of consolidation. Sulfadiazine was discontinued on January 30. He remained afebrile until February 4 when he had a sudden rise of temperature to 103 degrees associated with increased cough, which was unproductive. On the following day, the temperature remained elevated and the white blood count was 19,000, associated with sedimentation velocity of 160 mm. per hour. In view of the fact that there was marked systemic reaction to the disease which had seemingly been improving following a course of sulfadiazine, he was placed upon a penicillin regime, receiving 15,000 units every three hours intramuscularly. On the second day of penicillin therapy, the temperature remained elevated but he began to expectorate considerable mucopurulent sputum from which was culture non-typable pneumococci. The smear of the sputum did not reveal fusiform bacilli and spirilla. He became afebrile on the fourth day of penicillin therapy and remained afebrile thereafter. There was a gradual reduction in the sedimentation rate. On February 21 there was aeration of the lung adjacent to the abcess cavity which was difficult to outline. On March 13 there was complete disappearance of the lung abscess with only slight residual scarring and eight days later the lung x-rays of the chest were considered normal.

Streptococcal infections

The results following the use of penicillin in the treatment of the group of infections caused by streptococci of the alpha and beta types were uniformly satisfactory. Table VI shows the results in six such patients.

Case No. 043 with erysipelas involving the forehead made a rapid recovery from the disease.

The patient with chronic pansinusitis was of interest in that he had been subjected previously to an intranasal operation for the relief of obstruction caused by marked deviation of the nasal septum. However, the disease persisted and a streptococcus of the beta hemolytic type was cultured from the nose. Following the use of penicillin intramuscularly there was marked clinical improvement.

The patient suffering from tonsillitis was of interest in that he had recently recovered from scarlet fever and about the 23rd day following the onset of his disease he developed an acute suppurative tonsillitis due to hemolytic streptococcus of the beta type. This was sulfathiazole and sulfadiazine resistant. The disease rapidly responded to penicillin and there was a disappearance of the infecting organism as evidenced by repeated negative tonsil cultures.

Case No. 820 was one of severe bronchpneumonia with serofibrinous pleurisy due to hemolytic streptococcus of the alpha type. The process was diffuse throughout both lungs and was associated with marked tachycardia, fever, cyanosis and tachypnoea. There was no favorable response to the sulfadiazine administered for five days and to sulfanilamide for one day. Following the institution of penicillin therapy there was a gradual fall of temperature and an improvement in his general condition within 48 hours. Slight fever persisted, however, and

white, age 35, Case No. 563, was admitted to Gardiner General Hospital Dec. 11, 1943 complaining of extreme shortness of breath, cough, expectoration, pain in right chest, and marked prostration. Six days before entry he developed a chill with pain in the right chest, cough and expectoration of mucopurulent material. He was hospitalized in a civilian hospital where he was treated with sulfadiazine for five days. Four days before entry he expectorated blood. His fever remained elevated, the cough continued and he became progressively short of

TABLE VI
STREPTOCOCCI INFECTIONS

No.	Clinical Diagnosis	Source of Culture	Penicillin How Treated, Units	Total Dosage Units	Results	Comment
043	Erysipelas	Pharynx alpha? type	10,000 to 25,000 q. 3h I.M.	660,000	Satisfactory	Mild case involving forehead; rapid response.
026	Pan sinusitis, chronic	Nose, Beta type	15,000 q. 3h I.M.		Satisfactory	Previous surgery without cure; rapid clinical and bacteriological response to penicillin.
451	Tonsillitis, acute suppurative	Tonsils Beta type	10,000 q. 4h to 15,000 q. 3h I.M.		Satisfactory	A sulfathiazole and sulfadiazine resistant, penicillin sensitive organism; patient recently had scarlet fever and was clinically sensitive to sulfadiazine; excellent response.
563	Pneumonia and empyema	Sputum and pleural exudate Beta type	10,000 2. 4h to 12,5000 q. 3h I.M.		Satisfactory	Dramatic response in critically ill patient; clinically sulfonamide resistant; extensive empyema with cardiac shift; cured without thoracotomy.
820	Pneumonia, broncho; pleurisy, serofibrinous	Sputum Alpha type	65,000 to 100,000 q. 24h continuous I.V. for 5 days; 7,500 to 12,500 q. 3h I.M.	700,000	Satisfactory	Sulfadiazine and sulfanilamide resistant clinically severely ill patient; gratifying response; therapy supplements with sulfathiazole with results difficult to evaluate.
497	Cellulitis, acute suppurative, face	Pus from surgical drainage Beta type	15,000 to 20,000 q. 3h to q. 4h I.M.	1,315,000	Satisfactory	Sulfonamide therapy and surgical drainage ineffective; dramatic response to penicillin in the face of a rapidly spreading infection.

sulfathiazole was administered to supplement the penicillin therapy, with the result of an acceleration of improvement. It is difficult to correctly evaluate the role of penicillin in the recovery of this patient.

Case No. 497, a severe, acute, suppurative cellulitis of the face was first treated with sulfonamides and surgical drainings. The infection spread in spite of these measures and from the pus was obtained a streptococcus of the beta type. The response to penicillin was dramatic in that the spread of the infection was interrupted and there resulted a rapid diminution of redness, edema, and drainage from the wound.

Penicillin administered by the intramuscular route exerts a favorable effect upon pneumonia complicated by empyema due to a sulfonamide resistant hemolytic streptococcus. This is illustrated in Chart No. 3. Male,

breath. Examination showed moderate cyanosis, limitation of expansion of the right lower chest with flatness and suppression of breath sounds over the right lung posteriorly. The pulse was 130, temperature 102 degrees, respirations 24. There was displacement of the heart to the left, the apex being in the anterior axillary line and a soft systolic apical murmur was audible. There was marked abdominal distention. On admission and one week later cultures of sputum showed great numbers of hemolytic streptococcus of the beta type. On December 17, culture of the pleural exudate showed hemolytic streptococcus of the beta type. An x-ray of the chest showed homogeneous density obscuring the entire right lung. The white blood count was 18,000. It was the impression that he had pneumonia and empyema due to hemolytic streptococcus. He was given oxygen therapy with other supportive measures and sulfadiazine was administered. Repeated aspirations of the chest provided only a few drops of thick pus. His course was stormy as indicated in Chart 3, and on De-

See p 306

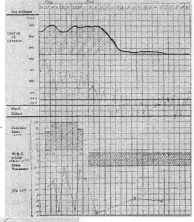

BETA HEMOLYTIC STREPTOCOCCUS PNEUMONIA AND EMPYEMA AND TYPE VIII PNEUMOCOCCUS PNEUMONIA

See p. 06

CHART 3, Case No. 563: Showing the temperature curve, the results of bacteriological examinations of the blood, sputum and pleural exudate, the penicillin dosage, the leucocyte count and the sulfadiazine dosage charted chronologically.

cember 17 cultures of the causative organism were subjected to sulfathiazole and sulfadiazine sensitivity tests in vitro. The organism grew on media containing both of these drugs, but did not grow on media containing penicillin. Because of the failure to improve and the seriousness of the disease, penicillin therapy was begun as indicated in Chart 3 on December 24, 1943 and continued through January 1, 1944. His response was most satisfactory. A thoracotomy was considered on several occasions, but since the progress was consistently favorable, surgical intervention was not instituted. X-ray on January 15 showed only pleural thickening.

In addition to this case we have seen favorable response in the treatment of a few infections associated with the Streptococcus viridans.

In summary all cases of streptococcus infections which have been treated with penicillin have responded favorably.

Pneumococcus pneumonia

Four patients with pneumococcic pneumonia have been treated with satisfactory results in all cases, and the results are shown in Table VII.

In Case No. 765 the response to penicillin was so striking that it resembled the crisis seen following the use of type specific antisera. This is illustrated in Chart No. 4. Male, white, age 20, was admitted to Gardiner General Hospital February 3, 1944 complaining of cough, chill, fever, and pain in the left chest. On admission he was acutely ill; the temperature was 104 degrees; pulse 120 per minute. Signs of consolidation of the lower third of the lowerlobe of the left lung were confirmed by x-ray examination. The sputum examination showed Type 11 pneumococcus. The white cell count was 30,-000 and the sedimentation rate 30 mm. per hour. Treatment with penicillin was immediately instituted using 15,000 units every three hours intramuscularly. Except for the development of a small amount of pleural fluid and the persistence of slight pleural thickening, the course of the illness was uneventful following an immediate and dramatic response to penicillin.

Chart No. 3 demonstrates the dramatic response of Type VIII pneumococcus pneumonia to penicillin. On January 17 this soldier developed a slight sore throat with temperature of 101.6 degrees, but within 48

PNEUMOCOCCUS. PNEUMONIA TYPE II

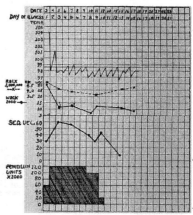

CHART 4, Case No. 765: Showing the changes in temperature, white and red blood cell counts, the sedimentation velocity and the daily dose of penicillin charted chronologically.

hours the temperature was normal and remained so until January 23 when he suffered a chill, shortness of breath, marked tachycardia, and tachypnoea. X-rays at this time showed consolidation of a small area in the periphery in the middle portion of the upper left lobe. From the bloody sputum pneumococcus Type VIII was recovered. The white blood cell count was 17,000 with 93 per cent polymorphonuclear cells. Penicillin therapy was immediately instituted as indicated in the chart, following which he made a striking recovery, the temperature reaching normal within 48 hours and remaining so thereafter. His convalescence has been slow. There remains some thickening of the pleura in the right cardiophrenic angle.

Thus, the response to penicillin was satisfactory in pneunomia due to Type VIII pneumococcus, Type II pneumococcus, and two cases in which the pneumococcus was not typable.

Infections caused by fusiform bacilli and spirochetes

Major Paul L. Shallenberger, M. C., a member of the Penicillin Board, suggested that since the effectiveness of penicillin in causing a rapid disappearance of treponema pallidum from primary lesions of syphilis has been shown, penicillin might be of value in the treatment of infections thought to be due to fusiform bacilli and spirochetes of Vincent's. The Dental Department of this hospital, under the direction of Lt. Colonel K.

TABLE VII
PNEUMOCOCCUS PNEUMONIA

No.	Clinical Diagnosis	Pneumococ-cus, Type	Penicillin How Treated, Units	Total Dosage, Units	Results	Comment
563	Pneumonia, lobar	VIII	15,000 q. 3h I.M.	810,000	Satisfactory	Dramatic response in 48 hours in patient who had recently recovered from sulfa resistant Beta haem. Strep-pneumonia with empyema.
765	Pneumonia, lobar	II	15,000 q. 3h I.M.	1,000,000	Satisfactory	Afebrile within 12 hours with slight fever on second day of treatment, thereafter remaining afebrile. Clinical response dramatic.
251	Pneumonia, lobar, middle lobe, with interlobar effusion	Unclassified	10,000 to 25,000 q. 3h I.M.	660,000	Satisfactory	Penicillin started following 7 days unsuccessful sulfonamide therapy; afebrile 39 hours after starting treatment; rapid clearing of pneumonia and absorption of interlobar effusion.
025	Pneumonia, lobar, left upper and lower; later, upper right	Unclassified	120,00 continuous I.V. first 18 hours; then, 15,000 q. 3h I.M.	765,000	Satisfactory	Both left lobes on admission involved; fourth hospital day disease spread to right upper while on sulfadiazine; dramatic response and afebrile 24 hours after start of I.V. penicillin therapy.

The third patient of this group was especially interesting in that on admission pneumonia of both lobes of the left lung resisted sulfadiazine therapy. In fact, on the fourth hospital day the disease had spread to the right upper lung. There was a dramatic clinical response within 24 hours after penicillin therapy was begun. Unfortunately, the pneumococcus was not typable.

The fourth case of this group had lobar pneumonia involving the middle lobe and was associated with an interlobar effusion. Pneumococcus isolated from the sputum was not typable. He was placed on sulfadiazine therapy for seven days and the response was not satisfactory. Sulfadiazine was discontinued and penicillin was begun. Within 39 hours after administering penicillin, the temperature was normal and there was rapid clearing of the pneumonia with subsequent absorption of the interlobar effusion.

R. Cofield, began using penicillin in the treatment of trench mouth and Vincent's infections.

The following case abstracts are fairly representative of the effect of penicillin on cases of Vincent's angina.

A white soldier was admitted with a history of severe throat of three days' duration. Examination of the throat revealed marked injection, edema, hypertrophy of the tonsils, and a grayish white membrane covering both tonsils and their fossae. The admission smear was positive for Vincent's organisms. He received local applications of penicillin in a concentration of 250 units per cc. by swabbing the throat four times daily with this solution. Treatment was continued for three days. At the end of two and one-half treatment days the smear was negative for Vincent's organism, and the edema had subsided and the grayish white membrane disappeared. He received no other medication and there was no recurrence.

Another patient who had a severe sore throat of 24 hours' duration on admission showed Vincent's organisms in a stained smear. The same therapy as described above was applied and his smears were negative for Vincent's organisms after three and one-half days' treatment. There was a rapid symptomatic improvement during the first 48 hours of treatment.

An interesting case was that of a soldier who had a history of chills and fever associated with sore throat for two days prior to admission. There was moderate injection of the pharynx, but no membrane was present. The smear on admission was positive for Vincent's organism. He received 16 grams of sulfadiazine over a period of four days and at the end of this time the smear was still positive for Vincent's organisms. Sulfadiazine was discontinued and penicillin was begun. There was definite clinical improvement during the succeeding three days and the smear became negative on the third day of penicillin therapy.

Another patient had a history of upper respiratory infection associated with sore throat of four days' duration. There was marked hypertrophy, redness, and swelling of the tonsils, and marked hyperemia of the posterior pharynx and fossae. No membrane was visualized. The admission smear. was positive for Vincent's organisms. He was given four and one-half grams of sulfadiazine daily over a period of four days at the end of which time smear was still positive for Vincent's organisms and there was only moderate improvement in the clinical picture. Penicillin was then applied locally to the pharynx and tonsils over a period of three days. The smear became negative on the third day of treatment. There was marked clinical improvement within the first two days at the end of instituting penicillin therapy.

A soldier was admitted to the hospital with a history of sore throat of three day's duration. On admission the tonsils were hyperemic and on the left tonsil an ulcer covered with a grayish membrane was observed from which a smear was obtained and found positive for Vincent's organisms. Topical applications of penicillin were initiated. Within 24 hours there was less hyperemia but the smear was still positive for Vincent's organisms. At the end of 48 hours there was marked clinical improvement and again the smear was positive for fusiform bacilli and spirilla. Clinical improvement was marked by the end of the third day of treatment, at

which time the smear was negative for Vincent's organisms.

A 22 year old officer was admitted March 10, 1944 with history of a sore throat of two days' duration. This became progressively more severe, and was associated with generalized malaise and progressive weakness. He appeared acutely ill, his face was flushed and he was obviously having marked pain with talking. He also had severe pain on swallowing and movement of his jaws. His temperature was 102 degrees and pulse 110 on admission. There was marked edema of the pharynx associated with redness of the pharyngeal mucosa and both tonsils. On the right tonsil there was a grayish exudate in which Vincent's organisms in great numbers were demonstrated by smear. There was also a thick grayish white film involving the gums. The white blood count was 17,800 with 90 per cent polymorphonuclear cells. A culture of the tonsils showed beta hemolytic streptococcus. Because of the marked edema of the pharynx associated with difficulty in swallowing, penicillin therapy was initiated, using an initial dose of 25,000 units followed by 15,000 units every three hours intramuscularly. The treatment was continued for a total dosage of 520,000 units. Within 24 hours there was marked reduction of the edema and hyperemia of the fossae, tonsils, and pharynx. The maximum temperature was 98.6 degrees. The smears were negative for Vincent's organisms at this time. By the end of the second day there was very little distress on swallowing, the temperature was normal and improvement continued. Slight bilateral anterior cervical adenopathy developed, but this rapidly subsided. The response to penicillin therapy was dramatic as evidence by the rapid improvement in the appearance of the infected gums, tonsils, and pharynx, and the rapid disappearance of Vincent's organisms from the lesions.

The response has been so dramatic and the results so striking that there can be little doubt that penicillin is the most effective agent that has as yet been discovered in the treatment of this group of infections. At present, penicillin solution in a concentration of from 100 units to 250 units per cc. is being applied locally to lesions of the gums, pharynx, and tonsils, both in the Dental Department and on the contagious ward.

Actinomycosis

One patient with this disease is being treated with penicillin at present. Although a final statement cannot be made of the value of penicillin in this patient, it is our impression that the drug may be of value. Although lesions of the lung disappeared and lesions involving the caecum were improved by the use of sulfadiazine in approximately 12 gram daily doses, an additional lesion developed in the soft tissue of the right lumbar region resulting in abscess formation while the patient was on sulfadiazine. It was at this time that penicillin was instituted and was used as a supplement to sulfadiazine. Subsequent to the institution of penicillin therapy the abscess receded in size and the drainage from the sinus tract ceased. The patient has gained approximately 35 pounds in weight over a period of three months.

TOXIC REACTIONS

We have encountered no severe toxic reactions. In one patient (Case No. 950) following the 36th and 37th injection of 12,500 units of penicillin, there was headache and dizziness. These reactions lasted but for a few moments and there was no subsequent untoward effect Slight fever has been observed in a few patients. Urticaria has not been noted in a single patient. One medical officer (Major H. D. P.)[10] who has been working with penicillin experienced a mild contact dermatitis involving his face and hands. Patch tests, using 5,000 units per cc. of regular penicillin and 3,000 units of purified penicillin, were positive.

SUMMARY AND CONCLUSIONS

Two hundred and seventy-six patients have been treated with penicillin. From our observations it is apparent that penicillin is highly effective in the treatment of sulfonamide resistant gonorrhea, as evidenced by the fact that 98.7 per cent of 243 patients were cured with 50,000 and-or 100,000 units. There was a satisfactory response to penicillin in all patients who were suffering from infections caused by streptococci of the beta and alpha types, and pneumonia caused by pneumococcus. In the patients suffering from infections due to staphylococcus aureus, the results were satisfactory in those whose lesions were superficial, or in which adequate drainage was instituted, or in whom the disease was relatively acute. In contrast to this group those in whom the disease was chronic, in which drainage was incomplete, or in which a foreign body or sequestrum existed, the results have been unsatisfactory.

No conclusions can be drawn from our observation in the treatment of acute rheumatic fever in view of the fact that relatively small doses were used in four patients. Further observations in the treatment of acute rheumatic fever with large doses of penicillin seems warranted. Our clinical and bacteriological observations indicate that penicillin is highly effective in the treatment of Vincent's infection.

FOOTNOTE

The following officers of the Medical Corps, Army of the United States, advised and assisted in this study, and their cooperation made its completion possible: Captain Louis A. Schneider; Captain Francis E. West; Captain William E. Lange; Lieutenant Erik Eselius.

[1]Herrell, W. E.; The Clinical Use of Penicillin, an Antibacterial Agent of Biological Origin, J.A.M.A. 124:627, Mar. 4, 1944.

[2]Abraham, E. P.; Chain, E.; Fletcher, C. M.; Gardner, A. D.; Heatley, N. G.; Jennings, M. A.; and Florey, H. W.; Further Observations on Penicillin, Lancet 11, 177. 1941.

[3]Abraham, E. P., and Chain, E.; An Enzyme from Bacteria able to Destroy Pencillin, Nature, 146:837, December 28, 1940.

[4]Bloomfield, A. L., Rantz, L. A., Kirby, W. M. M.: The Clinical Use of Penicillin, J. A.M.A., 124, No. 10:627. March 4, 1944.

[5]The Surgeon General: Letter, December 18, 1943.

[6]Rammelkamp, C. H., and Keefer, C. S.: The Absorption, Excretion and Distribution of Penicillin, J. Clin. Investigation, 22:425. May, 1943.

[7]Dawson, M. H.; Hobby, Gladys L; Meyer, Karl; and Chaffee, Eleanor; Penicillin as a Chemotherapeutic Agent, Ann. Int. Med. 19:707. November, 1943.

[8]Rammelkamp, C. H., and Keefer, C. S.: The Absorption, Excretion and Toxity of Penicillin Administered by Intrathecal Injection, Am.J.M.Sc. 205:342. March, 1943.

[9]War Department: Penicillin, War Department Technical Bulletin No. 9, February 12, 1944.

[10]Pyle, H. D., and Ratner, Herbert: Contact Dermatitis from Penicillin. To be published.

DISCUSSION

IAN MACKENZIE, M.D.,

TULSA, OKLAHOMA

I am very happy to have this opportunity of discussing this excellent paper by Colonel E. R. Denny. I have had the opportunity of reading this paper before it was presented and there were many points which Col. Denny did not have time to elaborate upon.

I represent the Orthopedic Specialty and I am glad to show you, that in spite of all the miracles accomplished by the sulfa group of drugs, there is still work for us to do. Also to show you that we are still working in spite of the wonderful results obtained in the treatment of infantile paralysis which have been treated by the 'much discussed' Kenny treatment. With the development of all the new alloys for the manufacture of bone plates, it looked for a while as though open reductions were going to be very easily done. However, the orthopedic man still sees some cases of non-union and osteomyelitis. I feel that Penicillin is giving us one more active agent to help us in treatment of many infectious conditions which we see in our practice.

Several cases in Col. Denny's paper were patients in whom a foreign body, such as vitallium plate had to be removed before Penicillin accomplished any results. He also reported another case, but did not have time to elaborate upon it, of a chronic cyst of the shoulder which had had repeated incisions in drainage. There was excessive scar tissue, and the Penicillin did not help much in this case. Similar experience has been found in certain cases of pneumonia and other infections, that, unless there was satisfactory circulation to distribute the Penicillin, no results were obtained. The Penicillin is a natural immunological development. We are here because our ancestors developed a certain resistance to bacteria, and it is alleged that the dinasours and other pre-historic animals became extinct because they did not develop any immunity. The molds and spore forming organisms are a higher development of the evolutionary process of life and have had to overcome many other organisms and infections in order to exist.

I feel that Penicillin will be the precursor of many other antibiotics which will be developed when conditions for research and careful study will be more normal, and I also feel, and I think this point was brought out in Colonel Denny's paper, that Penicillin is an aid, just as sulphonamides are aids, to treatments of diseases, but there is still no substitute for careful examination and good surgery.

I think we, as civilians, are fortunate that the Medical Corps of the Armed Services are doing such a thorough study of Penicillin before it is made freely available, because we will know how to use it properly when it is made available to the civilian population.

I am sorry that Colonel Denny could not have more time for the presentation of this paper and I am glad to see that Colonel Denny is continuing his same fine, thorough work in the Army as he did when he was practicing in Tulsa.

Cancer of the Prostate

ALFRED R. SUGG, M.D.

ADA, OKLAHOMA

Until recently there was little progress in the management and care of cancer of the prostate. The uniformly poor results, regardless of the method of treatment, has had a tendency to lessen the interest of urologists in the subject and to dampen the enthusiams of workers in this field. The one phase of the subject about which there is all but unanimous opinion is the bad prognosis.

Cancer of the prostate, like cancer in general, is a dreaded disease. X-ray and radium, together with surgery have constituted the methods of attack. There has been considerable difference of opinion as to which of these is the most effective. Irradiation has been disappointing and the attending discomfort to the patient from its use has discouraged many from attempting it. There is some difference of opinion as to the type of surgery that should be employed in cancer of the prostate, but this has about as much to do with geography as with pathology. North by Northeast perineal attack would seem to be the method of choice; while to the North transuretheral approach is in vogue; and in the Southwest, the attitude is "catch as catch can, and no holds barred." In the matter of palliation, which in a great majority of patients has been all that was left for the surgeon to do, the suprapubic catheter has been satisfactory to the surgeon, but terrible on the patient. Removal of enough of the gland by transurethral resection to permit a good uninary stream seemed at first to be a distinct advance in this direction. However, it has turned out that the resulting irritation, infection and ulceration leave much to be desired. Recently an inquiry was made to the Editor of the Journal of the American Medical Association as to what was the best thing to be done surgically for cancer of the prostate. The anonymous reply indicated that when a diagnosis of cancer of the prostate was made that it ceased to be a surgical problem. Several distinguished urologists of this country branded the above statement as untrue, misleading and harmful. Young, Hinman, Lowsley and others supported their resentment by producing a number of cured cases of cancer of the prostate by surgery. Their replies merit a little consideration here. Many surgeons have reported a few cured cases with surgery, but these have uniformly been in the very earliest cases, those that could not well be diagnosed by ordinary physical examinations. The plea is made regularly for doctors to be more alert in making rectal examinations and thus discovering these lesions early. Such advice is well in order, for it remains that even urologists are not sufficiently alert in this particular and certainly physicians in general are far too prone to overlook the rectal examinations. Still it is a fact that most of the cases reported as cured were diagnosed only after a biopsy was made and a frozen section reported. It is a radical operation with a high mortality and a higher ratio of serious complications, incontinence, etc. This is not to suggest that the radical operation for early cancer of the prostate should not be attempted. It should be, but as a matter of practical application in everyday use, the anonymous authors reply to the criticism of his statement remains true that when cancer of the prostate has been diagnosed by ordinary methods, it is not a surgical problem. It certainly will never solve the problem for the good and sufficient reason that the patient will not submit to a radical prostatectomy because the surgeon informs him that there is a small hard nodule palpable. He has no symptoms, he feels well, is urinating without difficulty and he will simply not submit to this type of surgery even though the diagnosis is made early enough to cure him. It becomes a matter of salesmanship rather than surgery and I do not believe we will succeed in a general way in this direction. There is some doubt that radical surgery should be generally employed even if the patient were willing to have it done. Cancer of the prostate is notoriously slow to metastasize and many men have several years of active life after the first nodule becomes palpable and I doubt that many of us, realizing the hazards of the surgery involved, knowing the possibilities of considerable time left to us, would take the gamble. We can therefore not complain too much if our patients do likewise. As for me, I have not had too good luck in selling a prostate operation to my friends, even though

they are sick, emaciated, in constant pain and with sleep continually broken by ferquently getting up, and days described best by the skeptic's remark about the first steamboat, "She will never start" and a few minutes later by the equally pungent phrase, "She'll never stop."

With this gloomy outlook then, there is little wonder that the profession was electrified with a new hope when Huggins and his associates presented their paper before the A. U. A. recently, laying the basis for a new method of attack. It has long been known that cancer of the prostate is often a mature type of cell; that serum phosphatase, an enzyme, is present in large quantities in this type of cell. Huggins demonstrated that injection of androgens produced a sharp rise of the serum phosphatase, while on the contrary, the elimination of the antigen or its decrease, shows a sharp decrease in this enzyme and that concomitant with this decrease, the tendency of the neoplasm to grow was specific. The problem seems to be then to eliminate the androgen. While androgens are thought to be produced by other tissues than the gonads, they are chiefly produced here. Castration, either surgical or by x-ray, or by the excessive use of estrogens has been tried and some encouraging reports have been made. There was naturally a marked tendency toward skepticism among physicians when a totally new and radical procedure was proposed. Testosterone had not lived up to its press agent's report and many other types of treatment in medicine have been found wanting, when weighed in the balance of experience and close scientific scrutiny, even though enthusiastic reports had reached the literature.

Castration is a safe and simple expedient of eliminating the gonadal androgen, but again the matter of salesmanship pops up when one starts investigation in this direction. The Orchid to the prostate of 75, is like that etheral flower by the same name to the debutante, it is of tremendous importance sentimentally though equally as valueless in a material and practical way. This is so true that we find only a small number who will consent to parting with these monuments to a spent life that it will take some

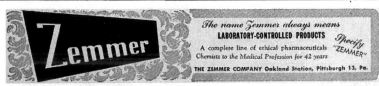

time for us to report a very large series of cases. It is well known that sufficient x-ray to the gonads will inhibit the hormonal activity of the testicles, and Munger has reported that while the best results are produced by large doses of hard irradiation, that as little as 500 R is effective. Stilbestrol, most potent of the estrogenic substances available, has been reported to produce atrophy of the testicles and to decrease the size of the prostate and in general to serve the same purpose as x-ray and castration in diminishing the activity of neoplasms of prostate. To test out these theories is the part of my mission. With this in view, I will therefore skip any discertation on the theory of the production of carcinoma of the prostate, and shall attempt no scientific proof of my findings and will confine my report to a short clinical study of a few cases.

I have four cases, treated sufficiently long and with sufficient observation to perhaps be of some small value in judging the efficiency of the therapy as outlined.

CASE NO 1

Age, 78 years. Admitted to the hospital in July, 1939, with the provisional diagnosis of being prostatic hypertrophy. He had all of the usual symptoms of the prostatic, (obstruction, infection, etc.). The prostate at that time was large, grade 3, and there was four to six ounces of residual urine. No nodules could be felt in the prostate and it certainly was not a carcinoma, clinically. There was no x-ray or neurological signs of metastasis. A suprapubic, two stage operation was done at that time, and the patient was discharged in thirty days in good condition. He was voiding well. He was seen several times after the operation, sounds were passed and rectal examination done and it appeared that the prostate had all been removed and that he was on his road to recovery. The microscopic examination of the resected glands showed very early carcinoma, in fact, it was so early that there was some doubt as to whether it was malignant or otherwise. About six months after the patient's discharge from the hospital, he returned to the office complaining of a recurrence of his urinary symptoms, dysuria, frequency, nocturia, etc. In addition he had definite root pain, backache and pain referred down his

leg so severe that he was a semi-invalid. Rectal examination at this time revealed a large, hard, irregular mass in prostate bed that no one would mistake for anything except prostatic cancer. He had a large amount of residual urine, the catheter passing with difficulty. These symptoms and signs became gradually but progressively worse without any treatment until he returned in October, 1941, at which time he had complete urinary retention. He was acutely ill and was suffering from intense pain. X-rays at this time show metastatic lesions in the pelvic bones. He was taking morphine at least twice daily from his family physician to make the pain bearable. He was losing weight rapidly; had marked constipation and anorexia. A small rigid catheter was the only instrument that would pass into his bladder. He was taken to the hospital and an attempt made to remove enough of the gland with the transuretheral instrument to relieve his retention. It was found that the resectoscope could not be passed on account of the density of the growth at the bladder neck. A retention catheter suprapubically through a Duffy Trochoscope was inserted for drainage and he was castrated. He remained in the hospital one week and after the third day it was not necessary to administer further narcotics. He was not seen for thirty days after he left the hospital and at this time examination revealed little if any change in the size or density of the tumor, but his clinical appearance was almost unbelievable. He was voiding without difficulty, his appetite had improved and in his words he "felt like a new man." There was two ounces of residual urine at this time. He has been seen at regular intervals to date, that is, about once a year after the castration. He has gained twenty pounds in weight. He sleeps all night without the necessity of voiding and has no pain or discomfort either in the bladder or in his back or legs. The tumor by rectal examination has become progressively smaller until at this time there is only an indurated area comparable to the usual bladder neck fibrosis. There is no residual urine and the patient is making a hand on the farm and does as much as a man of his age could usually do. X-ray of the pelvis taken recently still shows the metastatic lesions in the pelvis, but they seem to me to be distinctly less in size and density.

CASE NO. 2

J. G. K., age 70 years. Was first seen in 1938 with a moderately enlarged prostate with severe urinary symptoms, that is, urgency, frequency, dysuria, burning, slow stream, nocturia, etc., but with little residual urine and no other constitutional symptoms. He was not seen again until 1940, two years later, when he had all of the above symptoms together with some loss of weight and general malaise and the retention had reached five ounces. The prostate was suspected of malignancy, but on rectal examination this could not be confirmed. In fact, the prostate was large, soft, tender and no areas of palpable induration, but on attempting a suprapubic prostatectomy, it was apparent that the gland was malignant and this was confirmed by the pathologist. We were able in spite of the usual difficulties to effect a fairly complete removal of the gland. The pathologist's report says the specimen consists of three lobes of prostate gland. The tissue is moderately firm in consistency, but is not stony hard. No evidence of malignancy found. Microscopic report was "small alveolar carcinoma of the prostate". This patient was discharged after five weeks in the hospital and returned to his home in Iowa and was not seen again for almost a year. He was not told of his condition, but his family was advised. He had complete relief from his urinary symptoms for about nine months following the operation, at which time he began to have a recurrence of all of his symptoms which progressed rapidly and he began to have hematuria and at times passed rather large quantities of blood. He was seen early in 1942, when he had two ounces of residual urine and a No. 26 sound passed with great difficulty and with much bleeding. Prostatic capsule was fixed, firm, and irregular. X-ray of the bone showed no gross metastasis. His general condition was fairly good. He was castrated at that time and left shortly thereafter for his home in a distant state. I have heard from him regularly since that time. He has had no other medication or treatment, all of his symptoms having disappeared and he reports that he is in the best of health and is more active in

business than he has been for ten years. He was advised to consult an urologist for periodic check-ups at home, but in a letter recently he says he refuses to visit a doctor when he is feeling entirely well.

CASE NO. 3

J. D. W. This patient was admitted in October, 1941, with a provisional diagnosis of benign prostatic hypertrophy but some question of malignancy. The prostate on palpation was slightly firm but without definite nodules or areas of induration. Prostate was extremely large and with 500 c.c of residual. He had all the symptoms of obstruction together with extreme pain in his back and hips. He had catheterized himself for years but in spite of infected urine, there was no loss of weight, appetite was good and he was leading an active life. There was no x-ray evidence of metastasis. Bladder drainage was secured by the use of the suprapubic catheter through the Duffy Troscope. There was so much suspicion of carcinoma without proof, that we elected to remove at least a portion of the gland for biopsy since our transuretheralscope at that time was "hors de combat", with the idea of castrating him if our suspicions were confirmed. Our suspicions were confirmed, but a larger part of the gland was removed. This patient refused, on second thought, to have castration, but he did consent to x-ray of the testicles. There is not a deep therapy machine available in our city, so he was given a skin tolerance dose in three treatments, approximating ——R. This was given about four months post-operative, and then we were able to secure his cooperation only after he had had a marked recurrence of his urinary symptoms, and progressive pain. He was also given 5 mg. doses of stilbestrol every other day for sixty days. There was in this case also an almost immediate ceasation of pain and it has not recurred. The induration in the prostatic bed definitely decreased. There is at this time no residual urine and the patient has gained fifteen pounds and is leading an active life. An interesting observation in connection with the stilbestrol was his development of mammary glands. He is a very small man with no subcutaneous fat and the usual vestigal mammary glands. After two months of stilbestrol, he blushingly removed his shirt and asks me the cause of such unwanted development in this locality. It was amusing to see an old man with a spare frame with definitely hypertrophied mammary glands. There had been no pain or soreness in the mammary glands as has been reported by others.

CASE NO. 4

Briefly put, his story is: Age, 75 years, Admitted to the hospital May, 1941, acutely ill with phelonephritis from urinary retention. The prostate was extremely large, smooth and hard and for some reason the bladder was thick-walled and contracted. He could not tolerate catheter drainage so a suprapubic was done as an emergency measure. The majority of the prostate was enucleated, relieving the obstruction after which he made an uneventful recovery except for continued dribbling. In a few months all of his symptoms had returned and he was losing weight and suffering considerable pain. He refused either castration or x-ray, so he was accordingly given stilbestrol for a trial. He was given 500 mg. in four months, after which he became so nauseated that it was discontinued for a few weeks and he has taken the drug intermittently since. A recent examination revealed that he is clinically improved. That is, his pain is less severe and he feels well. However, he still dribbles and on rectal examination the mass in the prostatic bed has not decreased appreciably.

CONCLUSION

In conclusion I have not attempted to present a scientific paper on this interesting subject but we have recorded some clinical observations that indicate to me that we are on the right track and should pursue this matter of castration in cancer of the prostate further; that castration is probably the method of choice and for those patients who have androgens formed in other tissues than the testicles, stilbetrol maybe a satisfactory adjunct. Much more statistical study is necessary before conclusions can be definite, but it seems as if we have all to win and nothing to lose and the observation so far makes the situation more hopeful for the prostatic condemned by cancer. In fact, the work started by urologists in this field may have opened up a complete new line of approach to the cancer problem in general and the pioneers should be given all honor.

The above reported cases have been followed at regular intervals since they were operated. They are all alive, all are engaged in their usual occupations, and are clinically well. One of them complains of suprapubic pain at intervals. There is no evidence of metastasis in any of the cases. We feel that without castration these men would have been in a hopeless condition or dead by this time.

Since the paper was written we have five additional cases under similar circumstances and with the same favorable results today. Some of them, however, have been too recent to judge the results.

Congenital Defects of the Sternum[*]
With the Report of a Case

JOHN F. BURTON, M.D.

OKLAHOMA CITY, OKLAHOMA

Defects of the sternum are not common. Greig reviewed the literature in 1926 and reported:

1. Simple cleft sternum—20 cases.
2. Cleft sternum with ectopia cordis—19 cases.

These congenital defects vary from simple notching of the manubrium and irregularities in shape of the xiphoid to complete absence of the entire structure. The minor defects are not usually recognized and their discovery is used incidental to radiographic studies of the chest. The larger defects are brought to attention at birth because of their effects upon the thoracic and mediastinal contents. These effects may be varied depending upon the extent of the defect. Herniation of the lungs will cause marked disturbances of respiration. Lack of normal restraint of the heart and associated large vessels may cause profound circulatory phenomena.

In reviewing the literature, I was impressed by two facts, namely: the high mortality and the attitude of hopelessness of the medical attendants for such cases.

I wish to present a case of cleft sternum with ectopia cordis which has recently come

*Read before the Annual Meeting of the Oklahoma State Medical Association, May 11, 1943, at Oklahoma City, Oklahoma.

to our attention and which shows that these cases can be benefited if treated surgically with proper preparation and in stages as indicated.

CASE

J. S., white male, age seven weeks. Patient entered the hospital on January 14, 1943. Chief complaint: Paroxysmal attacks of rapid heart beat, accompanied by cyanosis.

Physical examination:

Head and scalp: Normal.

Neck: There was bulging of the anterior

The child was placed under an oxygen tent temporarily and during the next week a formula was supervised with definite improvement of the child. The second week the oxygen tent was removed but the child continued to have paroxysms of cyanosis and difficulty in breathing.

X-Rays were made showing the defect. Consultants of the general surgical service were of the opinion that surgical therapy was not indicated. Because of the unusual character of the congenital defect and the grave prognosis, surgical intervention was

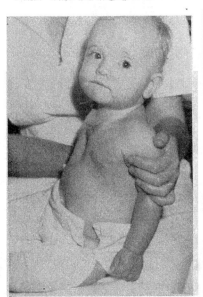 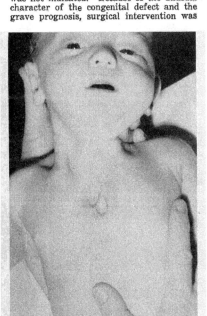

Fig. 1 Fig. 2. Age 2 months. Showing defect of sternum.

surface of the neck between the two sternocleidomastoid muscles, this became larger at times.

Chest: Anteriorly, the ribs did not meet in the midline and there was an absence of the entire manubrium and the body of the sternum. Only a thin layer of skin lay over the defect and with each pulsation of the heart, the cardiac structures raised the skin above the level of the chest wall. When this act took place, the large vessels leading from the heart could be seen. The lower end of the sternum showed the xiphoid present.

Abdomen: Normal.

Probable diagnosis: Congenital defect of the sternum with partial ectopic cordis.

chosen as a possible means of relief.

On February 11, 1943, under nitrous oxide and ether anesthesia, an incision was made on the right side of the lower chest. A block of cartilage which included the eighth and nineth costal cartilages, measuring one and one-half inches in diameter, was removed en masse. About 25 minutes was required for this procedure and when the child's pulse became somewhat irregular the wound was closed. The cartilage was placed in plasma and refrigerated. The wound healed by primary union.

On February 18, 1943, again under nitrous oxide and ether, the anterior chest was prepared and with Dr. Rix holding the heart in the chest cavity by direct pressure, a four inch transverse incision was made across the mid-portion of the hiatus. By sharp dissection, the cardiac structures were dissected loose from their attachment to the skin and surrounding cervical muscles, thus permitting their descent into the chest cavity. There was no definite pericardium. The soft structures were then mobilized. The piece of cartilage previously removed and prescribed in the plasma, was laid across the hiatus and two silver wire sutures were placed through the costal cartilages pulling the lateral sides of the opening medially and also serving to anchor the cartilage graft. The muscles were then pulled over about one-half way on each side. These were sutured with interrupted black silk sutures. The skin and subcutaneous tissues were closed with buried silk and interrupted black silk in the skin.

The convalescence was satisfactory, in that the paroxymal attacks of cyanosis did not recur and the pulse rate was reduced. The healing was clean, with the exception of two small sinuses leading down to the wires. On March 22, 1943, under nitrous oxide and ether anesthesia, the wires were removed. The wounds were filled with sulfanilamide powder. Healing was prompt and the child was discharged from the hospital on April 16, 1943 in good condition. Weight upon entrance to the hospital was nine pounds,

seven and one-fourth ounces and upon discharge was twelve pounds, three and one-half ounces.

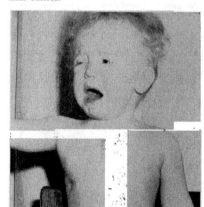

Fig. 3. Age 16 months. Weight 22 lbs, 6 oz. Crying and showing firm repair of anterior chest wall.

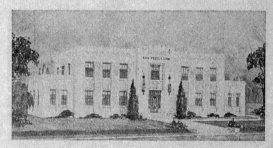

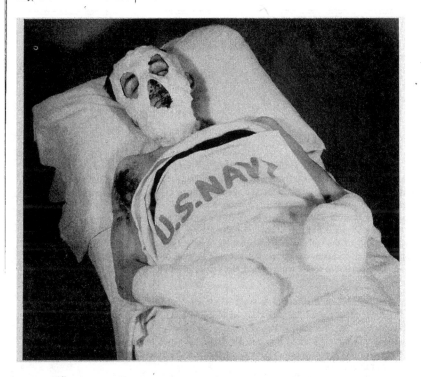

WHAT ARE A CASUALTY'S THOUGHTS?

"This may be it . . . no pain though . . . hope the folks back home don't know for a while . . . lucky to be alive."

Yes, lucky to be alive . . . but with an excellent chance of staying alive, thanks to research and the best medical care in the world.

We, at Warren-Teed, salute the busy physicians of America on the fighting front and on the home front.

WARREN-TEED
Medicaments of Exacting Quality Since 1920

THE WARREN-TEED PRODUCTS COMPANY, COLUMBUS 8, OHIO

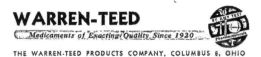

• THE PRESIDENT'S PAGE •

The Oklahoma State Medical Association has completed one of its most successful years. The Past President, Dr. James Stevenson, has set a noble example of fine leadership and unselfish devotion to duty. We are well aware of the numerous trips he made from Tulsa to Oklahoma City and the many hours of work in connection with this office; to say nothing of the time away from his private practice, which he gave in order to serve the physicians of this State. For all of this and more too, we take this opportunity, on behalf of the Oklahoma State Medical Association, to express our thanks and appreciation . In his new office as Delegate to the American Medical Association we are assured of leadership which will promote the best interest and welfare of organized medicine.

It is the earnest wish of the present administration that each and every member of the Association realize his obligation in connection with the welfare of the organization as a whole. We shall endeavor to keep you informed of the problems of economic and legislative nature in order that you may form your own intelligent opinion. We hope that you will feel free to come to your Councilor and the State Office with any problem which you may have.

This is your Association and its facilities are at the disposal of every member whenever he or she cares to utilize them. We shall expect your active support in advancing the cause of medicine. Constructive criticism is always welcome and will be received in the same good spirit as it is given, therefore, if all of us take an active interest in the affairs of the Association and fulfill the obligations assigned, we shall accomplish much, otherwise, this will be just another year.

President.

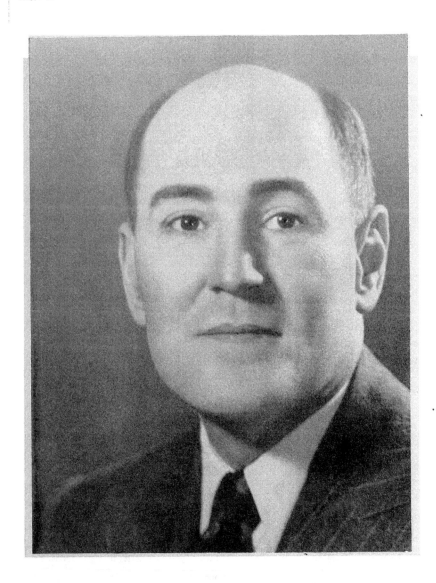

The JOURNAL Of The
OKLAHOMA STATE MEDICAL ASSOCIATION

EDITORIAL BOARD

L. J. MOORMAN, Oklahoma City, Editor-in-Chief

E. EUGENE RICE, Shawnee   BEN H. NICHOLSON, Oklahoma City

MR. PAUL H. FESLER, Oklahoma City, Business Manager

CONTRIBUTIONS: Articles accepted by this Journal for publication including those read at the annual meetings of the State Association are the sole property of this Journal.

The Editorial Department is not responsible for the opinions expressed in the original articles of contributors.

Manuscripts may be withdrawn by authors for publication elsewhere only upon the approval of the Editorial Board.

MANUSCRIPTS: Manuscripts should be typewritten, double-spaced, on white paper 8½ x 11 inches. The original copy, not the carbon copy, should be submitted.

Footnotes, bibliographies and legends for cuts should be typed on separate sheets in double space. Bibliography listing should follow this order: Name of author, title of article, name of periodical with volume, page and date of publication.

Manuscripts are accepted subject to the usual editorial revisions and with the understanding that they have not been published elsewhere.

NEWS: Local news of interest to the medical profession, changes of address, births, deaths and weddings will be gratefully received.

ADVERTISING: Advertising of articles, drugs or compounds unapproved by the Council on Pharmacy of the A.M.A. will not be accepted. Advertising rates will be supplied on application.

It is suggested that members of the State Association patronize our advertisers in preference to others.

SUBSCRIPTIONS: Failure to receive The Journal should call for immediate notification.

REPRINTS: Reprints of original articles will be supplied at actual cost provided request for them is attached to manuscripts or made in sufficient time before publication. Checks for reprints should be made payable to Industrial Printing Company, Oklahoma City.

Address all communications to THE JOURNAL OF THE OKLAHOMA STATE MEDICAL ASSOCIATION,
210 Plaza Court, Oklahoma City. (3)

OFFICIAL PUBLICATION OF THE OKLAHOMA STATE MEDICAL ASSOCIATION
Copyrighted May, 1944

EDITORIALS

SULFAMERAZINE

Anderson, Oliver and Keefer[1] have reported a clinical evaluation of sulfamerazine as compared with sulfadiazine. Previously reported studies show that sulfamerazine is more soluble than sulfadiazine and more readily absorbed from the gastrointestinal tract and more slowly excreted by the kidneys. When given in equal doses the blood level for sulfamerazine was 50 per cent higher than that obtained with sulfadiazine. These observations led to the conclusion that the desired blood level in the case of sulfamerazine can be maintained with a greatly reduced dose and that it can be maintained with a longer interval between doses. Also, because of greater solubility it was thought fewer kidney complications might occur.

The above mentioned authors set about to determine relative efficiency, dosage and reactions. In this study they employed sulfamerazine in 278 patients including 210 adults and 68 children. With some exceptions the initial dose in adults was 2 gm. followed by 1 gm. every eight hours. In children under 60 pounds, 0.5 gm. and a daily maintenance dose of 0.5 gm. for every 10 pounds of body weight given in three equal doses

eight hours apart. The duration of therapy varied but in general the drug was continued from 48 to 96 hours after the disappearance of fever.

The following conditions were among those treated: pneumococcal lobar pneumonia; lobar pneumonia—type undetermined; streptococcal pneumonia; broncho-pneumonia; primary atypical pneumonia of unknown etiology; meningitis; hemolytic streptococcus meningitis; pneumococcal meningitis; erysipelas; subacute bacterial endocarditis; infections of the urinary tract; acute otitis media; acute tonsillitis, peritonsillitis and cervical adenitis; staphylococcal infections; acute sinusitis; gonococcal urethritis.

In primary atypical pneumonia and subacute bacterial endocarditis the treatment was wholly ineffective. Under toxic reactions the authors state; "excluding uncomplicated crystalluria, toxic reactions were observed in 70 (25 per cent) of the patients treated. For the most part, these reactions were mild and not of a character to jeopardize the patient's health or cause severe discomfort. Nausea, 6.5; Vomiting, 4.3; Headache, 1.1; Psychosis, 1.8; Anemia, 1.1; Leukopenia (below 4000), 2.9; Granulocytopenia (below 50 per cent), 3.2; Crystalluria, 21.5; Microscopic hematuria, 0.7; Gross hematuria, 0.7; Renal colic, 0.7; Anuria, 0.4; Drug rash, 5.0; Drug fever, 5.0; Joint pains, 0.4; Conjunctivitis, 0.4.

In conclusion it is shown that "sulfamerazine was clinically effective in total doses that were on the average one-half to one-third smaller than the amounts of sulfadiazine usually administered for similar conditions.

"Toxic reactions to sulfamerazine were in general of the same character and occurred with about the same frequency as those caused by sulfadiazine. A greater tendency for sulfamerazine to produce leukopenia and to cause drug rashes and drug fevers constitutes a possible exception to this statement.

"It may be concluded that sulfamerazine is a potent chemotherapeutic agent and a valuable addition to the sulfonamide derivatives in general use."

1Anderson, Donald G.; Oliver, Charles S.; Keefer, Chester S. A Clinical Evaluation of Sulfamerazine. The New England Journal of Medicine, Vol. 230, No. 13, pp. 369-379. March 30, 1944.

"HOW CAN WE PROVIDE MEDICAL CARE FOR EVERYONE"*

Only our good friend Schwitalla can tell us what we know and feel about the impossible solution of good medical care for everyone. The following editorial appeared in the April 24, 1944 Jackson County Medical Society Weekly Bulletin of Kansas City, Missouri:

"If I give a direct answer to this question, it will not be acceptable to many people. My answer would simply be: In the same way as we provide food and clothing and shelter for everyone. We do not always succeed in doing that. Neither must we expect greater success in providing medical care for everyone. But I know that such an answer is not what is expected of me.

"The public has been aroused to expect medical care through social security legislation. Before I comment on that, may I make a few simple straightforward statements. Under today's conditions, you know what a loaf of bread costs, and if you have the price, you can get a loaf of bread; if you do not have the price, you can go without humiliating yourself to one of the recognized agencies that has made it their business to provide loaves of bread for those who do not have the price. You know what a suit of clothes costs, a ton of coal or the rental price of a flat. But let me ask you, how much are you willing to pay for your mother's love or your child's affection? Medical care is not a loaf of bread. To me, medical care is more related to a mother's love or a child's affection than it is to a loaf of bread or a ton of coal.

"Under this way of thinking, we have developed the most pretentious and comprehensive system of medical care in the world's history. Why must we now change? Where has our system broken down? On what score is the medical profession really open to legitimate criticism? We are living better and healthier lives than any other nation. Of course, there are short-comings in the system. It is a human system and no matter what you do, it will remain a human system subject to error and carelessness and even malice. If you own a baseball team that is a pennant winner but has a weak shortstop, do you fire the whole team or do you attempt merely to get a better shortstop? Medicine has been a pennant winner for humanity. Keep your team and strengthen the shortstop by more public health, for example. It has won the victory in most of the games that it has played with disease.

"My answer, therefore, to the question is very brief. Support medicine more strongly than you have ever supported it, if necessary, even by a government subsidy in those few places in the United States where we need more hospitals, doctors, and nurses. Provide people with adequate wages, reduce indigency and everyone will be able to secure medical care when it is needed. Don't blame medicine for your economics. If medicine "goes economic", it may have no time to be good medicine and then "God Help America."

*Schwitalla, Alphonse M., S. J., Dean, St. Louis University School of Medicine.

THE STATE MEDICAL ASSOCIATION VS.
STATE MEDICINE

The 52nd Annual Meeting of the Oklahoma State Medical Association has passed into history with its 52nd appeal in behalf of public weal. Its official negotiations in the Council and The House of Delegates and its scientific program in the interest of individual and public health stand high above the designing purposes of those who desire to bring medicine under the rule of so-called social and economic security.

The House of Delegates' appeal for a nonpartisan State Board of Health designed to take public health out of politics and give it to the people with no thought of votes is a good example.

God grant that we may have 52 more unsullied State Meetings before we take orders from the bureaucrats.

THE PROGRAM OF THE NATIONAL PHYSICIANS COMMITTEE

The following is lifted verbatum from the report of the National Physicians Committee entitled "The American People—What They Think About Doctors, Medical Care and Prepayment Plans."

"The Management Committee has been instructed by the Board of Trustees to: secure office facilities, additional personnel, and take all necessary steps designed to

"a. Encourage the medical profession to active participation in the development of plans and the more general use of existing facilities to provide for easy payment of insurance against unusual or prolonged illness;

"b. Educate the people to the importance, nature and value of pre-payment facilities (within the framework of principles approved by the medical profession), now available for meeting the costs of unusual illness;

"c. Investigate conditions relating to and inform industry concerning the principles underlying sound participation with employees in prepayment plans for meeting the cost of unusual and prolonged illness and hospitalization;

"d. Inform private insurance underwriters of the opportunity that is being offered through cooperation in nationwide efforts to provide group insurance policies for those needing or desiring insurance against the hazards of unusual illness;

"e. Encourage and provide state or local financial aid rather than Federal subsidies to insure effective medical care for the indigent;

"f. Encourage contributors and friends to a greater degree of participation in the efforts of the National Physicians Committee in this constructive program.

"With the active cooperation of the individuals and the groups directly affected—the Professions, the Manufacturers, the Distributors, American Labor, and Insurance Industry, and American Industrial Concerns—steps can be taken which will bring relief to 100,000,000 people and provide a method of meeting the cost of unusual and prolonged illness and of hospitilization."

To an old timer in the practice of medicine, the thought that 100,000,000 of our people are ready for a change in the type of medical care they are receiving constitutes a sad commentary on both the American people and the medical profession. But even though American medicine measured up to its full duty, the mass psychology of the people, unfortunately uninformed as to relative merit, and always presenting a ready ear for the promise of something allegedly better, could hardly escape the influence of ten years of government policy and political agitation, plus the selfish and exploiting activities of organized labor, in favor of some form of socialized medicine. The incessant political hammering over a period of years has welded a wicked chain which binds us to the alternative of accepting socialized medicine under government control or the lesser evil, except for the very low income groups, of the prepayment plans proposed by the National Physicians Committee. It is embarrassing for good American citizens to realize that, through political expediency the people and their physicians have been cast upon unfriendly seas where they must cling to the improvised raft thrown out by the National Physicians Committee or be picked up by the ship of state with nothing to look forward to except totalitarian resuscitation.

The National Physicians Committee is doing a grand job but the fact that it is faced with the necessity of making such far reaching plans that it causes serious minded citizens to wonder if we are still truly American; if we have not forgotten the principles of our honored forefathers and thereby trampling our immortal souls under our feet.

ASSEMBLING THE WISE MEN

According to Thomas Jefferson our Nation was created by "assembling the wise men instead of assembling armies."

Bismarck's method of building an Empire was with "blood and iron." His way of perpetuating the position of those in possession of power was through social legislation, including socialized medicine. By placing the common people under obligation to the government, he was able to exercise another check upon their independence.

Bismarck has his followers in Washington. What has become of our wise men; what can we do to safeguard our liberties?

Medical School Notes

A refresher course in Parasitology has been given by Dr. Donald B. McMullen at the University of Tulsa. Eighteen technicians and five physics completed the course.

Dr. McMullen has been selected by the American Society of Parasitology as one of a committee of three to compile a national list of common names of parasites which is hoped to be accepted as the standard common names of these parasites. This committee is composed of a veterinarian, a zoologist, and a medical scientist. Dr. McMullen is serving to compile the list of medical parasites.

Dr. H. A. Shoemaker, Assistant Dean and Professor of Pharmacology, will read a paper on "Socialized Medicine" at the annual meeting of the State Pharmaceuticals Association in Tulsa, Friday, April 21.

Antirabic Vaccine

SEMPLE METHOD

U. S. Government License No. 98

1. Patients bitten by suspected rabid animals, on any part of body other than Face and Wrist, usually require only 14 doses of Antirabic Vaccine.

    Ampoule Package................$15.00

2. Patients bitten about Face or Wrist, or when treatment has been delayed, should receive at least 21 doses of Antirabic Vaccine. (Special instructions with each treatment.)

    Ampoule Package................$22.50

Special Discounts to Doctors, Druggists, Hospitals and to County Health Officers for Indigent Cases.

Medical Arts Laboratory

1115 Medical Arts Building
Oklahoma City, Oklahoma

ASSOCIATION ACTIVITIES

52ND ANNUAL MEETING
WELL ATTENDED

The Annual State Meeting was well attended despite the flood conditions prevailing in the northern part of the State. Due to the weather it was impossible for Dr. Alfred W. Adson, guest speaker, to reach Tulsa. Dr. Walter C. Alvarez, Rochester, Dr. Duff S. Allen, St. Louis, Dr. Harry Mustard, New York and Dr. Cecil K. Drinker, Boston, were enthusiastically received. It was necessary for Dr. Alvarez to return by plane as train travel was suspended for two or three days due to weather conditions.

The younger men were greatly missed but there was a definite determination on the part of those at home to see that medicine is kept on a good scientific basis for the men now serving their Country in the Armed Forces.

After a buffet supper, sponsored by the Tulsa County Medical Society, on Monday evening, the House of Delegates met. One of the features of the Meeting was the discussion of the Prepaid Medical Plan. The Committee, headed by Dr. John F. Burton of Oklahoma City, presented a report which involved a thorough study of the Plan in all phases with the explanatory report to the effect that this Plan was not compulsory but could be tried out in any County Society or Community. Some felt that this Plan would lead to socialized medicine, others contended that, while the Plan might be acceptable, if conditions were to remain as they are, the medical profession should inaugurate some plan which would off-set government controlled medicine.

After considerable discussion an outline of the Plan was read by Dr. John F. Burton and a motion was made that the members of the House of Delegates consider it the following morning. In the Tuesday morning meeting, the House voted to commend the Committee for the work that they had done, that the Committee be continued, and that the Plan be submitted to the members of the Oklahoma State Medical Association with a ballot in which they could express their opinion as to the Plan or make suggestions for another Plan. There seems to be a concensus of opinion throughout the State that some plan of this kind should be set up, but there is much opposition in Oklahoma City.

Dr. McLain Rogers, Clinton, a former president of the Association, stated that he felt that while this might be obnoxious to the members of the profession, it seemed to be the indication that something of this kind would have to be inaugurated by the medical profession to off-set political control.

Another important subject was the passage of a law providing for a State Board of Health. Dr. Harry S. Mustard, Dean of the School of Public Health, Columbia University, New York, in a discussion before the Council called attention to the fact that Oklahoma, Nebraska, and Idaho were the only states in the Union which did not have a Board of Health and in a conference with the Council he also pointed out the advantages of such a Board. At present, the State Health Commissioner is appointed by the Governor and in times past has been changed with the administration, all of which has kept Oklahoma more or less in the background in modern health control.

The physical set-up of the House was different than it has been in previous years. Tables were provided for the Delegates and it was much easier to recognize those who were active in the proceedings.

There was an interesting meeting of the Alumni Association of the University of Oklahoma at which special honors were conferred upon Dr. E. S. Lain and Dr. W. A. Howard. Also, Dr. Byron E. Williams inaugurated a scheme for an endowment fund for the Medical School which received the approval of the group.

Approximately 375 physicians, wives, military personnel and guest speakers attended the President's Inaugural Dinner Dance that was held Tuesday, April 25 in the Crystal Ballroom of the Mayo Hotel in Tulsa. Dr. W. A. Snowman, Tulsa, General Chairman, presided and presented the guests. The Address of Welcome was delivered by Dr. Ralph A. McGill, President of the Tulsa County Medical Society. Dr. James Stevenson, Tulsa, President for 1943-44, then introduced President C. R. Rountree and presented him with the gavel.

Since Dr. Alfred W. Adson, the scheduled speaker, was unable to reach Tulsa, Dr. Walter C. Alvarez of the Mayo Clinic substituted and delivered a very interesting address.

The interest of the crowd was indicated by the large attendance until the close of the meeting on Wednesday afternoon.

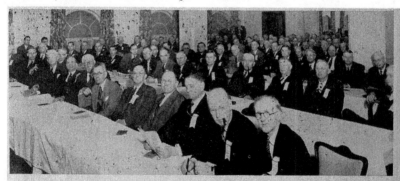

House of Delegates
Monday Evening, April 24, Tulsa

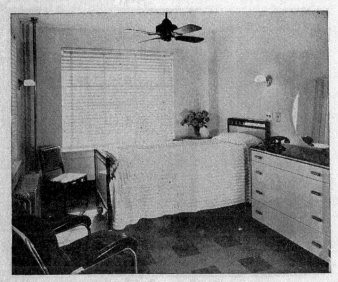

NEW OFFICERS ELECTED AT ANNUAL MEETING

Officers of the Association elected by the House of Delegates are as follows: V. C. Tisdal, M. D., Elk City, President-Elect; F. W. Boadway, M. D., Ardmore, Vice-President; George H. Garrison, M. D., Oklahoma City, succeeding himself, Speaker of House of Delegates; H. K. Speed, M. D., Sayre, succeeding himself, Vice-Speaker of House of Delegates. Out-going president, James Stevenson, M. D., Tulsa, was elected to serve as Alternate Delegate to A.M.A., Dr. A. S. Risser, Dele-

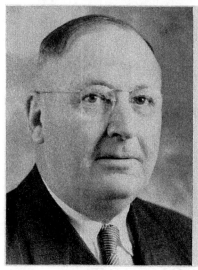

V. C. Tisdal, M.D.,
President-Elect

gate having been elected at the meeting last year to succeed himself.

J. William Finch, M. D., Hobart, was elected as Councilor for District No. 2 to replace Dr. V. C. Tisdal who was elected President-Elect. John A. Haynie, M. D., Durant, was elected as Councilor for District No. 10, succeeding Dr. J. S. Fulton, Atoka. The following Councilors were elected to succeed themselves: O. E. Templin, M. D., Alva, District No. 1; C. E. Northcutt, M. D., Ponca City, District No. 3; Tom Lowry, M. D., Oklahoma City, District No. 4; Clinton Gallaher, M. D., Shawnee, District No. 7; L. C. Kuykendall, M. D., McAlester, District No. 9.

Oklahoma City was elected as the meeting place for 1945.

BEN H. NICHOLSON APPOINTED TO EDITORIAL BOARD

Dr. Ben H. Nicholson, Oklahoma City, was appointed by the Council for the place on the Editorial Board left vacant by the resignation of Dr. Ned Smith, Tulsa.

PRESIDENT OF SOUTHERN MEDICAL ASSOCIATION DIES

Dr. William T. Wooton of Hot Springs, Arkansas, President of the Southern Medical Association died of a heart attack in a St. Louis hospital on May 3. Funeral services were held in Hot Springs on May 5.

ANNUAL RE-REGISTRATION FEE DUE

All physicians should bear in mind that under the Annual Registration Act they must register annually with the State Board of Medical Examiners. The registration fee is $3.00 and must be paid on or before June 10 of each year. All checks or money orders should be made payable to the Oklahoma State Board of Medical Examiners and should be sent to J. D. Osborn, M. D., Secretary, Frederick, Oklahoma.

LEWIS J. MOORMAN TO NATIONAL TUBERCULOSIS ASSOCIATION CONVENTION

Dr. Lewis J. Moorman, Oklahoma City, who is President of the National Tuberculosis Association, left on May 7 to attend the Fortieth Anniversary Meeting of the National Tuberculosis Association, held in Chicago on May 9 through May 12. In connection with the Meeting, the American Trudeau Society and the National Conference of Tuberculosis Secretaries were in session. The American Trudeau Society succeeded the old American Sanitarium Association and has increased the membership from approximately 300 at the time of replacement to over 2,000 members.

Dr. Moorman's Presidential Address was entitled "Our Knowledge of Tuberculosis—4,000 Years Accumulation—40 Years Application."

THE NEW COVER

For a number of years the front of the Journal of the Oklahoma State Medical Association has carried advertisements. You will notice that this issue carries a new design on the front. The design, made up in our Executive Office, was presented to the Council at the State Meeting and accepted.

We wish to express our thanks to Dr. E. S. Lain, Dr. W. E. Eastland and Dr. John H. Lamb of the Lain-Eastland-Lamb Clinic of Oklahoma City and to Dr. T. C. Terrell of Terrell's Laboratories of Ft. Worth, Texas, for so kindly relinquishing their former advertising space so that the new cover could become effective at once.

PAUL FESLER ELECTED TO COMMITTEES OF CHAMBER OF COMMERCE

Mr. Paul Fesler, Executive Secretary of the Association, has been been elected to serve on the Public Health and Safety Committee and the Medical Center Committee of the Public Welfare Division of Oklahoma City's Chamber of Commerce.

The Medical Center Committee cooperates with all interested groups of the community in the promotion of Oklahoma City as an outstanding medical center, and the development of the community resources for that purpose.

The Public Health and Safety Committee is engaged in the coordination of the various health organizations and agencies, and cooperates with them in the elimination of health hazards and other threats to public and individual safety, in making Oklahoma City a healthy and safe place in which to live.

NEW PROCUREMENT AND ASSIGNMENT APPOINTMENTS MADE BY C. R. ROUNTREE, STATE CHAIRMAN

Dr. J. Wm. Finch, Hobart, has been appointed Procurement and Assignment Chairman of Kiowa County, replacing Dr. B. H. Watkins who has moved to Trementina, New Mexico. Dr. Finch was appointed by Dr. C. R. Rountree, State Chairman.

Dr. G. R. Booth has moved to Wilburton to take the place of Dr. J. M. Harris who has moved to MidWest City. Dr. Booth was appointed Councilor Chairman of the Procurement and Assignment Service for District 9.

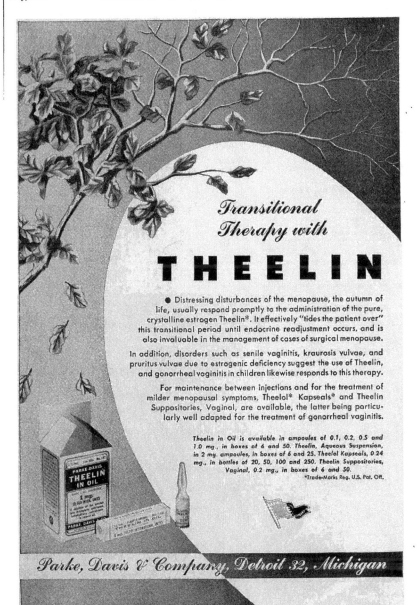

• OBITUARIES •

J. Fred Bolton, M.D.
1880-1944

Dr. J. Fred Bolton, prominent Tulsa obstetrician and gynecologist, died on March 27. Dr. Bolton came to Tulsa in 1923 after having practiced a number of years at his home in Eureka Springs, Arkansas. He was a graduate of the Washington University School of Medicine at St. Louis, Class of 1904.

Dr. Bolton was very active in civic affairs in Tulsa, serving with the Cooperative Club and as chairman or member of a number of committees in the Tulsa County Medical Society. He was a member of the Oklahoma State Medical Association and the American Medical Association.

Services were conducted by the First Presbyterian Church of Tulsa and burial was at Eureka Springs, Arkansas.

William L. Taylor, M.D.
1878-1944

Dr. William L. Taylor, Holdenville, died April 16 at Wesley Hospital, Oklahoma City, following a long illness. Dr. Taylor received his degree from the University of Oklahoma School of Medicine in 1910 with the first class of seven members. Since 1902 he has been the official state physician attending every execution at the McAlester State Penitentiary. Dr. Taylor came to Holdenville in 1934 after 33 years of service in Gentry. The pioneer physician was a member of the Calvin

Masonic Lodge, the Order of the Eastern Star, the York Rite Masonic Lodge in Holdenville and the Indian Scottish Rite Lodge in McAlester. He was a Shriner, being affiliated with the Bedouin Temple at Muskogee and was a member of the Holdenville Chapter of the Royal Arch Masons. Dr. Taylor was a veteran President of the Hughes County Medical Society and at the time of his death was to be Delegate to the Annual State Meeting of the Oklahoma State Medical Association.

Survivors include his widow, Mrs. William L. Taylor, two sons, Galen Taylor of San Jose and Sgt. Dale Taylor who is stationed in Washington State; five daughters, Mrs. Dewey Smith, Mrs. Faye Delude, Mrs. Gerald Mackrill, Mrs. Carra May Gorman and Miss Corrine Taylor; three brothers, one sister, eleven grandchildren and two great-grandchildren.

Charles E. Hales, M.D.
1874-1944

Dr. Charles H. Hale, Boswell, died in his office Tuesday, April 25 of a heart attack. He was born in Union Parish, La., received his degree at the University of Kentucky School of Medicine and moved to Texas for a short time before coming to Boswell. Dr. Hale was the oldest resident doctor in service in Choctaw County, having come to Boswell some 32 years ago.

Dr. Hale was highly respected in the profession by his fellow physicians, his patients and friends. For the past few years he has carried on despite failing health.

Survivors include his widow, Mrs. Belle G. Hale, one son, Hugh Hale and two daughters, Mrs. J. A. Still and Mrs. O. L. Watson, Jr. Also surviving are five brothers and three sisters.

DISTRICT COUNCILOR MAP

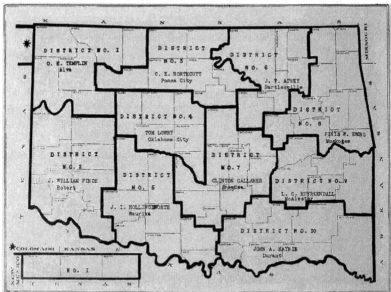

Councilor Districts and Councilors. Extra copies of this map available through Journal office. You will find this convenient in connection with legislation.

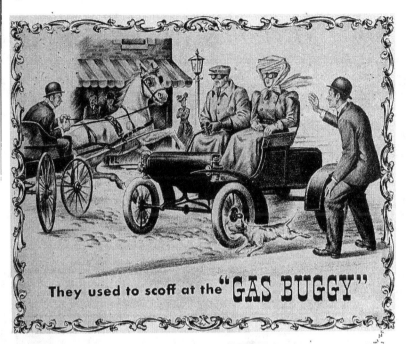

★ FIGHTIN' TALK ★

LT. COMDR. R. G. JACOBS, Enid, has recently returned from the South Pacific Combat Area where, he states that he was 'occupied with urgent problems due to our nasty Jap neighbors.'' Lt. Comdr. Jacobs is now stationed at the Mayo Foundation in Rochester, Minnesota.

CAPT. RALPH D. TURNER, Muskogee, has been ordered to active duty.

HAROLD LEROY BEDDOE, Tulsa, has been appointed a first lieutenant in the medical corps and is awaiting assignment to active duty.

MAJOR RICHARD J. BRIGHTWELL, Oklahoma City, has recently been promoted from captain. He is now serving at Patterson Field, Ohio, where he is Plans and Training Officer in the Medical Corps in the rehabilitation of wounded soldiers who have returned from combat duty. Before entering the service, Major Brightwell served his internship at St. Anthony Hospital in Oklahoma City.

MAJOR BERTRAM A. WEEKS, Oklahoma City, recently received his promotion to Major on his second wedding anniversary. He is stationed at Camp Maxey, Texas.

MAJOR HOWARD SHORBE, Oklahoma City, was wounded in the shelling of an American hospital on the Anzio beach in March. He was performing an operation when a shell fragment entered his abdomen. Major Shorbe is reported recovering in a base hospital.

CAPTAIN HAROLD B. WITTEN, Harrah, has been on the Italian battlefront for the past two years. Recently he was selected to attend Flight Surgeon's Training and was returned to the United States. He was unable to inform his wife of the move until he reached Jones where he called her long-distance. Captain Witten has a new son whom he had never seen.

MAJOR BLAIR POINTS, United States Public Health Service, is Director of the County Health Unit at Boise, Idaho. Major Points graduated from the University of Oklahoma School of Medicine in 1911.

MAJOR PATRICK S. NAGLE, Oklahoma City, has been transferred to Camp Polk, La. He was a recent visitor in Oklahoma City and made arrangements to take Mrs. Nagle and the three babies back to Louisiana with him.

CAPTAIN J. R. HUGGINS, Oklahoma City, has arrived in New Guinea according to word received by Mrs. Huggins.

The following information has recently been released although the action took place during September of last year. LT. COL. EVERETT G. KING, Duncan, landed before dawn at Lae, New Guinea, established a dispensary and had a hospital in operation in two days. Col. King served as supply officer for the entire organization, supervising the landing, storing and distribution of supplies—ordnance and quartermaster as well as medical. He was responsible for the evacuation of all cas-

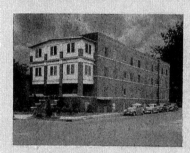
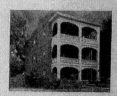

ualities and for a time, acted as executive officer of the base, a responsibility virtually without precedent for a medical corps officer, according to the announcement from the General Headquarters of the Southwest Pacific area.

Col. King is now Chief of the Evacuation and Hospitalization Section at Headquarters and provides adequate hospital facilities for troops stationed throughout the Southwest Pacific area.

CAPTAIN DONOVAN TOOL, Edmond, writes that he has been wounded in combat duty on the Italian front. He states that he has received several small chunks of 'made in Germany' scrap iron in arms, legs and back. He is recovering very nicely after the removal of the shell fragments and the only difficulty seems to be that he is tired of lying on his stomach.

CAPTAIN HARL D. MANSUR, graduate of the Class of 1939, has written that the practice of medicine in India is a lot different than in Oklahoma. He relays the information to Dr. Tom Lowry that "there are a lot of diseases over here that he did not tell us about in his medicine classes."

The following was received from CAPTAIN, R. J. REICHERT, Moore:

"I consider myself a garrison soldier. We are in —— —— and have most of the luxuries including a fresh egg about three times per week. We do get a limited liquor supply once per month so our morale does not get too low.

"We have plenty of time to think about the past and I recall how we used to go quail hunting and then when we got home my wife had hot buckwheat cakes and honey. We have all the necessities of life over here but it may be a few more years before we can again enjoy home and the things we are fighting to retain."

After an absence of 29 months and one day, LT. COL.

L. G. LIVINGSTON, Cordell, returned home. Col. Livingston was in the service before Pearl Harbor and when the news was received, the ship he was on was about a week southwest of Hawaii. A stop was made in the Fiji islands before the landing in Australia. Col. Livingston is awaiting new assignment.

Classified Advertisements

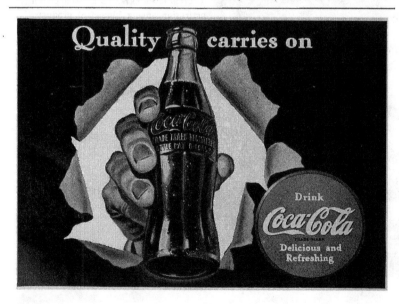

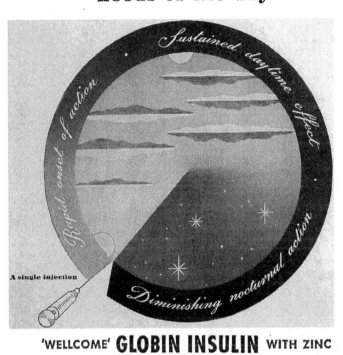

MEDICAL ABSTRACTS

"PENICILLIN AND TYROTHRICIN IN OTOLARYNGO-LOGY: BASED ON A BACTERIOLOGICAL AND CLINICAL STUDY." S. J. Crowe (et. al.) Annals of Otology, Rhinology and Laryngology. Vol. 52, pages 541-561. September, 1943.

Penicillin and tyrothricin are two new antibacterial drugs, which in some respect are superior to the sulfonamides. The two new drugs supplement each other to a certain extent.

Penicillin is produced by the growth of certain strains of Penicillium notatum on suitable liquid culture media. The original observations were made by Fleming in England; further studies were carried out by Clutterbuck and others in 1932. These authors found that the mold could be grown on a synthetic medium and the active principle extracted by ether. From successive research it has been established that penicillin is active mainly against gram-positive cocci but also against gonococci, meningococci, Clostridium welchii, anaerbic streptococci, and others. The purified extract is active in a very high dilution, and is not inhibited by pus, exudates, tissue cells, and is nontoxic even in large doses. Its extraction requires a great deal of crude material; therefore, it is not available for general distribution.

It is possible for one with knowledge of bacterial methods to prepare crude penicillin, which can be kept active for several months either in rubber-stoppered bottles or frozen. It was found to be nontoxic to animals both by local and parenteral administration. Its mechanism of action is not definitely known, but it is bactericidal in the more concentrate form, and bacteriostatic in higher dilutions.

Tyrothricin is the other bactericidal substance that was isolated by Dubos in 1939 from peptone cultures of the aerobic soil bacterium, bacillus brevis. From this substance two crystalline components have been separated; gramicidin and tyrocidine. Gramicidin is bactericidal for gram-positive organism only: Tyrocidine only aids the solubility of gramicidin. For experiments, the mother substance tyrothricin can be used, the activity of which is inhibited by phospholipids, which may explain its relative inactivity in the intestinal tract. Its activity is rapidly lost also in acid medium. Tyrothricin has a strong hemolytic action that prohibits its intravenous and subcutaneous use. If it comes into direct contact with gram-positive aerobic and anaerobic bacteria it kills them with great rapidity, without any damage to the tissues. It is for local use only. It is usually diluted with double distilled water to make a 1:10,000 or 1:20,000 suspension. It is used for irrigation of wounds after operations. In case of frontal sinus operation it is used as follows:

After the usual preliminary intranasal operation the frontal sinus may be entered through an external incision in the eyebrow not more than 2 or 3 cm in length. All infected mucous membrane together with the entire floor of the frontal sinus and all orbital ex-

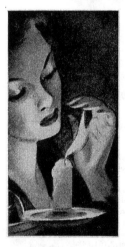

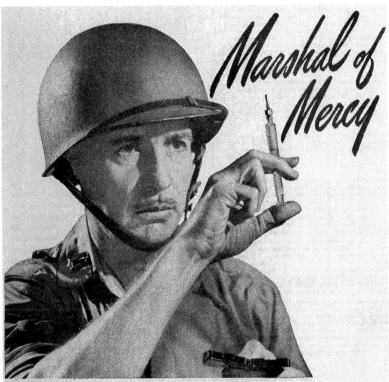

Marshal of Mercy

In war, even more than in peace... dispenser of blessed relief... his the precious power over pain.

Long hours the medical officer toils... routinely yet heroically... without thought of citation... grateful for brief moments of relaxation ... for the cheer of an occasional smoke. And likely as not, his cigarette is Camel, the favorite brand in the armed forces*... first choice for smooth mildness and for pleasing flavor. It's what every fighting man deserves... that extra measure of Camel's smoking pleasure.

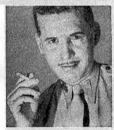

1st in the Service

*With men in the Army, Navy, Marine Corps, and Coast Guard, the favorite cigarette is Camel. (Based on actual sales records.)

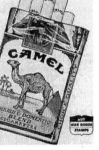

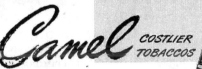

Camel COSTLIER TOBACCOS

New reprint available on cigarette research—Archives of Otolaryngology, March, 1943, pp, 404-410. Camel Cigarettes, Medical Relations Division ,One Pershing Square, New York 17, N. Y.

tensions of the ethmoidal cells are removed and a large opening made into the nose. The wound and surrounding soft parts are then thoroughly washed with 1:5,000 tyrothicin, and the frontal sinus packed with gauze saturated with tyrothricin. The external incision is closed and the end of the pack brought out through the nose. There is rarely any edema of the eyelid and the incision heals per primam. The pack is removed under light vinetheme anesthesia 24 hours later. The frontal sinus is rendered so sterile by this procedure that excessive growth of granulations is prevented and therefore the opening into the nose does not close, provided the operation has been through and the sinus is irrigated daily for ten days with 1:10,000 suspension of tyrothricin. After the first ten days, the frontal sinus irrigations should continue at longer intervals for another two weeks.

Tyrothricin is more valuable for prevention of wound infection than is penicillin. But if the infective organisms are sensitive to both drugs, the best results are obtained by using tyrothricin and penicillin, diluted with an equal amount of normal saline, for the postoperative irrigation.

Tyrothricin used as drops or irrigations for chronic infection of the sinuses or ears is of little value. Often penicillin is more effective in these cases because it is more soluble and therefore penetrates the tissues more than tyrothricin. It is assumed that bacteria are growing on or near the surface in acute infections, while they are deeply embedded and inaccessible to any locally applied bactericidal agent in chronic infections.

Many of the bacteria in chronic mastoid and sinus infections are resistant to the sulfonamides. In addition these powders are poorly soluble and act as foreign bodies. The chief objection to their use is that some individuals become so sensitized by local application in fresh operative wounds that the use of sulfonamides is precluded if the patient should develop pneumonia, meningitis or a general infection, even several years later.

To use the sulfonamides, tyrothricin and penicillin to the best advantage thorough bacteriological study is essential. Neither tyrothricin, penicillin nor the sulfonamides have any effect on the growth of Escherechia coli, Proteus, Pseudomonas aeruginosa and Friedlader's bacillus, which are often present in chronic infections of the ears and the sinuses. Tyrothricin is now prepared by most of the larger American pharmaceutical laboratories.
—M. D. H., M.D.

KEY TO ABSTRACTORS

M.D.H., M.D. ....Marvin D. Henley

Commercial Exhibits

The following companies were represented and their attractive booths added much to the meeting: Mead Johnson and Company; C. V. Mosby Company; Schering Corporation; Burroughs-Wellcome and Company; Merkel X-Ray Company; Smith, The Coca-Cola Bottling Company; General Electrical X-Ray Corporation; E. R. Squibb and Sons; Pet Milk Sales Corporation; J. A. Majors Company; Western Electric Audiphone Company; Camel Cigarettes; Parke, Davis and Company; The Borden Company; White Laboratories; Warren-Teed Products Company; A. S. Aloe Company; Ortho Products, Inc.; The Smith-Dorsey Company; Sharp and Dohme, Inc.; Petrogalar Laboratories; Philip Morris and Company, Ltd.; Holland-Rantos Company; John Wyeth and Brother, Inc.; Max Wocher and Son Company; Caviness-Melton Surgical Company; Lederle Laboratories, Inc.

Auxiliary to Decorate Association Office

Mrs. Gerald Rogers, Oklahoma City, has been appointed representative from the Woman's Auxiliary Committee for Extension and Redecoration of the Executive Offices in Oklahoma.

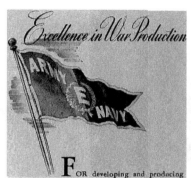
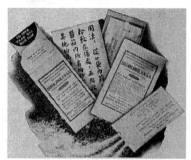

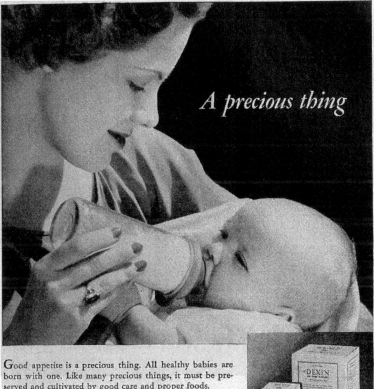

A precious thing

Good appetite is a precious thing. All healthy babies are born with one. Like many precious things, it must be preserved and cultivated by good care and proper foods.

'Dexin', a high dextrin carbohydrate food for infant feeding, is not oversweet and will not dull a good appetite—a major consideration for any baby's well being. Following the early use of 'Dexin', the addition of other bland foods to the diet is more easily accomplished.

The high dextrin content of 'Dexin' promotes (1) the formation of soft, flocculent, easily digested curds, and (2) diminishes intestinal fermentation and the tendency to colic and diarrhea. 'Dexin' is readily soluble in hot or cold milk.

'Dexin' Reg. U. S. Patent Office

'Dexin' does make a difference

COMPOSITION	Dextrins 75%	Mineral Ash . 0.25%
	Maltose 24%	Moisture . . 0.75%
	Available carbohydrate 99%	115 calories per ounce
	6 level packed tablespoonfuls equal 1 ounce	

'DEXIN'
HIGH DEXTRIN CARBOHYDRATE

Literature on request

BURROUGHS WELLCOME & CO. (U.S.A.) 9-11 E. 41st St., New York 17, N. Y.

Learn something about your War Bonds

from this fellow!

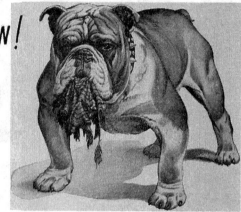

THE BEST THING a bulldog does is HANG ON! Once he gets hold of something, it's mighty hard to make him let go!

And that's the lesson about War Bonds you can learn from him. Once you get hold of a War Bond, HANG ON TO IT for the full ten years of its life.

There are at least two very good reasons why you should do this. One is a patriotic reason ... the other a personal reason.

You buy War Bonds because you know Uncle Sam needs money to fight this war. And you want to put some of your money into the fight. But ... if you don't hang on to those War Bonds, your money isn't going to *stay* in the battle.

Another reason you buy War Bonds is because

you want to set aside some money for your fami' future and yours. No one knows just what's going happen after the War. But the man with a fistfu War Bonds *knows* he'll have a roof over his h and 3 squares a day no matter *what* happens!

War Bonds pay you back $4 for every $3 in years. But, if you don't hang on to your Bonds the full ten years, you don't get the full face val and ... you won't have that money coming in la on when you may need it a lot worse than you n it today.

So buy War Bonds ... more and more War Bor And then *keep* them. You will find that War Bo are very good things to have ... and to hold!

WAR BONDS to Have and to Hold

The Treasury Department acknowledges with appreciation the publication of this message by

Oklahoma State Medical Association

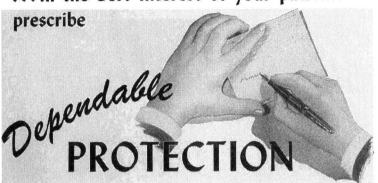
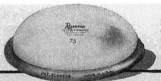

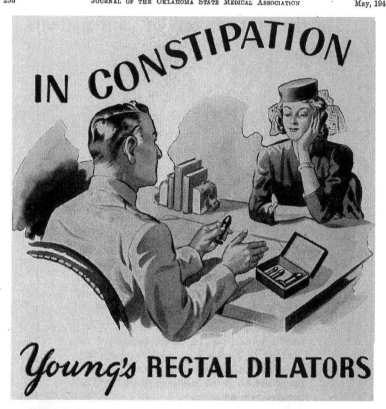

IN CONSTIPATION

Young's RECTAL DILATORS

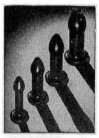

. . . have been used by the profession for more than 40 years to provide rectal dilation and aid in restoring normal tone where tight or spastic rectal sphincter muscles have brought about a constipated condition. Mechanical Rectal Dilation often succeeds when other modalities fail. Sold on prescription only—not advertised to the laity. Set of 4 graduated sizes $3.75, at ethical druggists or surgical supply houses. Write for literature.

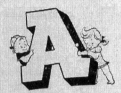
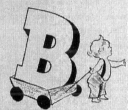
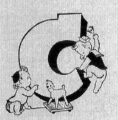

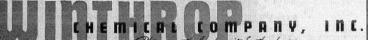

OFFICERS OF COUNTY SOCIETIES, 1944

★

COUNTY	PRESIDENT	SECRETARY	MEETING TIME
Alfalfa	H. E. Huston, Cherokee	L. T. Lancaster, Cherokee	Last Tues. each Second Month
Atoka-Coal	R. C. Henry, Coalgate	J. S. Fulton, Atoka	
Beckham	G. H. Stagner, Erick	O. C. Standifer, Elk City	Second Tuesday
Blaine	L. R. Kirby, Okeene	W. F. Griffin, Watonga	
Bryan	John T. Wharton, Durant	W. K. Haynie, Durant	Second Tuesday
Caddo	F. L. Patterson, Carnegie	C. B. Sullivan, Carnegie	
Canadian	P. F. Herod, El Reno	A. L. Johnson, El Reno	Subject to call
Carter	J. R. Pollock, Ardmore	H. A. Higgins, Ardmore	
Cherokee	P. H. Medearis, Tahlequah	W. M. Wood, Tahlequah	First Tuesday
Choctaw		E. A. Johnson, Hugo	
Cleveland	F. T. Gastineau, Norman	Iva S. Merritt, Norman	Thursday nights
Comanche	George L. Berry, Lawton	Howard Angus, Lawton	
Cotton	A. B. Holstead, Temple	Mollie F. Scism, Walters	Third Friday
Craig	Lloyd H. McPike, Vinita	Paul G. Sanger, Vinita	
Creek	J. E. Hollis, Bristow		
Custer	F. R. Vieregg. Clinton	C. J. Alexander, Clinton	Third Thursday
Garfield	Julian Feild, Enid	John R. Walker, Enid	Fourth Thursday
Garvin	T. F. Gross, Lindsay	John R. Callaway, Pauls Valley	Wednesday before Third Thursday
Grady	Walter J. Baze, Chickasha	Roy E. Emanuel, Chickasha	Third Thursday
Grant	I. V. Hardy, Medford		
Greer	R. W. Lewis, Granite	J. B. Hollis, Mangum	
Harmon	W. G. Husband, Hollis	R. H, Lynch, Hollis	First Wednesday
Haskell	William Carson, Keota	N. K. Williams, McCurtain	
Hughes	Wm. L. Taylor, Holdenville	Imogene Mayfield, Holdenville	First Friday
Jackson	C. G. Spears, Altus	E. A. Abernethy, Altus	Last Monday
Jefferson	F. M. Edwards, Ringling		Second Monday
Kay	J. Holland Howe, Ponca City	G. H. Yeary, Newkirk	Second Thursday
Kingfisher	A. O. Meredith, Kingfisher	H. Violet Sturgeon, Hennessey	
Kiowa	J. William Finch, Hobart	William Bernell, Hobart	
LeFlore	Neeson Rolle, Poteau	Rush L. Wright, Poteau	
Lincoln	W. B. Davis, Stroud	Carl H. Bailey, Stroud	First Wednesday
Logan	William C. Miller, Guthrie	J. L. LeHew, Jr., Guthrie	Last Tuesday
Marshall	J. L. Holland, Madill	J. F. York, Madill	
Mayes	Ralph V. Smith, Pryor	Paul B. Cameron, Pryor	
McClain	W. C. McCurdy, Sr., Purcell	W. C. McCurdy, Jr., Purcell	
McCurtain	A. W. Clarkson, Valliant	N. L. Barker, Broken Bow	Fourth Tuesday
McIntosh	Luster I. Jacobs, Hanna	Wm. A. Tolleson, Eufaula	First Thursday
Murray	P. V. Annadown, Sulphur	J. A. Wrenn, Sulphur	Second Tuesday
Muskogee-Sequoyah			
Wagoner	H. A. Scott, Muskogee	D. Evelyn Miller, Muskogee	First Monday
Noble	C. H. Cooke, Perry	J. W. Francis, Jerry	
Okfuskee	C. M. Cochran, Okemah	M. L. Whitney, Okemah	Second Monday
Oklahoma	W. E. Eastland, Oklahoma City	E. R. Musick, Oklahoma City	Fourth Tuesday
Okmulgee	S. B. Leslie, Okmulgee	J. C. Matheney, Okmulgee	Second Monday
Osage	C. R. Weirich, Pawhuska	George K. Hemphill, Pawhuska	Second Monday
Ottawa	Walter Kerr, Picher	B. W. Shelton, Miami	Third Thursday
Pawnee	E. T. Robinson, Cleveland	R. L. Browning, Pawnee	
Payne	H. C. Manning, Cushing	J. W. Martin, Cushing	Third Thursday
Pittsburg	P. T. Powell, McAlester	W. H. Kaeiser, McAlester	Third Friday
Pontotoc	A. R. Sugg, Ada	R. H. Mayes, Ada	First Wednesday
Pottawatomie	E. Eugene Rice, Shawnee	Clinton Gallaher, Shawnee	First and Third Saturday
Pushmataha	John S. Lawson, Clayton	B. M. Huckabay, Antlers	
Rogers	R. C. Meloy, Claremore	Chas. L. Caldwell, Chelsea	First Monday
Seminole	J. T. Price, Seminole	Mack I. Shanholtz, Wewoka	Third Wednesday
Stephens	W. K. Walker, Marlow	Wallis S. Ivy, Duncan	
Texas	R. G. Obermiller, Texhoma	Morris Smith, Guymon	
Tillman	C. C. Allen, Frederick	O. G. Bacon, Frederick	
Tulsa	Ralph A. McGill, Tulsa	E. O. Johnson, Tulsa	Second and Fourth Monday
Washington-Nowata	K. D. Davis, Nowata	J. V. Athey, Bartlesville	Second Wednesday
Washita	A. S. Neal, Cordell	James F. McMurry, Sentinel	
Woods	Ishmael F. Stephenson, Alva	Oscar E. Templin, Alva	Last Tuesday Odd Months
Woodward	H. Walker, Buffalo	C. W. Tedrowe, Woodward	Second Thursday

*(Serving in Armed Forces)

THE JOURNAL
OF THE
OKLAHOMA STATE MEDICAL ASSOCIATION

VOLUME XXXVII	OKLAHOMA CITY, OKLAHOMA, JUNE, 1944	NUMBER 6

Acute Surgical Abdomen

V. C. TISDAL, M.D.

ELK CITY, OKLAHOMA

In discussing the acute surgical abdomen it is not my policy to bring out any new ideas as to the diagnosis, but to refresh our minds on some of the symptoms that will enable us to make a diagnosis as early as possible, for we all realize that there is no one part of the anatomy that demands more alertness or accuracy in practice than does the acute abdomen.

For the past few years, the medical profession has been somewhat dilatory in keeping in mind these facts, possibly accounted for by the reason that most of us think we can diagnose an acute surgical case without any great effort. But when we realize that appendicitis, oopheritis, salpingitis, ectopic pregnancy, stone in the ureter, gall bladder disease, with or without stones, common duct stone, Dietl's Crisis, dilated ureter, perforating ulcer of the stomach, diverticulitis, and trauma to the abdominal viscera, with intussusception, volvulvus, all must be differentiated from one another, we realize that the diagnosis of appendicitis and other acute abdominal troubles may present serious diagnostic difficulties.

In my opinion every Medical Society should have one or two papers each year to refresh our minds on the importance of making an early diagnosis of appendicitis. Only a few years ago the surgeon who suspected an acute abdomen and said, "This case must be operated immediately", was termed a radical. The reverse is true now; for we all consider the man who says to the patient, "We will wait until morning and see what your condition is then," when he is suspecting an acute abdomen, surely must be considered the radical of today. The history is very important in all abdominal troubles and, of course, should be one of the first things considered. As a rule the first statement made by the patient suffering from abdominal trouble should assist us materially in making a diagnosis.

I wish now to mention a few of the symptoms found in the above mentioned maladies.

APPENDICITIS
Symptoms
1. Pain
   a. epigastric
   b. umbilical
   c. diffused
   d. localized
2. Nausea and vomiting seldom oftener than one to four times.
3. Fever of 99 to 100½.

The blood count is important and the differential is of more importance as to the character of your risk than is a high leukocyte count. The tenderness over Morris Point and the gas pressure on the appendix means almost as much to me as does the tenderness over McBurney's Point.

Abnormally located appendeces.
1. The Retrocecal Appendix
   Pain in the back with very little tenderness over McBurney's Point, due to the cushioning of the cecum over the appendix.
2. Low Hanging Appendix
   This lays across the ureter, simulating ureteral stone.
3. The Appendix turned up and attached to the under surface of the liver, which simulates gall bladder disease.

TUBE AND OVARY
1. Symptom of acute tubo-ovarian trouble is a history of discharge.

2. Pain below the umbilicus in the tubo-ovarian region.
3. Chills and high fever.
4. Onset slow, except in the case of twisted ovarian pedicle.
5. Nausea and vomiting may be present. When present, vomiting is much more persistent than in appendicitis.
6. Bimanual examination reveals tume-faction and tenderness.
7. The white blood count is high.

OOPHERALGIA

1. Constant pain, not paroxismal. Location, tubo-ovarian region.
2. No elevation of temperature or pulse.
3. Menstruation may be disturbed.
4. Position of uterus revealed by bimanual examination.
5. Temperament of patient.

TWISTED PEDICLE OF OVARY

1. Onset sudden.
2. Pain severe.
3. Nausea and vomiting.
4. Shock.
5. Tumefaction on bimanual examination, or possibly by palpation through abdomen.
6. Abdomen not rigid in the beginning.
7. Blood count negative.

ECTOPIC PREGNANCY—RUPTURED

1. Pain, sharp and severe which lasts a short time.
2. Shock.
3. Relaxation of the abdominal walls.
4. History
   a. Missing one or more periods.
   b. A sense of uneasiness and discomfort a few days preceeding rupture.
   c. Fainting and falling to floor if up and around when rupture occurs.
5. Symptoms of palor and hemorrhage.

STONE IN URETER

1. Pain
   a. Very severe, radiating to back in kidney region.
   b. Pain radiating to head of the penis, vulva, testicle, and down inner surface of limb of corresponding side.
2. Urinary disturbance
   a. Nocturia.
   b. Frequent Urination.
   c. Urinalysis shows blood and pus.
3. Nausea and vomiting, the latter may be persistent.
4. The first few hours temperature unchanged.

DIETL'S CRISIS

1. Pain in the back.
2. Urinary disturbance.
3. Frequency of urination.
4. Urinalysis negative.

5. Shock, and after a few hours, symptoms of uremia.

TWISTED OR DILATED URETER

1. Pain, severe and constant, most often located at the brim of the pelvis.
2. Lack of rigidity of abdominal muscles; no elevation of temperature; no change in the pulse. Blood findings, negative.

This disease is one that causes more appendices to be removed than any other of the above mentioned maladies, and it is only through the use of the cystoscope and pyelegrams that a definite diagnosis of this malady can be determined. I have personally experienced some very disappointing results in removing an appendix, when on awakening from the anesthetic the patient complains with the same pain as before the operation.

GALL BLADDER

1. Digestive disturbance
   a. Belching.
   b. Spitting up food.
   c. Uneasiness and fear on taking food.
2. Pain
   a. Location, upper right quadrant of abdomen.
   b. Radiating to the shoulder blade.
   c. Aggravated by eating.
3. Repeated attack of nausea and vomiting.
4. Jaundice may or may not be present, depending on whether or not there are stones present and also the location of the stone.
5. In cases of pyemia, blood counts are important.

COMMON DUCT STONES

1. Pain.
2. Chills and fever.
3. Jaundice.
4. Rigidity over seat of infection.
5. Nausea and vomiting with more chills and fever.

Unless there is some occlusion of the ducts of the gall bladder due to the stones, adhesions or plugging by mucoid material, you do not find jaundice.

ULCER OF THE STOMACH—PERFORATED

1. Pain
   a. Burning.
   b. Excruciating.
   c. Shocking.
2. Collapse.
3. Shock.
4. Pain going to lower right quadrant of abdomen asimulating appendicitis.
5. Continuous vomiting.
6. Patient looks as though he is going to die within a short time.
7. Marked rigidity of the abdominal muscles, boardlike. This is due to the

emptying of the gastric acids into the abdominal cavity.

DIVERTICULITIS

1. Pain.
2. Constipation or obstipation.
3. Tumefaction.
4. Vomiting and other symptoms of an obstructed bowel.
5. Very hard to make a diagnosis unless abdominal wall is thin.
6. Past history very important.

INTUSSUSCEPTION

1. Pain.
2. Nausea and vomiting.
3. Tenesmus.
4. The bowels fail to move and there is no passage of gas.
5. Blood and mucous discharge.
6. Tumefaction.
7. Usually occurs in children.
8. Shock and relaxation of the whole system of the patient.

VOLVULUS

1. Constipation.
2. Vomiting.
3. Pain.
4. Tumefaction.
5. History of the case usually following an operation or some marked gastro-intestinal disturbance, (case of Worms as example).

TRAUMATIC INJURIES TO THE ABDOMEN

1. History of trauma which may or may not be violent.
2. Pain, location of pain, shock or may or may not be severe.

Other symptoms will be influenced by the location of the upper gastro-intestinal tract we will bring about immediate rigidity of the abdominal wall with shock following.

PNEUMONIA

Pneumonia is one of the diseases that has to be differentiated from appendicitis and for this reason especially in the winter the lungs of all patients in whom appendicitis is being considered should be examined carefully before operation because a pleuretic irritation associated with pneumonia may cause a marked rigidity of the right abdomen with pain over McBurney's Point. The need of this differentiation happens more often in children than in adults. The laboratory findings are very similar and differentiation can be determined only by a careful examination of the lungs with definite attention given to the posterior and lower lobe of the right lung.

DISCUSSION

LOUIS H. RITZHAUPT, M.D.

Dr. Tisdal has refreshed our memory on the most common conditions that produce an acute surgical abdomen. It is impossible to bring out more than the salient points of diagnosis in the time allotted. The same is true in regard to the discussion.

The contents of the abdomen and their diseases are the cause for a large per cent of the major surgery performed on the human body. This necessitates making a serious and thorough attempt at diagnosis and the importance of reaching a decision early, especially of cases with severe abdominal pains which attack a patient previously well and which lasts as long as five hours. It is important to make a thorough routine examination of every patient with an acute abdomen, applying our knowledge of anatomy of this part of the body, as well as the points of referred pain. This is true of inflammatory lesions in the abdomen, while other conditions require a physiological knowledge and familiarity with medical diseases which may simulate acute abdominal conditions.

Permit me to call your attention to the true abdominal colic which is always caused by the violent peristaltic contraction of one of the involuntary muscular tubes, whose normal peristalsis is painless. The most common of these is the stomach, intestines, cystic, hepatic and common bile-ducts. The ureters, uterus and the pancreatic duct. We must not forget embolism of abdominal argon blood vessels.

Some of the general diseases which may produce acute symptoms in the abdomen and certainly do not indicate surgery are: influenza, diabetes, especially when impending coma produce severe abdominal pain and vomiting, typhoid fever and malaria, tubercular peritonitis, also lead and food poisonings. In some instances spleno-medullary leukemia, acute cardiac diseases, acute osteomyelitis of the dorsal or lumbar vertebrae, and in children, Pott's disease of the spine.

Posterior to the peritoneum we sometimes find conditions whose symptoms simulate intra-peritoneal diseases. They are rare but probably should be borne in mind in connection with this paper. As an illustration:

1. Rupture of aneurysm of aorta. In one case I call to mind, a dissecting aortic aneurysm in the lumbar region gave the patient considerable acute attacks of abdominal discomfort lasting from 15 minutes to five hours over a period of five years before a proper diagnosis was finally made. This patient was not operated.

2. Retro-peritoneal hemorrhage from injury of kidney; or spontaneous bleeding from renal growth. Kinked ureter with kidney engorgement.

3. Pelvic superitoneal infection or extravasation of fluid injected into the peri-rectal

tissue may produce considerable acute discomfort.

Although the diagnosis of an acute abdominal condition must be early, if satisfactory results are to be obtained, precaution should be taken and the surgeon should be sure of the diagnosis before surgery is done. "A Stitch in Time Saves Nine", and this works both ways, and may save hours of worry.

Common Orthopedic Conditions in Childhood[*]

D. H. O'DONOGHUE, M.D.

*Department of Orthopodic Surgery,
Crippled Children's Hospital*

OKLAHOMA CITY, OKLAHOMA

When your chairman favored me with an invitation to speak to you as guest of your section and suggested the subject of "Common Orthopedic Conditions in Childhood," I was somewhat at a loss as to the best method of considering such a comprehensive subject. It seemed to me presumptuous to try to give you, in a limited time, any material of value on a matter of which you are as familiar as I. Such a discussion must of necessity be superficial since it would be impossible to present sufficient detail to be stimulating.

There is one particular group of cases, however, about which little has been written and too little done. I refer to the condition which I call reverse club foot, but which is more commonly called congenital flat foot. The latter title is to my mind misleading, since the flat foot is essentially the result of an untreated deformity and not the original condition. On the other hand, the condition is entirely anologous with true club foot, with the one exception of direction of deformity, the reverse club foot showing a calcaneo valgus, the direct club foot an equino-varus. Otherwise, etiology, pathology and particularly treatment are the same.

Without doubt, this condition has been more often overlooked than recognized, in the past and, I am sorry to say, in the present. The consequences of its neglect are so grave that I feel fully justified in confining this discussion entirely to this one condition. It is largely academic whether the etiology be considered a reversion to a previous primordial state (ie., other primates have no longitudinal arch), or whether it be position in utero. There would seem to be a definite hereditary trend, but may be more apparent than real. Since all babies' feet are held one

*Read before the Annual Meeting of the Oklahoma State Medical Association, May 11, 1943 at Oklahoma City, Oklahoma.

way or another in untero, one must predicate some factor in addition to position as a predisposing factor. Kahns states that five per cent of all babies have this deformity at birth!. This is certainly a larger number than are ordinarily diagnosed. In the clubfoot clinic at Crippled Children's Hospital, the proportion between direct and reverse is about ten to one, certainly not a proper proportion. This is explained, I believe, by the fact that babies of this particular group are not brought in early unless they present an obvious and crippling deformity. When they come in late, they are called "flat foot". In our private practice, the story is very different and we are currently treating these in proportion to one direct to three reverse. In checking over cases for the past several years, in our office, the figure runs about two to three, which would indicate the general trend in favor of the reverse foot.

The deformity is essentially a calcaneo-valgus and in most instances, the forefoot can easily be opposed to the lateral side of the leg. Two distinct types are noted, the most severe presenting a fixed deformity; that is, the foot not only presents itself in calcaneo-valgus, but cannot readily be pulled into equino-varus because of contracture of the dorsal and lateral structures of the foot, together with a relaxation of the plantar and medial group. The second is the relaxed type with a flail type foot easily placed in almost any position. Since most babies' feet are, at birth, relaxed, it requires some diagnostic nicety to determine the exact condition. If one foot only is involved, a comparison of the two feet is of value. If both are involved, a few days of observation will be of value since a normal infant's foot tightens up fairly rapidly. The condition often accompanies a direct club foot and it is very common to have the parents report for treatment of the direct club foot when the opposite foot may present the more major problem.

From the standpoint of treatment, the analogy with direct club foot is even more noticeable. These feet are very commonly undertreated, and a little consideration will explain this readily. In the first place, the actual deformity is easily corrected; secondly, the feet do not look deformed unless under the stress of weight bearing; and, thirdly, the foot must be supported until the arch is formed and stable enough to support weight. After correction is obtained, weight bearing actually tends to correct a direct club foot; the deformity of a reverse club foot is never improved by weight bearing.

Treatment consists of correction of deformity and maintenance of overcorrection until overlong ligaments contract and deformed cartilage conforms to its proper shape. I think correction is best carried out by plaster casts, made very light. The position is gradually improved by weekly reapplications of casts, until an extreme equinvarus josition is obtained. Ordinarily this is promptly done, a few weeks sufficing to obtain complete over-correction. Then the battle begins. The feet look good, the parents become impatient and want to terminate treatment, nevertheless, it is imperative that this overcorrected position be maintained for weeks and months until the foot cannot be forced into its previous calcaneo-valgus position. This may require six, nine, or twelve months, but the goal can be attained if persistence and patience are employed. After several months the casts can be left off a few days between each change, gradually increasing the vacation period until they are left off entirely. By that time the patient is ambulatory and one must proceed with arch supports, wedged shoes, etc. until all tendency toward recurrence is gone. An ambitious program you say; over treatment? Well, possibly so, in an occasional case. The result of undertreatment is so dire that the price of an infrequent case of excess treatment is cheap, indeed, if it insures against the sequela which I know you have all seen, namely, the extreme flat, rocker-bottom foot which after weight bearing is hardly amenable to any type of successful treatment.

With proper treatment of these babies at the optimum time, within a few days of birth, we can materially reduce the number of children requiring drastic treatment, surgery, etc., which, at best, offers but an imperfect foot as the reward. You men, as pediatricians, can aid in early recognition of these cases; urge prompt and adequate treatment and so add another step to the long stairway of preventive medicine.

1. Kahns, John G., American Medical Journal. Vol. 120, No. 5, page 329.

Intramedulary Transfusions in Infants

Charles M. Bielstein, M.D.

Department of Pediatrics, Crippled Children's Hospital

Oklahoma City, Oklahoma

During recent years, transfusions and infusions in infants have become increasingly more important in pediatric therapy. With this increase in importance it has become apparent that, if possible, a route of introduction which requires smaller amounts of the physician's time should be employed. In addition, there are patients who have diseases such as nephritis or nephrosis with edema to whom it is impossible to give blood or other fluids via the intravenous route. It has been our experience that premature infants prove the most difficult to give intravenous fluids, due to both the size of the veins and to the fragility of the tissues.

With these factors in mind, Tocantins and O'Neil have investigated the possibilities of giving fluids into the bone marrow, or rather into the cancellous portion of the diaphysis. They demonstrated that adrenalin given into the bone marrow of dogs produced the same effects in the same length of time as did adrenalin given intravenously and they devised a technique by which blood given into the bone marrow of a dog, which had had blood withdrawn previously, caused a rise in blood pressure in approximately the same time as blood given intravenously. They also introduced a method by which blood could be given human beings by the bone marrow route with results comparable to those obtained by giving the same amounts intravenously. Tocantins, O'Neil and Jones[2] reported a series of 49 cases who had been given solutions by this route with no untoward sequelae and stated that they felt the method was indicated in patients to whom blood or other nonsclerosing fluids could not be given by the usual routes.

At the Crippled Children's Hospital there are many patients admitted who are suffering from anemia over long periods of time and who require multiple blood transfusions. It is relatively easy to give the first few intravenously, but as the number required increases, so does the difficulty in giving the blood. We have alternated the methods of giving the blood in hope that at least a portion of the difficulty might be eliminated. Our aim at first was to find a method which could be used in hospitals or clinics with a minimum amount of equipment and assistance.

The usual places of administration of fluids into the bone marrow are the sternum, the distal end of the femur, and the proximal end of the tibia. In infants and children under three years of age, the sternal marrow cavity is much too narrow to accommodate fluids. Since that is true, and since the femur and tibia offer very adequate cavities, we have given all our intramedullary transfusions into these bones. The method is based on the principle that the bone marrow has adequate drainage into the venous circulation and thus allows the fluids to leave the marrow cavity in a very short time.

Since September 1, 1942, there have been 75 attempts to give intramedullary transfusions or infusions to 28 patients. The ages ranged from a 48 hour old, seven months premature, to a 30 months old child. Twenty, or 70 per cent, were less than one year old. The number of transfusions given has varied from one to eight for each patient. The amount of fluid given has not exceeded 10 cc per pound, body weight, in any 25 hour period of time, except in two instances, one

of which was a 12 months old child with severe burns over the face, neck, and upper extremities, who was admitted in apparent extremis and received 400 cc of plasma over a period of two and a half hours. The other patient was a four day old premature infant who had very severe melena secondary to hemorrhagic disease of the newborn. The patient received 30 cc of plasma and 120 cc of blood in divided doses over a 16 hour period of time.

The fluids given have been restricted to citrated whole blood, plasma, or isotonic solutions of normal saline which contain no sclerosing substances.

Twenty attempts, or 26 per cent, were classed as failures for various reasons, the principal one being the use of needles too small to allow the fluids to enter the cavity fast enough to consider the attempt successful. In several instances we could find no explanation for the failure, therefore, in these cases it was considered to be due to faulty technique. In the remaining 58 attempts, or 74 per cent, the method was considered successful, in that the desired amount of fluid was given with a minimum amount of assistance and a decreased amount of discomfort on the part of the patient. We feel that in many cases an undetermined amount of benefit caused by transfusion is nullified by the struggling of the patient from discomfort.

In view of the place of administration we have been careful to observe any untoward effects of the transfusion given and especially have we been careful to note any types of infection. In one instance, in a patient on whom an attempt was made to enter both tibias with the same needle, a subqutaneous abscess developed over the proximal end of both bones. Repeated x-rays did not reveal the expected osteomyelitis, though the second attempt was successful and 50 cc of citrated whole blood was given. There was no evidence of a septicemia. The abscesses were incised when they became fluctuant and the recovery was uneventful. In none of the cases have there been evidences of emboli.

The technique which we have used is essentially a modification of the method described by Tocantins and Jones. Special needles have been designed and have been made available by one of the surgical houses*, but we were able to obtain some obsolete spinal puncture needles which were of large enough gauge to be used. These were shortened to varying lengths of three-fourths of an inch to one and one-fourth inches and have proved suitable for the purpose. We find that an 18 guage needle is as small as can be used with any degree of success except in rare instances which will be described.

We have used two techniques of giving the blood depending on the size and age of the patient and on the amount of fluid to be given. If the patient is very small and is to receive less than 50 cc of fluids, we insert the needle and then, using a syringe, force the blood into the marrow cavity very slowly, at the rate of approximately 5 cc a minute. When more than 50 cc is to be given, we have used the drip method.

In each case, premature infants excepted, the patient is securely restrained to a circumcision board to avoid struggling and we have found, by the use of this method that much less help is required in all transfusions. The site of injection is scrubbed and then prepared with tincture of merthiolate and the adjacent area is draped with sterile towels. In larger infants, small amounts of local anesthesia is used. The operator, using sterile technique, then inserts the 18 gauge needle, except in very small infants when a 20 gauge needle is used. When the site of injection is the tibia, the needle is inserted anteriorly at the inferior margin of the tibial tuberosity or into the medial surface of the tibia at the same level. The insertion is in such a direction as to have the shaft of the needle form an angle of 70 degrees with the knee joint. If the femur is the site of injection, the needle is inserted either into the lateral condyle or into the anterior surface as near the midline as possible just proximal to the epiphyseal line. The depth of insertion is guided by the resistance that is met. As soon as the cortex is penetrated there is a sensation of sudden decrease in resistance which signifies that the point is within the cancellous portion of the bone. With the needle in place, the stillete is withdrawn and a 10 cc syringe containing normal saline solution is attached. By withdrawing the plunger, marrow fluid can be obtained which verifies the position of the needle. Then from 5 cc to 10 cc of the saline is gently injected. The blood being injected either by syringe or by the open drip method. If the latter method is employed, the apparatus is supplemented by a three-way stopcock to which a Luer-lok syringe may be attached, thus the needle may be irrigated with normal saline intermittently to prevent stoppage of the flow of blood into the cavity.

In discussing, the patient is securely restrained to a well-padded circumcision board. This prevents excessive struggling and the attending nurse may go about her duties, returning at intervals to be sure the fluids are still running. The patient may be fed if still receiving fluids at feeding time. Each sterile package of bone marrow needles contains three needles for infant transfusions and one for sternal punctures. The Luer-lok syringe is attached to the three-way stopcock and is used to irrigate the system and prevent clotting. The needle is inserted into the anterior border of the left tibia, the stillete still being in place. The patient may move to a certain extent without danger of removing the needle.

SUMMARY

Intramedullary transfusions have been discussed and a series of 28 patients has been reported.

A modification of the technique of Tocantins and O'Neil has been presented and illustrations have been supplied. It is our belief that this method is worthy of a trial in cases in which no other route of administration is available.

DISCUSSION
W. B. MULLINS, M.D.
SHAWNEE, OKLAHOMA

The intramedullary route of fluid administration is proving to be a valuable therapeutic agent, and seems particularly applicable to pediatric practice, especially for infants. As the author of the paper under discussion has pointed out, the intramedullary method is not offered as one to supplant intravenous administration of fluids, but merely as an alternative in certain cases where the rapid administration of fluids is desired and the intravenous route is not available.

According to work previously done and reported, the intramedullary method seems to have a high safety factor, both as far as contamination of fluids and the probability of reaction are concerned. However, as has been pointed out, the intramedullary route is not advisable in cases of Bacteremia of any type as the site of puncture may offer favorable conditions for the development of a suppurative process and osteomyelitis.

Another question that may arise is the possibility of a "fat embolus". In the writer's opinion there is a very remote possibility of this based on the fact that the fat content of bone marrow in infants and children is relatively low, and that the type of bone marrow into which the fluids are given is the red bone marrow in which the fat content is very low. Also, there is apparently no extensive involvement of bone marrow tissue in the technique of the administration.

One should also consider the possibility of bone marrow or tissue injury by the sclerosing action or chemical irritation by the fluids used. It has previously been stated that no hypertonic fluids should be given by this method. The reports up to date have shown that there has been no ill effects on the bone marrow from the administration of whole blood, blood plasma or isotonic solution.

The technique of intramedullary fluid administration has been fully described and leaves little for discussion. There will, no doubt, be various modifications developed, however, the principle will remain the same and the type and amount of fluids to be given will always remain at the discretion of the physician in any case.

BIBLIOGRAPHY

1. Tocantins, L. M.: Rapid Absorption of Substances Injection into the Bone Marrow. Proc. Soc. Expr. Biol. and Med., Vol. 45, page 292. Oct., 1940.

2. Tocantins, L. M. and O'Neil, J. F.: Infusion of Blood and other Fluids into the Circulation Via the Bone Marrow. Proc. Soc. Exper. Biol. and Med., Vol. 45, page 782. December, 1940.

3. Tocantins, L. M. and O'Neil, J. F.: Infusion of Blood and Other Fluids into the Circulation Via the Bone Marrow. Technic and Results, Surg., Gynec. and Obst.; Vol. 73, page 287. September, 1941.

4. Tocantins, L. M., O'Neil, J. F., and Jones, H. W.: Infusions of Blood and Other Fluids Via the Bone Marrow. Jour. A. M. A., Vol. 117, page 1229. October, 11, 1941.

*Needles used by Tocantins and co-workers were made by George Pilling Company, Philadelphia, Pennsylvania.

A new name is herewith presented medical men for the dazed mental condition of citizens who have made out their income tax. They are intaxicated.—*Washington Evening Star.*

A huge fee (for an operation) was mentioned. "Ah, well then," said Oscar, I suppose that I shall have to die beyond my means."—*E. H. Sherard, Life of Oscar Wilde.*

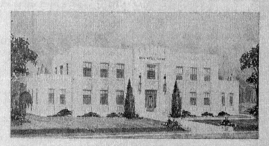

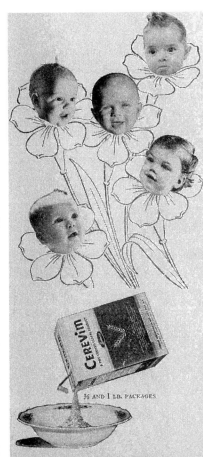

· THE PRESIDENT'S PAGE ·

Elsewhere in this issue of The Journal you will find a list of the Committees, both Standing and Special, which will serve during the ensuing year. The duties and activities of some of them, as for example the Standing Committees, are outlined in the Constitution, and we have endeavored to supply each member of these committees with an excerpt giving a synopsis of the scope and activities of the respective committee.

Special committees have no stipulated function or outline of activities. It is left to the members to determine the character and scope of their work. We have investigated the procedure relative to committee work that is followed in other states. We find in a considerable number of states that the functions of each committee are outlined. This idea has impressed us as being sound in principle and practical in effect and we are endeavoring to codify the duties of the Special Committees in order that each one may work toward a definite goal.

We know that each committee member will do his or her full duty in fulfilling his obligations, in order that the sum total of the work of all committees may be of such force and effect as to advance the cause of medicine not only in our own state but also as a contribution to organized medicine in the nation at large.

Since the Annual Meeting several committees have met and transacted business of considerable importance to the welfare of the State Association. Among these are the Public Policy Committee, meeting jointly with the Public Health Committee for the purpose of discussing a suitable public health law which will be presented at the next legislature.

Representatives of the Medical Economics Committee, together with your President and Executive Secretary, met with representatives of the Farm Security Administration, relative to a medical program for the State of Oklahoma. Regardless of what one thinks of the activities of the Farm Security Administration, we feel that they have a right to state their case and after all facts are available, a proper decision can be reached. Some interesting facts and figures were presented which are at present being studied by the Medical Economics Committee. A further report of this activity will be made later.

We plan to attend the meeting of the American Medical Association and I am sure that there will be many problems discussed which are of vital interest to the profession of Oklahoma. We shall endeavor to bring you a comprehensive report of the proceedings of this important body.

President.

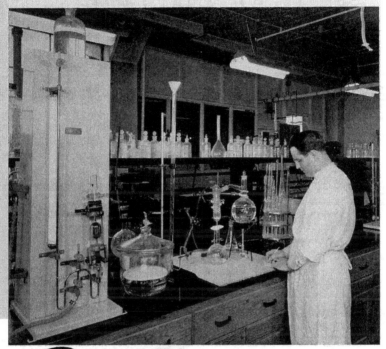

Research FOR TOMORROW

While we are supplying the home front today with reliable drugs and medicines, our research departments are delving into the realm of tomorrow.

We shall be ready for Peace . . . and the world to follow . . . with the most modern, up-to-date developments science has ever known.

Warren-Teed representatives realize the importance of keeping physicians and pharmacists supplied quickly and efficiently at all times.

WARREN-TEED

Medicaments of Exacting Quality Since 1920

THE WARREN-TEED PRODUCTS COMPANY, COLUMBUS 8, OHIO

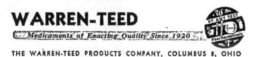

Visit Our Booth — No. 80 — At The American Medical Association Convention

The JOURNAL Of The
OKLAHOMA STATE MEDICAL ASSOCIATION

EDITORIAL BOARD
L. J. MOORMAN, Oklahoma City, Editor-in-Chief

E. EUGENE RICE, Shawnee   BEN H. NICHOLSON, Oklahoma City

MR. PAUL H. FESLER, Oklahoma City,   Business Manager

CONTRIBUTIONS: Articles accepted by this Journal for publication, including those read at the annual meetings of the State Association are the sole property of this Journal.

The Editorial Department is not responsible for the opinions expressed in the original articles of contributors.

Manuscripts may be withdrawn by authors for publication elsewhere only upon the approval of the Editorial Board.

MANUSCRIPTS: Manuscripts should be typewritten, double-spaced, on white paper 8½ x 11 inches. The original copy, not the carbon copy, should be submitted.

Footnotes, bibliographies and legends for cuts should be typed on separate sheets in double space. Bibliography listing should follow this order: Name of author, title of article, name of periodical with volume, page and date of publication.

Manuscripts are accepted subject to the usual editorial revisions and with the understanding that they have not been published elsewhere.

NEWS: Local news of interest to the medical profession, changes of address, births, deaths and weddings will be gratefully received.

ADVERTISING: Advertising of articles, drugs or compounds unapproved by the Council on Pharmacy of the A.M.A. will not be accepted. Advertising rates will be supplied on application.

It is suggested that members of the State Association patronize our advertisers in preference to others.

SUBSCRIPTIONS: Failure to receive The Journal should call for immediate notification.

REPRINTS: Reprints of original articles will be supplied at actual cost provided request for them is attached to manuscripts or made in sufficient time before publication. Checks for reprints should be made payable to Industrial Printing Company, Oklahoma City.

Address all communications to THE JOURNAL OF THE OKLAHOMA STATE MEDICAL ASSOCIATION, 210 Plaza Court, Oklahoma City. (3)

OFFICIAL PUBLICATION OF THE OKLAHOMA STATE MEDICAL ASSOCIATION
Copyrighted June, 1944

EDITORIALS

FULTON'S FULL LIFE

Dr. J. S. Fulton has voluntarily retired from the Council of the Oklahoma State Medical Association after more than 30 years service.

Dr. Fulton, a native of Texas, graduated from the Kentucky School of Medicine in 1890 and entered the practice of medicine in Atoka, Oklahoma the early part of 1891. In June of that year he became a member of The Indian Territory Medical Association and was elected president of that Organization in 1893. During that eventful year he went on to New York for postgraduate work in the Polyclinic Hospital. Dr. Fulton was a member of the Joint Committee from the Indian Territory and the Oklahoma Territory Medical Associations resulting in the amalgamation of these two Associations in 1905 to form the Oklahoma State Medical Association. He was elected president of The State Association in 1926. With the exception of this one year he served on the Council almost continuously from the time the State Medical Association was organized.

In 1941 Dr. Fulton's friends in the Southeastern Medical Society at the regular Annual Meeting, with the late LeRoy Long, Sr., as master of ceremonies, honored him by the presentation of a bronze plaque.

Dr. Fulton's loyalty to organized medicine is shown by the fact that he has missed only three out of 54 Annual Meetings of his State Association since 1891. In addition to the services he has rendered his profession, he has to his credit 53 years of unfailing loyalty and service day and night to the people of his community. In terms of labor union time schedules, he has worked in and out of Atoka approximately 175 years.

All honor to the vigorous, hard-hitting, kindly gentleman who, in behalf of humanity, continues to coax his coronaries toward the occlusions of the highways and byways of his own useful life.

NEWS AND NERVES

Long before we entered the present war, a tuberculous patient who had to chase the cure month after month for two years said, "Do you know what is the matter with the world? We know too much! In addition to reading the newspapers I listen to thirteen news broadcasts every day and what Japan is doing to China is about to drive me nuts.

Wish I was back on the old homestead digging ginseng."

The following, from Margaret Kennedy's "Where Stands a Winged Sentry," published by the Yale University Press of New Haven, Connecticut, tends to confirm the above statement and offers a fine example of medical wisdom:

"I still cannot sleep so I went to Dr. Middleton to ask for a bromide. He used to attend all our family in the old days. He asked:

"'Are ye worrying about anything?'

"When I said I was worrying about Hitler coming, he said, 'He won't,' so firmly that I almost believed him.   He looked up and down very crossly and said:

"'I suppose ye've been reading the newspapers?'

"I pleaded guilty.

"'What d'ye want to do that for?'

"'I like to know what is happening.'

"'Aw! The newspapers don't know.' ·

"He said if I must read a newspaper I should stick to The Times because I would find there any news there was, put in a way that would send me to sleep instead of keeping me awake. He said that when a war broke out once in the Balkans the headlines said: 'Activity in Europe.'

"He asked me how often I listened to the wireless.

"'Four times a day.'

"'And that's three times too often. I'm sure I wish that infernal contrivance had never been invented. When I think of all the insanity that's poured out over the ether every minute of the day, I wonder the whole human race isn't in a lunatic asylum. And what good does it do ye to know what's happening? Ye aren't responsible. Ye don't like it. Ye can't stop it. Why think about it? Go home and fly kites with your children.'

"'How many other patients have you said all this to?'

"'You're only the twenty-seventh this week'."

IMMUNIZATIONS

Fifteen years ago I listened in on an indignation meeting held because of a health department program of immunization in the local schools. After many heated words against the incursions of public health services into the domain of private practice, one timid soul got up and faintly addressed the group as follows:

"When children for whose care I am responsible have not been protected against the communicable diseases by the time they reach school age, I do not feel that I have any kick coming."

These words aptly answer any criticism of this particular function that the health departments have assumed. The primary concern of the Oklahoma State Health Department is to see that the children are protected, not so much for the sake of the individual as for the protection of the group. The department's very extensive educational program makes parents acquainted with the possibility and desirability of such procedures. Most parents are already sold on the idea. All the family physician needs to do is to say when.

There are people who are unable or unwilling or for various other reasons unlikely to seek medical counsel. The health department must make provision for these people, which it does among other ways by making the material available to doctors whose patients need help. Diphtheria in a poor child or in a child whose parents do not believe in the germ theory of disease is no less communicable to other children.

The medical profession must assume the responsibility of instituting preventive measures to protect the very young in whom the mortality rate is so high. Lest the lying-in period end the physician's contact with the child, it would seem wise to mention to the mother during that time the diseases that the child can be protected against and when the immunization should be carried out.

The following are the recommendation of the American Academy of Pediatrics:

1. Smallpox—vaccinate at any age during an epidemic, but routinely between 3 to 12 months. Repeat at 6 and 12 years of age and during an epidemic. Re-vaccinate if necessary.
2. Pertussis—vaccinate at 8 months or any subsequent age.
3. Diphtheria — immunize against diphther between 9 and 18 months.
4. Tetanus—tetanus toxoid has been used in combination with diphtheria toxoid (recommended by the Oklahoma State Health Department.)
5. Typhoid—typhoid vaccine may be given at any age when indicated. (Also recommended.)—B. H. N., M.D.

POETIC VISION

In 1849 the following verse by Ralph Waldo Emerson was employed to introduce his famous essay "Nature."

"A subtle chain of countless rings
The next unto the farthest brings;
The eye reads omens where it goes,
And speaks all languages the rose;
And striving to be man, the worm
Mounts through all the spires of form."

This ten years before Darwin published the "Origin of the Species" and at least twenty years before the publication of "The Descent of Man." Oliver Wendell Holmes says,

"It seems as if Emerson had a warning from the poetic instinct which, when it does not procede the movement of the scientific intellect is the first to catch the hint of its discoveries."

As we read Emerson's Essays "Nature" and "The American Scholar" and contemplate the past century's mill-run, we are impressed with his own reflections upon the naive way we utilize and assimilate the results of other men's labors. "They sun themselves in the great man's light, and feel it to be their own element."

During Food Shortages

It is well to bear in mind that dried brewers yeast, weight for weight, is the richest food source of the Vitamin B Complex. For example, as little as one level teaspoonful (2.5 gm.) Mead's Brewers Yeast Powder supplies; 45 per cent of the average adult daily thiamine allowance, 8 per cent of the average adult daily riboflavin allowance, 10 per cent of the average adult daily niacin allowance.

This is in addition to the other factors that occur naturally in yeast such as pyrodozin, pantothenic acid, etc.

Send for tested wartime recipes, the flavors of which are not affected by the inclusion of Mead's Brewers Yeast Powder. Mead Johnson & Company, Evansville, Ind., U. S. A.

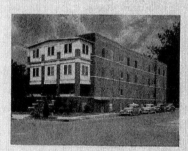
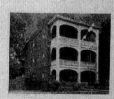

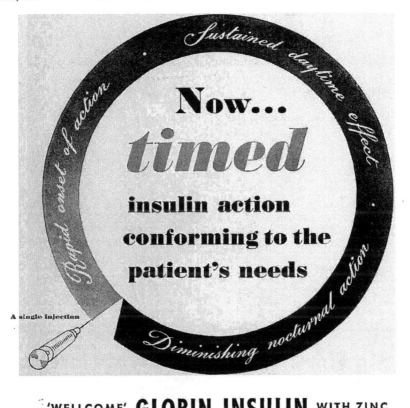

ASSOCIATION ACTIVITIES

NEW COUNCIL ON MEDICAL SERVICE AND PUBLIC RELATIONS DISCUSSES NEW WASHINGTON OFFICE

Dr. James Stevenson, Tulsa, Dr. A. S. Risser, Blackwell and Mr. Paul Fesler, Oklahoma City, attended the meeting of State representatives with the New Council on Medical Service and Public Relations at the Palmer House on Sunday afternoon, June 11 .

Dr. Louis H. Bauer of Hemstead, New York opened the meeting. He stated that Dr. Joe Lawrence who had been in charge of legislative work for the New York Society in Albany, was to be in charge of the Washington office. Dr. Bauer outlined the purpose of the Council and emphasized the importance of organization of the State and Local Societies so that direct contact would be maintained at all times with the Congressmen. He said that the office would work two ways—one to keep the members of the profession informed relative to activities in Washington and the other for the profession to keep the Washington office alive to local problems.

The State representatives present at the meeting all agreed that the office in Washington is a step in the right direction and all pledged support. Dr. Risser expressed gratitude that the resolution as presented by Oklahoma last year had finally been put into effect. All seemed to agree that the office should be provided with sufficient funds. and personnel to function effectively. It was explained that this was not a lobby but a Bureau of Information for the benefit of the members of Congress.

The importance of the Public Relations Program was emphasized and it seemed to be the unanimous opinion that this action on the part of the American Medical Association was late. It was stated that "it should have happened 25 years ago." It was explained that the Wagner Bill is not dead by any means and that if the freedom in the practice of medicine is to survive, much greater activity on the part of members of the medical profession is essential.

DR. D. H. O'DONOGHUE HONORED BY MORNINGSIDE COLLEGE

Dr. D. H. O'Donoghue, Oklahoma City, has just returned from Sioux City, Iowa, where he and his brother Dr. Arch F. O'Donoghue of Sioux City, were honored by receiving the honorary degree of Doctor of Science. The degree was bestowed upon Dr. O'Donoghue and his brother by their father, Dr. J. H. O'Donoghue of Storm Lake, who has the distinction of having once served on the faculty of Morning Side College.

The fiftieth anniversary of the founding of the College was celebrated on Tuesday, May 30, when the degree was conferred upon Drs. O'Donoghue. Rarely does a family boast so many physicians, and still more rarely does a father have the honor and pleasure of acting officially for a College in its bestowal of honorary degrees upon his two sons.

OKLAHOMANS ATTEND A.M.A. CONVENTION IN CHICAGO

Dr. C. R. Rountree, President of the Oklahoma State Medical Association; Dr. Tom Lowry, Dean of the University of Oklahoma School of Medicine; Mr. Paul Fesler, Executive Secretary of the Oklahoma State Medical

Association; Dr. James Stevenson, Tulsa and Dr. A. S. Risser, Delegates; Dr. V. C. Tisdal, President-Elect of the Association and Chairman of the Public Policy Committee and Dr. J. D. Osborn, Secretary of the State Board of the Medical Examiners and Member of the Public Policy Committee attended the meeting of the American Medical Association in Chicago the week of June 12.

HEALTH SECTION OF OKLAHOMA SOCIAL WELFARE ASSOCIATION CONFERENCE HELD JUNE 15-16

The opening subject of the Conference of the Health Section of the Oklahoma Social Welfare Association was the "Desirability of a State Board of Health." Dr. Carl Puckett, Oklahoma City, Managing Director of the Oklahoma Tuberculosis Association presided and the principal speaker was Dr. Lewis J. Moorman, President of the Oklahoma County Health Association.

The second meeting covered "Modern Concept of Mental Diseases," Dr. Puckett also presided at this meeting. Dr. Hugh M. Galbraith, Oklahoma City, Instructor of Neurology at the University of Oklahoma School of Medicine, spoke on the subject and the matter was discussed by Dr. Felix Adams, Vinita, Medical Director of the Eastern Oklahoma Hospital.

"Trends in the Practice of Medicine" was the principal topic of the Friday meeting and L. M. Jones, Oklahoma City, President of the Oklahoma Social Hygiene Association, presided. The speaker was Dr. Leo J. Starry, Oklahoma City, Chairman of the Committee on Medical Economics of the Oklahoma State Medical Association, and Dr. John W. Shackelford, Oklahoma State Health Department was the discussant.

L. M. Jones again presided at the session on "Social Hygiene After the War." Major Bascom Johnson, Dallas, Associate Director of the American Social Hygiene Association spoke on the subject which was discussed by Dr. Charles B. Taylor, Oklahoma City-County Venereal Disease Clinic; Mrs. Eileen Harrison Wilson, Social Hygiene Director Oklahoma County Health Association, Inc. and Dr. John A. Cowan, Director, Venereal Disease Control of the Oklahoma State Department of Health.

COUNCIL APPROVES NEW COUNCIL ROOM AND LIBRARY IN OFFICE OF STATE ASSOCIATION

Work is progressing on the new Council Room and Library in the Office of the Oklahoma State Medical Association in Oklahoma City. Authority was given for the remodeling at a recent meeting of the Council.

The Library will be set up with the idea of supplying complete information on the subject covered by the membership committees. There will be special sections on Public Health, Industrial Medicine, Medical Economics, Hospitals, and a complete file of Medical Journals of other States as well as Journals from professions allied to the medical profession. It is also planned to have a Library of motion pictures which will be available to various county medical societies. This motion picture library will be supplemented by the similar library of the State Health Department.

Announcement will be made as to the progress of the remodeling.

S. G. HAMM, M.D., HASKELL GIVES $100,000.00 TO TIPTON ORPHAN'S HOME

Dr. and Mrs. S. G. Hamm, Haskell, have bestowed on the Tipton Orphan's Home of the Church of Christ the largest benevolent gift ever given to an institution in eastern Oklahoma. The gift consisted of valuable property and other considerations approximating $100,000.00, and was unsolicited by the institution.

Dr. and Mrs. Hamm will see their gift transformed into blossoming lives of men and women as the Tipton Orphan Home will be one of the largest in the United States when their building program is completed. Six new buildings are planned and the Hamm's gift will make three of these possible, namely, an auditorium-dining room wing, a nursey and a home for larger boys.

Dr. Hamm came to Haskell in 1923 after having practiced for twelve years in Searcy County, Arkansas.

(Editors Note: *The following news story and editorial are reprinted from the Tulsa County Bulletin, Vol. 10, No. 6, June, 1944.*)

REREGISTRATION FUND AVAILABLE

BOARD OF MEDICAL EXAMINERS OFFERS USE OF FUND IN LOCAL DRIVE ON MEDICAL FRAUDS. FINANCIAL BASIS FOR EMPLOYMENT OF AN ATTORNEY-INVESTIGATOR QUESTIONED BY STATE ATTORNEY-GENERAL

Prospects of a stringent drive to rid Tulsa County of medical frauds were seen last month as the State Board of Medical Examiners assured the Tulsa County Medical Society of its cooperation in employing an attorney to investigate and prosecute local violators of the Medical Practice Act of Oklahoma as soon as certain legal difficulties can be surmounted.

Seen as the only stumbling block to the much needed project was a difference of opinion between the Board and the Attorney-General of the State of Oklahoma as to the financial basis on which such an attorney could be employed under the terms of the Annual Reregistration Act.

Dr. James D. Osborn, secretary-treasurer of the Board of Medical Examiners, told a special committee of the Tulsa County Medical Society that the Board was willing to make the Reregistration Fund available in any county for the definite need for clean-up if fraudulent practitioners existed. Speaking for the Board, Dr. Osborn stated that the Attorney-General of Oklahoma had advised him that it would be necessary to employ an investigating attorney on an annual basis, and that employment on a cash basis was not possible under the law. Attorneys of the Tulsa County Medical Society disagreed with this contention and announced they would seek to have the Attorney-General's opinion modified.

The satisfactory outcome of the conference between the Board and the local Society brought to an end long-standing differences in regard to the Annual Reregistration Fund. For more than a year the Tulsa County Medical Society has worked to obtain a series of investigations in Tulsa County of certain medical frauds, employing funds set up for that purpose by the Annual Reregistration Act of 1941. These funds are derived from the collection of an annual fee of $3.00 from each Oklahoma doctor for renewal of his medical license.

Representatives of the Board of Medical Examiners pointed out certain conditions which have made it difficult to place the Annual Reregistration Fund into operation. In addition to the contested point of the basis for the employment of investigating attorney, war conditions have made it difficult to secure a reliable attorney for this purpose. With many attorneys now in service, the problem is made unusually difficult. Furthermore, it is preferable to obtain the services of an attorney who has some knowledge of medico-legal procedure.

Income to the fund, which normally approximates $6,000.00 annually, has also decreased as the Board of Medical Examiners has suspended payment of the fee for all Oklahoma doctors now in the armed services. The amount collected in 1943 was the smallest amount during the three years of the fund's existence, and it is anticipated that the 1944 income may set a new low. Such collections are subject to statutory deductions of ten per cent for the general fund of the state and for necessary expenses in administering the law. At the end of 1943, approximately $10,000.00 was on deposit, this sum also including income from sources other than the Annual Reregistration Act.

If, and when, the legal difficulties are ironed out, the Tulsa County Medical Society hopes to secure investigations of alleged violators of the medical practice act of this state who are now residing within Tulsa County. It is believed that the successful prosecution of a few such suits will be sufficient to discourage other medical frauds from further activity.

The committee representing the Tulsa County Medical Society in the matter included Dr. H. B. Stewart, Chairman, Dr. W. A. Showman, and Dr. Ralph A. McGill.

GOOD INTENTIONS

Elsewhere in this issue of THE BULLETIN appears a news story devoted to a recent conference between representatives of the Tulsa County Medical Society and the State Board of Medical Examiners of Oklahoma relative to the Annual Reregistration Act. Every doctor in Tulsa County will be pleased to learn that action is being taken to effectively combat medical frauds in this area through the use of the Annual Reregistration Fund.

For more than a year, the Tulsa County Medical Society has sought an adjustment of this matter with the State Board of Medical Examiners. Some critical articles and editorials have appeared, in various numbers of THE BULLETIN during that period. It should be said here that it was not the intention of the Tulsa County Medical Society to criticize the actions of the State Board of Medical Examiners in any manner except in relation to the Annual Reregistration Fund. The Society wishes to hereby go on record as being thoroughly appreciative of the efforts of the State Board of Medical Examiners

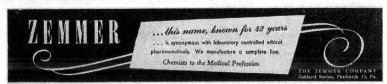

in other matters. It has been efficiently and competently administered to the satisfaction of the doctors of Oklahoma.

In the matter of the Annual Reregistration Fund, many of the comments made in these pages were not justified. These comments arose partially through a misunderstanding of certain circumstances and partially through inadequate information. If the Tulsa County Medical Society has occasioned any embarrassment to the State Board of Medical Examiners on unjust accusations, the Society take this means of apologizing and rectifying the error.

Following the recent conference, it is anticipated that the Society will be privileged to work in close cooperation with the State Board of Medical Examiners in effecting the investigation and possible prosecution of certain medical frauds in Tulsa County. It is desirable that a maximum of understanding exist between the State Board and the Society if best results are to be obtained in this project. Consequently, let it be understood that the Tulsa County Medical Society entertains a high regard for the State Board of Medical Examiners and its individual members, and that it rejoices that certain misunderstandings existing between the Society and the State Board have been eliminated to the satisfaction of both parties.

J. D. OSBORN SPEAKS FOR BOARD

The above news story and editorial are self-explanatory. Dr. J. D. Osborn, Frederick, Secretary for the State Board of Medical Examiners, speaking for the Board expresses deep appreciation of the time given by the Tulsa County Medical Society in getting the doctors together in order to iron out any differences of opinion on the above discussed subject.

POST WAR AIMS IN MEDICINE
JOHN F. BURTON, M.D.
OKLAHOMA CITY, OKLAHOMA

To my mind the days of the "rugged individualist" in any capacity, in this our great United States, are over. Especially do I feel that this is true of the Profession of Medicine. The science of medicine has become so complex, new discoveries have been, and will continue to be, so far reaching, that it will be a physical impossibility for one individual's mind to encompass all of modern medical knowledge.

Secondly, both Mr. and Mrs. John Q. Public, not neglecting Junior, who reads the latest periodicals, have become health conscious. They will be demanding preventive medicine to a degree that will be startling as considered in the light of today's practice. In their expectations regarding therapy, they will consider only the ideal, and although there may be now and then some mention of the personal relations between the patient and his medical attendant, these will be quickly sacrificed or forgotten in their zeal for results approaching the ultimate of perfection.

Thirdly, society as a whole is becoming more social minded. People are troubled and concerned about the future. With this trend, they are realizing that "they are their brother's keeper," and that what ill befalls their neighbor can easily happen to them. They are concluding that society as a whole must begin to think in terms of betterment of the entire group.

How will these trends affect the Post War Practice

of Medicine? In my opinion they will bring about the following:

1. An extensive and far reaching Public Health Program, which will be administered by the Federal Government.

2. The establishment of Institutions of Medical Research, supported by public funds.

3. The endowment or actual government support of first class medical schools, without tuition and having faculties of the best personnel obtainable.

4. A unified system of examination and licensure based upon the applicant's ability and competency, with appropriate designations as Doctor of Medicine, or any designated specialty of the practice of medicine.

5. A group association or organization in the actual practice of medicine. A group organized to give the individual complete diagnostic as well as therapeutic service.

6. Medical and Surgical Insurance Associations.

Woods-Alfalfa Medical Society
Meeting, May 23

The Woods-Alfalfa Medical Society met at Cherokee on Tuesday, May 23 with thirteen physicians and ten nurses present. Dinner for the physicians, their wives, and guests preceded the program.

Mr. Paul Fesler, Executive Secretary of the Oklahoma State Medical Association gave a short talk on the work of the State Association and on Medical Insurance. Colonel Ritzhaupt, Oklahoma City, spoke on "Procurement and Supply" and gave the percentage of rejections for a number of conditions, psychotic conditions and illiteracy being the highest. Lt. Charley E. Wysong, Enid Army Air Field, read a paper and gave a demonstration on "Caudal Anesthesia."

Guests included: Colonel L. H. Ritzhaupt, Oklahoma City; Paul H. Fesler, Oklahoma City; Captain E. M. Kimbrough, Captain D. H. McDonald, Lt. Charley E. Wysong, all of Enid Army Field; Captain W. H. Sweet, of the Alva Prisoner of War Camp; Nurses from Alva General Hospital included Mrs. Lois Martin, Mrs. Gladys Kerisher, Miss LaVee Waller, Miss Freda Dick, Mrs. Laura Edwards, Mrs. Eva Ammons and Miss Helen Leeper.

Blue Cross Reports

Fifteen Million members are now enrolled in the 77 approved Blue Cross Plans in the United States and Canada. Continued spontaneous acceptance of this voluntary health program is resulting in an ever increasing enrollment which is rapidly approaching one million new members every three months. A major problem in extending this service to a greater amount of the population is today being solved by the hospitals and the Blue Cross Plans, by conducting community enrollments in the smaller towns and employing procedures whereby the service is made available to the farmers throughout the country.

The Oklahoma Blue Cross Plan has recently completed a very satisfactory community enrollment in the city of Woodward. Here the Stock Exchange Bank and the Bank of Woodward cooperate with the people of their community by accepting remittances for dues without remuneration. Employing the same procedure as was used in Alva, Oklahoma. Through the cooperation of the city officials in Granite, the Plan is being offered community-wide, with the remittances made through the municipally owned utility system. The Bule Cross Plan

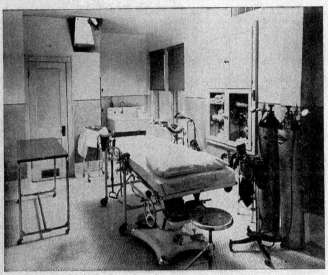

also had a very satisfactory enrollment recently in Ada, Oklahoma.

Several other community enrollments have already been completed and it is the desire of the hospitals and their "service arm"—the Blue Cross Plan, to make this health program available where the local leadership expresses a willingness to sponsor an enrollment. More than 8,000 Oklahoma Farmers and members of their families are today protected by the Blue Cross Plan by enrolling through the cooperation of the Farm Security Administration. The Farm Security Borrower group constitutes only the farmer who is ineligible for a loan through regular banking channels. As yet, the plan has been made available to only one of the four units in the State. The Farm Bureau is now conducting a state-wide enrollment in the Blue Cross Plan, for the members of their association.

More and more firms throughout the State are providing this health service without cost to the employees since the War Labor Board has ruled that payment for this service by the employer does not constitute a salary increase and is deductible for income purposes.

Blue Cross Promotes Distribution of Medical Care, Says Nathan B. Van Etten, M.D.

Blue Cross prepayment of hospital expense is an important factor in promoting a better distribution of medical care, according to Dr. Nathan B. Van Etten, former president of the American Medical Association. Doctor Van Etten expressed this opinion as the guest speaker on "Every 40 Seconds," regular weekly feature of WNYC, at 8:00 P.M. Monday, May 29. A public service feature of the Municipal Broadcasting System, the series is presented in cooperation with the Greater New York Hospital Association, the United Hospital Fund, and Associated Hospital Service.

Doctor Van Etten said in part, "Blue Cross Plans in the United States now include some 15 million people who have learned that they may provide for catastrophic illness without any real strain upon their pocket books. In New York this movement is approximately ten years old. It has developed from a small beginning to a subscription list of more than one and one-half millions. The knowledge of the availability of such service to the people of New York is causing more and more people to ask for this service, so that the number of subscribers is growing every day at a very remarkable rate.

"As a physician, I think the prepayment hospital service exemplified by Blue Cross Plans is one of the most valuable things that has ever happened in this country. The greatly enlarged interest of the people in prepayment of hospital and medical care gives a greater opportunity for the medical profession to promote a better distribution of medical care, which is one of the important objects of the medical profession at the present time. The wider the distribution of good medical care, the better the position of the practicing doctor. The medical profession desires the standards of medical care to be kept at as high a level as possible, and the quality of medical care may well be promoted by the ability of such a large number of people to prepay their hospital and medical bills.

"For another thing, there is no doubt about the diminution of the number of charity cases as evidenced at this time by the low census in the free wards of the city's hospitals, and this must be credited at least in part to the Blue Cross movement. In addition, Blue Cross has also made a large number of people conscious of the fact that they have provided for their hospital care, thus releasing them from worry over hospital bills. The self-respect of these people has been bolstered by the knowledge that when they enter the hospital they have already paid their bills.

"The physician is pleased over such a situation because when people have already paid their hospital bills, the physician in a measure is sure of the payment of his bills. Many times people without this protection will pay the butcher, the baker and the candlestick maker and take care of their doctor last. This splendid Blue Cross movement, which is sponsored by the hospitals of the American Hospital Association, gives the doctor a ready opportunity to meet his own financial obligations as well as to utilize in the care of his patients the resources of the community hospitals."

• OBITUARIES •

G. P. Cherry, M.D.
1861-1944

Dr. G. P. Cherry, Mangum, honorary member of the Oklahoma State Medical Association, died at his home on May 14 of a heart attack.

Born at Clarksville, Texas, June 16, 1861, Dr. Cherry came to Mangum in 1889 from Garland, Texas. He attended medical school at Trinity University, Tehuacana, Texas, and began practice in 1884 in Dallas, Texas. In 1902 Dr. Cherry went to Texas, but returned to Mangum in 1912 where he lived until his death.

In the early days of medicine in Oklahoma Dr. Cherry made many hard and tiresome trips by horseback and on foot to treat the people who lived in the territory near Mangum. He followed medical science through its many steps of development and lived to make use of science's latest discoveries. Beloved by his patients, Dr. Cherry combined a homely philosophy of simplicity with his professional treatment. Before his death he said: "Today, people are unable to enjoy themselves unless they are in violent motion. We need to return to simplicity in our living to enjoy the repose of the early days."

Survivors include his widow, a daughter, Gary June, both of Mangum; two sisters, Mrs. Alma Callahan, Clayton, N. M., and Mrs. Clara Wilson, Dallas.

R. O. Early, M.D.
1880-1944

Dr. Ralph O. Early, nose and throat specialist of Oklahoma City, died June 6, 1944 at St. Anthony Hospital following a cerebral hemorrhage at his office in the Medical Arts Building.

Dr. Early was born in Alvia, Iowa, moved to Ardmore, Oklahoma and then to Oklahoma City in 1920. He was a graduate of Rush Medical College in Chicago and took postgraduate work in Vienna, Austria and other medical centers. In World War No. 1 he served as a Captain in the medical corps.

Dr. Early stood high in his specialty and was prominent in civic affairs. He was a member of the Oklahoma State Medical Association, the American Medical Association and the Oklahoma City Academy of Medicine. He belonged to the American Legion and was a Mason and a Shriner.

Services were held Thursday, June 8 in Oklahoma City and burial was in Fairlawn mausoleum. Surviving are his wife, Mrs. Sue A. Early; a daughter, Mrs. Helen Klingaman, Omaha, Nebraska; two brothers, Ben C. Early, Alvia, Iowa and Ed Early, Tulsa.

Buy An Extra Bond!

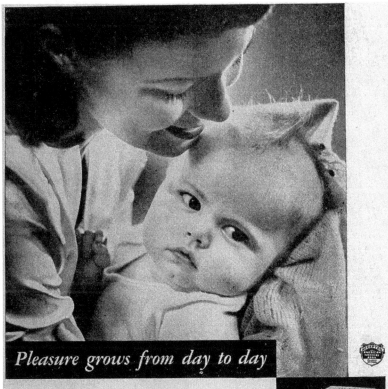

Pleasure grows from day to day

Mother's delight in her baby grows from day to day when a smooth feeding routine helps to keep him healthy and happy.

'Dexin' formulas are easily taken, for 'Dexin' is exceptionally palatable, not over-sweet, and does not dull the appetite. Supplementing the diet with other bland foods is facilitated.

'Dexin' helps assure uncomplicated digestion and assimilation. Its high dextrin content promotes the formation of soft, flocculent, easily digested curds. Distention, colic and diarrhea are avoided because of the relatively non-fermentable form of carbohydrate. 'Dexin' is readily soluble in hot or cold milk.

'Dexin' Reg. U.S. Patent Office

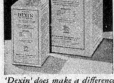

'Dexin' does make a difference

COMPOSITION	Dextrins 75%	Mineral Ash . 0.25%
	Maltose 24%	Moisture . . 0.75%

Available carbohydrate 99%   115 calories per ounce
6 level packed tablespoonfuls equal 1 ounce

'DEXIN'

HIGH DEXTRIN CARBOHYDRATE

Literature on request

BURROUGHS WELLCOME & CO. (U.S.A.) INC. 9-11 E. 41st St., New York 17, N.Y.

THE PHYSICIAN AND THE FIFTH WAR LOAN DRIVE

If each physician in the United States would subscribe $400.00 for War Bonds during the Fifth War Bond Drive this would mean a total of $40,000,000.00 which would equip 1,000 First Aid Stations. The doctors know better than anyone else how much it means for the members of the armed forces to have good medical care.

At the suggestion of the War Finance Division of the Treasury Department, the American Medical Association is asking that subscriptions for War Bonds be reported to the Secretaries of the various County Medical Societies and the totals will be tabulated and sent to the State Medical Association and the information will be sent to the American Medical Association so that the amount of Bonds purchased by doctors in the United States will be known.

The services rendered by the medical profession to the civilian population as well as to the Armed Forces can not be fully appreciated by the public but concrete evidence such as the amount of money subscribed for Bonds will be understood and will create favorable impressions.

It is not necessary to give names in the report but doctors subscribing for bonds should be reported to the Medical Societies at once. It goes without saying that no one can make a better investment even from a purely selfish standpoint.

What Did You Do Today My Friend?

What did you do today, my friend, .
From morn until dark?
How many times did you complain
The rationing is too tight?
When are you going to start to do
All of the things you say?
A soldier would like to know my friend
    What Did You Do Today?

We met the enemy today
And took the town by storm,
Happy reading it will make
For you tomorrow morn.
You'll read with satisfaction
The brief communique.
We fought, but are you fighting?
    What Did You Do Today?

My gunner died in my arms today
I feel his warm blood yet;
Your neighbors' dying boy gave out
A scream I can't forget.
On my right a tank was hit,
A flash and then a fire;
The stench of burning flesh
Still rises from the pyre.
    What Did You Do Today, My Friend?

To help us with the task.
Did you work harder and longer for less?
Or is that too much to ask?
What right have I to ask you this,
You probably will say;
Maybe now you'll understand
    You See, I Died Today.

(*Lt. Dean Shatlain, tank commander, wrote this poem on the battlefield of Africa. He amputated his own foot with a jackknife and thought he was dying when he wrote this poem. He was rescued by Americans after about two hours of hiding, and is now in a hospital in England.*)—from St. Louis Co. Med. Soc. Bulletin.

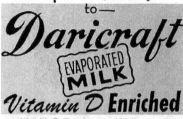
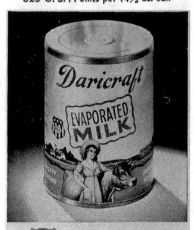

This American is not expected to buy an extra War Bond in the 5TH WAR LOAN

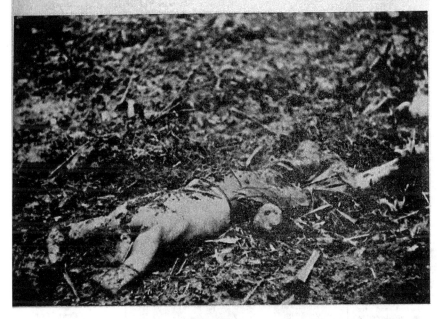

But we are.

For each of us here at home, the job now is to buy extra Bonds—100, 200, even 500 dollars worth if possible.

Many of us can do much more than we ever have before.

When the Victory Volunteer comes to you and asks you to buy extra Bonds, think how much you'd give to have this War over and done.

Then remember that you're not *giving* anything. You're simply *lending* money— putting it in the best investment in the world.

Let's Go . . . for the Knockout Blow!

Oklahoma State Medical Association

STATE HEALTH DEPARTMENT

THE OKLAHOMA PLAN FOR A HEALTH EDUCATION PROGRAM FOR THE SCHOOL YEAR

The State Superintendent of Public Instruction, the Commissioner of the State Health Department, and various staff members of these two organizations h a v e formulated a Plan for for Health Education for the coming School Year. It is planned to organize committees for the Health Program on the local level at the appropriate time.

As a preliminary step in developing the Program for the State of Oklahoma, it is planned to conduct workshops in Health Education for superintendents, principals, teachers, directors of physical education, public health personnel, other professional personnel, and lay people in general who may be interested in promoting individual and community health. These workshops are to be conducted at four centers, from June 12 to June 23, namely: Northeastern State College, Tahlequah, East Central State College, Ada, Southwestern Institute of Technology at Weatherford and for negroes at Langston University, Langston.

At the close of the year we plan to make a definite evaluation of the achievements of the health education program for the entire year. Plans for records during the year and for final evaluation of the program will be one of the projects to which attention will be given during the workshop program. Copies of all plans for school health records and evaluations will be sent to the W. K. Kellog Foundation at Battle Creek, Michigan, and to the Michigan State Department of Education, with a request for suggestion for their improvement. During the progress of the workshops, special attention will be given to the formation of committees for the purpose of outlining a syllabus and

THE CHILD AND IMMUNIZATION

In a recent survey of a group of school children it was found that less than 10 per cent had been immunized against smallpox. These schools offer fertile fields for epidemics of this disease. Responsibility for this condition goes back to the physician who delivered the child, to the lack of education of parents, or to an effective public health program.

The general concensus of opinion in medical circles and among interesting groups, is that children should be immunized at an early date against smallpox, whooping cough, diphtheria, typhoid fever, etc. Doctors recommend smallpox vaccination preferably about three months of age. At six months of age the child should receive whooping cough vaccination. This may be given alone or as a combination with diphtheria. The very young child is quite susceptible to whooping cough and the disease carries its highest mortality in the first few years of life. Diphtheria, like whooping cough, is a more serious disease in young children. A greater number of cases of fatality occur in the preschool age group than any other age year period during life. Diphtheria immunization is ordinarily given between the sixth to ninth month. Approximately a few months after the last injection of diphtheria toxoid, a Schick test is advised to determine whether sufficient protection was obtained from the toxoid injections.

Before the child enters school, a reinforcing dose of diphtheria toxoid should be given. Some time during the first year of life tetanus toxoid should be given. This toxoid, like diphtheria toxoid, gives lasting immunization against disease. Although this is a relatively new procedure, the safety and effectiveness of immunization have been well demonstrated and its use is now routine in the Army.

Typhoid fever is primarily a problem of sanitation and the administration of typhoid fever vaccination is a matter to be determined in individual cases. In communities where sanitation is poor, where milk and water supplies are of doubtful quality and particularly if typhoid fever is present or frequently occurs in the area children should be given the vaccine.

Any child having been exposed to measles, should receive the modifying dose of convalescent serum or immunizing globulin. The modifying dose of this biologic is quite advisable as it greatly lessens the severity of measles and reduces the frequency of complications which have labelled measles as a very dangerous disease.

Physicians are shouldered with the responsibility and obligation to see that all children under their medical supervision receive these undeniable rights and privileges. It is the duty of every citizen to concern himself with these matters and to take it upon himself both as an individual and member of the community to do something about it.

Oklahoma State Health Department

other materials necessary to the success of the Oklahoma plan for health education. The plan in general is to bring about a consciousness on the part of local communities of a need for better health practice and more knowledge of health needs. It is planned to make this program function as a program for better relationships in health education between school and community.

OKLAHOMA INDUSTRIAL SAFETY CONFERENCE

The Meeting of the Oklahoma Industril Safety Conference was held May 17 and 18 at the Mayo Hotel in Tulsa. The meeting was of great interest to the medical profession, in fact, there is scarcely a part of the Safety Program that does not in some way effect the members of the medical profession.

Dr. Hough of the State Health Department delivered a most interesting address on "Pre-E m p l o y m e n t P h y s i c a l Examinations" and Dr. T. J. Lynch of Tulsa delivered a paper on "The Problem of Industrial Medicine and Health." These papers were well received by the members of the Conference, most of whom were Safety Officers f o r large industrial organizations. Additional information wil be found in the State Health Department News in this issue. These papers indicated that the medical profession should take an active part in the Safety Program in every County.

OPPORTUNITIES FOR INDUSTRIAL PHYSICIANS

The American Medical Association has officially recognized industrial practice as one of the specialties. Oklahoma physicians have not, to any extent, taken advantage of the opportunities and responsibilities offered through their contacts (as in injury work) with the business concerns of the state, to build up a favorable reputation in this

· type of special work. Dr. Cary P. McCord, Detroit, has given an outline of the qualifications of an industrial physician.

1. The industrial physician should have some experience in general practice in order that he may know man and his foibles.

2. He should have a knowledge of medical practice, of the fundamentals of industrial relations, of applied preventive medicine, of occupational diseases, of psychopathic medical investigations of recreation, and of accident prevention methods.

3. He should have a knowledge of the special problems relating to the employment of women and children; some knowledge of pensions and insurance, including liability and group some knowledge of plant organization, which is likely to prove effective in dealing with the problems of labor.

4. He should have a knowledge of employment methods; some notion of job analysis, physical and mental tests to determine the fitness of applicants; a knowledge of race problems, industrial training, apprenticeship, continuation schools for training in particular jobs, and at least some knowledge in relation to the cost of living according to the local standards.

5. He should have knowledge of the hours of work in relation to fatigue and output; knowledge of shift systems, rest periods, regularity, absenteeism, turnover and its cost.

6. He should have at least a superficial knowledge of security and continuity of employment in slack seasons, while convalescing from accident or disease, in case of labor-saving improvements, as well as with the advent of old age.

7. He should have a general knowledge of physical working conditions, safeguards, disagreeable gases and dusts, heating, lighting, ventilation, locker rooms, wash rooms, rest rooms, resturants, hospitals, laundries, toilets, showers, plant beautification, drinking water, etc.

8. He shouuld be qualified to carry out physical examinations of applicants, and periodic re-examinations of employees.

9. He should have a very definite knowledge of housing, transporation, recreational and educational facilities; and the transfer and replacement of misfits—how to ''fit the square peg into the round hole.''

10. He should be familiar with the follow-up work, especially among new employees and with the injured; and familiar with the replacement of injured and crippled employees.

From the foregoing, it would appear that there is a need for many doctors to seek after and possess a knowledge of a great many sujects, which do not usually come within the scope of the private practitioner's daily work. A great demand from workers and industrial management for more adequate medical service in factories, offices and stores, et cetera, is developing Oklahoma. To deal with the many complexities and perplexities where people work, requires special attention and skill. So many have said ''the doctor should spend more time in, or going through the plant.''

Industrial Division

Oklahoma State Health Department

Buy An Extra Bond!

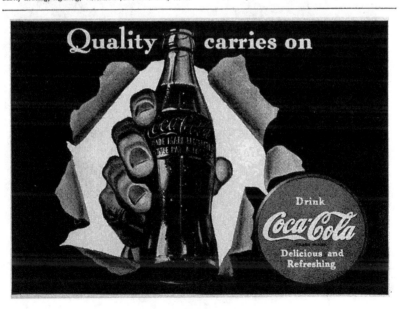

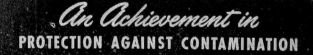

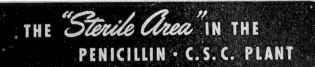
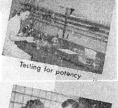
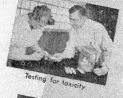
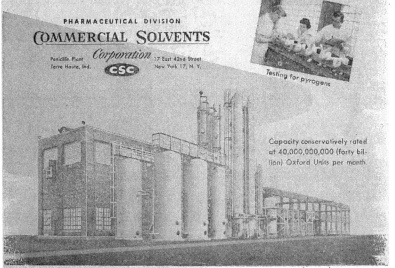

★ FIGHTIN' TALK ★

LT. COMDR. G. H. HENRY, Tulsa, reports from the Southwest Pacific Area and states that he is receiving his Journal and News Letters O.K. He says that he has recently seen DON BRANHAM, Oklahoma City, and LOGAN A. SPANN, Tulsa.

LT. CLEVE F. BELLER, Stigler, has been commissioned and is now awaiting orders at St. Luke's Hospital, Chicago where he is serving his internship. On June 17 he will be married to Miss Kathleen Neal of Oklahoma City.

MAJOR L. H. CHARNEY, Oklahoma City, is now serving with the medical corps in England. Major Charney is doing some very interesting work in research and has had a paper published by the Irish Medical Society .

MAJOR ANDREW RITAN, Tahlequah, has recently been promoted from Captain. He is a division artillery surgeon of an infantry division on the Fifth Army Front in Italy. Before entering the service he was senior physician at Hastings General Hospital in Tahlequah.

CAPTAIN J. G. WOOD, Weatherford, has returned from England where he has spent several months. Before joining the army two years ago Captain Wood was surgeon at the Weatherford Emergency Hospital of which he was owner .

MAJOR JOHN MUNAL, Holdenville, has recently been promoted from Captain. He is now stationed at Ft. Sam Houston, Texas .

From the Fifth Army in Italy comes news of CAPTAIN ROBERT KAHN, Lawton, who is commander of a medical detachment with the 45th "Thunderbird" division. Going gets rather rough at times and the medics are kept pretty busy taking care of the wounded, however, there is still time to play cards and keep up spirits in the usual American way.

MAJOR MEREDITH M. APPLETON, Oklahoma City, writes from overseas and calls our attention to the fact that we reported in a previous Journal that LT. COLONEL T. A. RAGAN, Fairfax, was a Captain. Our humble apologies to Lt. Colonel Ragan. He has recently been promoted to Lt. Colonel from Major and is in command of a Station Hospital overseas.
Major Appleton says that they are "itchin'" to see or be home.

LT. COLONEL COLE D. PITTMAN, Tulsa, recently promoted from Major, is in command of a Station Hospital in Great Falls, Montana. Lt Colonel Pittman entered the Army as a 1st Lt. and his advancements have come as a result of hard work.

MAJOR E. R. MUNTZ, Ada, has been stationed in the Hawaiian Islands for many months and has been kept busy. His assignment has been in general surgery. Major Muntz says that he has seen Lt. (sg) JOHN CUNNINGHAM, Oklahoma City, and spent some enjoyable time with him. (Editors Note: Since receiving this letter, we have had a visit from Lt. Cunningham who has returned to the States and is now stationed at the Norman Naval Base.)

LT. COLONEL W. H. AMSPACHER, Norman, 1936 graduate of the University of Oklahoma School of Medicine, is now stationed in England. Lt. Colonel Amspacher has previously had assignments in North Africa and Sicily.

MAJOR C. G. STUARD, Tulsa, Class of 1937, is Chief of the Eye Department in the Station Hospital at Greensboro, North Carolina. This month Major Stuard is going to New York to assist with the examinations of the American Board of Ophthalmology and hopes to see some of the Sooners there.

LT. (jg) RALPH ANDERSON, Tonkawa, has returned to the States after having spent some time in the Aleutians. He is visiting in Tonkawa before returning to San Francisco for reassignment.
Lt. Anderson graduated from the University of Oklahoma Medical School in 1942 and was called to active duty in July, 1943, leaving for overseas duty shortly thereafter. He says that most of the boys in the Aleutians were from Oklahoma, Texas and Louisiana and that all were very glad to get away from the chill breezes and back to a more temperate climate.

Home from the Anzio Beach Head is CAPTAIN CARSON L. OGLESBEE, Purcell. He is very glad to be back and says that he is "tired—dog tired." The days and nights of constant work have proved to be a great strain. Captain Oglesbee says, "But remember, we medics had an easier time than the boys in the actual fighting. Even though we were under shell fire often just like the others, they are the fellows . . . those men who attacked, who have suffered."

MAJOR D. J. LYONS, Seminole, was given an emergency leave to be at the bedside of his mother who is critically ill. Major Lyons has spent 28 months overseas and has participated in major combats on Guadalcanal. Recently he has been based in Australia .

MAJOR ROBERT E. ROBERTS, Stillwater, is stationed at a hospital in England. He states that he has an interesting assignment and is enjoying the country over there despite the fact that he is homesick.

CAPTAIN LAL D. THRELKELD, Oklahoma City, now serving with the medical corps in England, has a new daughter, Ann Margaret, born May 31.

DR. W. L. SHIPPEY, Poteau, has been retired from the Armed Forces because of ill health. Dr. Shippey has spent many months in India and it was there that he became ill. After spending some time in the hospital in India he was brought to the States where he was retained in an eastern hospital several weeks before his discharge.

CAPTAIN A. E. CULMER, JR., Oklahoma City, is on the staff of a hospital unit that recently had an ill fated landing in the South Pacific. Captain Culmer says that the boat ran aground and they were stranded many hours in South Pacific waters. Some of the men fished while waiting for transfer to other craft and none seemed excited over the situation despite the possible danger.

CAPTAIN PAUL S. ANDERSON, graduate of the University of Oklahoma School of Medicine in 1933, writes from his overseas assignment to say that he is receiving the Journal and letters and is enjoying them. He says that it seems to be the concensus of opinion that an Oklahoman should either be an Indian or a renegade cowboy.

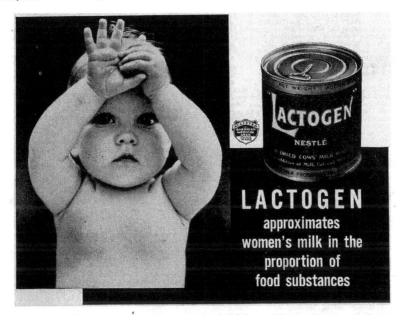

LACTOGEN
approximates
women's milk in the proportion of food substances

The cows' milk used for Lactogen is scientifically modified for infant feeding. This modification is effected by the addition of milk fat and milk sugar in definite proportions. When Lactogen is properly diluted with water it results in a formula containing the food substances—fat, carbohydrates, protein, and ash—in approximately the same proportion as they exist in women's milk.

One level tablespoon of LACTOGEN dissolved in 2 ounces of water (warm, previously boiled) makes 2 ounces of LACTOGEN formula yielding 20 calories per ounce.

No advertising or feeding directions, except to physicians. For feeding directions and prescription blanks, send your professional blank to "Lactogen Dept." Nestle's Milk Products, Inc., 155 East 44th St., New York.

> "My own belief is, as already stated, that the average well baby thrives best on artificial foods in which the relations of the fat, sugar, and protein in the mixture are similar to those in human milk."
>
> John Lovett Morse, A. M., M. D.
> Clinical Pediatrics, p. 156.

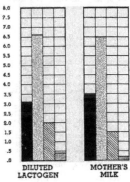

DILUTED LACTOGEN   MOTHER'S MILK

Fat   Carb.   Protein   Ash

NESTLÉ'S MILK PRODUCTS, INC.
155 EAST 44TH ST., NEW YORK, N. Y.

From "Somewhere in India" comes the following word from CAPTAIN R. O. SMITH, Hominy: "I hope the fight against the Wagner Bill is successful. It will be difficult enough to get readjusted to practice after the War, without having socialized medicine to contend with. I have not yet seen any of the Oklahoma 'docs' in this theatre. Have pretty well covered this country from stem to stern and the U.S.A. still looks awfully good to me."

LT. COMMANDER GEORGE M. DAVIS, Bixby, brother of Dr. Karl T. Davis, Pryor, has been commended by Admiral Chester W. Nimitz for his work during the recent Marshall Islands invasion. The citation was for "Exceptionally meritorious conduct in the performance of outstanding service to the government of the United States while serving on the division staff of the—censored—on Roi-Namur, Marshall Islands."
Lt. Commander Davis is a graduate of the University of Oklahoma School of Medicine and has been in the service since 1939.

CAPTAIN W. C. TISDAL, Clinton, has been transferred from the Prisoner of War Camp at Boswell, New Mexico, to Camp Fannin, Texas.

MAJOR RAYMOND H. FOX, Altus, is now Commanding Officer of the Station Hospital of Red River Ordnance at Texarkana, Texas.

University of Oklahoma School of Medicine

Dr. Anderson Nettleship, Associate Professor of Pathology, is attending a course in Tropical Medicine in the Army Medical School, Washington, D.C., during the months of May and June. This course is given under the auspices of the Association of American Medical Colleges.

Dr. Charles Allen Winter, Ph. D., has recently been appointed Assistant Professor of Physiology. Dr. Winter comes from the University of Iowa College of Medicine.

Capping Services were held in the auditorium of the Medical School on May 12. The following students received their caps: Virginia Allen, Weatherford; Mary Helen Brown, Ada; Alice Bryant, Seminole; Elizabeth Carpenter, Oklahoma City; Vera Dean Dick, Vinita; Ruth Eldridge, Skiatook; Helen Habr, Hanover; Mildred Hester, Oklahoma City; Helen Hinz, Camas; Leona Hollingshead, Blackwell; Mary Kincaid, Blackwell; Shirley Marrs, Oklahoma City; Patricia Miller, Hinton; Lillian Nagel, Lawton; Betty Lou O'Mara, Seminole; Marcene Peeler, Lone Wolf; Mildred Pillow, Oklahoma City; Mary Anna Paymer, Oklahoma City; Etta Vee Reeves, Disney, Billie Joe Rickerson, Durant; Bettye Savage, Oklahoma City; Shirley Shire, Medford; Carol Slaughter, Fairhope; Blanche Southwell, Custer; Margaret Strader, Oklahoma City; Velda Wilson, Okeene. Following the ceremony a reception was held in Cadet Hall for students, relatives and friends.

The first semester of the school year on the accelerated program was finished on May 5. Registration for the second semester took place on May 12 and 13. Class work began at 8 A.M., Monday, May 15.

Dr. O. Boyd Houchin, Instructor in Pharmacology, has recently resigned to accept the position of Assistant Professor of Biochemistry at Loyola University.

Dr. P. M. McNeill, Professor of Clinical Medicine, recently attended the College of Physicians Post-Graduate Course held in Columbus, Ohio, and Boston, Massachusetts.

At an early date the Library of the School of Medicine will have for distribution a list of books received since December 1, 1943. A copy of this list may be secured upon request. Following is a list of a few of the new books recently received in the Library:

Beaumont, G. E. & Dodds, E. C.—"Recent Advances in Medicine—11th Edition." 1943.

Bourne, A. W. & Williams, L. H.—"Recent Advances in Obstetrics and Gynaecology." 1942.

Bowden, A. E. & Gould, George—"Summary of State Legislation Requiring Pre-Natal Examinations for Venereal Diseases." 1944.

Dyke, C. G. & Davidoff, L. M.—"Roentgen Treatment of Diseases of the Nervous System." 1942.

Geckeler, E. O.—"Fractures and Dislocations for Practitioners." 1943

Grant, J. C. B.—"Atlas of Anatomy." 1943.

Higgins, C. C.—"Renal Lithiasis." 1943.

Hill, Justina—"Silent Enemies; Story of the Diseases of War and Their Control." 1942.

Hollander, Eugene—"Die Karikatur Und Satire in der Medizin. 2nd Edition." 1921.

Kolmer, J. A.—"Clinical Diagnosis by Laboratory Examinations." 1943.

Kretschmer, Ernest—"Textbook of Medical Psychology." 1934.

Landon-Brown, Walter and Hilton, R.—"Physiological Principles in Treatment—8th Edition." 1943.

Leonardo, R. A.—"History of Surgery." 1943.

McLester, J. S.—"Nutrition and Diet in Health and Disease—4th Edition." 1944.

Pattison, H. A.—"Rehabilitation of the Tuberculous." 1943.

Rowbotham, G. F.—"Acute Injuries of the Head." 1942.

Smout, C. F. V.—"Anatomy of the Female Pelvis." 1943.

Truby, A. E.—"Memoir of Walter Reed." 1943.

Wharton, L. R.—"Gynecology." 1943.

White, W. A.—"William Alanson White, the Autobiography of a Purpose." 1938.

Since January 1 the following articles have been published by members of the Faculty of the School of Medicine:

John H. Lamb, M.D., "Dermatomyositis." Journal of the Oklahoma State Medical Association. January, 1944.

Gregory E. Stanbro, M.D., "Cancer of the Breast." Journal of the Oklahoma State Medical Association. January, 1944.

Joseph M. Thuringer, M.D., "Histoplasmosis." Archives of Pathology. February, 1944.

Peter E. Russo, M.D., "Spontaneous Gastrocolic Fistula." Journal of the Oklahoma State Medical Association. February, 1944. Also, "Acute Suppurative Arthritis of the Hip in Childhood." American Journal of Roentgenology and Radium Therapy. April, 1944.

Alfred J. Ackerman, M.D., "Pulmonary and Osseous Manifestations of Tuberous Sclerosis, with Some Remarks on Their Pathogenesis." The American Journal of Roentgenology and Radium Therapy. March, 1944.

O. Boyd Houchin and Paul W. Smith, "Cardiac Insufficiency in the Vitamin E Deficiency Rabbit." The American Journal of Physiology, Vol. 141, No. 2. April 1, 1944.

E. Lachman, M.D., "The Anatomical Pathways for the Metastatic Spread of Cancer of the Breast." The Journal of the Oklahoma State Medical Association. April, 1944.

Gerald Rogers, M.D., "Surgical Complications of Pregnancy and Their Management." Journal of the Oklahoma State Medical Association. April, 1944.

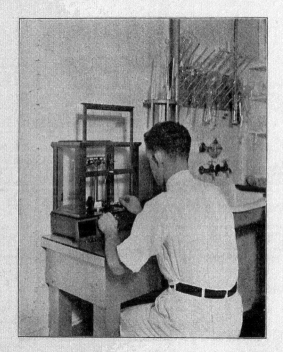

Woman's Auxiliary

State Officers of the Auxiliary 1944-1945

President ....Mrs. C. C. Young, Shawnee
Vice-President ....Mrs. Grider Penick, Oklahoma City
President Elect ....Mrs. J. W. Rogers, Tulsa
Secretary ....Mrs. Chas. W. Haygood, Shawnee
Treasurer ....Mrs. Clinton Gallaher, Shawnee
Historian ....Mrs. R. H. Mayes, Ada

The annual Oklahoma State Medical Association Convention was held in Tulsa, Oklahoma, April 24, 25 and 26 and arrangements for the Auxiliary Meeting was made by members of the Auxiliary to the Tulsa County Medical Society. Mrs. J. W. Rogers, Tulsa, was the general chairman of the entertainment committee for the wives of several hundred physicians from various parts of the State who attended the meeting. Mrs. John C. Perry, president of the Tulsa County Medical Auxiliary, entertained the State Executive Board at a buffet supper in her home, Monday evening. A business meeting of the State Board followed the supper.

Following the general 9:30 A.M. Tuesday session held on the mezzanine floor of the Mayo Hotel, a luncheon was given at 1 P.M. in the First Methodist Church. Ben Henneke, Director of the University of Tulsa Experimental Theater, assisted by Mrs. Ellen Eaves Henneke, presented a one-act play entitled ''Gas Light.'' The Past Board meeting was held following the luncheon.

Mrs. C. P. Bondurant, 1943-44 Treasurer, reported the purchase of nine Series F $100.00 War Bonds at the cost of $666.00 to mature in 12 years.

Mrs. Hugh Perry, Chairman of the Tray Committee reported the final award of the silver tray to Oklahoma City. This is the third year the Oklahoma County Auxiliary has been awarded the tray and it will remain the property of that Auxiliary.

Oklahoma County Annual Report

Mrs. Gregory Stanbro, President of the Annual County Auxiliary reported 115 paid members for 1943-44. Wives of service men who have temporarily moved from Oklahoma City are carried on the roster as of last year, without dues. Six regular meetings and two executive board meetings were held for the year, the average attendance being 30 to 35.

Social Service project for the year has been the making of surgical supplies for University Hospital. A total of 2,989 surgical dressings and 132 garments were completed. Fifteen scrap books were given to the patients at Crippled Childrens Hospital, the scrap books not being stressed this year due to the real need of surgical supplies. Four layettes were made from left over material. For the Thanksgiving shower fifty jars of home canning were given to one of the members whose home had been destroyed by fire. Forty-one subscriptions to Hygeia were reported. Money gifts for the year were: War Chest, $10.00; Red Cross, $15.00; Piano Fund, $10.00; Jane Todd Crawford Fund, $5.00. The Auxiliary manned a booth for six weeks for Bond Sales with a total of $25,450.00 in sales. The Auxiliary financed the buying of candy, cigarettes and other gifts for the inductees which were distributed by members of another organization meeting the troop trains, the total amount being expended was $35.00. A detailed report was given by Mrs. Joseph Kelso on other war activities with the total of 15,506 hours. A report of the purchase of $400.00 in War Bonds from the Auxiliary Funds. Doctors' Day was observed by the Auxiliary by members writing to a doctor in service and the setting aside of $60.00 for charitable purposes.

Pottawatomie County Report

The Auxiliary to the Pottawatomie County Medical Society completed its 37th year of activity. The membership consisted of 20 members with 16 being eligible for State membership. Of 11 subscriptions to Hygeia sold, nine were placed in the City Schools of Shawnee,

Oklahoma. War activity hours for the year totaled 5,280: Mrs. R. M. Anderson, County Chairman of Red Cross Surgical Dressings; Mrs. C. C. Young, WAVE Recruiter, Chairman of Old Clothes Drive; Mrs. Clinton Gallaher, Staff Assistant of Red Cross; Mrs. H. E. Hughes, Chairman of Activities of Army and Navy Women. Some members helped with Well Baby Clinics held each month.

Pontotoc County Report

The Pontotoc County Medical Auxiliary has a membership of 14 members with an average attendance of 12. The programs during the year have been educational. The superintendent of the Valley View Hospital discussed the ''Blue Cross Plan for Hospitalization.'' A speaker from the Public Health Unit presented a plan for a Well Baby Clinic and several of the members attended a clinic. The Wagner-Murray-Dingell Bill has been discussed in order to be better informed as to its purpose. Also discussed were the Articles in Hygeia Magazine.

Practically all of the members are engaged in some kind of War Work. During the past year the Auxiliary During the past year the Auxiliary has put in a total of 2,041 hours. Mrs. C. F. Needham is Chairman of Pontotoc County Red Cross Surgical Dressings and of course, leads the way for us by putting in many hours at that work. One member is back on full time duty at the hospital to relieve the acute shortage of nurses. Three members are helping in their husbands offices. We have placed the Hygeia in the Valley View Hospital and the U.S.O. reading room and have purchased one War Bond.

Cleveland County Report

Cleveland County has a paid membership of 18, five of this number being honorary, i. e., State and National dues paid by the Auxiliary for the wives of Doctors who are serving overseas. Fourteen Hygeia subscriptions were given to rural schools, Norman City Library and the Norman U. S. O. Club.

One of the projects is the sponsoring of Red Cross Home Nursing classes. A classroom in McFarland Memorial Church is equipped by Auxiliary members. We organized and supervised the classes. This year we have had classes in Noble Highschool and in Norman Highschool.

Five dollars was donated to the Blood Plasma Fund, and the March of Dimes; helped with the Greek Relief and Russian Clothes Drive; helped with the repairing and packing for shipping of these garments. The approximate number of hours total 820.

Tulsa County Report

Mrs. John C. Perry, President of the Tulsa County Auxiliary reported 121 members, of which eight members, whose husbands are with the Armed Forces, we exempt from all dues. There has been an average attendance of 43.

Meetings are held monthly but on account of our gas rationing and surgical dressings, half of the meetings were held in the homes following a luncheon served by five hostesses. The rest were held at the Oklahoma Natural Gas and Public Service Clubrooms, with each member bringing sandwiches and cookies. Coffee was served by two hostesses.

An executive board meeting has been held each month preceding our regular Auxiliary meeting. The board meetings have been well attended, committee reports and plans for the coming meetings were discussed. Programs have been most timely and helpful, and have been subjects to include our wartime needs.

The Philanthropic Committee had for their project the collection of the toys for the Children's Christmas parties at St. John and Hillcrest Hospitals and also made investigation and found the cost to be $50.00 which the Auxiliary voted to give to bring to date the loose leaf book in medicine by Tice for the Doctor's Library.

The Public Relations Committee presented their annual Program. A very enlightening talk from the layman's point of view on Bill 1161, the Wagner-Murray-Dingell Bill, was given by our own Dr. Donald L. Mishler. George Sarimento spoke on ''Relations between

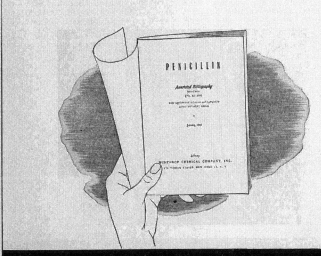

North and Latin Americans.'' Principals of the Senior and Junior High Schools were guests for the luncheon and program.

A donation was made to the Babies Milk Fund in memory of Dr. C. E. Bradley. Also financial gifts to Tulsa D.A.R. for Blood Plasma Bank in memory of Drs. Fred Cronk and Fred Bolton.

The Hygeia Comittee has placed 59 subscriptions to Hygeia in the schools all over the city and county. The War Aid Committee worked very efficiently in distributing and collecting questionaires, which made a splendid report for the year's work. Sixteen members are filling jobs, thereby releasing someone for War Work. One member has graduated over 700 people in Home Nursing classes since Pearl Harbor. Another member, a graduate dietitian, was Chairman of the Red Cross Nutrition Committee of Tulsa County, teaching Nutrition and Canteen classes which include over 3,000 women. She is Vice-President of the Oklahoma Dietetic Association and Treasurer of the Oklahoma Home Economics Association.

We have sent boxes to soldiers in hospitals at Christmas and some members have been continuing this. Several members are following a study of our International Relations and Peace Planning. By such study we hope to be more intelligent and helpful in the year to come. Also for the March of Dimes, a demonstration of the Hot Pack System was given to 1,800 girls and a sum of $350.00 was raised. This year for the first time a team was selected among the doctors and the Auxiliary for the Tulsa Community Drive to call upon their own members. This was most gratifying as they secured $2,077.00 in pledges and cash. The Auxiliary responded to the call of Mrs. Lahah of the Army Mothers and sent Christmas boxes to the wounded soldiers at Chickasha.

During the year the Auxiliary suffered the loss of one of its oldest members, Mrs. W. Albert Cook.

AMERICAN MEDICAL ASSOCIATION JOURNAL LISTED 20 PHYSICIANS KILLED IN ACTION DURING 1943

Out of 3,156 obituaries of physicians published in The Journal of the American Medical Association during 1943, there were 20 physicians who died in action in World War II and 105 of those who died while in military service, The Journal announces in its January 1 issue. The Journal says, however, that it believes that the military deaths listed represent a small percentage of those recorded in Washington but not yet released for publication. Analyzing the data on the published obituaries The Journal says that whereas 3,156 were published 'The American Medical Directory Report Service, including the United State, possessions and Canada, recorded 3,582 deaths. Of this total, 189 were Canadians, a group omitted this year from the regular obituary columns. Deducting the Canadians, a total of 237 deaths more is shown in the Report Service than were included in the published notices in The Journal.

''The introduction of the accelerated program for medical students during 1942 precludes an attempt at this time to estimate accurately the net increase to the profession. An increase, however, can be assumed. As of August 14 the graduation of 5,223 students had been recorded. The expected annual average total of students to graduate under the three year accelerated program is 7,000, the heaviest total falling in 1943, when two graduations a year launched the program. On January 1, 1944 the estimated physician population of the United States, exclusive of possessions and temporary foreign, is 188, 159.

''*Age*—The average age at death was 65.2 in 1943, as compared with 65.0 in 1942 for 3,211 deaths published in The Journal. Thirty-nine physicians died between the ages of 25 and 29. Forty-nine between 30 and 34, 71 between 35 and 39, 93 between 40 and 44, 126

between 45 and 49, 158 between 50 and 54, 270 between 55 and 59, 396 btween 60 and 64, 545 between 65 and 69, 543 between 70 and 74, 371 between 75 and 79, 265 between 80 and 84, 173 between 85 and 89, 46 between 90 and 94, 9 between 95 and 99 and 2 of 100 or over.

''*Causes*—Heart disease continues to lead the causes of death among physicians. As is customary, when a contributary factor was returned with a primary cause, both conditions were recorded. Coronary thrombosis and occlusion accounted for 598 deaths, of which 218 occurred in the age group 60 to 69. Angina pectoris and other coronary diseases totaled 136, chronic heart valvular disease and rheumatic heart disease 35, subacute bacterial endocarditis (except rheumatic fever) 11, diseases of the myocardium and pericardium 213, and other diseases of the heart 401 . . .

''*Accidental Deaths*—Of 117 accidental deaths, automobile accidents accounted for 41. Falls were involved in 33 deaths, airplane accidents 22, trains 6, burns 6, bullet wounds 4, drowning 2, asphyxiation 1 and drugs 1. Fractures, which were also included under falls, were of the skull, hip and femur, 13 being recorded for the hip alone. There was one unexplained fracture. Of the unusual accidents which have been entered under a general classification, 1 physician was killed in a fall from a horse, 1 tripped over a rifle when hunting, 1 died of a skull fracture received during the Detroit race riot and 3 from burns received when they fell asleep while smoking.

''*Suicides and Homicides*—Forty suicides were recorded. Bullet wounds led in the method selected with 16, poison 7, drugs 5, cut arteries 4, carbon monoxide 2, drowning 2, hanging 2 and illumination gas 1. One suidice was unexplained. Shooting was the method in the 4 homicides in the civilian group of physicians.

''*Miscellaneous Positions*—Among the decedents were 253 who had been teachers in medical schools, 150 of whom had reached the professional rank;; there were 5 deans, 1 associate dean, 1 president of a university and 1 teacher in a public school. One hundred and ninety-one had been health officers, 127 members of boards of health, 116 members of boards of education, 66 coroners, 65 mayors, 63 pharmacists, 45 authors, 35 bank presidents, 33 legislators, 24 members of city councils, 20 editors, 11 members of police department, 9 clergymen, 9 postmasters, 8 missionaries, 8 lawyers, 6 dentists, 3 members of fire departments, 3 judges, 2 justices of the peace, 2 village presidents, and 1 each had been governor, intern, sheriff and alderman. One had been a member of the Austrian army, 1 chief medical officer of the Supreme Bench of Baltimore, 1 vice consul of Argentina, 1 U. S. minister to Liberia, and 1 a commercial flight surgeon.

''Of the total of 3,156 physicians, 558 had served in World War I, 6 in the Spanish American War, 7 in the Civil War and 2 each in the Boxer Rebellion (China), the Boer War and the Philippine Insurrection. Thirty-two were members of the U. S. Public Health Service, 26 of the U. S. Army and 17 each of the Navy, Veterans Administration and Indian Service. Four were in the Air Corps. Twenty-seven were classified in the Army Medical Reserve Corps and 57 not on active duty, 21 were listed in the Navy Medical Reserve Corps, 2 not on active duty. Ten were in the Public Health Service Reserve. Fifty-two were classified in the medical corps of the Army of the United States, 11 not on active duty. Thirty-four were reported in the National Guard; 2 Navy men were assigned to the Marine Corps. Thirty-nine had been members of draft boards in World War I and 84 in World War II . . .

''*Military Service*—Twenty physicians died in action in World War II and 105 while in military service. One, aged 26, who died in the unexplained explosion of the Escanaba, was classified as 'killed while in military service.' One, aged 29, serving with the medical corps of the Royal Army, died in action while serving in the front line during the advance in Egypt. Five died in the Pacific, 9 in the Solomon Islands, including

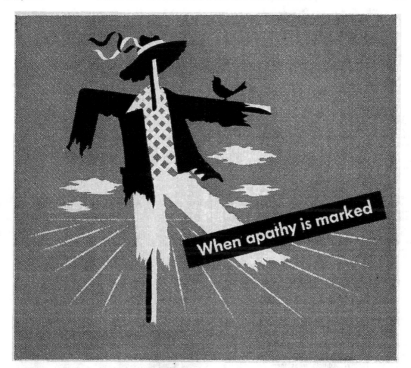

In patients with marked apathy and associated low muscle tone and low resistance, dramatic response may often be effected by adrenal cortex therapy when these symptoms are due to adrenal cortical insufficiency.

Adrenal Cortex Extract (Upjohn) used as replacement therapy in these cases often restores alertness and a healthy outlook. It relieves asthenia, strikingly increases resistance to infection, improves capacity for work, and strengthens muscle tone. Available for subcutaneous, intramuscular, and intravenous therapy.

Adrenal Cortex Extract (Upjohn)

Sterile solution in 10 cc. rubber-capped vials for subcutaneous, intramuscular and intravenous therapy

ANOTHER WAY TO SAVE LIVES . . . BUY WAR BONDS FOR VICTORY

4 in Guadalcanal, 4 in the North African area, 1 in Sicily and 1 in a torpedoing off the coast of Cape May, N. J. Of 2 merchant Marine causalties, both died in torpedoings, 1 in the North Atlantic and 1 off Iceland. Of those killed in action, 8 were between the ages of 25 and 29, 6 between 32 and 34, 1 between 35 and 39, 2 between 40 and 44, 1 between 40 and 54, 1 between 55 and 59, and 1 in the age group 60 to 64. Of those who were classified under military service, 21 died between the ages of 25 and 29, 18 between 30 and 34, 25 between 35 and 39, 15 between 40 and 44, 10 between 45 and 49, 4 between 50 and 54, 6 between 55 and 59, 5 between 60 and 64 and 1 between 65 and 69. Of the deaths in military service, 12 were attributed to coronary thrombosis or occulusion 7 to heart disease, 1 to cerebral embolism, 5 to bullet wounds, which are also included in 6 recorded sucides, 24 to airplane accidents, 2 to burns, 4 to automobile accidents, 1 to virus pneumonit, 2 to encephalitis, 7 to some form of pneumonia, 1 to alcoholism, 1 in a bomber crash, 2 to homicide, 1 to drowning, 2 to brain tumor, 3 to meiningitis, 1 to carcinoma of the brain, 4 to other types of cancer, 2 to malaria and 1 to bacterial endocarditis. The rest were classified under various physical conditions. In 1942 the obituaries of 11 physicians who died in action were publish in The Journal and 37 of those who died while in military service. Thus The Journal notices the record 31 physicians who died in action during the two year period 1942-43 and 142 who died while in military service. The Journal does not believe that the analysis of the military deaths reflects a true picture of the situation as a whole and believes that the group represents a small percentage of those recorded in Washington but not yet releases for publication.

"The total of 3,156 physicians includes 1 who died in Missouri but who had been a missionary in the Belgian Congo, 1 in Alaska, 1 in Switzerland, 1 in Edmonton, Canada, and 1 in Newfoundland. An editorial entitled 'When and How Physicians Die,' published in 1903, was the first review of deaths of physicians by The Journal. A total of 1,400 physicians gave an average age of death of 58.

NARCOTIC "DONT'S FOR THE PHARMACIST

Don't leave prescription pads around. Caution the doctors you supply. Addicts want them for effecting narcotic forgeries.

Don't leave narcotics exposed near your wrapping counter. Drugs disappear this way. Check receipts on your order forms.

Don't accept a narcotic prescription written in pencil. It is not a valid order even when written by a physician.

Don't fail to scrutinize prescriptions when written thus: Morph. HT ½ oN. X or Morph. HT ¼ No. 10. Several X's or zeros can be added to raise amounts. Spelling or brackets obviate this possibility.

Don't carry a large stock of narcotics. Only a three months' supply is good practice. Addicts are breaking into pharmacies and hospitals to get their drug needs.

Don't leave the key inserted in the lock of your narcotic cabinet. Keep cabinet locked. Make it harder to effect robberies. Keep excess stock in a safe if possible.

Don't place your narcotic stock where it is accessible to others. Avoid storage near sink or toilet. Customers may ask to use these.

Don't leave anyone alone in the back of your store if you can avoid it. Cabinets have been pilfered this way. Addicts pose as salesmen or ask to use your back room.

Don't become rattled by a rush request to fill a narcotic prescription. Claim for emergency use may be made to create confusion and pass a forgery.

Don't be taken in by a person wearing a white uniform presenting a narcotic prescription. Addicts have posed as nurses to mislead pharmacist and place them off guard.

Don't fill telephone orders for narcotics unless you are assured that prescription will be available upon delivery. Bogus doctor calls are made to effect delivery to addicts. Watch change racket along with this method.

Don't fill prescriptions for unusual quantities of narcotics unless checked with physician. Diversion to addicts is a profitable business, as much as $1 for ¼ grain MS.

Don't refill narcotic prescriptions without getting a new prescription. Fairly large shortages eventually occur through this practice.

Don't hesitate to call the physician about a narcotic prescription you may be questioning. The pharmacist is held responsible for filling forgeries. The doctor's cooperation should be sought.

Don't supply a doctor with his office narcotic needs on a prescription blank (except solutions on order forms) The law requires him to use an Official Order Form filled by a wholesaler.

Don't dispense any exempt narcotics without keeping a record. You must account for the distribution of your purchases.

Don't break the law to accomodate others or for business expediency. Explain the regulations. The customer or physician will cooperate if he sees the point.—*New York State Journal of Medicine, May 15.*

A man moved to a new boarding-house. After a week, he confessed to a fellow boarder that he could never remember the landlady's name. Said the other, "That's easy. Her name is Womack. Rhyme it with stomach. Here's where you get your stomach fed. Womack stomach."

The new boarder was grateful and the next morning when he came down to breakfast, he called out cheerily, "Good morning, Mrs. Kelly."—Eleanor M. Garrett.

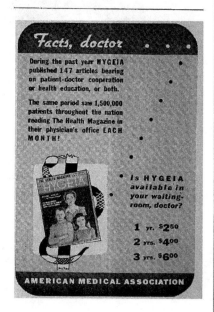

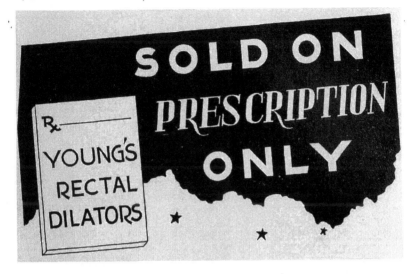
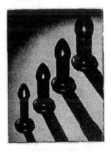

BOOK REVIEWS

"The chief glory of every people arises from its authors."—Dr. Samuel Johnson.

CIVILIZAION AND DISEASE. Henry E. Sigerist, M.D., D. Litt., LL.D. Cornell University Press, Ithica, New York. 255 pages. Price $3.75.

This is an engaging chronicle of civilization, conditioned by the fitful friction of abnormal stimuli resulting in many facinating facets. The introduction is a masterpiece in orientation. It identifies man with his origin, properly places him in history, relates his life to heredity and environment and aptly depicts the conditioning influence of each of these two factors.

The scope of this interesting volume is to some extent indicated by the following list of chapters; Civilization as a Factor in the Genesis of Disease; Disease and Economics; Disease and Social Life; Disease and the Law; Disease and History; Disease and Religion; Disease and Philosophy; Disease and Science; Disease and Literature; Disease and Art; Disease and Music; Civilization Against Disease.

In the opinion of the reviewer the book might have taken on a more facinating role if the author had supplemented the historical facts with a bit of justifiable romancing with reference to the conditioning influence of disease upon important personalities and upon the course of civilization.

This is a book every doctor should read. In the closing chapters the author expresses a broad viewpoint with reference to universal medical service to the rich and poor in keeping with the optimism of those doctors who have never had general professional contact with either the rich or the poor.—Lewis J. Moorman, M.D.

HANDBOOK OF NUTRITION. A Symposium Prepared Under the Auspices of the Council on Foods and Nutrition of the American Medical Association. 586 pages. American Medical Association, Chicago, 1943. $2.50.

This particular handbook represents the reprinting of a series of articles which appeared in various issues of the Journal of the American Medical Association. It is fortunate that these articles on the various phases of nutrition have been collected and compiled into one single volume.

Inasmuch as nutrition is the most important factor of life during both health and disease, the contents of this single volume should appeal to all of those interested in this widely discussed, present-day subject. The articles are written by a group of 28 contributors, professors of medical schools and men directly engaged in research work—all outstanding figures in the world of nutrition. "The advances which have been made in the science of nutrition during the past few years fire the imagination. . . . Finally, there has developed a clearer understanding of the deficiency states with a fuller appreciation of the frequency with which these states impair man's usefulness and destroy his happiness. This marks an era of signal achievement."

It is worthy of consideration to note that protein is characterized as "unquestionably the most important of all known substances in the organic kingdom. Without it no life appears possible on our planet." In addition, other topics discussed include the role of fat in the diet, calories, mineral elements and vitamins. There are also chapters on foods of plants and animal origin, food processing, feeding of children and the aged, and principles of diet in the tretatment of disease. The follow-

ing is an interesting observation with reference to the American diet: "Food habits vary from place to place and from season to season. They differ from family to family too, reflecting economic circumstances and cultural backgrounds. Even within a single family group diets of individuals vary more than is generally realized."—Anne Betche.

CECIL'S MEDICINE—NEW SIXTH EDITION. Edited by Russell L. Cecil of Cornell University, written by 154 American authorities. W. B. Saunders Company. Illustrated. 1566 pages. Price $9.50.

If science were as stagnant now as it was when the teachings of Hippocrates and Galen were above question, this book could not have run through six editions in such a short time. The modernization of medicine necessarily requires new and revised editions of important tests in order to keep up with the rapid progress of medicine.

The First Edition of Cecil's Medicine appeared in 1927 with numerous collaborators under the editorship and authorship of Russell A. Cecil, and now comes the Sixth Edition with Cecil still editor but with 154 collaborators, all men chosen because of their particular interest, experience, and reputation in the field allocated to them. These co-authors could be readily recognized as belonging to "Who's Who" in American medicine.

This new tome has changed considerably in format. It is larger, both in length and breadth (7"x10"). It has 1566 pages, while the Fifth Edition had 1744 pages. A most striking innovation is that each page has two columns. This seems to be an idea which publishers of educational books think is less confusing and easier to read with these shorter lines. The type is not smaller but more printing can be done on the same number of pages. Bibliography follows each article, so that further research is made easier. Dosage is by the metric system, in keeping with newer pharmacopedias, but most of the authors give the apothecaries equivalent in parenthesis. There are three pages of normal values for values for laboratory reports, which makes it easily accessible when the reader is not clear about the facts.

In keeping with war medicine, quite a few new and revised articles are added, such as aviation medicine, seasickness, and air sickness. Disease from animal parasites, which will be introduced to many doctors with patients from the far-flung battle lines. Internationalism is confronting the medical profession in many ways now, and these new diseases must be diagnosed and treated.

Since heart diseases are coming on more with the stress of war and the length of life, this section is revised and increased so that the busy practitioner can get a good nosology in the terse handling of the subject. The elucidation of peripheral vascular diseases of both arteries and veins, have been considered and integral part of circulatory troubles, and handled under one authorship. The sections devoted to mental disorders and somatic neurology have been enriched and increased.

Many new authors appear in this edition and much of the text has been rewritten. I would think it favorable for every student of medicine, either in college or active practice, to have this edition.—Lea A. Riely, M.D.

The health of the people is really the foundation upon which all their powers as a State depend. — Benjamin Disraeli.

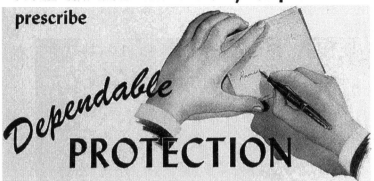
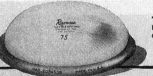
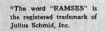

CHICAGOAN SAYS BASIC FACTS BEING IGNORED IN EVALUATION OF POLIOMYELITIS

The amount of ultimate recovery from acute infantile paralysis depends primarily on the degree of initial involvement of the central nervous system rather than on the type of treatment, Mary S. Sherman, M.D., of the Departmnt of Surgery, Division of Orthopedic Surgery, University of Chicago, declares in The Journal of the American Medical Association for May 13. She reports a study of 70 unselected patients during the 1943 epidemic in Chicago who received only supportive treatment. Fifty-one, or 72.8 per cent, had no residual weakness or such slight weakness that it was barely detectable.

Dr. Sherman believes that consideration of some obvious basic facts about infantile paralysis seems lately to have been abandoned. She points out that back in 1913 attention was called to the high incidence of nonparalytic poliomyelitis which, after a study of 1,025 European records. was conservatively estimated at 25 to 56 per cent of all cases.

"This group, which varies with the epidemic," Dr. Sherman says, "obviously affects the recovery rate, and no appraisal of results of any treatment can be made without an accurate statement as to the number of cases which were of this type.

"It has also been known for years that epidemics vary not only as to geographic but also as to the attack rate, the severity of general symptoms, the incidence of bulbar involvement (affecting the muscles of breathing). the incidence and severity of paralysis and, of course, the mortality. . . . In general, the death rates in recent years have been always lower than in the older epidemics. This appears to be due to the recognition of abortive cases (in which no symptoms of parlysis appear), which formerly were not usually reported even when they were recognized.

"Until recently there has never been any disagreement with the idea that the percentage of recovery, depending as it does on the factors just outlined, also varies with the epidemic rather than with the treatment. This is borne out by reports from many locations. . . ." She cites several reports of recovery rates ranging from 70 to 85 per cent, all of them in groups receiving the so-called orthodox treatment.

Discussing the 70 Chicago patients, Dr. Sherman says her paper is a report of the group six months after their acute attack. She explains that "Obviously this is too short an interval to permit a conclusive study. However, it can surely be assumed that the nonparalytic will not change, and since all the other survivors of this group seem now to be stationary or progressing satisfactory it is unlikely that future examinations will reveal much change except for improvement. . . .

"All patients . . . were kept at absolute bed rest with as nearly normal a diet as possible. . . . They were disturbed only for rapid physical examinations, and often these were done several times daily. These examinations apparently had no effect on the extent or duration of muscle weakness. . . . As 'spasm' and stiffness of the back and hamstrings appeared to be present in all cases, and since they seemed of no significance except as symptoms, no treatment was directed toward them. These manifestations disappeared spontaneously in every case within a few weeks, . . ."

Ten per cent of the 70 patients had enough residual weakness to require braces or future surgery; 86 per cent had functionally significant weakness which does not require further treatment and which does not constitute a handicap to normal life. There were six deaths (8.6 per cent). The average hospital stay, excluding the fatal cases, but including readmissions for supervised physica lactivity, was 17.9 days.

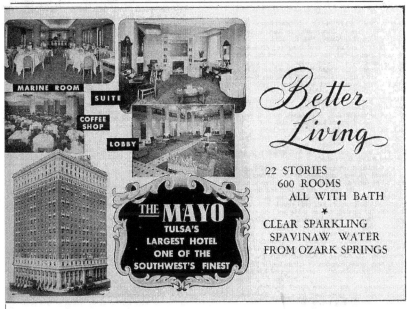

MEDICAL ABSTRACTS

"TRAUMATIC SURGERY. A REVIEW OF SOME BONE AND JOINT INJURIES IN WARTIME." A. G. Ord. Ralph Shackman, and H. L. M. Toualle. Surgery. XIV. 651. 1943.

Injuries treated by the authors occurred in service men during training, or, together with some that occurred among women, while in action on the home front. During the years 1940 to 1941, a total of 258 fractures of all types and 21 dislocations came under observation of these British surgeons. Standing methods of splinting, with or without skeletal traction, were used.

The authors advocated:

1. Early excision of the radial head where irregularity of the articular surface may lead to a progressive arthritis.

2. Grafting fractures of the scaphoid bone where they have been untreated for six months or longer.

3. Reconstruction of the coraco-acromial joint in severe displacements, rather than simply attempting to restore the acromioclavicular ligaments.

4. Ambulatory treatment in fractures of the lower limbs.

5. Taking repeated roentgenograms, and using a rapid developer, in preference to using the fluoroscope during manipulations or bone-grafting operations.—E. D. M., M.D.

"FRACTURAS EXPUESTAS (COMPOUND FRACTURES)." Juan B. Carpanelli. La Revista de Medicina y Ciencias Afines. Vol. 6. 1943.

The author begins by explaining the difference between open, compound, and other forms of fractures. A fracture is compound when bone fragments protrude from the edge of the wound or are found on its surface. The particular types of compound fractures the author mentions are those caused by firearms, vehicular collisions, and industrial accident.

Due to gravity of compound fractures, emergency treatment, consisting of anti-infection therapy, reduction, and immobilization, is essential. Chronic suppuration is the most frequent local complication of compound fractures. Infection is successfully combated, if treatment is started within six to eight hours after the occurrence of the accident. In a compound fracture, the wound can be closed, if the anti-infection procedure is started within that period.

Good treatment requires that the degree of shock and the general physical condition of the patient be determined as early as possible. The anesthetics to be used must depend on the age of the patient and the type of fracture. Foreign bodies should be removed; deep sutures should be avoided; and only vessels of heavy caliber should be ligated, torsion being used in all others. Caustic antiseptics should be avoided, and wherever possible, use should be made of the antiseptics suggested by Albert Key, and Frankel. These suggestions include the use of powered sulfonamides for connective tissues, muscles, and joints, while solutions of sulfonamides are recommended for pleurae and peritoneum.

It is best to use mixtures of sulfanilamide and sulfathiazole when available. Roentgenographic control is as indispensable as are frequent and complete physical examinations, for the success of the treatment.

Good circulation is favored by appropriate position, adequate warmth, and active movement of distal seg-

ments. The fracture should be immobilized for as long a time as may be necessary to obtain the best results, consideration being given to the possible existence of soft callouses. Local immobilization serves best the healing process of wounds and fractures, but there can be no objection to accelerated general mobilization and respiratory gymnastics, which may be begun at the bedside of the patient. The patient is encouraged to get up as soon as his condition permits.—E. D. M., M.D.

"THE VALUE OF ROENTGEN THERAPY IN CARCINOMATOUS METASTASES TO BONE." Edward C. Koenig and Gordon J. Culver. Radiology. Vol. XLI. No. 38. 1943.

Roentgenotherapy in metastatic carcinomata to bone is justified by the relief of pain and prolongation of life. Borak classifies these lesions into two groups:

1. Those which involve bone alone, producing local pain through periosteal involvement;

2. Those which involve the paraskeletal lymphatics or bone in such a way as to press on nerves, producing neuritic pain. Thus skeletal changes can be present without pain, and pain can be present without skeletal changes. Routine roentgenography of the skeleton, particularly of the pelvis and lower spine in breast lesions, is indicated, even when symptomatic. Also, in a case without roentgenographic findings, where it is felt that pain is a result of skeletal changes, roentgenotherapy is indicated.

The pathological processes are described:

1. The local destructive effect of the neoplastic cells.

2. The reaction of the inflammatory zone.

Borak's thesis, that the effect produced is only upon the non-specific inflammatory reaction and on the malignant process, is considered more likely than Leddy's additional proposition of action on nerves, since hyperaesthesia of the skin is often a result of the exposure of non-pathological tissue to roentgen rays. The immediate relief of pain is attributed to the effect of the roentgen ray on the inflammatory reaction. This may be seen in five to ten days after the first treatment. A later effect, attributable to the action on the malignant cells, is also seen.

The authors feel with Borak that bone metastases are not as radio-resistant as supposed. They have noted recalcification following irradiation. The measure to be used, however, in treating the patient, is his general condition and not the roentgenographic findings. Patients in good health, even with extensive lesions, represent better risks than the cachectic patient. The effect to be expected are regression of the lesion, alleviation of pain, improvement in the general condition, and prolongation of life.—E. D. M., M.D.

"VITAMIN E (WHEAT GERM OIL IN THE TREATMENT OF INTERSTITIAL KERATITIS. Simon Stone. Archives of Ophthalmology. Vol. 30, page 467- 475. October. 1943.

Interstitial keratitis remains one of the most frequently encountered complications of late congenital syphilis. The fact that it is most resistant to antisyphilitic therapy has brought fourth the suggestion that other factors besides spirochetal invasion of the cornea are responsible. Many contributing factors have been considered. Success with sulfanilamide treatment and with

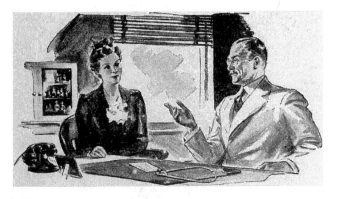

IN THE *Progressive*
NUTRITIONAL NEEDS OF GESTATION

While it is not strictly true that the gravid woman must "eat for two," nutritional requirements nevertheless are higher during pregnancy. As the fetus increases in size, its nutritional demands increase. In consequence, food consumption must be progressively raised to prevent catabolic breakdown of maternal tissue to satisfy these needs.

Ovaltine proves of real value as an aid in satisfying the greater nutritional needs during pregnancy. This delicious food drink proves appealing during this period when anorexia may seriously curtail food consumption. It supplies the nutrients especially required for proper fetal growth—minerals, vitamins, and biologically adequate proteins. Prescribed during the second and third trimesters, Ovaltine helps promote a state of optimum nutrition in the mother and optimum development of the fetus.

THE WANDER COMPANY, 360 North Michigan Avenue, Chicago 1, Illinois

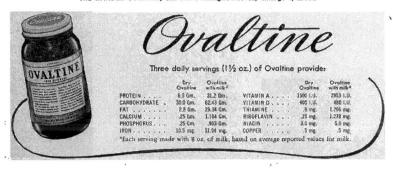

Three daily servings (1½ oz.) of Ovaltine provide:

	Dry Ovaltine	Ovaltine with milk*		Dry Ovaltine	Ovaltine with milk*
PROTEIN	6.0 Gm.	31.2 Gm.	VITAMIN A	1500 I.U.	2953 I.U.
CARBOHYDRATE	30.0 Gm.	62.43 Gm.	VITAMIN D	405 I.U.	480 I.U.
FAT	2.8 Gm.	29.34 Gm.	THIAMINE	.9 mg.	1.296 mg.
CALCIUM	.25 Gm.	1.104 Gm.	RIBOFLAVIN	.25 mg.	1.278 mg.
PHOSPHORUS	.25 Gm.	.903 Gm.	NIACIN	3.0 mg.	5.0 mg.
IRON	10.5 mg.	11.94 mg.	COPPER	.5 mg.	.5 mg.

*Each serving made with 8 oz. of milk; based on average reported values for milk.

the use of riboflavin suggested a mixed infection as well as a possible dietary deficiency.

The authors, based upon reports of increased absorption of tissue exudates after Vitamin E treatment, began to experiment with Vitamin E treatment in cases of resistant interstitial keratitis. The Vitamin E was administered in the form of 50 mg. mixed tocopherol capsules, one capsule once or twice daily, usually in combination with one or two capsules of Vitamin B complex. With improvement in the patient's condition this dose was gradually reduced, so that in the end a maintenance dose of 50 to 100 mg. of mixed tocopherols weekly appeared ample. Several patients received this combined vitamin therapy for twelve to eighteen months.

Ten patients were treated; all had received ample antisyphilitic therapy in the past. Four had received artificial fever therapy a number of months earlier because of associated involvement of the central nervous system without its markedly affecting the course of the keratitis. Two patients were given artificial fever treatments shortly after therapy with Vitamin E was begun.

Vitamin E was effective in hastening absorption of superficial and deep corneal exudates; it helped to relieve the associated photophobia and reduce excessive corneal vascularization and circumcorneal congestion. In cases of longstanding involvement with extensive opacities and corneal scarring, its administration for a period of months has produced a gradual and continuous clearing of the cornea with a return of normal vision. In one case complete clearing of the cornea occurred after eighteen months of vitamin therapy although only perception of light was present in one eye and perception of fingers in the other when therapy was begun. Absorption of corneal exudates and return of normal vision took place in another case after four weeks of vitamin therapy alone.

Riboflavin when administered alone or in combination with Vitamin E was effective primarily in relieving some of the photophobia and reducing the extent of circumcorneal injection and capillary proliferation. It had no effect on the absorption of corneal opacities and scars.

From these experiments it seems that Vitamin E combined with Vitamin B Complex is a most valuable adjunct in the treatment of interstitial keratitis. If the patient has received ample treatment in the past, antisyphilitic therapy is apparently not needed to produce complete disappearance of the visual symptoms and corneal opacities of interstitial keratitis. Artificial fever therapy is of value mainly in preventing relapses and in producing more rapid amelioration of acute symptoms. It has little effect when administered alone on the rate of absorption of corneal opacities of long standing.—M. D. H., M.D.

"CLINICAL EVALUATION OF TENDERNESS OF THE MASTOID. Harry Rosenwasser. Archives of Otolaryngology. Vol. 38, pages 447-452. November, 1943. Tenderness is one of the most important and most constant signs of disease of the mastoid. Yet, it may be absent in some cases, and it may be modified by general and local factors in others.

Patients may be hyposensitive or hypersensitive. Pressure over the styloid process may show how a person reacts to pain. Past history is another guide to evaluate a patient's sensory make-up. A hyposensitive person minimizes his symptoms, and the surgeon may find a far greater destruction than suspected. In a hypersensitive individual even pressure exerted on the normal scalp or over the uninvolved mastoid process may cause great pain.

Tenderness is best elicited by using the same degree of pressure on both mastoids. The pressure should be slowly applied with the pad of thumb, with avoidance of the use of the finger nail, and the facial expression

of the patient watched. Not infrequently tenderness will be manifested by wincing, if the attention of the patient tested is distracted elsewhere. Tenderness, if real, should be persistent. One should remember that pain is frequently anticipated and the prospect causes flinching to occur before significant pressure is made. The confidence and cooperation of the patient must be secured; otherwise it is safer to minimize the significance of this sign and attempt to establish the diagnosis from other available data.

Neurosis can exist side by side with serious organic disease and at times the serious organic disease may cause a latent neurosis to come to the surface. If the history and the clinical signs and symptoms give reason to suspect neurotic simulation of tenderness over the mastoid, in the absence of other urgent indications for intervention, one should not hesitate to resort to the aid of a trained psychiatrist.

During the administration of sulfanilamide and its derivatives, certain changes in the classic signs and symptoms of mastoiditis have been observed. One of the most stricking is the effect of sulfanilamide on tenderness of the mastoid. It is, therefore important to know whether a patient has had or is still receiving chemotherapy. Modified criteria of diagnosis must be established in order that administration of the drugs can be continued for their best effort when complications are imminent and not discontinued, as seems too commonly done, for fear of masking symptoms.

Tenderness occasionally disappears or becomes greatly diminished after irradiation of the mastoid. This is a temporary masking effect similar to that caused by sulfanilamide, and consequently it must be considered in evaluating mastoid tenderness. Many roentgenologists feel that the irradiation which results during making one or two roentgenograms is totally inadequate as a therapeutic agent.

Small circumscribed inflamed lymph nodes over the tip or antrum of the mastoid process may frequently be extremely tender. In such cases, the pressure on the mastoid should be made as far removed as possible from the site of the nodes. Wet dressings could be also applied to see whether the tenderness disappears with the subsidence of lymphadenitis.

It is also known that diabetic patients with extensive disease of the mastoid have no evidence of mastoid tenderness. On the other hand, repeated pressure over the mastoid bone of a person can cause a mild traumatic periostitis which may account for tenderness, independent of the underlying process in the mastoid bone. External otitis and furunculosis of the canal may also cause tenderness of the mastoid.—M. D. H., M.D.

KEY TO ABSTRACTORS

E. D. M., M.D. .... Earl D. McBride
M. D. H., M.D. .... Marvin D. Henley

SUMMER DIARRHEA IN BABIES

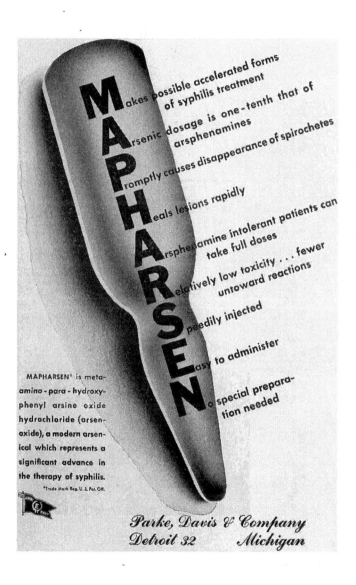

OFFICERS OF COUNTY SOCIETIES, 1944

★

COUNTY	PRESIDENT	SECRETARY	MEETING TIME
Alfalfa	H. E. Huston, Cherokee	L. T. Lancaster, Cherokee	Last Tues. each Second Month
Atoka-Coal	R. C. Henry, Coalgate	J. S. Fulton, Atoka	
Beckham	G. H. Stagner, Erick	O. C. Standifer, Elk City	Second Tuesday
Blaine	L. R. Kirby, Okeene	W. F. Griffin, Watonga	
Bryan	John T. Wharton, Durant	W. K. Haynie, Durant	Second Tuesday
Caddo	F. I. Patterson, Carnegie	C. B. Sullivan, Carnegie	
Canadian	P. F. Herod, El Reno	A. L. Johnson, El Reno	Subject to call
Carter	J. R. Pollock, Ardmore	H. A. Higgins. Ardmore	
Cherokee	P. H. Medearis, Tahlequah	W. M. Wood, Tahlequah	First Tuesday
Choctaw		E. A. Johnson, Hugo	
Cleveland	F. T. Gastineau, Norman	Iva S. Merritt, Norman	Thursday nights
Comanche	George L. Berry, Lawton	Howard Angus, Lawton	
Cotton	A. B. Holstead, Temple	Mollie F. Scism, Walters	Third Friday
Craig	Lloyd H. McPike, Vinita	Paul G. Sanger, Vinita	
Creek	J. E. Hollis, Bristow		
Custer	F. R. Vieregg. Clinton	C. J. Alexander, Clinton	Third Thursday
Garfield	Julian Feild, Enid	John R. Walker, Enid	Fourth Thursday
Garvin	T. F. Gross, Lindsay	John R. Callaway, Pauls Valley	Wednesday before Third Thursday
Grady	Walter J. Baze, Chickasha	Roy E. Emanuel, Chickasha	Third Thursday
Grant	I. V. Hardy, Medford		
Greer	R. W. Lewis, Granite	J. B. Hollis, Mangum	
Harmon	W. G. Husband, Hollis	R. H. Lynch, Hollis	First Wednesday,
Haskell	William Carson, Keota	N. K. Williams, McCurtain	
Hughes	Wm. L. Taylor, Holdenville	Imogene Mayfield, Holdenville	First Friday
Jackson	C. G. Spears, Altus	E. A. Abernethy, Altus	Last Monday
Jefferson	F. M. Edwards, Ringling		Second Monday
Kay	J. Holland Howe, Ponca City	G. H. Yeary, Newkirk	Second Thursday
Kingfisher	A. O. Meredith, Kingfisher	H. Violet Sturgeon, Hennessey	
Kiowa	J. William Finch, Hobart	William Bernell, Hobart	
LeFlore	Neeson Rolle, Poteau	Rush L. Wright, Poteau	
Lincoln	W. B. Davis, Stroud	Carl H. Bailey, Stroud	First Wednesday
Logan	William C. Miller, Guthrie	J. L. LeHew, Jr., Guthrie	Last Tuesday
Marshall	J. L. Holland, Madill	J. F. York, Madill	
Mayes	Ralph V. Smith, Pryor	Paul B. Cameron, Pryor	
McClain	W. C. McCurdy, Sr., Purcell	W. C. McCurdy, Jr., Purcell	
McCurtain	A. W. Clarkson, Valliant	N. L. Barker, Broken Bow	Fourth Tuesday
McIntosh	Luster I. Jacobs, Hanna	Wm. A. Tolleson, Eufaula	First Thursday
Murray	P. V. Annadown, Sulphur	J. A. Wrenn, Sulphur	Second Tuesday
Muskogee-Sequoyah			
Wagoner	H. A. Scott, Muskogee	D. Evelyn Miller, Muskogee	First Monday
Noble	C. H. Cooke, Perry	J. W. Francis, Jerry	
Okfuskee	C. M. Cochran, Okemah	M. L. Whitney, Okemah	Second Monday
Oklahoma	W. E. Eastland, Oklahoma City	E. R. Musick, Oklahoma City	Fourth Tuesday
Okmulgee	S. B. Leslie, Okmulgee	J. C. Matheney, Okmulgee	Second Monday
Osage	C. R. Weirich, Pawhuska	George K. Hemphill, Pawhuska	Second Monday
Ottawa	Walter Kerr, Picher	B. W. Shelton, Miami	Third Thursday
Pawnee	E. T. Robinson, Cleveland	R. L. Browning, Pawnee	
Payne	H. C. Manning, Cushing	J. W. Martin, Cushing	Third Thursday
Pittsburg	P. T. Powell, McAlester	W. H. Kaeiser, McAlester	Third Friday
Pontotoc	A. R. Sugg, Ada	R. H. Mayes, Ada	First Wednesday
Pottawatomie	E. Eugene Rice, Shawnee	Clinton Gallaher. Shawnee	First and Third Saturday
Pushmataha	John S. Lawson, Clayton	B. M. Huckabay, Antlers	
Rogers	R. C. Meloy, Claremore	Chas. L. Caldwell, Chelsea	First Monday
Seminole	J. T. Price, Seminole	Mack I. Shanholtz, Wewoka	Third Wednesday
Stephens	W. K. Walker, Marlow	Wallis S. Ivy, Duncan	
Texas	R. G. Obermiller, Texhoma	Morris Smith, Guymon	
Tillman	C. C. Allen, Frederick	O. G. Bacon Frederick	
Tulsa	Ralph A. McGill, Tulsa	E. O. Johnson, Tulsa	Second and Fourth Monday
Washington-Nowata	K. D. Davis, Nowata	J. V. Athey, Bartlesville	Second Wednesday
Washita	A. S. Neal, Cordell	James F. McMurry, Sentinel	
Woods	Ishmael F. Stephenson, Alva	Oscar E. Templin, Alva	Last Tuesday Odd Months
Woodward	H. Walker, Buffalo	C. W. Tedrowe, Woodward	Second Thursday

(Serving in Armed Forces)

THE JOURNAL

OF THE

OKLAHOMA STATE MEDICAL ASSOCIATION

| VOLUME XXXVII | OKLAHOMA CITY, OKLAHOMA, JULY, 1944 | NUMBER 7 |

The Restoration of Breathing in Emergencies and the Maintenance of Respiration in Non-Breathing Patients

CECIL K. DRINKER, M.D.

*Professor of Physiology in the Harvard
School of Public Health
From the Department of Physiology*

BOSTON, MASSACHUSETTS

INTRODUCTION

The association of breathing with life itself is a natural one for man and runs through the beliefs and writings of the ages. You remember that in the Biblical creation, "God formed man of the dust of the ground, and breathed into his nostrils the breath of life and man became a living soul." Death and the taking away of the "breath of life" are two eventualities which all must face and which have been easy to consider one.

We know today that the "breath of life" is in reality the giving of oxygen to all the tissues of the body, a process far more complicated than the obvious movements of breathing. We know, too, that death is a procession of events in the human body and that the movements of breathing may cease as much as 15 minutes before the heart stops beating. Furthermore, it is often the fact that the heart beat is so feeble near the end of asphyxia as to be difficult of detection, but even this does not preclude the possibility of recovery if breathing is supplied artificially. It is impossible to have much experience with these familiar phenomena and with the age-long belief that breathing and life are practically synonymous, without realizing how inevitable it is to find instances of the miraculous raising of the dead in the ancient literature of many different races. All of us have seen instances of transient revival and even recovery in patients apparently dead, to whom nothing in the way of resuscitation was done at the time the change occurred, and we are equally aware of how little in the way of turning or moving the body may occassionally just serve to produce the minimum of respiration to preserve life and permit recovery to follow.

Today, it is our task to examine what may be happening during the few critical moments following failure of breathing and then what is best to be done. In the first place, how many minutes may pass after a man, in previous good health, stops breathing before the heart beat ceases and the chance for recovery is gone? In Figure 1, I have constructed a curve from my own experience and the writings of others which expresses my personal judgment. If breathing stops at O upon the abscissa and artificial respiration is applied at the same time, the chances of recovery are placed at 100 per cent. From the second to the sixth minute the curve falls abruptly, and from the sixth to the twelfth minute the chances of regaining breathing are possible but slight. It is perhaps true that revival has been achieved after twelve minutes, but it is exceedingly rare. This is out of accord with many accounts of drowning, where it is often stated that persons have been under water for half an hour and life has been restored as a result of artificial respiration. If anything so extreme as this has certainly been achieved, I have been unable to authenticate it. At the same time, it is far from my desire to discourage the practice of continuing artificial

*Read before the General Session. Annual Meeting, April 25, 1944 in Tulsa.

respiration uninterruptedly for at least two hours, particularly in cases of submersion and electric shock. In these emergencies asphyxia is abrupt and the victim is usually in good health. There is no long period of advancing oxygen lack, so that nervous and other vital tissues are minimally damaged. Furthermore, under artificial respiration the circulation may recover so slowly that only by repeated and careful examination can one be sure whether or not the heart is beating. Spontaneous breathing may not be re-established for even twelve hours, but it is certain it will never occur if oxygenation of the blood is not steadily maintained by artificial respiration.

THE PROGRESSIVE NATURE OF ASPHYXIAL DAMAGE

The nerve impulses which activate the respiratory muscles originate in the respiratory center and are apparently due to carbon dioxide produced in the normal oxidative metabolism of the nervous tissues making up the center. When carbon dioxide accumulates locally to a sufficient degree it acts as a chemical excitant and nerve impulse inducing inspiration are the result. We thus depend upon oxygen use by living tissue to produce carbon dioxide through whose agency we in turn obtain oxygen. Truly Miescher was right when, in 1885, he said, "Over the oxygen supply of the body carbon dioxide spreads it protecting wings!"

It is the fact that the sensitivity of the respiratory center, that is, the capacity to originate the impulses resulting in breathing, is depressed by a number of agents and enhanced by very few. Thus alcohol, ether, chloroform, morphine, the barbiturates, and many other compounds, all depress breathing when taken in ordinary amounts and may readily pass beyond depression to paralysis. But of all the agencies diminishing the efficiency of the respiratory center, lack of oxygen is the commonest and the most insidious. It is, therefore, the fact that as the supply of oxygen to the center falls, which it does very rapidly when breathing stops, the functional efficiency of the center falls with it. It is as though lack of oxygen dampened this nervous tissue so that a greater blaze is necessary to set it off. There are no histological changes in the cells of the respiratory center which we are able to associate with the physiological effects of anoxia. When oxygen is cut off slowly and goes on to fatality, it is possible to find vacuolation of nerve cells and changes in staining characteristics, but these relatively gross alterations mean enormous damage and are far more prevalent in cells of the cerebral cortex than in the medulla.

There is subtle effect of anoxia on capil-laries throughout the entire body which is of especial importance to us in the nervous system. It is the dilation and increased permeability which may result from asphyxia. Edema is a condition which requires time for development and for removal. It will not be of moment when breathing stops abruptly, but if, as is so often the case, asphyxia develops slowly, edema of the brain and medulla with increased cerebro-spinal fluid pressure will surely be prominent when final functional breakdown takes place. Swelling and edema do not cause the failure of the respiratory center but they are certainly handicaps to recovery and they may exist for a long time. In carbon monoxide poisoning the victim may lie unconscious in a low concentration of the gas for many hours; when found alive, breathing is almost invariably present but may be so feeble as to be barely perceptible. Such patients, if they survive, may show permanent cerebral and mid-brain damage, and it is noteworthy that they may have suffered damage to cerebral capillaries which results in increased cerebro-spinal fluid pressure persistent for a whole month following the accident.

Let me also call attention to two special instances of respiratory failure which are unfortunately frequent. First, in electric shock, if the current passes through the medulla, breathing may stop instantly. The effect upon the respiratory center is probably similar to that upon other nervous tissue. I have talked with many men who have received an electric shock which has passed through the cerebrum and never have encountered one who could tell anything of the experience. Cerebral function apparently ceases instantly as evidenced by unconsciousness, often only momentary, but sufficient to blot out any perception. From complete unconsciousness, recovery may occur at once and without the slightest evidence of damage. If the shock is more severe, prolonged unconsciousness and after effects indicating destruction of brain tissue may result. In the medulla it is right to expect the same consequences from the passage of the current. Owing to the fact that the respiratory center expresses normal activity by rhythmic discharge of impulses resulting in breathing, one is instantly aware of the effect of the current upon this collection of nerve cells. Just as in the cerebrum, the result may be a temporary suspension of activity with no damage which does not disappear completely if artificial respiration is applied promptly. Or, if the shock is severe, there may be cell death, not the suspension of animation, which characterized the first and milder accident. The dominating influence of the respiratory failure in electric shock and, indeed, in other forms of asphyxia causes us to forget the medulla is a small bit of tissue which contains the vaso-motor and cardiac vagal centers in addition to that for respiration. One must not forget that complications from these control points may easily complicate what seems to be a simple suspension of breathing. Thus, in non-fatal electric shock, there may be great and persistent slowing of the heart and a shock-like fall in blood pressuer and these accessory problems must be met in the struggle for the recovery of the patient.

The second, and by long odds the most distressing failure of breathing we encounter, is that in poliomyelitis. The site of the paralysis in this disease is more diverse than in the emergencies so far discussed. In simplest form, only the lower neurones originating in the anterior horns of the spinal cord are affected. These elements innervating the diaphram and respiratory muscles are no different from the motor nerves to the voluntary muscles which are the classical points of attack in the disease and they are affected, recover, or are permanently destroyed in every conceivable variation. There is no doubt that the purely spinal form of poliomyelitis respiratory paralysis is the one most susceptible to treatment by prolonged artificial respiration. A fair number of these patients recover. But let me again call your attention to the fact that asphyxia causes capillary dilation and capillary leakage and that the local inflammation in the anterior horns of the spinal cord will be increased by freer leakage of exudate if anoxia is allowed to progress before artificial respiration is used.

When one encounters the second type of poliomyelitic respiratory paralysis, that attacking the bulbar centers, the problem becomes far worse on account of simultaneous involvement of other bulbar mechanisms, most notably that of swallowing. There is no satisfactory way of giving these patients the oxygen they must have and at, the same time keeping them from drowning in profuse secretions which they cannot swallow. If the disease is of combined type beginning in the cord and extending slowly into the medulla, every effort should be made to supply breathing since one never can tell how far the bulbar involvement will progress, and if the disease ceases before the paralysis is too great, there may be a chance for recovery. Again, it must never be forgotten that the anoxia, which the disease brings on through gradual reduction in the breathing, of itself adds directly to the severity of the disease and must be combatted from the very first.

THE TREATMENT OF RESPIRATORY FAILURE
Emergency Artificial Respiration

Since the beginning of time there has been no disagreement about the fact that if breathing stops, the effectiveness of whatever is done depends on no delay in doing it. That fact is the essential lesson of Figure 1.

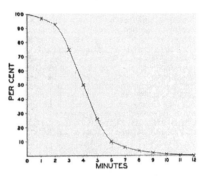

Figure 1. The chances of recovery after cessation of breathing, provided competent artificial respiration is given. Abscissa time in minutes. Ordinates percentage chances of recovery.

In spite of this conviction, there is virulent argument about what should be done. That has been true since the end of the 18th century and, I believe, depends upon two things; first, the place and cause of the failure of breathing, and second, the knowledge, training, and experience of those at hand when the emergency occurred. It would be a fortunate circumstance if any single method of procedure could be prescribed for the use of lifeguards upon a bathing beach and for the surgical staff of a modern hospital in the operating room! It is inevitable that every year large numbers of people requiring instant application of artificial respiration be treated first by laymen, and I believe that the prone-pressure method of artificial respiration described by Schafer in 1903 is the best for lay use. It is easily taught and millions of persons have received training. The face-down position, coupled with the pressure used, provides more certain and better drainage of the air passages than is possible for the layman provided with any sort of mechanical device. It produces lung ventilation not only adequate for a few minutes but capable of sustaining life for twelve hours in a man incapable of breathing[1]. A long experience in the training of the employees of a large gas and electric company has caused me to add a brief description of the Silvester method, since occasionally these laymen have had to perform artificial respiration on individuals who have an open wound of the abdomen or upon women in the last stages of pregnancy, where increased pressure on the abdomen may be harmful and the patient must lie upon the back and gain lung ventilation by the indirect increase and decrease of chest size incident upon rhythmic complete extension of the arms above the head and return over the chest.

These simple methods have given excellent emergency service in the field and often in the hospital with physicians as the operators.

In patients under anesthesia and upon the operating table artificial respiration is sometimes imperative and must be given without the interruption and loss of sterility which often accompany the use of the classical Schafer and Silvertown method. Waters[2], on the basis of long experience with such emergencies, advises the simple procedures shown in Figure 2. Mouth to mouth insufflation is the most ancient of all types of artificial respiration and has place in the miraculous

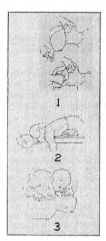

Figure 2. In 1, the bag is filled with oxygen and by squeezing it the operator forces the gas into the lungs. When he is sure this has happened, the bag is released thus allowing expiration to take place. In 2, the position used provides drainage from the lungs and throat. In 3, mouth to mouth insufflation is carried out, a layer of gauze being placed over the patient's mouth to prevent infection. Note the position of the right hand for determining the success of lung inflation. (From J.A.M.A., October 30, 1943, 123, 559.)

restorations of life described in both the Old and New Testaments. The other procedure employs the ordinary mask and rubber bag of the anesthetist and the lungs are inflated by gentle squeezing of the bag. Waters makes a particular point of the necessity to watch and to feel the chest in order to be sure that the oxygen from the bag is actually entering the lungs and advises the prone position with the head down to permit drainage of the air passages. These simple procedures making use of what is immediately at hand and allowing expiration to occur passively, that is without suction, must commend themselves to all.

Protracted Artificial Respiration

The fact that in far the greater number of cases artificial respiration must be continued for some time furnishes many problems and also many ways of solving them.

A. Manual Methods

There are many variants of the prone pressure method. All cause forcible expiration by manual pressure which decreases the size of the chest by forcing the contents of the abdomen up against the diaphragm and by narrowing the lower part of the thoracic cage through inward and upward movement of the lower ribs. When pressure is released, the elastic recoil of the parts involved causes inspiration. The success of the manoeuvre depends pre-eminently on the efficiency of the elastic recoil and this in its turn depends upon the condition of the tissues in which there is a large factor of muscular tone. By tone I mean the slight but constant tension under which quiescent living muscle normally exists. It is a property lost rapidly as muscles are badly circulated and die. This accounts for the fact that if one measures the ventilation secured through the Schafer method, a small amount of air may be moved in and out of the lungs during the first few efforts, but it rapidly falls to little or nothing. On several occasions I have made this trial upon individuals immediately after they were certainly dead. Almost at once the body feels dead and the fruitlessness of the effort is apparent. In the Silvester method, in which the chest is stretched into fullest possible passive expansion by bringing the arms into full extension above the head, the patient is served more by the inherent elasticity of all the tissues and less by muscle tone. Very fair ventilation in a cadaver can be obtained in this way, since the arm extension enlarging the chest and putting the tissues on stretch during inspiration is followed by recoil which provides expiration. The physiological soundness of the Silvester method is, however, negated by the position of the patient on his back which does not favor drainage from the mouth and throat, and even more by the fact that the inspiratory expansion of the chest attained by arm extension may be too slight to provide an adequate minute volume.

B. The Tilting Method of Eve

In 1932, a British physician, Frank C. Eve[3], was called in an emergency to attend a child of two with post-diphtheritic paralysis of the diaphram. The child was dying of asphyxia. He at once tilted it head down, thus clearing the throat of mucus which was "rattling" there in the ineffective respiratory movements. This clearance was beneficial, but Eve noticed that the tilt produced expiration. Commandeering a long rocking chair which was at hand, the child was laid in it and rocked by the parents slowly and fairly continuously over two and a half days, during which the paralysis passed off and recovery was complete. This dramatic experience, the result of the best sort of clinical acumen on the part of an active practitioner, has had an impressive effect. There was no doubt it had saved a life.   It was easily carried out, since any sort of see-saw arrangement could be used. It could not harm the patient, even if continued for a long time. From the physiological point of view, respiration by the tilt technique is due to forcing air out of the chest through an upward push of the diaphragm by the abdominal contents followed by maximum passive descent of the diaphragm when the head-up swing causes the abdominal contents to slide downward. If, while the head-down position is being achieved, pressure is applied as in the Schafer method, ventilation will be even greater and clearance of the air passages still better. There is, furthermore, no doubt that the rhythmic head-down position is exceedingly beneficial to the circulation. In my opinion this is the best, easily accomplished means of continuous artificial

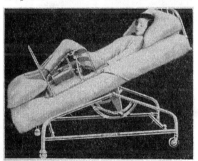

Figure 3.   A subject arranged for artificial respiration by the tilting method. The greatest angle of tilt is 45 degrees and at the start all of this is essential. A slightly higher trestle permitting even larger swings would be better. The rate of tilt should be 12 times a minute. (From Report of the Respirators (Poliomyelitis) Committee, Special Report Series No. 237. Medical Research Council, London, 1939. "Breathing Machines" and Their Use in Treatment.)

respiration we possess.   Figure 3 shows a convenient arrangement of a patient upon tilter. It is equally possible to use a door or plank upon a trestle, but do not forget that the tilting movements must be at least 45 degrees .each way in order to make real use of gravity.

Eve's enthusiasm for his measure and the almost lyrical praises of his followers are characteristic phenomena in the history of resuscitation. Any measure which saves life, as this has done, merits commendation and, never forget this, the most intensive

critical examination. This last is still lacking. We should be most unwise to swallow Eve's[3] statement, "Our old comfortable confidence in Schafer's method has been roughly shaken" other than as a stimulant. The prone-pressure technique has survived for 51 years and is thus a physiological experiment of tried competence. Eve's[3] final sentences, "Uncomplacently we must all 'go to school' again. More experiments are badly needed: resuscitation is in the melting pot" are true only in the sense that doctors must "go to school" through all their lives relative to every therapeutic suggestion. No one will ever develop a method for resuscitation competent in all situations. "More experiments" will always be "needed" and the "melting pot" boils no more furiously for this special therapy than for all other advance in the art of medicine.

C.   The Bragg-Paul Pulsator

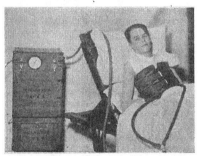

Figure 4.   The Bragg-Paul Pulsator in operation upon a patient. The boxes contain a pump, motor, and accessories to drive air into rubberized bag held under the broad belt. Inflation compresses the lower part of the chest and upper abdomen causing expiration.   Inspiration follows as a result of the elastic recoil of the parts. (From Report of the Respirators (Poliomyelitis) Committee, Special Report Series No. 237. Medical Research Council, London, 1939.   "Breathing Machines" and Their Use in Treatment.)

This mechanical appliance shown in Figure 4 is the best of the many methods which operate by mechanical imitation of the prone-pressure procedure. It was devised in 1933 by Sir William Bragg[4] to aid a friend, the victim of progressive muscular atrophy, who had simply become too weak to breathe successfully and was being kept alive by friends who assisted his ineffectual breathing by manual methods. In his own words, Sir William "thought that it might be possible to reduce the labour and inconvenience, and I arranged that a football bladder should be bound upon my friend's chest, connected with a similar bladder fixed between two hinged boards. By closing and opening the boards the chest was alternately compressed and allowed to recover by its natural elasticity." The device worked and was soon mechanized so that the patient lived for over three years, bedridden all the time but easily cared for and comfortable. The Pulsator has attained good results in the protracted treatment of respiratory arrest from poliomyelitis, post-diphtheritic paralysis, morphine, and barbiturate poisoning and other conditions[1]. The device is simple and inexpensive. It is well tolerated by conscious patients. Young children and adults learn to live in it readily. Eating, sleeping, nursing care, all become minor problems when compared with the situation provided by the body respirator which encloses all except the head of the patient. The sitting position favors diaphragmatic descent when positive pressure ceases. In reading the accounts of the cases treated, I gain the impression that the device is most useful for assisting the breathing of patients who are losing their power to breathe but who have not lost it entirely and retain some ability to assist the device. The Pulsator, like the prone-pressure method, is certainly capable of providing enough ventilation to sustain life but not much more, and over long periods of time will work best when it does not have to accomplish the whole task of breathing.

D. Blow and Suck Machines

There are several devices on the market in this country which aim to provide artificial respiration by alternately blowing air mixed with oxygen into a mask covering the mouth and nose and sucking it out again. In qualified hands a pharyngeal or laryngeal tube may be used instead of the mask. Appliances of this type have always had great appeal on account of the apparent reasonableness of getting air into and out of the lungs by means of a pump, just as one would do in the case of a rubber bag. The first such device, a double acting bellows, was recommended by John Hunter in 1776. The method and apparatus received prompt approval from the Royal Society, but within a few years experimental analysis caused its disappearance. In a sense, this history has been repeated three times in our own day and, unfortunately, a degree of feeling has developed which has made it hard to appraise the value or dangers of appliances operating on the blow and suck principle. At the onset it is certain that if air enters the pulmonary air sacs by excess pressure from a pump or under atmospheric pressure as in normal breathing, respiratory exchanges will occur, yet ventilation of the lungs secured by alternate blowing and sucking lacks every vestige of being normal physiologically. It is quite an assumption to believe that air forced into the lungs by positive pressure sufficient to stretch the thorax and force the dia-

phragm will reach the lung alveoli with the uniformity of distribution achieved by the normal expansion of the chest accomplished by the beautifully coordinated muscular act of breathing. If the trachea is cannulated and the chest opened, one may observe an apparently uniform expansion and contraction of the lungs as air is pumped in and sucked out. The condition of an anesthetized animal so ventilated remains excellent for an hour and may be apparently so far much longer. But from the very start, the lungs posteriorly, where they lie against the chest wall are less well ventilated than in the freely moving parts directly under the eyes of the observer. The pressure necessary to inflate the lungs alone, without the necessity to expand the chest forcibly, as is the case when the cavity is closed is very slight. The air goes to the alveoli most easily expanded and these are not those upon which the lungs filled with blood are resting. Every physiologist knows that the blood of a quiescent anesthetized animal can be aerated adequately by artificial respiration, but this is accomplished at the expense of the lungs themselves. There is far more lung tissue than is necessary to meet the requirements of the inactive body and in a laboratoy experiment of moderate duration, progressive loss of functioning lung tissue may do no harm for a time. But all of us know that in such experiments the excess lung tissue is gradually filled up by edema or lost through atelectasis and generalized anoxia of the body eventually results. In resuscitation, the chest is not open and to expand the lungs by blowing air in through the mouth and nose requires pressure. In the fear of lung rupture from excessive pressure it has been recommended that blow and suck devices be constructed so that positive pressure higher than 10 mm. of Hg. or 13.5 cm. of water cannot occur. Since these appliances are sold widely for operation by laymen, it is of course necessary to put some automatic limit upon the pressure they can develop. At the same time, few people realize the consequences of this safeguard. Let us see what happens if a dog is anesthetized, a tracheal cannula introduced, and artificial respiration instituted by means of a "blow and suck" appliance. In order that the animal may be entirely incapable of breathing but have a normal circulation, curare is giving intravenously. The arrangement of the experiment is shown in Figure 5. A motor-driven pump, P, delivers air or any gas mixture through a cannula, C, tied in the trachea of the dog. The pump, adjustable for rate and stroke, is set so that the respiratory needs of the animal are met adequately. A "T" tube, T, is inserted in the inspiratory line and is connected with a second tube, the lower end of which is open under water in the container, W. After curarization the overflow tube is pushed just far enough under water to prevent escape of the inspiratory blast from the lower orifice of the tube. Expiration is accomplished

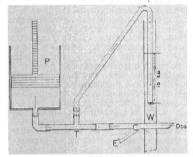

Figure. 5. Diagram to illustrate an experiment showing the course of events when a dog with normal circulation, but with breathing completely paralyzed, is given artificial respiration by the "blow and suck" technique. P, the pump, T, tube in line of inspiratory blast leading through the horizontal arm to C, the tracheal cannula, and through the upright arm and then down to a point 10 cm. below the surface of the water in a large tube, W. Expiration by suction takes place through a branch of the tracheal cannula, E. When the pump creates pressure above 10 cm. of water, air escapes by bubbling out through the water in W.

through a second limb, E, of the tracheal cannula and may be passive, as in normal breathing, or aired by suction, a fundamental feature of the appliances we are discussing. In an actual experiment upon a dog weighing 12 Kg., it was found that before anesthesia the animal breathed 2,490 cc. per minute at a rate of 19. Accordingly, the respiration pump was set to supply 2,610 cc. at the same rate and after curarization it was necessary to immerse the inspiratory tube 10 cm. to prevent a single bubble of air from escaping. During expiration, suction was applied, equalling —8 cm. The experiment lasted 4 hours and 49 minutes, when the animal was sacrificed. What happened to the air supply delivered absolutely steadily from the respiration pump? At the end of 7 minutes a bubble or two began to escape from the overflow tube constantly immersed under 10 cm. of water. After 2 hours and 35 minutes, 210 cc. of air per minute were being lost through this escape tube; at 3 hours and 40 minutes, 495 cc. per minute; at 4 hours and 40 minutes, 580 cc. per minute. This gradual loss of air is inevitable if the pump is supplied with a safety valve, which all agree it must have in order to prevent lung rupture by excess pressure. The loss is due to gradual atelectasis and exudation in dependent parts of the lungs where expansion is most difficult. It occurs more rapidly in a machine which sucks during expiration, than one in

which expiration is passive, as in normal breathing. At the start of the experiment cited, the animal was entirely normal. There was no antecedent period of asphyxia, no water or excess secretion in the air passages. The breathing of the dog was simply shifted from his usual method to ventilation by the blow and suck technique, arranged so as to meet respiratory requirements quite perfectly. It was an ideal situation for the adequate performance of the machine, but it failed slowly from the start. During the experiment the loss in minute volume was not serious, but it must be realized that this variety of artificial respiration will always create and leave behind an area of atelectatic and edematous lung tissue from which trouble may arise. If the air passages are blocked to any degree by water or exudate, or if the animal has been severely asphyxiated prior to instituting artificial respiration, the machine fails in air delivery even more rapidly. These, you understand, are my appraisals of principles basic in a certain type of resuscitating device. They are not directed at any special appliance and are directly at variance with the Council on Physical Therapy of the American Medical Association, which has endorsed such devices for use by physicians or under their direction. I have never been afraid that blow and suck machines as safeguarded today would do harm by rupturing the lungs. Their failure is through lack of air delivery. This is often hard to appreciate, especially since in most cases ventilation must be accomplished through a face mask.

I am quite sure that if such a machine is at hand when breathing stops and if the respiratory passages are clear of any sort of obstruction, one can ventilate a patient successfully for some time and may save life. Since the days of John Hunter this has certainly happened, but occasional successes and mechanical attractiveness do not overbalance physiological unsuitability, at least they have not done so through the first 150 years of this controversy. Relatively recently, Thompson and Birnbaum[1] have summarized their experiments upon the effects of intratracheal suction as causing stimulation of breathing and believe this to be strong reason for the employment of the blow and suck principle. This means making use of the vagal fibers in the alveolar walls, which excite inspiration when expiratory collapse of alveoli is excessive. Their contention may prove useful and will certainly receive trail, particularly in operating room practice, where it can be applied at intervals and properly evaluated. At the moment I am not convinced that the possible usefulness of suction outweighs the harm it can do if applied rhythmically for considerable periods, and the more severe the asphyxiation, the longer it may be before spontaneous breathing is resumed. It is noteworthy that blow and suck artificial respiration does not have to its credit the reports in medical journals of successful resuscitation after hours of use which are available for many of the other methods I have cited. While one cannot expect to perform continuous artificial respiration on a non-breathing conscious patient through a face mask, still unconsciousness may persist for many hours in patients requiring artificial respiration, and I am of the opinion that the lack of instances of successful restoration of breathing following hours of blow and suck artificial respiration is due to the fact that this procedure builds up its own ill-success if it is used beyond the first minutes of resuscitative effort.

E. Oxygen and Carbon Dioxide

I am very strongly convinced that pure oxygen, or air enriched with oxygen as much as possible, should be given to all cases of asphyxiation. If oxygen can be supplied to their blood, life may continue, and pure oxygen has 5 times the efficacy of air. It will have much wider use in the medicine of the future.

The use of carbon dioxide to stimulate breathing is wholly natural. When Henderson and Haggard[7] advocated an oxygen-carbon dioxide mixture for the treatment of carbon monoxide poisoning in 1922, the utility of the method was at once apparent. Its use spread to asphyxiation from other causes. As is the rule in medicine, there was an element of "if a little is good, more is better" in this wider application, and concentrations as high as 25 per cent were employed. Above 10 per cent, carbon dioxide begins to act as an anesthetic and depressant. I do not think there is any profit in employing it in concentrations above 7 per cent, which is that generally recommended for use in the treatment of carbon monoxide asphyxia. Oxygen rather than air should accompany the carbon dioxide.

F. Respirators

In 1925, when my brother, Philip Drinker, and our associate, Louis A. Shaw, first discussed the possibility of making a man breathe by sealing him in a box through a rubber collar about his neck and inducing lung ventilation by alternations of negative and positive pressure in the box, I was sure the plan would not work. My lack of acumen at that time has caused me ever since to examine and re-examine every idea and every appliance for resuscitation which has come to my attention. It was my good fortune to be at the Peter Bent Brigham Hospital when the first case of poliomyelitic respiratory paralysis was admitted for treatment. He was a junior in Harvard College and when

he was put in the respirator I thought him dead. In a matter of minutes he was speaking to us. For about 2 weeks he could not live without artificial respiration. He recovered completely. It seemed as if a way had opened for saving almost all of the victims of an acute disease. This has not proved to be the case and had the first patient been an instance of bulbar poliomyelitis instead of a spinal type ideal for treatment, enthusiasm for the respirator would have been less marked. The respirator will always save the lives of some patients. There are a larger number it will not save. The situation with the public is a troublesome one, since it is impossible to be sure what the outcome will be, and so when poliomyelitis is epidemic, access to a respirator is almost imperative.

Experience with the respirator has certainly taught us a great deal about the failure of breathing and about the treatment of ineffectual breathing. In this last relation the Cuirass Respirator shown in Figure 6 merits discussion. Devices of this type are

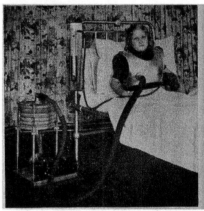

Figure 6. A type of Cuirass Respirator sealing around the arms, neck, and abdomen. A motor-driven diaphragm pump causes respiration by creating negative pressure in the space between the respirator and the chest and upper part of the abdomen. (From Report of the Respirators (Poliomyelitis) Committee, Special Report Series No. 237. Medical Research Council, London, 1939. "Breathing Machines" and Their Use in Treatment.)

fairly numerous. They give the patient freedom and they make nursing care far less difficult, but they do not work well unless some ability to breathe is retained. On the other hand the respirator enclosing the entire body is capable of giving good ventilation in the face of complete respiratory paralysis. I have made no experiments but believe the difference may be due to the fact that the lower seal of the Cuirass Respirator is usually around the abdomen. This interferes with the best inspiratory enlargement of the chest, particularly when the patient is in the sitting position. In experiments upon dogs I have found it easy to make the lower seal around the thighs and if the same method was used for human patients by putting the legs through elastic cuffs, it would seem that an efficient but less confining respirator could be constructed.

CONCLUSIONS

In concluding I must re-emphasize the fundamental necessity for no delay in the application of the simplest methods when treating cessation of breathing. Whenever possible, breathing should be aided as it weakens. Anoxia breeds anoxia and physicians often begin to use oxygen or artificial respiration when it is too late. If artificial respiration must be continued for some time, apparatus becomes important. The simplest effective method for hours of use is the tilting technique of Eve, the materials for which are at hand almost anywhere. Next to this, and deserving wider use in this country, is the Bragg-Paul Pulsator. As a last reliance we have the body Respirator or possibly a Cuirass Respirator of the sort suggested. We have no reason to be too well satisfied with any of these methods. Most of the best are relatively recent which, in a subject of so much medical importance, is, after all, a healthy and promising symptom of progress.

BIBLIOGRAPHY

1. Oldham, J. B. Continuous Artificial Respiration, With Maintenance of the Circulation for Twelve Hours after Apparent Death, The Lancet, Sept. 7, 1929, 497.
2. Waters, R. M. Simple Methods for Performing Artificial Respiration, J. A. M. A., Oct. 30, 1943, 123, 559.
3. Eve, F. C. Actuation of the Inert Diaphragm by a Gravity Method, The Lance, 1932, II, 995.
   See also Eve, F. C. Resuscitation of the Drowned Today, J. A. M. A., 1944, 124, 964; and Cordier, D. G. Methods of Artificial Respiration, British Medical Journal, Sept 25, 1943, 2, 381.
4. Bragg, W. H. British Medical Journal, 1938, 2, 254.
5. Report of the Respirators (Poliomyelitis) Committee, Special Report Series No. 237. Medical Research Council, London, 1939. "Breathing Machines" and Their Use in Treatment.
6. Thompson, S. A., and Birnbaum, G. L. Asphyxial Resuscitation; The Phenomenon and Its Mechanism, J. Thoracic Surgery, 1943, 12, 624. (This paper utilizes data in several which precede it and provides reference to them.)
7. Henderson, Y., and Haggard, H. W. The Treatment of Carbon Monoxide Asphyxia By Means of Oxygen plus CO 2 Inhalation, J.A.M.A., Sept. 30, 1922, 79, 1137.

Trends In Public Health*

HARRY S. MUSTARD, M.D., Director
DeLamar Institute of Public Health
College of Physicians and Surgeons
COLUMBIA, UNIVERSITY

It is not easy to discuss trends in public health. Among the many difficulties that one encounters in such an attempt is that there is no uniformly accepted or consistently observed definition of what makes up public health problems; nor is there any agreement as to the minimum and maximum boundaries of a public health program. As a matter of fact, there is considerable disagreement as to what constitutes health itself. On the one extreme are those who consider as healthy any individual who is not obviously sick. Those who are satisfied with this concept are not concerned with the possibility that the individual may be building up thumping high blood pressure, or getting hog fat; or that he is just one jump ahead of frank deficiency disease, or has a positive Wassermann. In this school of thought, the individual is healthy if he is able to get up on any particular morning and do a fairly de-cent day's work. On the other extreme are those who insist that the healthy man or woman must radiate vigor and well-being; must be one who, compared to ordinary mortals, shines and glistens and twinkles as a planet among dead stars. Such an individual, they say, possesses "positive health." Medical men, raised in the somewhat strict discipline of science, find it a little difficult to accept these euphoric and hyperkinetic manifestations as essential in health. Dr. Edward S. Godfry, Commissioner of Health of New York State, has expressed himself as unable to visualize these "positively" healthy individuals except as a crowd of back-slapping extroverts. He feels that a world so peopled would not necessarily be a pleasant place in which to live. In any event, somewhere between the preclinical case on the one hand and the manic-happy individual on the other, is to be found that health status which all physicians desire for their patients. To reach this goal, common sense and the practicabili-

*Read at the Annual Meeting of the Oklahoma State Medical Association, Section on Public Health, April 25, 1944, Tulsa, Oklahoma.

ty of applying an expanding medical knowledge must be relied upon.

Having disposed, in none too satisfying a manner, of the question of what constitutes health, it is necessary to proceed similarly vaguely with the word "public" as used in the phrase "public health." Here again, the connotation is confused. Does the word "public" refer to something that affects the public or something in which the public ought to take action? Is public health service to be rendered to the public or only by the public authorities? Does the public include all persons or only those who are indigent? In this country, one regards public schools as those supported by taxes and administered by public authorities for the public. In England a public school is really a private school. Because of these confusions in phraseology, perhaps the most sensible way to approach this whole question and to determine trends in public health is to do it in retrospect: To work from the past up to the current situation and, by analysis, attempt to discover the factors that have brought about the recognition of public health problems and the organization of public health services.

Looking now into the past, it would seem that one of the very first health problems to which the public and the public authorities gave attention was leprosy. This disease dates far back into the history of man, into that period when the milk of human kindness was rather a raw and sour product, there being little compassion with which to warm and pasteurize it. Doubtless, many other diseases were confused with leprosy, for clinical and epidemiological evidence suggests that elephantiasis, psoriasis, syphilis, and even scabies were sometimes caught in the term leprosy as then loosely used. However, the disease would appear to have been quite common in China, India, Egypt at least 500 years before Christ. The Bible contains many references to it, and it is a matter of record that it reached a peak in Europe and the British Isles in the thirteenth century, declining in the latter places fairly steadily after that. Significant in the history of this early, if not first recognized, public health problem, are certain points. First, leprosy was a disease that produced disfigurement and destruction in the individual; second, it was loathsome and repulsive from an aesthetic standpoint; third, it was believed to be highly contagious; and fourth, it was regarded as incurable: one who contracted the disease was considered doomed. The picture as a whole was such that it produced stark and traditional fear; individual fear, public fear, official and government fear.

Now fear, and its half-brother anger, is the emotion that is most likely to precipitate group action. This was true in those days as well as now; and the reactions of primitive societies in such circumstances is likely to be precipitate and harsh. The Babylonians, the Assyrians, the Jews, and Egyptians of early days, and the medieval Europeans, were primitive as regards medical knowledge and social conscience, and it is not therefore surprising that lepers were cast out, stoned, left to beg or starve, or even executed en masse. Actually, as late as the thirteenth century Philip IV of France suggested that all lepers be gathered and burned and that this be a regular procedure until the disease disappeared. He was known as Philip the Fair.

Out of these early experiences come two principles that must be recognized as of influence in originating and shaping public health practice. First, aesthetic considerations markedly influence the public and its officials in decisions as to the seriousness of a disease; and second, fear of a disease will impel public authorities to take action.

Important to bear in mind at this point is the fact that while the fear of leprosy produced quite definite procedures that it was hoped would protect the rest of the community, it did not give rise to any health mechanism as such. The action that was taken came from kings and priests, without direct judgment or decision of any authoritative medical group. It may be said, therefore, that the leprosy situation prepared the soil but did not plant the seed for public health service. For the latter, the events of the great epidemics must be examined. One does not have to go back very far to gain an appreciation of the confusion and terror of such tragedies. Just a quarter of a century ago, the United States suffered from an influenza epidemic recalling similar episodes of the Middle Ages. In the 19th century, great and lethal outbreaks of cholera occurred. Smallpox, yellow fever, diphtheria, scarlet fever have appeared as recurring waves in one place or another. Except in relation to smallpox, repulsiveness of these diseases was not a consideration as had been the case of leprosy. But epidemics of them involved a far greater proportion of the population than did leprosy at its worst, and in addition caused immediately a vast number of deaths. The civil authorities could not adopt the relatively simple measure of expelling the sick man or woman from the city. These people died right in the city and sometimes on the streets without the warning of a gradually developing leonine expression or of ulcers or autoamputations as in leprosy; and the authorities had to do something about it, and at once. In the meantime, however, the medical man had attained a place of respect in the community and his comparatively expert knowledge of disease had become recognized. It was not natural, in the circumstances, that the civil authorities should turn to the medical profession for guidance, and that designated groups of physicians be given authority to decide what measures might best be instituted for community protection. Within the limitations of their knowledge, they tried to prevent the disease from appearing in their community, and if the epidemic did occur, guided control measures. Thus was born the board of health, from which most of today's public health activities spring.

Without further belaboring the point, it may be said that out of the confusion, distress and terror of epidemics, two principles in public health practice were recognized and established. First, that control of epidemic diseases requires expert knowledge; and second, that in times of epidemics, or of threatened epidemics, action must be organized and communal rather than on an individual basis.

It should not be assumed that these actions and concepts developed simultaneously or in equal degree in all places. Nor may it be assumed that no other public health problems or practices were developing. Quite the reverse was the case. Measures for disease control were spotty and intermittent, with forward looking activities in one place, none at all in another, even as it is today. Other problems and approaches and newer knowledge that would shape public health practice were crowding into the picture in the nineteenth century. From a medical standpoint, a gradually established faith in the efficacy of vaccination against smallpox was giving a new vision of one phase of prevention of disease; and professional thought was commencing to focus itself upon another field. This was the newly-developing science of bacteriology. With micro-organisms recognized as a cause of the communicable diseases, it seemed quite logical to emphasize the control of the environment as the great hope for the prevention of epidemics. Thus was laid the foundation for environmental sanitation. Another great influence also arose in the 19th century, and this, too, tended to encourage programs for improvement of the environment. It came as one result of an investigation by the Board of Poor Law Commissioners of Great Britain, published in 1842 as the report on the Sanitary Condition of the Labouring Population of Great Britain. The interest aroused from these influences and the action taken over the next fifty years is too complex and far-reaching to present in any detail. Suffice to say that this was the age of sanitary reform, and fixed firmly on health agencies a responsibility for sanitation of the environment. For a

good many years, practically all health departments were preoccupied with this activity. Aside from this, they did little except for quarantine and occasional smallpox vaccinations when there was an outbreak of that disease.

Gradually, however, there was an evolution in the character of the public health program. As medical knowledge expanded, vaccines against other diseases became available and, in cities at least, sanitation became a part of good municipal housekeeping. Through these influences and others, the great epidemics became things of the past, and the endemic level of acute communicable disease reached new low points: typhoid from 31.3 per cent per 100,000 in 1900 to 1.0 in 1940. Diphtheria from 40.3 per 100,000 in 1900 to 1.1 in 1940. And now, a newly-awakened social consciousness began to make itself felt. Society's attitude had been that if an individual did not have the wit and the means of raising his children, it was no concern of the government if those children died, or if the individual died, provided it was a quiet and undramatic death, not a source of danger to the public and not harrowing to its sensibilities. But public sensibilities became more acute and there developed a gnawing disquiet that what happens on the wrong side of the railroad tracks is a responsibility of the community or the nation, as the case might be.

As a result, undertakings of a new sort became incorporated in public health programs. One was in relation to tuberculosis and venereal diseases; another concerned disabilities against which presumably the individual could take measures if informed: Problems of maternity and childhood, degenerative diseases, malnutrition. But these newer programs demanded another approach than had those relating to sanitation. The latter, and even quarantine and vaccination, had been carried out largely by enforcement. One could not, however, force a pregnant woman to report early and often to her doctor nor to sterilize bottles for the baby's formula. Nor could health authorities use strong-arm methods to get a case of tuberculosis to take treatment. These things obviously demanded an understanding on the part of the public, and to meet the need there arose that process known as health education, which has now become an important part of the work of every health agency. Incidentally, in a sort of bastard form, it has become the stock in trade of every commercial concern that has a patent medicine to sell.

Out of these considerations, which have been presented at some length, arise certain facts which it would seem well at this point to summarize. First, public health activities arise as a result of public disquiet; second, public disquiet is engendered by drama, fear, and aesthetic consideration; third, the diseases that in the past caused public disquiet are those that are repulsive or which occur in great and devasting epidemics; fourth, various influences early caused the public to look to sanitation of the environment as a means of controlling such diseases; fifth, as the threat of epidemics lessened and as newer knowledge and concepts arose, other activities were incorporated in the public health program; sixth, government created boards of health or health departments as its agent in protecting the community.

It will be remembered that previous reference has been made to boards of health in the very early days. It should be emphasized that at first such efforts were temporary and that, as the threat of the epidemic posted, the board of health went into abeyance. It should be emphasized, too, that such efforts arose locally, quite independent of and uncoordinated with efforts in other parts of a given state and without relation to the nation as a whole. Gradually, in first one place and then in another, these organized efforts for protecting community health became more firmly established. Petersburg, Virginia, is credited with having a local board of health in 1780. Other cities followed, but it was not until the middle of the 19th century that the first state board of health was organized. Those whose affiliations are below the Mason-Dixon line say that the first state board of health was established in Louisiana in 1855. Those with a New England background date the first state board of health as that of Massachusetts in 1869.

As the years passed, other states and smaller civil units developed permanent health agencies either in terms of departments of health or boards of health. Created as they were, boards of health and health departments form an integral part of government. This is a significant fact, for, because of this relationship, a national, state or local health program is inevitably limited, expanded, balanced or unbalanced by the laws, resources, and policies of that government from which it springs. Some must do certain things because of legal requirements; others may not undertake an obviously needed activity because there is no law authorizing it, or no funds available. Over and above this is another consideration; namely, that the organization of public health work in the United States is necessarily complex because of the interrelationships between national, state and local governments.

There is separation and, to some extent overlapping of authority and responsibility as between state and federal governments, with varying degrees of autonomy delegated by the several states to their respective local jurisdictions. One of the reasons for this is that the evolution of state and federal governments did not come about by delegation of authority to the states from an all-powerful central government. The process was rather the reverse of this: thirteen separate, independent and sovereign states created a federal government and by joint action invested that government with authority and responsibility in certain limited fields. Now one may have convictions as to the propriety or even the necessity of an all-powerful federal government or he may be equally determined to support state sovereignty. Regardless of this, so far as concerns public health, the states, in the establishment of the Constitution retained their respective responsibilities and authorities for maintenance of the public health except as concerns international and interstate relationships in this field. These, by implication, they ceded to the federal government, and that government, from a strictly legal standpoint, has limited to these fields the exercise of its authority in public health matters.

There is, however, in the Constitution another clause which can be interposed as implying additional federal obligations, if not authority, for the public health. This is found in Article 1, Section 8, where it is said that the Congress shall be responsible, among other things, for the general welfare. It is assumedly upon the implications of these Constitutional provisions that the states now receive rather generous federal grants which help them finance their routine public health activities. It should be noted that the federal government does not force the state to accept such aid nor does it supersede state health officers by federal ones. In effect, one who favors such a plan can with truth, in the present instance, say that there is no federal encroachment on the state. One who is opposed to such federal grants can reply by saying that there may be no overt encroachment but, that any agency that has millions of dollars to give away inevitably exercises definite authority. Regardless of whether one accepts this with favor or disfavor, health work in the states is more and more being stimulated, supported and indirectly guided by the federal government. Further there is an increasing tendency for states to aid and, more than previously, to direct local government. As a result, and for good or ill, whatever arises at a federal level seems likely, by this new and financially implemented federal-state relationship, to come hard and fast as an influence in state and local health programs.

This is important to remember, for in recent years the federal government has enacted rather far-reaching social security provisions that relate to public health; and still broader laws, buttressed with vast sums, are under consideration. This is not the time or place to argue the merits and soundness of these new trends. In some directions they will surely prove beneficial to the public health; in others, the implications are such as to make the thoughtful and practical citizen apprenhensive. But regardless of this, the federal shaping of public health practice is a factor to be considered in any analysis of trends in this field.

In summary, now, of these trends, one may say that the history has been somewhat as follows: arising early from fear of a repulsive disease, public health action commenced to take shape as a result of the great epidemics. Until the close of the last century, these programs were concerned essentially with the communicable diseases, and quarantine and sanitation were relied upon mainly for control. Expanding medical knowledge and its practical application has markedly lessened the communicable disease. At the same time, this increased knowledge has made apparent many new opportunities for the prevention of non-communicable conditions. Services in this field now form an integral part of public health programs. A greater participation in health matters by the federal government, plus far-reaching social security legislation may change markedly the character and extent of state and local public health practice.

Chronic Digestive Disturbance in the Elderly Patient[*]

D. D. PAULUS, M.D.

OKLAHOMA CITY, OKLAHOMA

Elderly patients with chronic digestive disturbances "coming in for a workout" often present a confusing array of symptoms that makes it difficult even for the experienced clinician to interpret and properly evaluate the same. It is our purpose in this paper not to go into the recognition of demonstratable disease by the usual clinical and laboratory methods but rather to dwell on some of the borderline cases in which laboratory methods of precision are not available at the present time to the average diagnostician. Also to touch on some other conditions which perhaps are purely functional in character.

In many cases the harrassed patient is very reluctant to come to the consultant and only does so at the persistent urging of a close relative or his family physician because she or he is beset by anxiety and fears that the investigation might reveal some serious condition such as a malignancy or other serious ailment that might require a major operation. Such patients usually present themselves because in addition to the digestive disturbance a rather marked distress, even amounting to definite pain, has come into the picture. In others, loss of weight, loss of appetite, strength or endurance, or a change of bowel habits, are the disturbing factors which make the patient uneasy about himself. This array of symptoms will immediately put the experienced clinician on the alert for a possible malignancy.

In the other extreme we have the elderly, more or less neurotic patient usually a woman who persists in telling a long drawn-out story of her ailments which are accompanied by such awful pains that she cannot see how she can go on much longer—although a casual look or first glance at the patient may reveal a pretty healthy-looking specimen.

In the first group of cases the patient is often found to be minimizing his symptoms or distress and perhaps unconsciously is not quite ready to divulge all the facts in his case. A conference with a near relative or his family physician may supply the missing link or additional facts in his case. While in the second group it may be necessary to cut short the interview by some well directed questions.

While the number of cases of functional digestive disturbances in the elderly patient is not as great as in the younger or middle-aged group, yet a not inconsiderable number will fall in this category. Others will be found to be due not to a disease of the di-

*Read before the Annual Meeting May 11-12, 1943, Oklahoma City.

gestive or associated digestive organs but rather the result of a primary cardiovascular degeneration with its consequent circulatory disturbance. It is to be remembered then that the elderly patient comes in at a period in his life when generalized arteriosclerosis is to be expected, often with advanced arteriosclerotic changes in many organs and extensive cardiovascular damage, to say nothing about the disease of the digestive organs.

To the patient gaseous indigestion generally means excessive belching and a feeling of fullness and bloating. True flatulence with bloating and an excessive amount of flatus is also a common trouble. Flatulence in the elderly patient may be simply due to poorly regulated bowel habits, since constipation is almost the universal rule at that age. This may be aggravated to some extent by the over-enthusiastic physician who prescribes a bulky diet. This leaves a considerable increase in the total cellulose in the colon upon which some bacteria may thrive, creating still more gas and causing an increase in gas pains. Many of these patients have difficulty in properly masticating their food, due to poor teeth or even lack of teeth, so they bolt their food, unconsciously swallowing a not inconsiderable amount of air with their food.

In most cases the gas that is expelled or flatus consists mainly of the nitrogen left over after the oxygen has been absorbed from swallowed air. Another factor may be the impaired circulation of the intestine due to arteriosclerotic and vascular changes, which brings about failure to re-absorb enough of the gas that ordinarily would be carried to the lungs and gotten rid of in that way.

Insufficient daily intake of fluid is a common fault at this age and so still further aggravates the problem of constipation. A marked relaxation of the perineum with pronounced rectocele is sometimes a very definite factor because of impaired expelling power. We have seen such patients operated on with marked improvement in their previous constipation. Occasionally I am sure that cases with hemorrhoids, especially those cases of fissure-in-ano accompanied by a sentinel pile, will show marked improvement in bowel habits after proper operative treatment has been carried out.

That the advent of a daily thorough satisfactory bowel action or lack of it often will materially influence the mental outlook of the senile patient for that particular day is well known to all physicians. Coming at a time in life when the pleasureable activities have long since ceased, the satisfactory functions of the urinary apparatus and bowel are of considerable importance to him. Therefore, the problem of constipation in the elder-

ly patient merits the careful consideration of all physicians who have this type of patient under their care.

The elderly man who has been getting up three or four times at night may complain of distress or pain in the abdomen running down both sides towards the midline in the pubic region. These pains usually are more pronounced in the evening or early part of the night and often accompanied by marked increase in his chronic constipation or a distended abdomen, especially the lower part, only partially relieved by enemas. These symptoms are often miraculously improved or eliminated entirely by an in-dwelling catheter preparatory to operation. In such cases resection of the prostate relieves the toxemia from the back-pressure of the retained urine in the bladder and affords permanent relief.

In every case of real flatulence, especially when the flatus is persistently foul, one must make sure that the difficulty is not due to some particular article of food to which the patient is sensitive. Measures directed toward elimination of the offended foods may go far toward making the patient happy again.

When such flatulence comes only in occasional attacks the patient should be instructed to keep track of the unusual foods eaten a few hours before each upset.

Gaseous indigestion with bloating may be a major complaint for many months before the onset of cardiac failure manifests itself in the chronic hypertensive heart case. Once dyspnea, edema of the ankle, liver engorgement and other evidences of disturbed circulation appear, the gaseous disturbance will fluctuate with the degree of circulatory deficiency. The elderly man who complains of gas which comes only when he tries to exercise, especially after a full meal or during cold weather, usually has a narrowed coronary artery and the flatulence may be the only symptom by which one may recognize this condition before the advent of more serious manifestations.

There is another group of cases in our experience which causes no end of confusion. They are the cases that have chronic gaseous indigestion with belching, colicy gas pains, flatulence, bloating, often with constipation, which are commonly labeled chronic cholecystitis or even biliary tract disease. When we advise operation in a chronic gall bladder diseases with stones or in those who have recurrent gall bladder colic we are assured of reasonably good results. Not so, however, with the third group; here we may anticipate symptomatic relief in less than half the cases. Under these circumstances one must conclude that the mildly diseased gall bladder was only a part of the biliary tract disease or that other conditions were responsible for the symptoms; namely a primary colon disturbance or some mild process in the associated digestive organs.

We know that chronic cholecystitis with. or without stones is extremely common, especially in women after the third decade. Rivers states it occurs in 24 per cent of those who complain of chronic dyspepsia and that it is present in over 9 per cent of men over forty with similar complaints. Autopsy records show that gall stones are found in more than 20 per cent of women and about 10 per cent of men after the age of 39, and that the percentage showing some evidence of cholecystitis is much higher. Thus we see that chronic cholecystitis is the most common cause of chronic dyspepsia in the elderly patient.

It should be stated that it is also true that gall bladder colic occurs only in a small fraction of people with gall stones, perhaps not more than 5 per cent. Equally important, however, is the belief among many good clinicians that symptoms not distinguishable from biliary colic may occur without evidence at operation or autopsy of any pathologic condition of the gall bladder and that the pain persists after cholecystectomy. The obvious explanation for some of these failures would be that the pain did not originate in the biliary tract. Many excellent observers believe otherwise. There is some evidence that the pain may originate in a normal biliary tract. That functional disturbance of the biliary tract can cause an attack of biliary colic in the absence of stone or inflammation seems fairly well established. These disturbances of secretion or absorption may depend on the character of the liver bile and good evidence exists today chiefly for the motor type of dysfunction, the so-called biliary dyspepsia.

There are many leading clinicians who believe that the syndrome of chronic gall bladder colic are not really due to gall bladder disease at all, but rather due to an irritable colon with associated pylorospasm at times. Certainly it is very difficult to differentiate between the two unless gall bladder disease is supported by evidence of a non-functioning gall bladder as shown by the cholecystogram.

It may be said as a general rule that patients in middle life who are troubled with an irritable, spastic colon will find that after the age of 50 this condition will gradually ameliorate and be far less troublesome to them; yet we know that many of them will continue to be plagued by an irritable colon. even as late as 70. Mucous colitis is not infrequently seen to continue even though the patient is past 60 years of age.

How then are we to judge the surgical indications in these chronic gall bladder dyspepsias without gall stones or colon? Often it is difficult to determine which cases should be operated and which ones should be continued under medical management even though results are only temporary.

It is my opinion that those cases in which a cholecystographic workout has revealed a non-functioning gall bladder, surgery may be indicated. It is well, however, to treat such cases medically for a reasonable time and then repeat the cholecystogram. If a non-functioning gall bladder is still present then one may be reasonably sure of the diagnosis, provided of course that a badly damaged liver is not the cause of the non-filling or non-concentrating gall bladder.

It is surprising that in some cases a second cholecystrogram will show a fairly good functioning gall bladder. It should be remembered that in the vast majority of cases suffering from advanced hepatic disease a non-functioning gall bladder will be revealed by the cholecystrogram.

There is still another group of cases in which the present laboratory methods are of limited value. This group is made up of patients suffering from chronic disease of the liver. They are usually due to some intrahepatic condition such as cirrhosis or fatty degeneration. They are most frequently associated with chronic gastritis and chronic gall bladder disease and they are more common than usually supposed.

Clinically, most of these cases give an indefinite history of indigestion over a relatively long period of time. Anorexia is frequently of long-standing, especially in those addicted to the use of alcohol. Clinical experience, however, has shown that an alcoholic history is found in only 30 to 40 per cent of cases in cirrhosis of the liver and so there must be many other causes for this condition. Nausea is another common symptom and is most noticeable in the morning. Distress after eating is common. Then intensity of the distress is seldom, however, as severe as in peptic ulcer, unless there is a considerable peri-hepatitis or swelling of the liver, when the pain will be found to be in the right upper quadrant. Belching, gas distention and an intolerance for fat are all common manifestations. There is usually a furred tongue, bad breath and chronic constipation. Evidence of bleeding may be present such as nose-bleed; hematemesis from esophageal varices, and intestinal hemorrhage are probably most prevalent, and icteric pallor is common. Actual jaundice only occurs in the terminal condition, such as cirrhosis.

Because of the diverse function of the

liver, no available tests are of absolute diagnostic value. It is the clinical picture which should be of paramount importance. The hippuric acid and bromsulfathalein tests are fairly good. The very nature of the symptoms in hepatic dysfunction are such that it is easy to confuse them with mild cases of gall bladder disease. Only too often in the absence of any appreciable enlargement of the liver the condition it thought to be due to some gall bladder condition until some time later when, much to our surprise, the patient turns up with ascites.

It is our experience that the ordinary cholecystographic workout always shows a practically complete absence of any dye in the gall bladder in advanced liver disease and that it is of definite value in making us at least think in terms of liver damage. Therefore I believe with our limited experience that the cholecystographic workout is one of the best liver function tests we possess to date.

Chronic gastritis is a disease which again has been forcibly brought to our attention with increasing emphasis during the past 10 years. Although we have reliable knowledge regarding this condition for at least 85 years, the diagnosis of chronic gastritis fell into disrepute until the use of the flexible gastroscope allowed a study of the mucosal pattern of the stomach by direct visualization.

The development of improved x-ray technique by the compression method which permits better visualization of the mucosa has also been a contributing factor.

Twenty-five years ago the diagnosis of chronic gastritis was limited largely to that of chronic alcoholic gastritis, syphilitic gastritis or the early mucosal atrophy associated with pernicious anemia or the environmental gastritis around ulcer or cancer discovered on operative interference. Today we are led to believe by many competent gastroscopists that chronic gastritis is a very common condition. It may be the pendulum has already swung too far in that direction. Those of us who have been in practice for 25 years or more are quite aware of the over-enthusiasm to which the profession so easily succumbs.

Nevertheless, as time goes on the diagnosis of chronic gastritis will be on a much firmer basis since we now possess an instrument of diagnostic precision. Unfortunately the technique of doing a gastroscopic examination requires considerable training and skill. Long experience is necessary in the proper evaluation of what is seen through a gastroscope and this limits its diagnostic use to a small number skilled in this procedure.

The symptoms of chronic catarrhal superficial and chronic hyperthophic gastritis simulate those of chronic gastric or duodenal ulcer in a considerable measure, even with respect to gross hemorrhage. Epigastric pain and discomfort which usually have some relation to meals and from which relief by food or antacid is less consistent than in ulcer cases are outstanding features of gastritis. In the past, in the absence of any x-ray evidence of ulcer, the physician labelled such conditions nervous indigestion, pseudo-ulcer, pseudo-cholecystitis, achylia gastrica or what-not. The competent gastroscopist of today very often finds the explanation for these symptoms in chronic inflammatory lesions of the mucosa of the stomach and so one should not lightly scoff at the gastroscopist's contention that the most common organic disease of the stomach is a chronic inflammatory lesion of the stomach.

Time will not permit the discussion of the many other causes for the chronic digestive disturbances in the elderly patient, among the most interesting of which are those due to psychoneurosis. Suffice it to say, that since no precision methods of laboratory study are available in most cases, a critical study of the clinical symptoms forms the basis for the differential diagnosis in these various conditions.

DISCUSSION

Minard F. Jacobs, M.D.

Dr. Paulus' discussion of chronic digestive disturbances in the aged patient is an excellent and timely paper because with the younger men in the service it will be necessary for those who are left behind to care for more old people proportionately. Furthermore, as statistics show people are living longer, hence there are more old people. The 1940 census showed an increase of 35 per cent over 1930 of folks over 65 years of age. The medical management of disease in individuals beyond the sixth or seventh decade of life presents unique problems and so is fast becoming a specialized field. In geriatrics, as the specialty is known, one is dealing with individuals whose tolerance is low and whose powers of regeneration are definitely limited. However, as he or she has so far withstood the stress and strain of life one must give special care in advising too drastic changes. The fact is that these individuals are not tolerant of changes and they often feel they know better what to do for themselves than the physician. Their ways of life have become fixed just as their organs have become less elastic. They quickly become dissatisfied if the remedies advised do not give immediate results. Hence it is well to discuss their problems simply and truthfully with them.

A most important decision that usually must be made at the start is whether or not the patient should be kept at absolute bed rest. In general one can say that they should be allowed up as much as is compatible with their condition and strength. Prolonged periods of bed rest may not only be harmful physically but psychologically. Drugs must be used cautiously. This applies particularly to sedatives. In cerebral arteriosclerosis capillary permeability is increased and so they diffuse more rapidly. There may frequently be some renal damage also and thus excretion is interferred with and this may easily result in a cumulative effect.

There has never been any extensive studies on the digestive enzymes in the aged. Is there a decrease with the physiological process of aging? One would think so. We do know there is a decrease in salivary ptyalin, but we do not know in how many the pancreatic amylase is likewise deficient. Meyer concluded after testing the carbohydrate digestion in a number of old people that there was probably a sufficient amount of pancreatic amylase to make up for the deficiency in salivary amylase. It has also been shown that fatigue in old folks causes a reduction in the ferments in the saliva and the stomach. By their own choice old people consume a diet heavy in carbohydrates. This is frequently due to the greater ease in eating this type of food. Likewise, they choose a diet low in fat and protein. Because of this type of diet they often obtain an insufficient amount of vitamins, chiefly the B group. Because of the high carbohydrate intake, additional B complex vitamins are required. A study made at the Laukenau Hospital revealed that the diet of old people was deficient in foods rich in Vitamin B, iron and calcium, and one result of this was anemia. By giving these patients a balanced diet, liver twice a week, injections of liver extract for one to three weeks and iron there was not only an increase in the blood count but a definite increase in vigor. Other studies have shown that the vitamin C intake is likewise inadequate. It should be realized that the body stores only small amounts of these water soluble vitamins and so they must be replenished from day to day. Hence giving these old people an adequate amount of vitamin B and C is definitely helpful. I do not mean to imply that this will stop the biological developments of senility yet certain features are changed chiefly in relation to the muscular, cardio-vascular, and mental systems and to some extent the gastro-intestinal.

Dr. Paulus made some pertinent remarks regarding roughage in the diet of old people. I heartily concur in this. Constipation is a frequent complaint and many times can be corrected by diet alone if the full co-operation of the patient can be had which as you all know is often difficult. In general these old people should eat a diet that is rich in fruits, vegetables, especially the green and yellow ones, milk and milk products such as cream, ice cream and cheese. Meat in small amounts is advisable. The vegetables should perferably be those that contain a low fiber content. We are deluged by the drug houses with various bulk producers to aid constipation and although in many individuals these hygroscopic agents are beneficial they must be used with caution in the elderly patient as they not infrequently cause an impaction. Good results may be had with an occasional small normal saline enema or at times oil retention enemas may be helpful. However, if the patient has been taking laxatives for forty or fifty years without any apparent harm, it seems somewhat foolhardy to advise stopping them. The patient will usually ignore the advice anyway.

• *THE PRESIDENT'S PAGE* •

The present policy of Selective Service of NOT deferring pre-medical students after July 1, 1944, has created a serious problem in connection with the supply of physicians for the future. It is felt by some that the output of doctors may be inadequate to meet the replacement demands of the army and civilian needs despite the fact that the medical schools are running at full capacity. It is obvious, therefore, that under no circumstances should the enrollment in the first year classes of the medical schools be allowed to fall below the maximum number that can be accommodated in each medical school.

According to the recent information supplied by the Procurement and Assignment Service and published in the Journal of the American Medical Association, June 10, 1944, estimates of medical students for 1945 are as follows:

Total number of places in entering classes—6,440.
    Army students, 28 per cent—1,790
    Navy students, 25 per cent—1,540—3,330
    Balance to be filled by women
and by men disqualified for general
military service ....   —3,110.

Granting that it is possible to fill 400 to 500 of these places with women students, this still leaves about 2,600 places which, according to present regulations, must be filled by physically disqualified men or ex-service men.

It is not possible to predict how far the schools can go in solving this problem without lowering their standards of admission, but it should be the concern of every physician to see to it that this situation is changed.

There has been introduced in the House of Representatives recently a Bill HR 5027, which would, under certain conditions, defer 6,000 medical and pre-medical students from induction. We earnestly urge that each of you immediately contact the Senator or Representative of your District and ask that he support this legislation. An adequate supply of doctors must be maintained and this can only be done by training a sufficient number of medical students.

The ruling of the Selective Service is apparently final. The matter is now up to the President and/or Congress.

President.

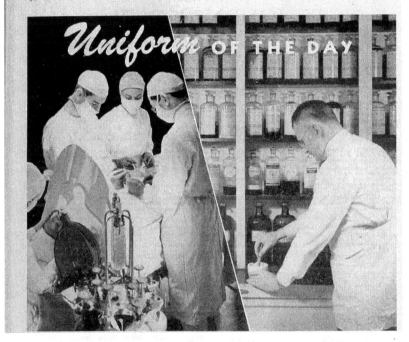

★ Many of our physicians are now wearing the Olive Drab . . . Navy Blue . . . and Khaki. Their absence greatly increases the responsibility of home front physicians — constantly demanding more time and energy, to keep civilians fit for strenuous war jobs.

We appreciate the long hours and many sacrifices necessary to keep the home front healthy, thereby speeding supplies and equipment to the fighting front. Warren-Teed is anxious to help these busy physicians at all times.

WARREN-TEED

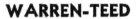
Medicaments of Exacting Quality Since 1920

THE WARREN-TEED PRODUCTS COMPANY, COLUMBUS 8, OHIO

The JOURNAL Of The
OKLAHOMA STATE MEDICAL ASSOCIATION

EDITORIAL BOARD

L. J. MOORMAN, Oklahoma City, Editor-in-Chief

E. EUGENE RICE, Shawnee

BEN H. NICHOLSON, Oklahoma City

MR. PAUL H. FESLER, Oklahoma City, Business Manager

CONTRIBUTIONS: Articles accepted by this Journal for publication including those read at the annual meetings of the State Association are the sole property of this Journal.

The Editorial Department is not responsible for the opinions expressed in the original articles of contributors.

Manuscripts may be withdrawn by authors for publication elsewhere only upon the approval of the Editorial Board.

MANUSCRIPTS: Manuscripts should be typewritten, double-spaced, on white paper 8½ x 11 inches. The original copy, not the carbon copy, should be submitted.

Footnotes, bibliographies and legends for cuts should be typed on separate sheets in double space. Bibliography listing should follow this order: Name of author, title of article, name of periodical with volume, page and date of publication.

Manuscripts are accepted subject to the usual editorial revisions and with the understanding that they have not been published elsewhere.

NEWS: Local news of interest to the medical profession, changes of address, births, deaths and weddings will be gratefully received.

ADVERTISING: Advertising of articles, drugs or compounds unapproved by the Council on Pharmacy of the A.M.A. will not be accepted. Advertising rates will be supplied on application.

It is suggested that members of the State Association patronize our advertisers in preference to others.

SUBSCRIPTIONS: Failure to receive The Journal should call for immediate notification.

REPRINTS: Reprints of original articles will be supplied at actual cost provided request for them is attached to manuscripts or made in sufficient time before publication. Checks for reprints should be made payable to Industrial Printing Company, Oklahoma City.

Address all communications to THE JOURNAL OF THE OKLAHOMA STATE MEDICAL ASSOCIATION, 210 Plaza Court, Oklahoma City. (3)

OFFICIAL PUBLICATION OF THE OKLAHOMA STATE MEDICAL ASSOCIATION
Copyrighted July, 1944

EDITORIALS

LET THE PEOPLE KNOW

If the people of the United States could be brought to an adequate understanding of what preventive medicine, including public health and sanitary engineering, both of which are based upon and sustained by medical knowledge, has done to safeguard them against the ravages of disease and disaster, they would rise up in arms against the false security of any revolutionary, government controled, regimented form of medical service, which would deal the death blow to medicine as a free enterprise. If the people knew how adequately the march of medicine has matched mechanistic progress, including the growth of industry and commerce, the present widespread criticism of medicine would be replaced by a just commendation.

If the people were fully apprised of the fact that they might have been wiped from the face of the earth by disease and pestilence as the world, on fast going wheels for the first time in history, cut all corners to get on with industry except for the saving grace of preventive measures; if they knew how medicine at the turn of the century, placed spiritual and humanitarian values far above material gain in the application of newly acquired knowledge, they would pile high their remonstrances on the desks of congressmen who might otherwise legalize some change in medical practice.

Finally, if the people knew to what extent congested areas of population are dependent upon preventive medicine; if, for instance, they knew that the withdrawal of all preventive measures provided by American medicine from the city of Washington today would soon make it necessary for all citizens to duck the shadow of death, and within a few months block the streets with the decaying dead bodies of men, women and children; converting the dome of the Capitol into a rendevous for carrion crazed vultures and causing the most beautiful city in the world to be spattered and blighted with the pale excrement of these filthy scavengers; if the people knew all this they would rise up and call the medical profession blessed.

Benjamin Franklin, statesman, scientist, friend of medicine and sponsor of hospitals and medical schools made the following broad statement which may be specifically applied to our present situation; "They that give up essential liberty to obtain a little temporary safety deserve neither liberty nor safety."

ON THE WITNESS STAND

As noted by an editorial in The New England Journal of Medicine, June 1, 1944, The Massachusetts Medical Society in 1936, appointed a Committee to consider "Expert Testimony." In the Journal of the American Medical Association of April 1, 1944 there is a discussion of action taken by the Minnesota State Medical Association through a similar committee appointed three years ago.

Often the medical profession is embarrassed by alleged "expert medical testimony." As a rule, the best physicians shun the witness stand because of the unbridled license in the choice of medical witnesses and the loose application and questionable meaning of the term "expert."

If such a committee could be counted on for the conscientious execution of its assigned functions, the Oklahoma State Medical Association should have one. We suggest that the officers and the Council take the matter under consideration. The following paragraph from the discussion appearing in The Journal of the American Medical Association clearly places the responsibility.

"Next to saving life and giving aid to the sick and injured no greater responsibility devolves on the medical profession than giving testimony in court or elsewhere. The right of a physician to continue in the practice of medicine is measured not only by his professional competence as a physician but also by what he says and does as a physician."

THE ART AND THE SCIENCE OF MEDICINE GO HAND IN HAND AT THE FRONT

Millions of mothers and fathers have had their hearts cheered by the widespread news that our brave sons wounded on the Normandy beaches in the morning were snugly tucked away in hospitals on the English shore by the following evening with the best medical and surgical care.

While this note of merciful efficiency and skill is most gratifying, the greatest spiritual uplift came through the knowledge that Major General Paul Ramsey Hawley according to published reports "paced the docks at a south-of-England port, making sure for himself that the wounded were comfortable." Also that the stretchers were handled with the tenderness and dexterity which the traditional art of medicine demands in the presence of sickness and suffering.

It is heartening to see how well the wisdom of William Osler wears in war as in peace. "The practice of medicine is an art, not a trade; a calling, not a business; a calling in which the heart will be exercised equally with the head."

CIVILIAN PENICILLIN

Through American ingenuity and industry Penicillin for civilian use has been made available sooner and in greater quantities than originally anticipated. Until recently it was to be had for emergency cases only when specific indications were established and then its use required the approval of a committee of The National Research Council and the War Production Board. Now that it is more readily available because more plentiful, its distribution is to be governed by W.P.B., the N.R.C., the U. S. Public Health Service and the A.M.A.

Certain hospitals in the State of Oklahoma have been designated as repositories and distributors of the precious product. All doctors should remember that the supply is still limited and that its more generous allocation places upon them heavy responsibility. They should strive for up-to-date information concerning specific indications, being quick to employ it when definitely indicated and badly needed, but equally quick to advise against its use in conditions already proven to be resistant to its curative powers.

Considering the limited supply, unwise or wasteful use of Penicillin is next to criminal. Always it should be employed with a reasonable hope of saving life and not for the purpose of satisfying curiosity or appeasing the clammering insistance of desperate patients or relatives.

THE FREEDOM OF MEDICINE

American medicine rests upon a tripod . . . the patient, the physician and God. Almost without exception the patient and physician are mutually helpful and pleased with the relationship. If they are not satisfied, they are free to tell each other to go to the hottest place that their religious inhibitions permit.

God seems interested in both the patient and the physician. He exacts no accounting except a reasonable exercise of conscience, and He presents no interminable, incomprehensible blanks to be filled out in triplicate.

Let's Keep American Medicine Free!

ASSOCIATION ACTIVITIES

REPORT OF AMERICAN MEDICAL AS-SOCIATION HOUSE OF DELEGATES CHICAGO, JUNE 14, 1944

It is not possible in the space alloted to give a comprehensive report of the meeting of the House of Delegates of the American Medical Association. A complete report will appear in the Journal of the American Medical Association beginning with the June 24 issue where it can and should be read by every practicing physician. If you have time for nothing more, read pages 573-576.

But the experiences of the meeting gave rise to some ideas which the Editor of the Oklahoma State Medical Journal has asked us to express. Unfortunately, it is evident at the onset that too few Oklahoma physicians will read the proceedings of the meetings of the House. The record shows that only 716 of our 1493 members of the Oklahoma State Medical Association are subscribers to the American Medical Association Journal. This is too small a proportion to prove that our Oklahoma physicians appreciate ''the best Medical Journal in the World.'' We are told that the Journal is to be made still increasingly useful in that more articles are to be printed which will be of special interest to the general practitioner. We would respectfully suggest that many more physicians become habitual readers of the American Medical Association Journal.

Hygeia is another magazine which should be found on every physicians office table—to be read by him as well as by his patients. This ''Health Magazine'' is a happy combination of the ''popular'' and the scientific in medicine. It can be read with profit by the physician, illustrating as it does so well, usually, avenues of approach to giving information which the laity so much needs.

The reports of the various councils and committees given at the meeting of the House of Delegates were most interesting. Even a mere list of them here would require too much space. The extent of the activities would be a revelation to most physicians. The many-sided activities for the advancement of scientific medicine and for its applications to the good of the people is too little understood by a large body of physicians.

It is a hopeful sign that there are many physicians who are willing to sacrifice of their own leisure and practice to do this necessary organizational and ''public relations'' work. If we are at times disposed to criticize them for apparent lack of progress we might frankly ask ourselves: ''How much have I done of this work?''

American medicine needs no defense either before intelligent people nor before the politicians. The record of its attainments are sufficient justification for its status and its methods. But, because of its scientific basis in which the laity is not trained, we the profession owe the people an intelligent and sympathetic explanation of good medicine and its social and political implications.

This is precisely the function which the House of Delegates, last year and again this year, desired as one of the primary functions of the new ''Council on Medical Service and Public Relations.'' The personnel of this council as decided in this years' election is perhaps as ''popular'' a choice as could well be made. Many of us who know these men and their attitude, believe a great improvement will be wrought in the ''public relations'' between organized medicine and the public- including the members of our legislative bodies.

This Council has achieved wonders in a short space of time, and its activities, which have been well supported by the Trustees of the Association, should end the criticism of the American Medical Association—that it is an organization without a positive program. Certainly the program as outlined on pages 573-576 of the June 24 Journal of the American Medical Association is very positive. Please read it carefully.

But this Committee, however efficient, cannot accomplish all that should be done in the education of the public. Each physician, in the course of his daily contacts with his patients and associates, has a most potent opportunity for forming and molding a favorable and intelligent attitude towards medicine as it relates to the public welfare, and the enactment of laws.

The American Medical Association form of organization is democratic and representative only to the extent to which the rank and file—members of the State Medical Associations exercise care in electing delegates to the American Medical Association and then ask an accounting of their actions in the House of Delegates.

Judging from signs of the floor of the House and from numerous remarks in the corridors, we can be encouraged to believe that the rank and file of the profession are becoming more and more aware of the need for cooperation in taking, adopting and continuing a progressive program.

A. S. Risser, M.D., Delegate
James Stevenson, M.D., Delegate

LEWIS J. MOORMAN GUEST SPEAKER AT DENVER MEETING

The Regional Meeting of the American College of Physicians was held in combination with the War College in Denver, Colorado, June 22-24. At the dinner meeting held on June 23, one of the guest speakers was Lewis J. Moorman, M.D., Oklahoma City, who spoke on ''American Medicine—Past and Future.''

APOLOGY

On page 220 of the May Journal the following statement appeared in the write up of the 52nd Annual Meeting: ''Also, Dr. Byron E. Williams inaugurated a scheme for an endowment fund for the Medical School which received the approval of the group.''

The scheme for an endowment fund for the Medical School was inaugurated by Dr. Wayman Thompson instead of Dr. Williams.

⌐CORRECTION

"Clinical Observations in the Use of Penicillin"
Published in the May issue of the Journal

In the paper entitled ''Clinical Observations in the Use of Penicillin.'' by Lt. Col. Earl R. Denny, M.C., A.U.S., Major P. L. Shallenberger, M.C., A.U.S., and Major H. D. Pyle, M.C., A.U.S., which appeared in the May issue of the Journal, the following changes should be made: The title and footnote on the chart appearing on Page 198 should appear above and below the chart in the left hand column on Page 202. The title and footnote of the chart appearing in the left hand column of Page 202 should appear above and below the chart presented on Page 199.

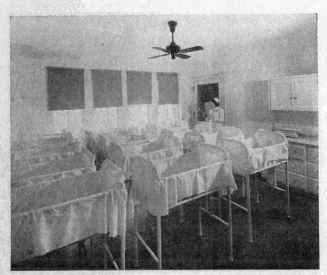

Official Proceedings of House of Delegates
Oklahoma State Medical Association
April 24-25, 1944, Tulsa

MINUTES OF FIRST SESSION
Monday, April 24, 1944

The first session of the House of Delegates at the 52nd Annual Meeting of the Oklahoma State Medical Association held at Tulsa was called to order in the Ivory Room of the Mayo Hotel, at 8:45 P.M., Monday, April 24, 1944, by the Speaker, Dr. George H. Garrison of Oklahoma City.

The Chairman of the Credentials Committee, Dr. Finis W. Ewing, Muskogee, stated that the records indicated a quorum was present.

A group photograph was taken of Dr. James Stevenson, Tulsa; Dr. C. R. Rountree, Oklahoma City; Dr. Ralph A. McGill, Tulsa; Senator E. H. Moore, Tulsa; also one of the Delegates, Alternates and guests who were seated on the floor of the House.

The President, Dr. Stevenson, presented Senator Moore who made several pertinent remarkes with reference to his attitude toward medicine.

The Speaker read the following telegram from Dick Graham, Executive Secretary of the Association on leave of absence with the Army: "Please convey to House of Delegates and all others present my sincere hope for a successful meeting. Only wish I could be present. Association is perhaps too near to me for its own good. I know House of Delegates will continue to lead rather than be lead."

On *motion* by Dr. J. S. Fulton, Atoka, *seconded* by Dr. J. G. Edwards, Okmulgee, and *carried*, the minutes of the meetings of the House of Delegates held on May 10 and 11, 1943 were *approved* as published.

Following the adoption of the above motion, the Speaker, in compliance with the provisions of Chapter III, Section 4, Subsection (a), of the By-Laws, appointed the following Reference Committees: Resolutions Committee—Dr. Clinton Gallaher, Shawnee, Chairman; Dr. H. M. McClure, Chickasha, and Dr. J. T. Phelps, El Reno. Advisory to the Resolutions Committee—Dr. G. L. Johnson, Pauls Valley, and Dr. J. G. Edwards, Okmulgee. Tellers and Judges of Elections—Dr. A. K. Cox, Watonga; Dr. H. C. Huntley, Atoka, and Dr. J. Hobson Veazy, Ardmore. Sergeant-at-arms—Dr. Mack I. Shanholtz, Wewoka, and Dr. S. A. Lang, Nowata.

At this time, the Speaker, in compliance with the provisions of Chapter VII, Section 3, of the By-Laws of the Association, called for the Annual Report of the Council.

Annual Report of the Council

In submitting the Report of the Council for 1943-1944 to the House of Delegates, your Officers desire to call attention to the fact that our Executive Secretary, R. H. Graham, is now on leave of absence from the executive office following his call to active service with the Army the first of October. It is further our desire to report that recently Paul H. Fesler has been employed as Acting Executive Secretary during his absence.

Your Officers, during the past year, have striven diligently to see that the activities of the Association were curtailed very little as was reflected in the reports of committees published in the March Journal and those reports that will be made during the sessions of the House of Delegates.

As has been the custom in the past, the audit of accounts, as prepared by the office of the public accountant, was published in the March Journal, and delegates and members are referred to this report for a detailed analysis of the finances of the Association.

The auditor's report for January 1, 1943, showed total assets of $5,392.46; the report for January 1, 1944,

shows a total of $8,115.05, an increase of $2,722.59. Of this total, $7,834.24 belongs to the Membership account. In studying the membership dues, we find there was a gain of $1,395.50 in 1943 as compared with the total for 1942. The income on the Journal shows an increase from its advertising of $460.47, the income for 1943 showing a total of $7,969.81 while the 1942 advertising totaled $7,509.34.

In addition to the above-mentioned balances, the Association owns $2,235.78 in United States Treasury and Savings Bonds payable to the Membership account, and $8,163.10 in United States Treasury and Defense Bonds payable to the Medical Defense account.

In 1943, the House of Delegates approved the Council's recommendation that the Medical Defense account be stabilized with an operating cash reserve in the amount of $500.00 and that should it become necessary to increase this total that this amount would be augmented from moneys in the Membership account. This recommendation was by virtue of the fact that during the past five years there had never been a single year when the fund had expended in excess of $300.00. As of January 1, 1944, the Medical Defense account showed a balance of $606.84. Inasmuch as the interest for the United States Treasury Bonds of the Medical Defense account totals $120.50 each year and is payable to no other account, the Council recommends that the bonds of this account in the amount of $8,163.10 be transferred to the Membership account.

At the present time, the total membership for 1944 is 1,447. Of this number, 1,121 are active Members, 298 Service Members, three of which were reinstated in 1944 by payment of 1943 dues; 24 Honorary Members and four Associate Members. This compares with the total membership of 1,498 for 1943 as follows: 1,179 Active Members; 287 Service Members paying $4.00 dues; 28 Honorary Members and four Associate Members. With further reference to statistics of 1943 memberships, nine Active Members have entered the Armed Forces, seven Active Members have moved out of the State, five Service Members have been retired from duty with the military forces and have re-entered civilian practice and 19 Active and four Honorary Members have passed away.

With the condition existing that the total amount of revenue from membership dues continues to decrease with additional physicians entering the service, the Council recommends that the dues for 1945 remain the same as for 1944 ($12.00), and that no dues be charged Service Members in 1945 provided they were members in good standing in 1944.

The budget of the Association for the coming year, as prepared by the Secretary-Treasurer, has been approved by the Council.

The Procurement and Assignment Service, under the direction of the State Chairman, Dr. Rucks, and with the advice and counsel of his Advisory Committee composed of a Vice-Chairman, County and Councilor Chairman, has been outstanding in its cooperative attitude and broad understanding of the many problems that are involved. The Procurement and Assignment Committee is to be highly commended for the untold hours of time and work given to personal interviews and careful consideration of each individual problem as well as to attention given to the requests of the military forces and the needs of individual communities with reference to medical care of civilians. Records of the Procurement and Assignment Service and those of the Association show over 500 Oklahoma physicians in the Armed Forces with 355 of these having been in active practice prior to their entrance into the various branches of the Armed Forces.

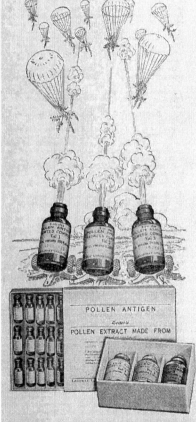

The Council recommends that committees as well as individuals continue to extend every possible cooperation in behalf of the Procurement and Assignment Service.

The House of Delegates at its 1943 meeting endorsed the report of the Prepaid Medical and Surgical Service Committee thereby approving the execution of proper instruments and the establishment of an experimental plan of prepaid medical and/or surgical service under the guidance of the medical profession for the citizens of Oklahoma in the lower income group. The Council meeting in regular session on February 20,1944, re-endorsed the plan as submitted by the Committee and instructed its individual Councilors in so far as possible to bring this plan before the membership of their County Societies for detailed discussion prior to this meeting. Your Council urges that Delegates give special consideration to the report of the activities of this Committee. The Council having endorsed the plan now refers it to the House of Delegates for further consideration and also goes on record as complimenting the Committee for its work and recommends that the Committee be continued.

During the past year, the Committee on Industrial Medicine and Traumatic Surgery has spent endless hours studying the present workman's compensation laws in Oklahoma. The Council recommends that the House of Delegates instruct the Public Policy Committee to work with the Committee on Industrial Medicine and Traumatic Surgery in an attempt to introduce proper legislation at the next Oklahoma State Legislative Session which would bring the above-mentioned laws up to date.

The two-year course in internal medicine conducted under the direct auspices of the Postgraduate Committee for the benefit of the physicians of Oklahoma was completed in February, and a course in surgical diagnosis is now in progress. Your Council recommends that the wishes of the Committee, as pointed out in its annual report published in the March Journal, be carried out in that resolutions expressing appreciation for cooperation and financial assistance be extended to The Commonwealth Fund of New York, the United States Public Health Service and the Oklahoma State Health Department. It is further urged that the members of the Association take advantage of the privilege extended them to gain new knowledge as is afforded through the means of postgraduate education.

Following the report of the Post-War Planning Committee at the Fourth Annual Secretaries Conference in October and which report was published in the November issue of the Journal, the Committee conducted the survey as suggested. The results will be given by the Committee in a report in the proper order of business. It is the recommendation of the Council to the House of Delegates that the work of this Committee be continued and that every assistance be extended by the members of the Association either individually or collectively in an effort to assist those who will be returning from the Armed Forces following the cessation of hostilities.

The Council in its afternoon meeting has gone on record and desires to recommend that the Speaker of the House appoint a Committee at this evening meeting to study the idea of a State Board of Health for Oklahoma and report its findings at tomorrow's session in order that definite recommendations might be referred to the Governor for his study prior to the meeting of the coming Legislature.

The Council recognizes the fact that physicians remaining at home are especially busy and have little available time for the attendance of meetings of medical societies, however, it urges that all county secretaries watch their membership lists and constantly remind their physicians of the vital need of maintaining society membership during these times. Each member should remember that he adds immeasurably to the influence of his profession on matters important to public welfare by maintaining membership in his county and state so-

cieties. The Council desires to remind the membership that a united front is vitally important at this time in view of the possibility of the passage of legislation by the National Congress that would affect our profession regarding its attitude toward the freedom of choice on the part of the people for the scientific services our physicians have been trained to give. Too, those of us on the home front should be constantly reminded that when our Service Members return from duty, it is important they find their medical society active in the affairs of state. County Societies are urged to continue with regular meetings, and where the membership is too small to hold frequent joint meetings with adjoining societies.

It is the desire of the Council to go on record as expressing appreciation for the undivided support given it by the individual members of the profession as well as commending the various committees for their work during the past year, and to assure the House of Delegates that it will render service to the Association to the best of its ability constantly keeping in mind the many obligations bestowed up it. Recognizing that the House of Delegates is the policy making body of our Association, the Council will continue to execute its mandates.

On *motion* by Dr. D. H. O'Donoghue, Oklahoma City, *seconded* by Dr. G. S. Baxter, and *carried*, the Report of the Council was *accepted*.

Following this action, the Speaker states that the following Councilor Reports had appeared in the March issue of the Journal: District No. 1, Dr. O. E. Templin, Alva; District No. 4, Dr. Tom Lowry, Oklahoma City; District No. 7, Dr. Clinton Gallaher, Shawnee, and District No. 9, Dr. L. C. Kuykendall, McAlester.

On *motion* by Dr. J. S. Fulton, Atoka, *seconded* by Dr. J. G. Edwards,Okmulgee, and *carried*, the above-mentioned Councilor Reports were *approved* as printed in the March Journal.

Following this action, Dr. Garrison asked for the report of Councilor District No. 2, and Dr. V. C. Tisdal, Elk City, was recognized and presented his report.

Annual Report District No. 2

Officers and Members of the House of Delegates
Of the Oklahoma State Medical Association
Gentlemen:

I am pleased to report that the Second Councilor District is in a normal and healthy state of affairs considering the conditions under which we labor. The tarian attitude. The sense of gratitude for the many men in our District that are in service is being manifested by th men at home in that they are anxious to do everything to make their return home as welcome as possible, return to them their practice in good condition, to keep their profession on as high a plane as is possible while they are away, and to forestall any move that might be foreign to their form of practice of medicine as to the time when they left.

Our District has had representatives in Washington contacting our Senators and Congressmen regarding the legislative measures that have been proposed which we realize would change our entire form of practice. There have been numerous meetings discussing the Wagner-Murray-Dingell Bill, and the representative from our District who was in Washington received very definite information from our National Representatives that they would not vote for the bill in its present form or any other form to which it might be amended.

A rather careful survey was made of the membership of Councilor District No. 2, and the vast majority are in favor of some form of medical and hospital benefits, mutual iu character, which will give them free choice of medical and hospital services with the opportunity to buy or reject. It is also optional with the physician as to his participation—the same to be sponsored and endorsed by our State Association, giving each county in the state and each group in the state a chance to reject or affiliate with said organization.

Our District is fully aware of the fact that economic conditions, as they are today, do not demand that some relief be given to the lower income brackets as they

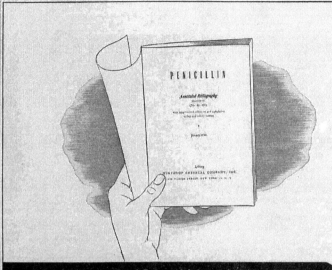

did during the depression or even in normal times. But we are of the opinion that they deserve some form of relief before conditions are such that they will make such request as they have in the past. We feel that the medical profession's first responsibility, of course, is to the people they serve and since the American Medical Association has endorsed many mutual plans that are operated under the supervision of the medical profession and since the medical profession, by sponsoring such service, can better make the experiment and cure its defects or faults and thereby curb any let down in the proper ethical relation between the doctor and the patient, they wish to endorse a trial of the benefits offered by the Oklahoma Physicians' Service (a mutual corporation) that was passed by the House of Delegates at its 1943 meeting.

Respectfully submitted,
V. C. Tisdal, M.D.
Councilor, District No. 2

On *motion* by Dr. W. S. Larrabee, Tulsa, *seconded* by Dr. L. Chester McHenry, Oklahoma City, and *carried*, it was moved that the Report of Councilor District No. 2 be *accepted*.

The Councilor of District No. 3, Dr. C. E. Northcutt, Ponca City, who was appointed by the Council on February 20, 1944, to replace Dr. C. W. Arrendell, Ponca City, who had been forced to resign because of ill health, was next granted the privilege of the floor and made his report.

Annual Report District No. 3

To the President and House of Delegates
Oklahoma State Medical Association
Gentlemen:

Due to the recent illness of Dr. C. W. Arrendell of Ponca City, who has been confined to bed for the last ten weeks, and who has been serving as Councilor for the Third District, it is necessary that I report his activities, as well as my own, during the past year.

I find that due to the present conditions and the reduced number of doctors in this District, which necessitates long hours for the remaining members, it is difficult to hold regular meetings with a satisfactory attendance.

Dr. Arrendell has visited a few of the counties and has written numerous letters to all of the counties trying to aid in establishing as nearly as possibly adequate medical care for all counties, more especially those counties having fewer doctors. He has cooperated in collecting the annual dues and aided with the work of the Procurement and Assignment Committee and has encouraged all the doctors to write to their representatives asking that they give their full consideration to the Senate Bill No. 1161. Dr. Arrendell has encountered the distribution of literature from the National Physicians Committee as well as other literature obtained through the State Association.

After my election as Councilor, I checked with Dr. Arrendell's activities and have proved to my satisfaction that each county is making every effort to render adequate medical service in an organized way as nearly as it is possible.

It is unfortunate that such a valuable member of our profession should become temporarily incapacitated at this time. I wish to take this opportunity to express my appreciation, as well as that of other members, for his work and splendid cooperation.

Respectfully submitted,
C. E. Northcutt, M.D.
Councilor, District No. 3

On *motion* by Dr. L. O. Kuyrkendall, McAlester, *seconded* by Dr. J. G. Edwards, and *carried*, the Report of the Councilor District No. 3 was *accepted*.

The Speaker next asked for the report of the Councilor from District No. 5, and inasmuch as Dr. J. I. Hollingsworth, Waurika, was not present, no report was given.

Next, the privilege of the floor was extended to the Councilor from District No. 6, Dr. J. V. Athey, Bartlesville, who made his report.

Annual Report District No. 6

To the President and House of Delegates
Oklahoma State Medical Association
Gentlemen:

Due to tire and gasoline shortage and to war conditions in general, your Councilor has been unable to visit all the Societies in the District; however, he has kept in touch with all and can report that all are holding regular meetings which are fairly well attended.

Two District meetings have been held—one in Bartlesville last May, with a good program furnished by Dr. O. R. Withers and Dr. Clifford C. Wilson, of Kansas City, and the other in Tulsa in March, addressed by Dr. P. S. Pelouze, of Philadelphia, in the interest of the campaign against venereal disease sponsored by the State Health Department.

Much interest is shown over the District in the fight against the bill for "Socialized Medicine," Senate Bill 1161, and addresses have been given showing the fallacies of this proposed legislation before doctors, nurses, dentists and many lay organizations.

It is hoped that travel conditions will improve during the coming year, so that your Councilor may be able to be more service to the Societies in the District.

Respectfully submitted,
J. V. Athey, M.D.
Councilor, District No. 6

On *motion* of Dr. J. T. Phelps, *seconded* by Dr. L. C. Kuyrkendall, and *carried*, Dr. Athey's report was *accepted*.

At this time, the Speaker called for the report of the Councilor from District No. 8, and the privilege of the floor was granted to Dr. Finis W. Ewing, who presented his report.

Annual Report District No. 8

Officers and Members of the House of Delegates
Of the Oklahoma State Medical Association
Gentlemen:

The Eighth Councilor District is in a very good condition. We, like all other sections of the state, have contributed to the Armed Forces. Those who are left are the older men but are carrying on in a most credible way. Meetings have not been held as frequently in the various County Societies as we would have liked, but considering the shortage of manpower, the unusual demand on the time of those who are left in private practice, the rationing of gasoline and tires, it is the opinion of your Councilor that they are doing an excellent piece of work.

A meeting of this Councilor District was held in the Red Cross rooms at Camp Gruber, March 2, at which time Dr. P. S. Pelouze was our guest Speaker. His address was well received and the attendance was very good.

Respectfully submitted,
Finis W. Ewing, M.D.,
Councilor, District No. 6

On *motion* by Dr. O. E. Templin, *seconded* by Dr. J. T. Phelps, and *carried*, Dr. Ewing's report was *accepted*.

Following the report of Dr. Ewing, Dr. Garrison called for the Report of the Councilor from District No. 10, Dr. J. S. Fulton. Dr. Fulton made the following remarks:

Annual Report District No. 10

Officers and Members of the House of Delegates
Of the Oklahoma State Medical Association
Gentlemen:

I have no written report to make. I am from the part of the state where there is definitely a scarcity of physicians. In many counties there are only three or four doctors of medicine.

Because of this existing condition and since all the doctors are extremely busy, it is very difficult to conduct regular county medical meetings. At Durant in Bryan County there is an active Society, however, I understand it has been necessary that they skip some meetings. In Atoka-Coal County we have nine members and attempt to meet regularly. In my section of the State, we are

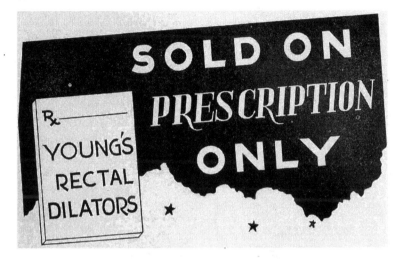
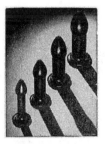

anxious to extend every cooperation to those doctors now in the various branches of the Armed Forces.

I am sorry that I have no written report to make, but I too have been very busy with my practice and often find it difficult to get away to attend meetings.

Respectfully submitted,
J. S. Fulton, M.D.
Councilor, District No. 10

On *motion* by Dr. Clinton Gallaher, *seconed* by Dr. J. G. Edwards, and *carried*, Dr. Fulton's report was *accepted*.

At this time, the Speaker of the House stated the next order of business would be the Report of the Standing Committees.

The first Committee to report was the Annual Session Committee, and Dr. James Stevenson, as Chairman, made the following remarks: "I did not know that I would be called upon to make a report, however, this is the Annual Session and if you like it thus far, I trust you will accept my report." Immediately upon completion of Dr. Stevenson's remarks, the Speaker stated "It stands approved."

The Speaker next requested the report of the Scientific Work Committee, and the privilege of the floor was granted to Dr. W. A. Showman, Tulsa.

Report of Scientific Work Committee

The Committee is hopeful that each and everyone of you will enjoy the meeting that has been prepared for you. We have run into some difficulty in the preparation of the program, but fortunately we have been successful in overcoming them. We have a good program in order for you and hope that it will meet with your approval.

Respectfully submitted,
W. A. Showman, M.D. Chairman
Ben H. Nicholson, M.D.
M. J. Searle, M.D.

On *motion* by Dr. W. S. Larrabee, *seconded* by Dr. W. E. Eastland, Oklahoma City, and *carried*, Dr. Showman's report was *accepted*.

The Speaker stated that the next report to be presented would be that of the Committee on Publicity. The Chairman, Dr. William A. Tolleson, Eufaula, was not in attendance, consequently, no report was given.

At this time, the Speaker requested the pleasure of the House concerning the disposition of the reports of the Committee on Judicial and Professional Relations, Chairman, Dr. S. A. Lang, and the Committee on Public Policy, Chairman, Dr. J. D. Osborn, Frederick, which reports had appeared in the March issue of the Journal. On *motion* by Dr. L. S. Willour, McAlester, *seconded* by Dr. O. E. Templin, and *carried*, the two above-mentioned reports were *approved*.

In order, the Speaker next called for the report of the Committee on Medical Education and Hospitals, and Dr. Tom Lowry, Oklahoma City, presented the following report:

Report of Committee on Medical Education and Hospitals

The Committee on Medical Education and Hospitals submits the following report to the House of Delegates:

The past year has brought many changes in medical education and some changes in hospital services. These have been made primarily to aid the war effort. Yet, it has made us study our methods of medical education. By lowering the requirements for admission to the School of Medicine to sixty hours, by accelerating and compressing the medical course into three years instead of four, we are increasing the output of physicians by 46.6 per cent and graduating doctors several years younger than heretofore. Also, the number of medical students accepted for admission to medical schools has increased about 10 per cent. The accelerated program will provide approximately 5,000 additional medical officers and physicians in the period 1942-1945.

Lowering the admission requirements for medical schools is bringing to us a group of students younger, less mature, with less diversity of preliminary training, and with fewer cultural interests than before. It seems advisable that as soon as possible we resume a longer premedical training for at least a considerable portion of our medical students. Acceleration in the elementary and secondary schools and telescoping the last year of high school with the first year of college may mature and prepare some students earlier and qualify them for admission earlier in the medical college.

Accelerating the medical curriculum allows a student to graduate a year earlier which is a decided advantage to him. He still has four to six weeks vacation each year. New courses such as military and tropical medicine and physical medicine should be stressed.

The maintaining of satisfactory standards of instruction during the war is somewhat difficult, due to the loss of members of the teaching staff, but those remaining are cooperating in every way. Because of the increased teaching load, the time for medical research is also probably reduced.

The financial support offered to medical students who are in the Armed Forces has probably opened the doors of medical education to some worthy students who would have been denied the privilege heretofore. When this financial aid is withdrawn, it would be well for us to consider the establishment of loan or aid funds to assist these worthy students who need financial assistance to carry on their medical education.

The nine-nine-nine intern service is meeting the condition for which it was adopted, but it offers adequate hospital training for less than 50 per cent of graduates of medical colleges. This will create a demand for more residencies for the post-war period, and we must be making every effort to raise our hospital standards so that we can increase the number of hospitals in our state which can supply residencies. By reducing the number of years required for premedical and medical school training, we hope that the number of years devoted to hospital training will be increased. We also should be making every effort to provide adequate diagnostic and hospital facilities to rural communities. These will provide better medical care to the communities and also be an inducement for well-trained young doctors to practice in these rural areas.

We must commend the Oklahoma State Board of Medical Examiners for conscientiously and rigidly upholding the highest standards to practice medicine in this State. Also the administration of the State of Oklahoma for their support in upholding the standards of medical education.

The post-war period will offer us an opportunity to re-evaluate, re-appraise and re-adjust our medical and hospital program. May we use wisdom in so doing.

Respectfully submitted,
Tom Lowry, M.D., Chairman
Sam A. McKeel, M.D.
Roscoe Walker, M.D.

On *motion* by Dr. D. W. Darwin, Woodward, *seconded* by Dr. O. E. Templin, and *carried*, the Report of the Committee on Medical Education and Hospitals was *accepted*.

In order, the Speaker announced that this completed the Reports of the Standing Committees and that the next order of business would be that of the presentation of Reports of Special Committees.

The privilege of the floor was granted to Dr. Tom Lowry, Chairman of the Post-War Planning Committee, who made the following report:

Subsequent Report of the Post-War Planning Committee

The first report of this Committee was presented at the Fourth Annual Secretaries Conference held in Oklahoma City in October, 1943. Subsequently, a report was published in the November, 1943, issue of the Oklahoma State Medical Journal. Briefly that report included several suggestions, among which were:

(1) That the Executive Secretary of the Oklahoma State Medical Association set up an information bureau or clearing house, which would include such information as would be of value to the doctor upon his return from military duty.

(2) That the Postgraduate Committee of the Oklahoma State Medical Association, the State Commissioner of Health and the University of Oklahoma School of Medicine be giving serious consideration to the feasibility of offering refresher courses in various branches of medicine to the doctors of the State after the cessation of hostilities.

(3) That a questionnaire be sent to each member of the Oklahoma State Medical Association who is serving in the Armed Forces. Also, that this questionnaire include the following questions: 1. Do you plan to return to Oklahoma after termination of the War; or do you plan on remaining in the Armed Forces; or do you plan on locating elsewhere? 2. Do you expect to return to your original location to practice? 3. Do you want a refresher course in some branch of medicine? If so, what branch? Do you want an internship, or do you want a residency? 4. Do you want information about other localities of the State in which you might be interested? 5. What do you want Amercian medicine to be like when you return? 6. What can the Oklahoma State Medical Association or your local County Medical Society do to help you to plan your future and help re-establish your practice?

(4) That every effort be made for the larger hospitals of the State to meet requirements for accredited internships and residencies, and other postgraduate facilities, which returning doctors may want and need.

(5) That efforts be made by rural communities to establish hospital and diagnostic centers in areas where these facilities are at present inadequate.

(6) That we make every effort to preserve so far as possible the privileges of the practice of medicine which the doctors enjoyed in this State at the time that they entered the Service.

The Committee wishes to report that the Executive Secretary of the Oklahoma State Medical Association has set up an information bureau or clearing house, covering such questions as were included in the original report concerning the status of various communities and that this information will be available and will be forwarded to those members of the Armed Forces who have requested such data.

Further, the Executive Secretary of the Oklahoma State Medical Association sent out a questionnaire to each member of the Association in the Armed Forces. This questionnaire included the questions enumerated above. 173 questionnaires were completed and returned to us. Out of the 173 returned questionnaires, 159 indicated that they expected to return to Oklahoma to practice medicine; three indicated they might remain in the Armed Forces; 122 that they intended to return to their original location; 18 that they were undecided about their future location; and 19 who had entered the Service after internship or residency before they had started practicing.

Out of the 173 returns, 114 stated that they desired postgraduate courses of study. The postgraduate specialties requested were listed as follows: Surgery 41, Obstetrics 21, Gynecology 19, Internal Medicine 18, General Medicine 5, Eye, Ear, Nose and Throat, or Ophthalmology 13. There were also requests for courses in 17 other specialties. There was one request for an internship, and 34 requests for post-war residencies.

Fifty-three men desired information concerning 21 different cities in the State of Oklahoma.

In answer to the broad question of What Do You Want American Medicine To Be Like When You Return, 135 reported (a free medicine, non-political, as pre-war,) or in other terms equally significant. Nineteen favored the establishment of well-directed prepaid medical plans. Two reported against hospital and medical insurance plans. Four favored adequate medical care for all income groups controlled by organized American Medicine.

In reply to the question of Ways that the Oklahoma State Medical Association and County Societies could be of assistance to them upon their return, there were numerous suggestions. Eighteen suggested that we prevent the passage of socialized medical laws. Twelve

suggested that we keep the State free of refugees and of the influx of physicians. Fourteen suggested more facilities for postgraduate refresher courses. The remaining 93 had various other interesting suggestions.

The Committee feels that this work which has been started should be continued by some committee; that as many of the questionnaires as is possible and feasible be answered by letter; and that if deemed advisable, other questionnaires which might be of value to this committee be sent out, and data accumulated. We also feel that we should cooperate so far as possible with the American Medical Association in their post-war planning for members of the Armed Forces.

Respectfully submitted,
Tom Lowry, M.D., Chairman
Gregory E. Stanbro, M.D.
Wann Langston, M.D.

On *motion* by Dr. V. C. Tisdal, *seconded* by Dr. J. G. Edwards, and *carried*, the subsequent report of the Committee on Post-War Planning was *approved*.

Following this action, the Speaker observed that the Annual Reports of nine of the 16 Special Committees; namely, Conservation of Vision and Hearing, Crippled Children, Malpractice Insurance, Maternity and Infancy, Medical Economics, Military Affairs, Public Health, Study and Control of Tuberculosis, and Medical Advisory Committee to the Department of Public Welfare, had been published in the March issue of the Journal and did not carry any controversial discussion.

On *motion* by Dr. W. S. Larrabee, *seconded* by Dr. C.B. Sullivan, Carnegie, and *carried*, the above-mentioned reports were *accepted*.

At this time, the Speaker stated that he desired to read a portion of the Report of the Committee on Industrial Medicine and Traumatic Surgery in order that it might be called to the attention of the Delegates. The portion read was taken from the Journal of the Oklahoma State Medical Association, March, 1944, page 135.

On *motion* by Dr. L. S. Willour, *seconded* by Dr. Ellis Lamb, Clinton, and *carried*, the entire Report of the Committee on Industrial Medicine and Traumatic Surgery was *accepted*.

Next; Dr. Garrison read the part of the Report of the Committee on Postgraduate Medical Teaching which appeared in the Journal of the Oklahoma State Medical Association, March, 1944, page 129.

On *motion* by Dr. A. S. Risser, Blackwell, *seconded* by Dr. S. A. Lang, and *carried*, the Report of the Postgraduate Medical Teaching Committee was *accepted*.

In order, the Speaker read the Report of the Committee on Necrology as published in the March Journal, and it was the request from various Delegates from the floor that the following additions be added to the list:

J. M. Pemberton	Okemah	February 21, 1944
W. G. Bisbee	Bristow	March 17, 1944
Fred J. Bolton	Tulsa	March 27, 1944
L. L. Wade	Ryan	April 1, 1944
W. L. Taylor	Holdenville	April 10; 1944

On *motion* by Dr. W. S. Larrabee that the names be added to the original report, *seconded* by Dr. V. C. Tisdal, and *carried*, the report was *accepted*.

At this time, the privilege of the floor was extended to Dr. Ralph A. McGill, Chairman of the Committee on the Study and Control of Cancer, who presented the report of his Committee.

Report of Committee on Study and Control of Cancer

The Committee on the Study and Control of Cancer submits the following report to the House of Delegates for the year 1943-1944.

The Cancer Committee during the past year has not been as active educationally as in some of the previous years. However, this does not mean that there has been a lack of interest on the part of the Committee nor does it indicate that there is a less need for such a program. As a matter of fact, there is a greater need now than ever before. As most of you know, cancer ranks second in the list of diseases causing death, and there were more than 163,400 deaths from cancer in

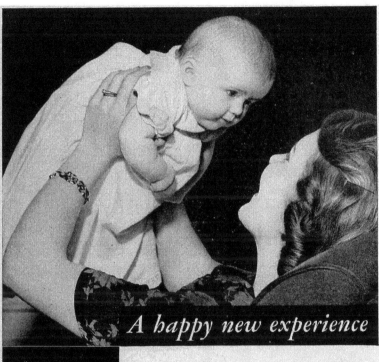

A happy new experience

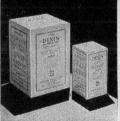

'Dexin' does make a difference

'DEXIN'

HIGH DEXTRIN CARBOHYDRATE

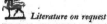
Literature on request

When mothers give 'Dexin' formulas in the early months, they find that baby's first experience with solid food is likely to be a happy one. Supplementary foods are easily added because 'Dexin' formulas are exceptionally palatable, not over-sweet, and do not dull the appetite.

'Dexin' also helps avoid disturbances that might otherwise interfere with the addition of other foods. Its high dextrin content (1) reduces intestinal fermentation and the tendency to colic and diarrhea, and (2) promotes the formation of soft, flocculent, easily digested curds. 'Dexin' is readily soluble in hot or cold milk.

'Dexin' Trademark Registered

COMPOSITION		
Dextrins 75%	Mineral Ash . 0.25%	
Maltose 24%	Moisture . . 0.75%	

Available carbohydrate 99%   115 calories per ounce
6 level packed tablespoonfuls equal 1 ounce

BURROUGHS WELLCOME & CO. (U.S.A. INC.) 9-11 E. 41st St., New York 17, N.Y.

the United States during 1942. Therefore, the prevalence of cancer in our state and nation emphasizes the continuing need for active intelligent efforts by the profession in the dissemination of all known knowledge concerning the prevention, recognition and treatments of this disease.

Dr. Thomas Parran, Surgeon General of the United States Public Health Service, makes this statement in his proclamation for 1944, declaring April as ''Cancer Control Month.'' ''No more challenging task faces the medical and public health professions than the conquest of cancer. Periodic examination of men and women in the susceptible ages, followed by prompt treatment, is still our most potent weapon for saving lives.''

Your Committee feels that a review of the work of the Cancer Committees of the past few years would be interesting and perhaps inspiring to this group. In reviewing the reports of the Committees, previous to 1934, it was noted that the educational work was carried on mostly by the State Chairman of the American Society for the Control of Cancer. Dr. Everett S. Lain was chairman for a number of years and carried on almost a one man campaign, and the Committee feels that the profession of Oklahoma is indebted to Dr. Lain for his untiring efforts.

In 1934, the American Society for the Control of Cancer asked that the State Chairman not be an active member of the State Cancer Committee but that he should act in an advisory capacity. It was in Tulsa, in 1934, that the Oklahoma State Medical Association appropriated $250.00 to defray the expenses of cancer programs of that year. The report shows that 21 counties throughout the state joined in the campaign with talks by doctors to lay groups. These meetings were followed by clinics conducted by the same group of doctors.

During the year 1935-1936, the report shows that several meetings and clinics with lectures were conducted by a number of the County Societies under the sponsorship of the local groups. The organization work, however, was done by Mr. Kibler of the Public Relations Department of the State University. It was largely through his efforts that the local Societies were encouraged to conduct clinics and to have progress on the subject of cancer.

Dr. C. C. Little, Director of the American Society for the Control of Cancer, has been of the opinion for a number of years, and once made the statement that ''if we can get the women to talking about cancer then our educational program will become much more effective.'' In 1936, he was able to persuade the American Federation of Women's Clubs to incorporate in their health program an intensive educational program on the subject of cancer. From that time on, the Woman's Field Army, which group is selected from the membership of the Federated Clubs of the various states throughout the country, was organized. Each state has its own organization, but its activities are conducted along the plan outlined by the American Society for the Control of Cancer. The State Cancer Committee in Oklahoma was very conservative and proceeded very carefully with the organization, and it was not perfected until the following year, 1937.

During the year of 1937-1938, an active campaign was conducted throughout the state. A State Speaker's Bureau was formed which met in February, 1938, in Oklahoma City to review all of the literature and film strips which were then available for lectures to lay groups. Forty-three Societies appointed cancer committees and had local speakers' bureau and conducted an active campaign. This same organization continued to function throughout the following year 1938-1939. During that year, Dr. Samuel Binkley, now Medical Director of the American Society for the Control of Cancer, in New York City, spent two months in the state. He spoke in forty-three centers throughout the state to a total of 12,702 lay people and 1,142 members of the medical profession. This work was sponsored by the State Cancer Committee, in cooperation with the Woman's Field Army and the American Society for the Control of Cancer and the Public Health Department of the State of Oklahoma. This program received nation-wide publicity and was noted as the Oklahoma Plan.

In 1940-1941, the Woman's Field Army became somewhat disorganized and did not conduct its usual enrollment campaign. However, your State Cancer Committee in cooperation with the State Health Department purchased and distributed 1,000 books entitled ''Cancer, A Manual for Practitioners.'' The purchase of these books and the distribution was made possible by the help of the State Health Department under the guidance of Dr. Grady Mathews. During the year 1941-1942, the program continued to function but only in local communities. The Woman's Field Army did not have its organization perfected and again it did not conduct its usual enrollment campaign. This lack of activity on the part of the Woman's Field Army was no doubt occasioned by the fact that many of the members of the Women's Field Army were actively engaged in projects and organizations now in existence with reference to war activities.

During the year of 1942-'43, Mrs. Lloyd D. McClatchey who had been State Commander of the Woman's Field Army, was forced to resign because of her moving to New York City. Mrs. McClatchey has been a very enthusiastic and untiring worker. Her resignation was a great loss to the woman's organizations. However, during that year, numerous lectures were given throughout the local communities, literature was distributed and a number of state-wide radio broadcasts were made.

During the past year 1943-1944, the Woman's Field Army again did not conduct an active enrollment campaign. However, there has been a number of meetings with doctors giving talks on cancer, a number of pamphlets on the subject have been distributed, and also a number of radio broadcasts have been made.

Early in the year, an effort was made to get all of the members of the State Committee, the Woman's Field Army and the State Representative of the American Society for the Control of Cancer together, in order to outline plans for an active campaign for the coming year. Mrs. E. Lee Ozbirn of Sentinel, Oklahoma, who was functioning as State Commander, was actively engaged in activities relating to the war efforts. Then our very efficient Executive Secretary, Dick Graham, went into the service and as a consequence, our group was not able to conduct a program such as we had hoped to do. However, this has not dampened our spirits and whenever

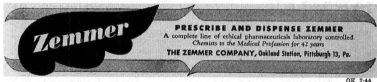

A Radio Program of Interest to All Physicians...

"THE DOCTOR FIGHTS"

starring RAYMOND MASSEY

HERE is a Report to the Nation on the wide-spread activities of America's doctors in a world at war, not only on the battlefronts, but on the home front as well. Documentary histories of medical heroism, carefully authenticated and ethically presented, should prove of interest to every physician, military or civilian. The comments or suggestions of the profession are welcomed.

Tuesday Evenings
COLUMBIA BROADCASTING SYSTEM
8:30 C.W.T.

two or more of our group got together on any occasion, the subject would soon turn to our cancer program.

The Committee met in Oklahoma City on Sunday, April 9, 1944, at which time Mrs. Ozbirn, State Commander of the Woman's Field Army; Dr. Everett S. Lain, a Director of the American Society for the Control of Cancer; and Dr. Wendell Long, State Chairman for the Control of Cancer, were present. A review of the work of the recent years and plans were discussed for the program for the coming year or years. Numerous proposals for the good of the program were discussed, such as, a state-wide campaign with lectures to secondary schools and colleges, showing movies which are now available together with lectures by representatives of our State Association. The question of diagnostic centers for facilities for treatment in different sections of the state was also discussed. The Committee is also urging the pathological group of the state to institute pathological conferences for the study of case histories and interesting slides. The question of setting up facilities for research in the field of cancer was also brought out and one member of the committee announced that he had been approached by one of our wealthy men of the State and that he also knew of other men who would do likewise. There are just some problems which the Committee has to consider and wishes to pass on to the Committee which will be appointed for next year.

The Committee wishes to express its appreciation to all individuals and agencies who have contributed their time and services toward the success of this program during the past year, and we wish to call your attention to the fact that this program has always been under the direction and absolute control of doctors of our Association, and we heartily recommend that this same policy be maintained.

In closing, we offer the following recommendations: (1) The continued active cooperation with the American Society for the Control of Cancer, the Woman's Field Army and the Health Department of the State of Oklahoma. (2) The encouragement of frequent programs and discussions on cancer in all of the County Medical Societies and that local cancer committees be appointed in each County Society to aid in this work. (3) Avoidance of radical changes in the personnel of this committee in order to maintain a continuity of the purpose and its activity. (4) While it is true the Association has not been called upon during the past year for funds, we recommend that the appropriation of $750.00 be made available if and when the expenses of the program requires such further expenditures. (5) A rigid adherence to the ethical principles outlined and followed by the Committee in cooperation with the American Society for the Control of Cancer.

Respectfully submitted,
Ralph A. McGill, M.D., Chairman
Joseph W. Kelso, M.D.
Paul B. Champlin, M.D.

On *motion* by Dr. S. A. Lang, *seconded* by Dr. G. S. Baxter, it was moved that the Report be accepted. The Speaker emphasized that the Report had mentioned the appropriation of certain funds and that it was not possible under the provisions of the Constitution and By-Laws for the House of Delegates to appropriate money but rather that this recommendation-must come from the Council. Dr. J. S. Fulton *moved* that the Report be accepted but that the appropriation be referred to the attention of the Council at its next meeting. The Speaker *ruled* that this motion was out of order since there was already one motion before the House. Dr. L. S. Willour *moved* that the original motion by Dr. Lang be amended to the effect that the Report be accepted and that the paragraph recommendation concerning money be referred to the Council. The amendment was seconded by Dr. McLain Rogers, Clinton. The amendment was accepted by Dr. Lang and his second Dr. Baxter.

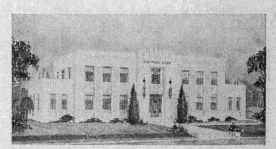

Now... *timed* insulin action, the <u>keynote</u> of control

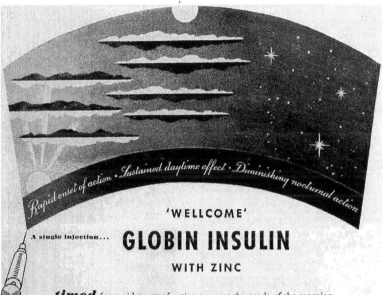

Rapid onset of action · Sustained daytime effect · Diminishing nocturnal action

A single injection...

'WELLCOME'
GLOBIN INSULIN
WITH ZINC

timed for rapid onset of action to meet the needs of the morning

timed for strong continuing daytime effect

timed for diminishing action during the night when the needs become less

While fulfilling these requirements for timed insulin action, the keynote of control in diabetes, this new type insulin also has the advantage of controlling many moderately severe and severe cases of diabetes with only a single injection daily. It is a clear solution and in its freedom from allergenic skin reactions is comparable to regular insulin.

'Wellcome' Globin Insulin with Zinc, an important advance in diabetic control, was developed in the Wellcome Research Laboratories, Tuckahoe, New York. U. S. Pat. 2,161,198.   Vials of 10 cc. 80 units in 1 cc.

Literature on request

'Wellcome' Trademark Registered

BURROUGHS WELLCOME & CO. (U.S.A.) INC. **9-11 E. 41 St. New York 17, N. Y.**

At this time, the Speaker stated the House would first vote on the *amendment* which *carried*. The vote was next on the original *motion as amended* which also *carried*.

The privilege of the floor was next granted to the Chairman of the Committee on the Study and Control of Venereal Diseases, Dr. David V. Hudson, Tulsa, who presented the Report of his Committee.

Report of Committee on Study and Control of Venereal Disease

A revised set of regulations has been issued by the State Health Department covering the management of venereal disease, and physicians who have not received copies may secure them from the State Health Department. These rules and regulations cover the question of quarantine of infectious individuals who are promiscuous or who fail to take treatment. Promiscuous females with infectious venereal disease may be quarantined to Rush Springs Rapid Treatment Hospital. For further information regarding this hospital, the physician should consult his local health officer.

It is recommended that physicians cooperate with the State and Local Health Departments in the control of venereal disease, especially in the instruction of patients with infectious lesions and the reporting of contacts of infectious cases.

Physicians have been active in the treatment of venereal disease, especially in industry. Lectures on venereal disease have been made available by the Medical Association and the State Health Department. Th lectures on Syphilis by Dr. U. J. Wile and the lecture on Gonorrhea by Dr. P. S. Pelouze were very instructive.

Respectfully submitted,
David V. Hudson, M.D., Chairman
John H. Lamb, M.D.
E. Halsell Fite, M.D.

On *motion* by Dr. W. S. Larrabee, *seconded* by Dr. Robert H. Akin, Oklahoma City, and *carried*, the report was *accepted*.

The Speaker next called for the Report of the Committee on Prepaid Medical and Surgical Service, and, Dr. John F. Burton, Oklahoma City, presented the Report of the Committee. Prior to reading the report of the Committee, Dr. Burton enumerated the names of the members of this Committee (Listed at end of report). Dr. Burton further remarked that it was his desire to point out that the House of Delegates at its 1943 Meeting had directed the President to appoint a Committee to prepare and set in motion a prepaid medical and/or surgical service plan on an experimental basis. He further observed that the Committee had prepared such a plan and that the following was the Report of the Committee:

Report of Committee on Prepaid Medical and Surgical Service

The Committee on Prepaid Medical and Surgical Service has had several meetings and has spent considerable time and thought on formulating a plan. They have sought the advice of the American Association and have been advised that this organization is quite anxious for various State Societies to establish a plan as well as individual county societies, and after diligent labor and careful thought have formulated a plan and now have it ready to be tried.

The Committee would like to call to the attention of the Association the following pertinent facts: (1) That this plan is prepared for state-wide application, but it would not be mandatory for every county to adopt. It would permit those counties that wish to participate freedom of action, and at the same time it would not be forced upon those which did not desire to join the plan. Likewise, it would not force any physician to become a participant. (2) This plan is designed to furnish aid to an income group that is now having difficulty in paying hospital and medical and surgical fees. It is a form of insurance but due to its low overhead and the fact that it would be under complete direction of the medical profession, it is possible to supply

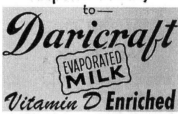
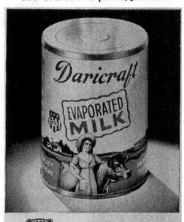

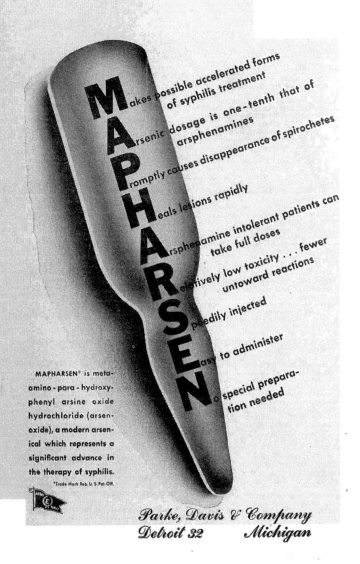

this at a cost cheaper than private insurance plans with many inherent advantages to the physicians.

Respectfully submitted,
John F. Burton, M.D., Chairman
V. C. Tisdal, M.D.
W. Floyd Keller, M.D.
A. S. Risser, M.D.
H. C. Weber, M.D.
Finis W. Ewing, M.D.
·A. W. Pigford, M.D.
Ben W. Ward, M.D.

On *motion* by Dr. W. S. Larrabee and *seconded* by Dr. O. E. Templin ,it was *moved* that 'the report of the committee be *accepted.*

Discussion followed by Dr. R. Q. Goodwin, Oklahoma City, who requested the action of the House of Delegates at its 1943 Meeting, and Dr. Burton observed that the report as presented in 1943 had been adopted.

Dr. T. H. McCailey, McAlester, remarked that in his opinion the report should be accepted and that the intent of the Committee was not to include the plan as a part of its report.

Dr. L. R. Kirby, Okeene, requested that the report of the Committee, as approved in 1943, be read. The Speaker read the report of the Committee which appeared in the Journal, May, 1943, (page 210).

Dr.L. R. Kirby remarked that the House of Delegates had already voted and accepted the report to the effect that this plan was to be enacted on an experimental basis, that it was not compulsory that the plan be put into effect in every county, but rather that it was optional and only to be tried on an experimental basis and further that before it was to be accepted on a state-wide basis it would receive final vote by the House of Delegates.

Dr. Garrison called attention to the two pertinent facts as set out in the Report of the Committee (listed above).

Dr. F. W. Boadway, Ardmore, observed that he failed to see how the House could act upon the Report without the presentation of the plan.

Following this observation, the Speaker stated: "The Chair would rule that in this instance the Report of the Committee does entail the plan and in all fairness to the Assembly an abstract of the plan should be presented."

Dr. W. S. Larrabee *withdrew* his motion with the approval of the second by Dr. Templin.

It was moved by Dr. J. V. Athey, seconded by Dr. J. G. Edwards, that further consideration of this plan be made the first order of business at the second session of the House of Delegates on Tuesday morning and *that the plan be read* at that time.

Dr. L. S. Willour *moved* that the above *motion* be *amended* to read that the plan be presented at this meeting and discussion and action deferred until the following morning. Dr. Athey and Dr. Edwards accepted the amendment which was *seconded* by Dr. D. H. O'Donoghue, and *carried.*

Dr. Burton head the prepared draft of a plan which is abstracted as follows:

Oklahoma Physicians' Service
A Mutual Corporation

1. That the State Association take steps to form a corporation to be known as The Oklahoma Physicians' Service.

2. Non-profit organization and statement of purposes: a. To inaugurate in the State of Oklahoma a Physicians' Service plan to subscribing members. b. To enter into contracts with physicians in the State of Oklahoma to furnish said care to members. c. To establish a system of payments to participating physicians. d. Oklahoma Physicians' Service will contract with Group Hospital Service, Inc., (a nonprofit corporation) to execute the mechanics of selling Oklahoma Physicians' Service membership agreements to eligible groups.

3. Income limitations—any salaried individual with an annual income up to $3,000.00 per year.

Terms and conditions of membership. a. Defining

Member and Dependent. b. Participating Physician means any Doctor of Medicine, who at the time of service is a party to an existing contract with Oklahoma Physicians' Service. c. The Term Surgical Care includes fractures, dislocations, cutting procedures, pathologist and anaesthetist as necessary in above services, and obstetrics after 10 months.

The term Surgical Care does not mean or include: Hospital service, nurse's care, diet, operating room, drugs, medicines, medical or surgical appliances, medications or dressings, x-ray therapy, ambulance service, whole blood, blood plasma or serum, oxygen tent or supply of oxygen, radium treatments, and services of any resident doctor of medicine or intern, nor any care or services of any kind or character rendered in connection with conditions existing prior to application, quarantinable diseases. certain chronic disorders, additonis, military or self-inflicted disability or physiotheraphy, and other conditions covered by Veterans' or Workmans'. Compensation.

Contract year and conditions of renewal. Freedom in choice of participating Physician. Provision for emergency care of accident by non-Participating Physician.

Limits of Benefits. During any contract year,·Single Person Agreement $300.00, One Dependent Agreement $600.00, and Family Agreement $1,000.00.

Annual Dues. The amount of annual dues shall be, Member $9.00, Member and One Dependent $16.20, and Member and All Dependents $24.00.

Limitation on Liability—in ·case of war or public disaster.

Participating Physicians. To be eligible as a physician to participate in the plan, a physician must (a) be a member in good standing in a local county medical society, (b) be acceptable to the Board of Trustees of Oklahoma Physicians' Service and must sign a service contract with the corporation, (c) bind himself not to join or emerge in any contract or agreement with any other competitive group physicians organization after the date of a contract with this organization, and (d) observe the rules and regulations of Oklahoma Physicians' Service in the By-Laws.

Physician's Contract. Settlement by the Oklahoma Physicians' Service and Participating Physician. On the first of each calendar month 75 per cent of the premium income accruing to Oklahoma Physicians' Service, earned during the previous month from premiums paid to it by its Members, and proportionate shares of annual premiums, shall be credited on its books to an account denominated "Participating Physicians' Account." ·

On the tenth day of each calendar month payment shall be made by Oklahoma Physicians' Service out of said Participating Physicians' Account of all statements rendered by all Participating Physicians, to Oklahoma Physicians' Service during the preceding calendar month. If such account be sufficient, then such statements shall be paid in full. Otherwise, the funds then credited to such Participating Physicians' Account shall be applied toward the payment, on a pro rata basis, of all statements of all Participating Physicians, received during such prior month. Any such pro rata payment shall constitute payment in full of Second Party's Account, and shall be accepted by Second Party as his sole, full, and only compensation for the rendition of such surgical care.

Second Party agrees that he will look solely to Oklahoma Physicians' Service for payment of his charges · and fees for any surgical care he may render any Member, or Dependent, during the time any such Member, or Dependent, is insured by Oklahoma Physicians' Service.

———

The Speaker remarked that amendments to the By-Laws to be acted upon at this session must be presented at this time. The Speaker presented three amendments to the By-Laws which had been approved by the Council

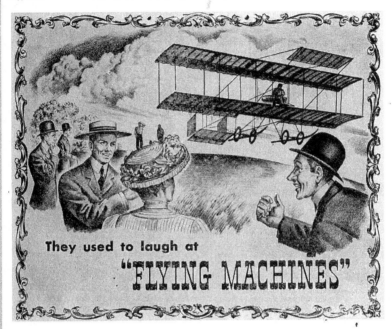

for approval of the House. (amendments in the proceedings of Tuesday morning, April 25.)

No amendments were presented from the floor.

The Speaker next recognized Dr. L. Chester McHenry: "I am in possession of a formal letter from the Oklahoma City Chamber of Commerce as well as a letter from the Oklahoma County Medical Society extending an invitation to the Oklahoma State Medical Association to hold its 1945 Annual Meeting in Oklahoma City."

On *motion* by Dr. Sam A. McKeel, *seconded* by Dr. F. W. Boadway, and *carried*, the invitation was *accepted*.

Under new business, the Speaker read the Official Call to the Officers, Fellows and Members of the American Medical Association signed by the President, Dr. James E. Paullin; the Speaker of the House of Delegates, Dr. H. H. Shoulders, and the Secretary, Dr. Olin West, that had been received in the executive office of the Association.

The next order of business was a communication petitioning for the creation of the Pontotoc-Murray County Medical Society. The Speaker presented the following resolution submitted to the office of the Association by the Pontotoc County Medical Society and which had been given Council approval at its meeting on February 20, 1944:

"The membership of the Murray County Medical Society in meeting assembled on December 15, 1943, respectively requests that the Pontotoc County Medical Society give consideration to the following proposal of the Murray County Medical Society, which has unanimously adopted the following resolution:

"*WHEREAS*, The Murray County Medical Society is composed of only four active members and

"*WHEREAS*, The maintenance of an active medical society is difficult to maintain with this listed membership from both a scientific and economic standpoint, and

"*WHEREAS*, Chapter VII, Section 5, Subsection (d), of the By-Laws of the Oklahoma State Medical Association, provides for the bringing together of county societies into one organization without the loss of individual identity or representation in the House of Delegates.

"*NOW, THEREFORE, BE IT RESOLVED*, That the Murray County Society, in the interest of scientific and economic medical relief for the communities of Murray and Pontotoc Counties and the scientific advancement of the medical profession of the two counties, requests consideration by the Pontotoc County Medical Society for the amalgamation of the two societies into a two-county society to be known as the Pontotoc-Murray County Medical Society, and

"*BE IT FURTHER RESOLVED*, That the Councilors of the Oklahoma State Medical Association representing the two societies be advised of this resolution and petitioned to interest themselves in the resolution to the end that their advice be secured upon the propitiousness of the proposed joining together of the two societies, and

"*BE IT FINALLY RESOLVED*, That should this amalgamation be consummated that the Council and House of Delegates be petitioned to place Murray County in the same Councilor District as Pontotoc County."

This action is recommended by the Councilors of both Districts.

On *motion* by Dr. D. H. O'Donoghue, *seconded* by Dr. J. G. Edwards, and *carried*, the above resolution was adopted.

Following this action, the Speaker stated that it would be necessary to *change* Murray County from District No. 5 to District No. 7 in order that both be in District No. 7.

On *motion* by Dr. A. S. Risser, *seconded* by Dr. J. V. Athey, and *carried*, it was moved that Murray County be placed in District No. 7.

The Speaker called for additional resolutions to be submitted to the Resolutions Committee other than those already in possession of the Chair. None were presented. (The resolutions appear in full in the proceedings of Tuesday morning, April 25.)

The Speaker, upon recommendation of the Council report, appointed the following Committee to present recommendations with reference to a State Board of Health at the second session of the House of Delegates: Dr. L. J. Moorman, Chairman, Oklahoma City; Dr. V. C. Tisdal, and Dr. Mack I. Shanholtz.

The Speaker then presented the names of the following physicians, as published in the March issue of the Journal for election as Honorary Members, all of whom were submitted by their respective County Societies; Dr. N. N. Simpson, Henryetta; Dr. J. M. Postelle, Oklahoma City; Dr. W. H. Livermore, Chickasha; Dr. Walker W. Beesley, Tulsa; Dr. J. E. Brookshire, Tulsa; Dr. Paul R. Brown, Tulsa; Dr. Gilbert H. Hall, Tulsa; Dr. Joel S. Hooper, Tulsa, Dr. James L. Reynolds, Tulsa, and Dr. Albert W. Roth, Tulsa.

On *motion* by Dr. J. G. Edwards, *seconded* by Dr. G. Y. McKinney, Henryetta, and carried, it was moved that these physicians be elected to Honorary Membership.

Following this approval, Dr. Garrison remarked that in compliance with the provisions of Chapter I, Section 3, Subsection (d), of the By-Laws of the Association, the names of the following physicians had been submitted to the office of the Association for election to Associate Membership: Dr. Ralph M. Alley, Shawnee, and Dr. David A. Myers, San Francisco, California, past President of the Oklahoma State Medical Association in 1910-1911.

On *motion* by Dr. O. E. Templin, *seconded* by Dr. V. C. Tisdal, and *carried*, the above-mentioned names were *approved* for Associate Membership.

On *motion* by Dr. D. H. O'Donoghue, *seconded* by Dr. J. V. Athey, and *Supported*, the House adjourned to recess until 8:30 A.M., Tuesday morning.

MINUTES OF SECOND SESSION
Ivory Room, Mayo Hotel, Tulsa, Oklahoma
Tuesday, April 25, 1944.

The final session was called to order by the Speaker, Dr. George H. Garrison.

The Credentials Committee announced a quorum present and upon *motion*, duly *seconded*, the report was adopted.

The Speaker called for unfinished business. The floor was declared open for discussion of the Prepaid Medical and Surgical Service Plan.

Discussion for the plan followed by Dr. McLain Rogers, Clinton; Dr. A. S. Risser, Blackwell; Dr. Carl Puckett, Oklahoma City, and Dr. S. A. Lang, Nowata. Dr. J. S. Fulton, Atoka; Dr. G. Y. McKinney, Henryetta, and Dr. H. K. Speed, Sayre, spoke against the plan.

Dr. R. Q. Goodwin, Oklahoma City moved that the Committee be commended for the work done and that it be continued and further that the members of the State Medical Association be given a printed copy of the abstract of the plan for study and that it be presented later to the House of Delegates for consideration. The motion was *seconded* by Dr. S. A. Lang.

Dr. L. Chester McHenry, Oklahoma City, moved that the motion be *amended* to the effect that some kind of ballot be included in the mailing in order that an expression with reference to the plan might be secured from the entire membership. This motion was *seconded* by Dr. O. H. Miller, Ada.

The Speaker stated the House would first vote on the amendment which *carried*, and next on the original motion as amended. Motion *carried*.

Dr. J. S. Fulton *moved* that the House of Delegates not be called together for at least a year for final action on the plan. The *motion was lost* for want of a second.

It seemed to the Delegates that it might be possible to determine from the ballot whether or not the plan might be put into effect in one town or community on an experimental basis in order that it might be given a fair trial.

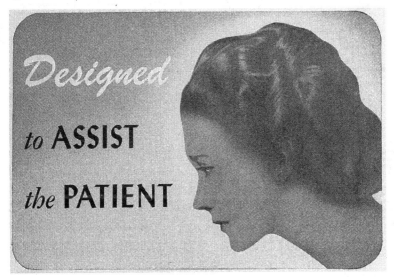
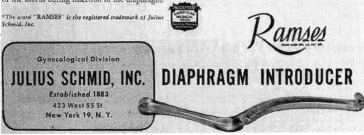

The Speaker called for the report of the Committee appointed with reference to recommendations concerning a State Board of Health for Oklahoma. In the absence of the Chairman, Dr. L. J. Moorman, Oklahoma City, Dr. James Stevenson, Tulsa, read the following report:

Report of Committee on State Board of Health

In view of the present status of health administration in the State of Oklahoma, your Committee recommends that the House of Delegates approve a plan for the appointment of a State Board of Health by the Governor and that the Committee on Public Policy be instructed to present the designated plan to the Governor in time for it to receive legislative consideration at the next session of the State Legislature.

Your Committee further recommends that the Board should be non-partisan with authority over all agencies and institutions concerned with the health of our citizenry. This would relieve the Governor of a heavy responsibility; serve as a guide to and check upon the State Health Commissioner; and prove a great savings to taxpayers.

The State Board of Health should consist of seven members with four representatives from the medical profession, one from the dental profession and the other representatives should be chosen because of special interests or qualifications from other professions or from the business world. The original appointment should be made in such a way that the retirement of individual members will be staggered. All subsequent appointments or re-appointments should be for a period of seven years. In this way, the Board will always have the services of seasoned members familiar with the established policies and practices, and thus escape the dangers of sudden changes consequent upon shifting political administration and executive policies.

Under this plan, the State Health Commissioner should be chosen by the Board and should be responsible to the same for the judicious and efficient performance of the functions of his office.

The functions of the Board should be broadly supervised in all matters having to do with the health of the citizenry of the State.

Further, the Board should have the power to promulate public health regulations based upon statutes that at present exist or may in the future be passed. And that in controversial matters relating to public health, the Board may in its discretion conduct hearings in an attempt to adjudicate.

The Board should have no power to nominate personnel for positions subordinate to the Commissioner of Health but should have the power of confirmation or rejection of the same. The Board shall have no executive authority, the administration of public health affairs shall remain under the direction of the Commissioner of Health within the policies that may be established by the Board.

Respectfully submitted,

Lewis J. Moorman, M.D., Chairman
V. C. Tisdal, M.D.
Mack I. Shanholtz, M.D.

Immediately following the reading of the above report, Dr. Stevenson observed that it might be necessary to make certain and proper changes at the advice of the Public Policy Committee of the Association and the Governor of the State to iron out and perfect minor changes and difficulties.

On *motion* by Dr. James Stevenson, *seconded* by Dr. G. S. Baxter, Shawnee, and *carried*, it was *moved* that the House of Delegates approve a plan for the appointment of a State Board of Health by the Governor and that the Committee on Public Policy be instructed to present the designated plan to the Governor in time for

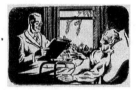
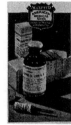

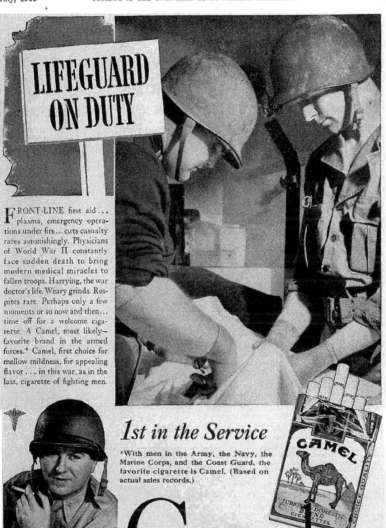

it to receive legislative consideration at the next session of the State Legislature.

The Speaker recognized the Chairman of the Committee, Dr. Clinton Gallaher, Shawnee, who reads the resolutions.

Birth Certificates

WHEREAS, Under the laws of the State of Oklahoma and procedure prescribed by the administrators of said laws, all official records pertaining to the birth of an individual within the State are matters of public record, available for original perusal, formal copying, and formal reproduction. Copies of birth certificates are available upon request in the exact form as officially contained in the public records, and

WHEREAS, Such copies do contain information regarding the legitimacy or illegitimacy of birth of the individual concerned, and

WHEREAS, Such information indicating illegitimate birth has been the source of much unhappiness, embarrassment, and mental suffering to the individual named and to his friends and associates, and

WHEREAS, Unhappiness, embarrassment, and mental suffering arising from this condition has been eliminated in many states of the union through the simple expedient of legal measures designed to restrict information of this character from public knowledge, and to make such information available only under exceptional circumstances and on the order of a duly qualified court of law, and

WHEREAS, Such a system would be of humane advantage to the citizens of this State, serving to eliminate the stigma of illegitimate birth from individuals who are not responsible for this circumstance, to promote continued happiness and mental well-being, and to simplify the procedure of issuing public copies of certificates of birth,

NOW, THEREFORE, BE IT RESOLVED, That the Oklahoma State Medical Association, by action of the House of Delegates of this resolution, endorses the principles set forth by proposed legislation of this character, and that it instruct the Public Policy Committee of the Oklahoma State Medical Association to foster such principles and work toward the enactment of such legislation to accomplish objectives as named and,

BE IT FURTHER RESOLVED, That the Public Policy Committee of the Oklahoma State Medical Association to secure the passage of such legislation at the next regular session of the State Legislature, and

BE IT FINALLY RESOLVED, That attention be called to model laws of this character now existing in the states of Texas, New York and Colorado, among others, and that any legislation to this effect in the State of Oklahoma be modeled on the laws of these states.

On *motion* by Dr. Gallaher, *seconded* by Dr. L. Chester McHenry, and *carried*, the resolution was *adopted*.

The Commonwealth Fund

The House of Delegates at the 52nd Annual Session of the Oklahoma State Medical Association desires to go on record and express appreciation to The Commonwealth Fund of New York for their liberal financial support in making possible the post-graduate instruction in obstetrics, pediatrics, internal medicine and surgical diagnosis in the State of Oklahoma.

From resolutions of County Medical Societies, comments of individuals, and the obvious enthusiasm in the course in surgical diagnosis now under way, it is apparent that hundreds of physicians throughout the state are appreciative of and have benefited by reason of these courses.

We request that a copy of this resolution be sent to The Commonwealth Fund of New York.

On *motion* by Dr. Gallaher, *seconded* by Dr. A. S. Risser, and *carried*, the resolution was adopted.

Postgraduate Education

The House of Delegates of the 52nd Annual Session of the Oklahoma State Medical Association desires to express appreciation and thanks to the Oklahoma State Health Department and the United States Public Health Service, Washington, D. C., for their financial support in making the postgraduate programs in internal medicine and surgical diagnosis in the State of Oklahoma.

It is the opinion of the House of Delegates from numerous letters, comments and resolutions from County Medical Societies, that hundreds of physicians in our medical profession have benefited by reason of the postgraduate programs in Oklahoma.

Further, we request that a copy of this resolution be sent to Dr. Grady F. Mathews, Commissioner, Oklahoma State Health Department, whose valued assistance to the profession in Oklahoma has been noted, also a copy be sent to the United States Public Health Service, Washington, D. C.

On *motion* by Dr. Gallaher, *seconded* by Dr. G. S. Baxter, and *carried*, the resolution was *adopted*.

Infectious and Contagious Diseases

WHEREAS, The Attorney General's office of the State of Oklahoma has given an opinion to the effect that syphilis and gonorrhea are not contagious, infectious or communicable diseases and consequently are not covered with our quarantine laws, and

WHEREAS, This interpretation would greatly jeopardize the health of our citizens and practically nullify our quarantine law relative to these two diseases,

NOW, THEREFORE, BE IT RESOLVED, That the Oklahoma State Medical Association in regular session assembled this 24th day of April, 1944, respectfully submit that gonorrhea has a definitely infective period and that syphilis, while there are any open lesions, is definitely communicable and recommend that the Attorney General's office give due consideration to the infectious and contagious nature of these two diseases in its interpretation of the law and that it be so changed or amended that our quarantine laws may be invoked in these two diseases.

On *motion* by Dr. Gallaher, *seconded* by Dr. J. T. Phelps, El Reno, and *carried*, the resolution was *adopted*.

Governor Robert S. Kerr

WHEREAS, The Honorable Robert S. Kerr, Governor of Oklahoma, has during the past year demonstrated a broad understanding of the problems of medicine, public health and general welfare of the people,

NOW, THEREFORE, BE IT RESOLVED, That the House of Delegates of the Oklahoma State Medical Association does hereby commend and express its appreciation for the continuance in office of Grady F. Mathews, M.D., as Commissioner of Health of the State of Oklahoma. The medical profession has the utmost confidence in this man as an administrator of the public health activities of our State.

BE IT FURTHER RESOLVED, That the heartiest cooperation of the Association is extended to Governor Kerr with respect to all matters pertaining to the health of the people of Oklahoma.

On *motion* by Dr. Gallaher, *seconded* by Dr. O. H. Miller, and *carried*, the resolution was *adopted*.

Amendments to the By Laws:

Chapter I, Section 3, Subsection (e)
Special Service Members

Chapter I, Section 3, of the By-Laws, to be amended as follows:

"Any physician who is in the Armed Forces of the United States, who has been licensed to practice medicine and surgery in Oklahoma, and who has not previously been a member of any county medical society may be recognized as a Special Service Member of this Association. Such physician shall first have been elected to membership as a Special Service Member by a component county society in accordance with the provisions of its Constitution and By-Laws, and the fact of such membership be certified to the Executive Secretary of the Association. Special Service membership shall include all the rights and privileges of Active membership except voting and holding office.

"No dues shall be assessed such member until the

month following his discharge from the Armed Forces of the United States and at which time he shall pay prorated dues for the balance of the calendar year following his discharge from active service. Special Service membership shall lapse at the close of the calendar year following the discharge of such member from service with the Armed Forces.''

On *motion* by Dr. McLain Rogers, *seconded* by Dr. W. Floyd Keller, Oklahoma City and *carried*, the amendment was *adopted*.

Chapter XI. Section 3. Subsection (b 1)
Membership

Chapter XI, Section 3, Subsection (b), of the By-Laws, to be amended as follows:

''Should the license of a member of a component society be suspended for any period, his name shall be automatically dropped as of the date of suspension, and he shall not be entitled to reinstatement of membership in the State Association until January of the year following his period of suspension.''

On *motion* by Dr. J. D. Osborn, Frederick, *seconded* by Dr. J. S. Fulton, and *carried*, the amendment was *adopted*.

Chapter XI. Section 3. Subsection (b 2)
Membership

Chapter XI, Section 3, Subsection (b), of the By-Laws, to be amended as follows:

''Should a case regarding the licensure of a physician be pending before the Oklahoma State Board of Medical Examiners, membership privileges in the State Association cannot be granted the physician in question until such time as a final determination has been reached by said Board.''

On *motion* by Dr. G. S. Baxter, *seconded* by Dr. William M .Gallaher, Shawnee, and *carried*, the amendment was *adopted*.

Following this .action, the Speaker stated that the Committee on Maternity and Infancy had requested that they be given an opportunity to offer a supplemental report. There being no members of the Committee present, the Speaker remarked that it was his impression that the report was with reference to the care of enlisted men's wives with the request that the House of Delegates go on record as favoring that the Government make the payment to the patient and, in turn let the patient make arrangements for payment to the attending physician.

On *motion* by Dr. J. G. Smith, Bartlesville, and *seconded* by Dr. J. S. Fulton, it was *moved* that the supplemental report be approved.

The *motion was lost.*

Dr. C. R. Rountree, Oklahoma City suggested that it might be wise that the election of new officers be set at a definite and certain time on .the agenda of business in order that everyone might be present to vote.

On *motion* by Dr. E. Halsell Fite, Muskogee, *seconded* by Dr. L. Chester McHenry, and *carried*, it was moved that the above arrangement be *effected* at the 1945 meeting.

Dr. D. H. O'Donoghue, Oklahoma City, *moved* that a vote of thanks and appreciation be extended to the Tulsa County Medical Society for the manner in which they had been hosts at the 52nd Annual Meeting of the Oklahoma State Medical Association. The motion was *seconded* by Dr. W. Floyd Keller, and *carried*.

The next order of business was the election of officers.

The Speaker announced that the first election would be that of President-Elect and recognized Dr. A. S. Risser, who nominated Dr. V. C. Tisdal, Elk City.

Remarks made by Dr. Risser were furthered by Dr. H. C. Weber, Bartlesville and Dr. McLain Rogers, Clinton.

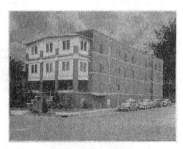
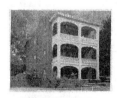

Dr. T. H. McCarley, McAlester, stated that the Pittsburg County Medical Society unanimously endorsed and recommended Dr. L. C. Kuyrkendall of McAlester.

Dr. O. C. Newman, Shattuck, endorsed and seconded the motion with reference to Dr. Tisdal.

Dr. O. E. Templin, Alva, then spoke, endorsing Dr. L. C. Kuyrkendall.

Dr. J. S. Fulton, Atoka, spoke, endorsing Dr. Kuyrkendall.

On motion by Dr. J. C. Matheney, Okmulgee, seconded by Dr. G. S. Baxter, and carried, it was moved that the nominations cease.

The Tellers and Judges of Elections reported that Dr. Tisdal had been elected.

Following his election, Dr. Tisdal made the following remarks to the Delegates: "Members of the House of Delegates of the Oklahoma State Medical Association: I assure you that I appreciate the confidence you have placed in me. I appreciate the responsibility and feel that there has never been a time in the history of our organization when more thought, more action and more deliberation should be given to the needs of organized medicine than today. This can only be accomplished by the cooperative effort of every man in our Society. I certainly solicit your cooperation and help and deliberation with regard to everything that will come before our Society during my tenure of office. I appreciate this honor more than anything that has ever been bestowed upon me. I most assuredly feel my limitations and know that I must have your support to give you what you deserve. I most heartily appreciate the attitude of Dr. Kuyrkendall and his co-workers, and I shall do everything possible to meet the requirements that you have imposed upon me."

The Speaker called for nominations for Vice-President. Dr. Ellis Lamb, Clinton, was recognized by the Speaker: "I would like to put before this House the name of a man who is worthy—Dr. Frank W. Boadway, Ardmore."

Dr. J. S. Fulton: "I move that the nominations cease and that Dr. Boadway be elected by acclamation." The motion was accepted by Dr. Sam A. McKeel, Ada, and carried.

After his election, Dr. Boadway made the following remarks: "This is really unexpected, and I certainly appreciate the nomination of Vice-President of this Association. I shall be happy to assist in every way."

The Vice-Speaker took the Chair as the next order of business was the election of the Speaker of the House .

Dr. S. A. Lang nominated Dr. George H. Garrison of Oklahoma City to succeed himself. The motion was seconded by Dr. A. S. Risser.

On motion by Dr. G. Y. McKinney, seconded by Dr. G. S. Baxter, and carried, it was moved that the nominations cease and that Dr. Garrison be elected by acclamation.

The next order of business was the election of Vice-Speaker. Dr. Sam McKeel moved that Dr. H. K. Speed, Sayre, be elected to succeed himself. The motion was seconded by Dr. F. W Boadway and to the effect that he be elected by acclamation. Motion seconded by Dr. J. S. Fulton, and carried.

The Speaker next called for nominations for Delegate to the A.M.A. to serve for 1944-1945. Dr. Finis W. Ewing, Muskogee, nominated Dr. James Stevenson. Dr. J. S. Fulton seconded the nomination.

It was moved by Dr. L. S. Willour that the nominations cease and that Dr. Stevenson be elected by acclamation. Motion carried.

Following his election, Dr. Stevenson remarked: "Thank you very much. I appreciate the honor and responsibility. I appreciate too that the House of Delegates is the policy making body, and I will endeavor to carry your mandates to the A.M.A. and to properly represent you."

The Speaker then called for nominations for Alternate Delegate to the A.M.A. Dr. J. D. Osborn, Frederick, nominated Dr. Finis Ewing, Muskogee.

It was moved by Dr. H. K. Speed, seconded by Dr. S. A. Lang, and carried that the nominations for Alternate to the A.M.A. cease and that Dr. Ewing be elected by acclamation.

At this time, the Speaker stated that the Delegates from District No. 1, District No. 2, District No. 3, District No. 4, District No. 7, District No. 9 and District No. 10 might retire in order to prepare their nominations for Councilors from their respective Districts. The Speaker further observed that the Delegate from District No. 2 would complete the unexpired term of Dr. Tisdal of until 1945, the Delegate from District No. 3 to complete the unexpired term (1946) for Dr. C. W. Arrendell, Ponca City, who had been forced to retire because of ill health, and that the term of the Councilor from District No. 9 would expire in 1946 since this election was supposed to have been in 1943 but because of floods no representative from that District had been able to attend the Annual Meeting.

Following recess, the Speaker called the House to order and requested nominations for Councilor from District No. 1. Dr. C. A. Traverse, Alva, nominated Dr. O. E. Templin, Alva, seconded by Dr. L. Chester McHenry, and carried, Dr. Templin was elected by acclamation.

In order, Dr. V. C. Tisdal nominated Dr. J. William Finch, Hobart, seconded by Dr. D. H. O'Donoghue, and carried, Dr. Finch was elected by acclamation to fill the unexpired term of Dr. Tisdal, upon his election as President Elect, as Councilor of District No. 2.

Next, Dr. L. A. Mitchell, Stillwater, nominated Dr. C. E. Northeutt of Ponca City as Councilor for District No. 3 to fill the unexpired term of Dr. Arrendell. The motion was seconded by Dr. D. S. Harris, Drummond, and moved that Dr. Northeutt be elected by acclamation. The motion was seconded by Dr. W. Floyd Keller, and carried.

Dr. J. T. Phelps, El Reno, was next recognized by the Speaker and moved that Dr. Tom Lowry, Oklahoma City, be re-elected by acclamation as Councilor for District No. 4. The motion was seconded by Dr. R. Q. Goodwin, and carried.

The Speaker next recognized Dr. M. E. Robberson, Wynnewood, who moved that Dr. Gallaher, Shawnee, be re-elected as Councilor for District No. 7 by acclamation. The motion was seconded by Dr. John H. Lamb, Oklahoma City, and carried.

In order, Dr. L. S. Willour, McAlester moved that Dr. L. C. Kuyrkendall be elected by acclamation to succeed himself as Councilor of District No. 9. The motion was seconded by Dr. J. C. Matheney, and carried.

The Chair next recognized Dr. O. J. Colwick, Durant, who moved that Dr. John A. Haynie, Durant, be elected by acclamation as Councilor for District No. 10. The motion was seconded by Dr. C. A. Traverse, and carried.

At this time, Dr. Garrison announced that the desk of the Speaker was cleared and unless there was other business to be transacted, a motion for adjournment was in order.

Dr. L. S. Willour was recognized: "There is a man, Dr. J. S. Fulton, Atoka, retiring from the Council this year who has served as a member of the Council, President-Elect and President of the Association for nearly 30 years. I sincerely hate to see him retire from the Council although I know it is at his request. The House of Delegates should express appreciation to this man for 30 years of service. I move that we express our appreciation by a rising vote of thanks."

The motion was seconded by Dr. Finis W. Ewing, and carried.

On motion by Dr. S. A. Lang, seconded by Dr. O. J. Colwick, and carried, a motion for adjournment was adopted.

Classified Advertisements

FOR SALE: Portable oxygen equipment; ediphone; Westinghouse X-Ray Machine. Address Key 51, care of The Journal, 210 Plaza Court, Oklahoma City 3, Oklahoma.

FOR SALE: One combination Fischer and Company R & T X-Ray Unit, No. 35L23 with Timer (tube No. 1261.) Good condition, entire unit like new. Also table No. 35178. Reasonably priced for quick sale. Doctor changing locations. J. T. Antony, Box 303, Lawton, Oklahoma or 430½ D. Avenue, Lawton, Oklahoma.

FOR SALE: Large attractive house, spacious grounds. Suitable for small hospital. County Seat town, 2,000 population, one block from Court House. Fifty miles any direction to nearest hospital. Want to retire. Write care of The Journal, 210 Plaza Court, Oklahoma City 3, Oklahoma.

FOR SALE: Twenty bed hospital, brick and concrete, modern, party equipped. Would be very desirable location for a good internal medicine man and surgeon. Write Key 50, care of The Journal, 210 Plaza Court, Oklahoma City 3, Oklahoma.

• OBITUARIES •

Hugh R. Shannon, M.D.
1885-1944

Dr. Hugh R. Shannon, Pond Creek, died recently at an Enid hospital after an illness of several months.

Dr. Shannon came to Oklahoma from Kingman, Kansas, residing first at Carrier. He also practiced medicine at Hillsdale and Pond Creek before moving to Enid. He was a member of the Oklahoma State Medical Association and the American Medical Association.

Surviving are his wife, Mrs. Ethel Shannon, a daughter, Mrs. Pope Strimple, Norfolk, Nebraska, two sons, Lowell H. Shannon, Camp Howze, Texas and Hugh Shannon, Fort Knox, Kentucky.

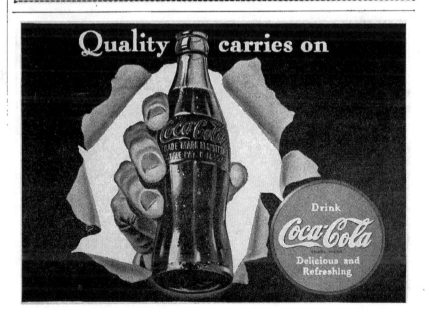

In Memoriam

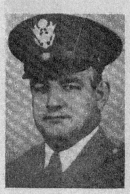

Bernard Bullock, M.D.
1912-1944

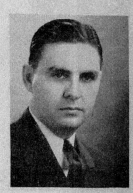

Frank M. King, Jr., M.D.
1911-1944

Lt. Colonel Bernard Bullock, Clinton, died on June 10 from wounds received in France on Invasion Day. Word was received by Mrs. Bullock in Clinton on June 6 that Colonel Bullock had been seriously wounded and that details would follow. Later word was received of his death and that other details would be sent at a later date.

Colonel Bullock left the United States in December, 1943. He was sent to England where he was commander of a medical battlion. He remained in England until Invasion Day, when it is assumed he went across to France with the Invasion Troops.

After graduating from the Baylor University College of Medicine in Dallas, Texas, Colonel Bullock came to Clinton where he began practice. He maintained offices with Dr. A. W. Paulson, also in the armed forces, and Dr. McLain Rogers. He served as City Health Officer for two years and directed advancement in public health practices in Clinton.

A Reserve Officer, Colonel Bullock entered the armed services as a first lieutenant in 1941, before Pearl Harbor, and was stationed at Fort Sam Houston at San Antonio, Texas. He and his family lived there for two years and then moved to the east coast where they remained for several months. Promotions came rapidly and he received his commission as a lieutenant colonel some time before going overseas.

Colonel Bullock was a member of the Junior Chamber of Commerce of Clinton, the Custer County Medical Society, the Oklahoma State Medical Association and the American Medical Association. He was well known in the State and was a popular and successful young physician.

Surviving are his wife, three sons, Jimmy, Jerry and Charles, who make their home at 411 South Seventh St., Clinton.

Word has been received that Captain Frank M. King, Jr., Woodward, was killed in action on January 10, 1944. Captain King was with an Armored Infantry Unit stationed in Italy at the time of his death.

In August, 1942, he entered active military service and departed for foreign service in February, 1943. After active duty in the Tunisian Campaign he went to Italy and was serving in a battalion aid station. His station was hit by a number of shells from enemy artillery fire.

Captain King was born September 23, 1911 in Crawford County, Illinois, moving to Keifer, Oklahoma in 1913. In 1922 he came to Ramona, Oklahoma where he graduated from Ramona High School in 1930. For two years he attended Kansas City Junior College, Kansas City, Missouri and then enrolled at St. Louis University for his third year of pre-medical training. He graduated from St. Louis University School of Medicine in 1937 at which time he received his commission in the Reserve Army. On October 2, 1937 he was married to Miss Ramona Bigham of Ramona, Oklahoma.

From 1937 to 1940, Captain King served two years of internship and one year of medical residency at the University and Crippled Children's Hospitals at Oklahoma City. In July, 1940 he went to Woodward, Oklahoma with the State Health Department as Director of that Unit.

Captain King was a member of the Woodward County Medical Society, the Oklahoma State Medical Association and the American Medical Association. He was held in high esteem by his many friends and his associates in the medical profession.

Surviving Captain King are his wife and five-year old daughter of Stillwater, Oklahoma, and his parents, Mr. and Mrs. Frank M. King of Ramona.

<u>This</u> American is <u>not</u> expected to buy an extra War Bond in the 5TH WAR LOAN

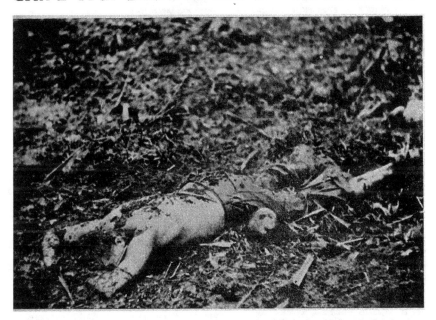

ut we are;

For each of us here at home, the job now is) buy extra Bonds—100, 200, even 500 ollars worth if possible.

Many of us can do much more than we /er have before.

When the Victory Volunteer comes to you and asks you to buy extra Bonds, think how much you'd give to have this War over and done.

Then remember that you're not *giving* anything. You're simply *lending* money—putting it in the best investment in the world.

Let's Go... for the Knockout Blow!

Oklahoma State Medical Association

MEDICAL ABSTRACTS

"THE PREVENTION OF PYOGENIC INFECTIONS OF THE NOSE AN THROAT." A. Fleming. The Journal of Laryngology and Otology. London. Vol. 58. Pages 296-304. July. 1943.

Infections of the nose and throat are probably responsible for more sickness than infections of any other region. Fungi, bacteria, or viruses may be responsible for these infections. The nose, apart from the anterior nares, is in health a relatively sterile cavity. The anterior nares is normally infected with a number of organisms, especially staphylococci and diphtheroid bacilli, the latter being but little pathogenic. At birth the nose is sterile, but after two weeks some 90 per cent of infants harbor staphylococcus aureus. With advancing age the number diminishes, being 20 to 40 per cent in young adults. In patients suffering from recurrent attacks of boils the percentage carrying pathogenic staphylococci is much higher and it may well be that this is a reservoir of staphylococci from which various parts of the skin are infected by the finger nails.

In a very large percentage of people the postnasal spaces are in a chronic catarrhal condition. In the ordinary "healthy" person the postnasal space harbors staphylococci, streptococci, pneumococci, gram-negative cocci, and bacilli of the type of the influenza bacillus. The tonsils are infected with large numbers of organisms.

In normal defensive mechanism of the nose the ferment called lysozyme plays an important role. The ferment is found in great concentration in nasal mucus, in sputum, and especially in tears; it is also found in cells such as leukocytes, and in cellular organs such as tonsils. Another protection is the presence of phagocytes. Both the lysozyme and the phagocyte are easily destroyed and inhibited in their actions by antiseptic solution.

The sources of infection and the spread of nose and throat infections have been studied for some time. The actual sources of the infection may be a clinical case of the disease, missed case, incubating case, and carrier. The methods by which a throat or nose patient may pass on an infection are very numerous. Infected material may be expelled from the nose or mouth in coughing, sneezing, etc. Fingers may be directly infected by contact with secretions. Handkerchiefs, certain parts of the clothing, or toys, may similarly become infected.

When a patient coughs or sneezes he expels droplets large or small, infected and uninfected. The larger ones drop quickly within a foot or two of the patient, on clothing, bedding, floors, books or toys. There they dry. The very small droplets evaporate in the air, and the dried residue may float for relatively large distances by currents of air before settling down as minute dust particles. The infected droplets which fall on floors or walls become part of the dust, and may infect the air again at time of daily dry sweeping, or bedmaking. It has been estimated that in floor sweepings of a nose and throat ward, 100 million hemolytic streptococci are present. The blankets of patients with upper respiratory tract infection may contain one million hemolytic streptococci each.

The fingers of the infected individual may become infected either by direct contact with the infective secretions or by droplets, especially since the mouth is covered up by the hand at time of coughing. The infected fingers may pass on the pathogenic organisms in a great variety of ways. The types of clinical disease these streptococci may produce are varying from sepsis to simple rhinitis. The streptococcus of scarlet fever may cause also skin infections, and may be carried into hospitals as such. The prevention of infection may be attempted in several ways. The infecting bacteria may be prevented from reaching a possible infectee. The resistance of possible infectees can be increased. Finally, the infected individual can be treated so as to render the infective period as short as possible.

Besides ward regulations and air sterilization, simple measures can accomplish much in this respect. Avoid dust raised by violent bedmaking and by dry sweeping of floors or dry dusting of walls. Efficient masking of medical and nursing attendants, or of the patient, is of obvious value. Nothing should be touched with the finger, but with the forceps. Possible infectees may be immunized against a particular infection, but it is impossible to immunize completely against all the nose and throat infections that may occur.

Chemotherapy may benefit the patient's clinical condition much more than his position as a distributor of infective bacteria. The sulfonamides may be good, but when a man is merely a throat carrier of hemolytic streptococci the general administration of the sulfonamide drugs has not had the same good results. Sulfathiazole snuff for treatment or prophylaxis seems to be a simple and practical method. In tonsillitis, gargling is useless, as the contact is very short and the action of sulfonamide is slow. Chewing gums incorporating sulfapyridine have been already used with success. It was found that during the chewing an appreciable amount of sulfapyridine was present in the saliva.

Active immunization by means of vaccines has in the past been extensively used in the treatment of chronic septic conditions, and this treatment was often successful. The advent of sulfonamides has made vaccine treatment of even greater importance. A combination of sulfonamide therapy with immunotherapy will give results far better than either alone. The ideal combination would be first an increase in immunity by vaccine, and then to give sulfonamide treatment. At present, it is unfortunately done in the reverse order: sulfonamide first, and vaccine afterwards.

In the prevention of these infections, education of the nursing staff is also highly important. Nurses should have some knowledge of bacteria in the air, on blankets, etc., methods of sterilization, the manner in which infections spread, and practical matters of this sort.—M. D. H., M.D.

"A SUMMARY OF EIGHTY LIVING CASES OF PERNICIOUS ANEMIA." Maurice Hardgrove, F.A.C.P., Lt. Col. M. C., A.U.S., Gorgas Hospital, Panama Canal Zone; Robert Yunck, M.D.; Hugo Zotter, M.D.; Francis Murphy, M.D., F.A.C.P., Milwaukee, Wisconsin. Annals of Internal Medicine. Vol. 20, No. 5. May, 1944.

The study of these 80 cases is summarized as follows:

A study has been made of 80 living cases of pernicious anemia who had been under treatment, 17.5 per cent for more than ten years. The highest incidence occurred in the seventh decade, although the age varied from 37 to 83 years. A possible family history was obtained in 12.5 per cent. A majority, 67.5 per cent, were derived from three national groups: German, Polish and Irish. One was a negress. Of the 80 cases, 28 were male and 52 were female patients.

In about 14 per cent of the cases the hair became gray before 30 years of age. In one case gray hair became dark under treatment. In 67.5 per cent the eyes were blue, gray or green, and in the rest brown.

A correct diagnosis was made during the first year of illness in only 36.25 per cent. In 53.75 per cent the diagnosis was not made by the first physician consulted, and in 86 per cent it was not adequately established until hospitalization.

The most common initial symptoms were weakness and fatigue. Sore tongue occurred at onset in 56 per cent; paresthesias in 71 per cent; disturbances of gait in 41 per cent; bladder disturbances in 32.5 per cent and gastro-intestinal complaints in 82.5 per cent. Heart disease of a degenerative type occurred in 33.7 per cent.

Treatment was designed to keep the red blood cell count between 4,500,000 and 5,000,000 and the hemoglobin above 80 per cent. Maintenance of weight also seemed to be an important guide as to efficiency of treatment. This was accomplished satisfactorily in 66 per cent of the cases by one injection of 3 cc of crude liver extract (15 units) every four weeks, and and in 11.5 per cent every three weeks. In individual cases more frequent injections were required.

Reactions to injections of liver extract, usually allergic in nature, occurred in 27.5 per cent of the cases and in five forced a change to oral therapy.

Nineteen patients discontinued treatment for periods of three months to five years, but all subsequently resumed it. The time elapsing before severe relapse occurred varied greatly in different cases.—H. J., M.D.

"GLOBIN INSULIN WITH ZINC IN THE TREATMENT OF DIABETES MELLITUS." Herman O. Mosenthal, M.D., New York. The Journal of the American Medical Association. Vol. 125, No. 7. June 17, 1944.

The author discussed "Globin Insulin," which has been made available for the market recently, but which has been studied since 1939.

He discusses the duration of the effect of globin insulin on the blood sugar and reports his experience on: 1. Cases with mild diabetes, requiring 30 units of insulin or less; 2. Cases with severe diabetes, requiring more than 30 units of insulin, and several individual cases illustrating points about the use of globin insulin. He calls it a 12 to 15 hour insulin and suggests that it is a distinct addition to the efficient management of diabetes.

"It is particularly valuable in regulating patients who have a rise in blood sugar after eating only and in the control of patients whose nocturnal fasting blood sugar is normalized by a given dose of protamine zinc insulin."

He recognizes the objections of increasing the number of available insulins, but at the same time indicates that its use may bring about further attempts in different forms of insulin which will eventually lead to better treatment and management of diabetes.—H. J., M.D.

KEY TO ABSTRACTORS

M. D. H., M.D. ....Marvin D. Henley
H. J., M.D. ....Hugh Jeter

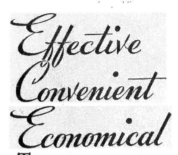
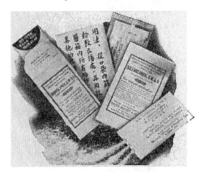

OFFICERS OF COUNTY SOCIETIES, 1944

★

COUNTY	PRESIDENT	SECRETARY	MEETING TIME
Alfalfa	H. E. Huston, Cherokee	L. T. Lancaster, Cherokee	Last Tues. each Second Month
Atoka-Coal	R. C. Henry, Coalgate	J. S. Fulton, Atoka	
Beckham	G. H. Stagner, Erick	O. C. Standifer, Elk City	Second Tuesday
Blaine	L. R. Kirby, Okeene	W. F. Griffin, Watonga	
Bryan	John T. Wharton, Durant	W. K. Haynie, Durant	Second Tuesday
Caddo	F. L. Patterson, Carnegie	C. B. Sullivan, Carnegie	
Canadian	P. F. Herod, El Reno	A. L. Johnson, El Reno	Subject to call
Carter	J. R. Pollock, Ardmore	H. A. Higgins, Ardmore	
Cherokee	P. H. Medearis, Tahlequah	W. M. Wood, Tahlequah	First Tuesday
Choctaw		E. A. Johnson, Hugo	
Cleveland	F. T. Gastineau, Norman	Iva S. Merritt, Norman	Thursday nights
Comanche	George L. Berry, Lawton	Howard Angus, Lawton	
Cotton	A. B. Holstead, Temple	Mollie F. Seism, Walters	Third Friday
Craig	Lloyd H. McPike, Vinita		
Creek	J. E. Hollis, Bristow		
Custer	F. R. Vieregg, Clinton	C. J. Alexander, Clinton	Third Thursday
Garfield	Julian Feild, Enid	John R. Walker, Enid	Fourth Thursday
Garvin	T. F. Gross, Lindsay	John R. Callaway, Pauls Valley	Wednesday before Third Thursday
Grady	Walter J. Baze, Chickasha	Roy E. Emanuel, Chickasha	Third Thursday
Grant	I. V. Hardy, Medford		
Greer	R. W. Lewis, Granite	J. B. Hollis, Mangum	
Harmon	W. G. Husband, Hollis	R. H. Lynch, Hollis	First Wednesday
Haskell	William Carson, Keota	N. K. Williams, McCurtain	
Hughes	Wm. L. Taylor, Holdenville	Imogene Mayfield, Holdenville	First Friday
Jackson	C. G. Spears, Altus	E. A. Abernethy, Altus	Last Monday
Jefferson	F. M. Edwards, Ringling		Second Monday
Kay	J. Holland Howe, Ponca City	G. H. Yeary, Newkirk	Second Thursday
Kingfisher	A. O. Meredith, Kingfisher	H. Violet Sturgeon, Hennessey	
Kiowa	J. William Finch, Hobart	William Bernell, Hobart	
LeFlore	Neeson Rolle, Poteau	Rush L. Wright, Poteau	
Lincoln	W. B. Davis, Stroud	Carl H. Bailey, Stroud	First Wednesday
Logan	William C. Milley, Guthrie	J. L. LeHew, Jr., Guthrie	Last Tuesday
Marshall	J. L. Holland, Madill	J. F. York, Madill	
Mayes	Ralph V. Smith, Pryor	Paul B. Cameron, Pryor	
McClain	W. C. McCurdy, Sr., Purcell	W. C. McCurdy, Jr., Purcell	
McCurtain	A. W. Clarkson, Valliant	N. L. Barker, Broken Bow	Fourth Tuesday
McIntosh	Luster I. Jacobs, Hanna	Wm. A. Tolleson, Eufaula	First Thursday
Murray	P. V. Annadown, Sulphur	J. A. Wrenn, Sulphur	Second Tuesday
Muskogee-Sequoyah			
Wagoner	H. A. Scott, Muskogee	D. Evelyn Miller, Muskogee	First Monday
Noble	C. H. Cooke, Perry	J. W. Francis, Jerry	
Okfuskee	C. M. Cochran, Okemah	M. L. Whitney, Okemah	Second Monday
Oklahoma	W. E. Eastland, Oklahoma City	E. R. Musick, Oklahoma City	Fourth Tuesday
Okmulgee	S. B. Leslie, Okmulgee	J. C. Matheney, Okmulgee	Second Monday
Osage	C. R. Weirich, Pawhuska	George K. Hemphill, Pawhuska	Second Monday
Ottawa	Walter Kerr, Picher	B. W. Shelton, Miami	Third Thursday
Pawnee	E. T. Robinson, Cleveland	R. L. Browning, Pawnee	
Payne	H. C. Manning, Cushing	J. W. Martin, Cushing	Third Thursday
Pittsburg	P. T. Powell, McAlester	W. H. Kaeiser, McAlester	Third Friday
Pontotoc	A. R. Sugg, Ada	R. H. Mayes, Ada	First Wednesday
Pottawatomie	E. Eugene Rice, Shawnee	Clinton Gallaher, Shawnee	First and Third Saturday
Pushmataha	John S. Lawson, Clayton	B. M. Huckabay, Antlers	
Rogers	R. C. Meloy, Claremore	Chas. L. Caldwell, Chelsea	First Monday
Seminole	J. T. Price, Seminole	Mack I. Shanholtz, Wewoka	Third Wednesday
Stephens	W. K. Walker, Marlow	Wallis S. Ivy, Duncan	
Texas	R. G. Obermiller, Texhoma	Morris Smith, Guymon	
Tillman	C. C. Allen, Frederick	O. G. Bacon Frederick	
Tulsa	Ralph A. McGill, Tulsa	E. O. Johnson, Tulsa	Second and Fourth Monday
Washington-Nowata	K. D. Davis, Nowata	J. V. Athey, Bartlesville	Second Wednesday
Washita	A. S. Neal, Cordell	James F. McMurry, Sentinel	
Woods	Ishmael F. Stephenson, Alva	Oscar E. Templin, Alva	Last Tuesday Odd Months
Woodward	H. Walker, Buffalo	C. W. Tedrowe, Woodward	Second Thursday

*(Serving in Armed Forces)

THE JOURNAL

OF THE

OKLAHOMA STATE MEDICAL ASSOCIATION

| VOLUME XXXVII | OKLAHOMA CITY, OKLAHOMA, AUGUST, 1944 | NUMBER 8 |

An Analysis of the Modern Treatment of Severe Burns[*]

CECIL K. DRINKER, M.D.

*Professor of Physiology in the Harvard
School of Public Health*

From the Department of Physiology

BOSTON, MASSACHUSETTS

INTRODUCTION

My interest in the treatment of burns arose three years ago while working with Dr. W. W. L. Glenn upon the physiological changes at the basis of inflammation. At the time, Dr. Glenn, one of the residents in surgery at the Massachusetts General Hospital, was spending a year in my laboratory and we were concerned with the effects of swelling as a problem in healing. We were anesthetizing dogs with nembutal and then cannulating a lymphatic craining one of the feet, so that we could collect normal lymph and compare it with lymph from the foot after causing severe, sterile inflammation. The lymph under such circumstances is in reality the inflammatory exudate with which the inflamed tissue becomes turgescent.

It was necessary to use a method of cuasing inflammation which would not be subject to infection for some time, which would not break the skin and lose inflammatory exudate through the surface, which could be precisely limited in extent and repeated with reasonable accuracy upon other animals or upon other feet of the same animal. The simplest and most satisfactory method for meeting these requirements was immersion of the parts in hot or boiling water for precise periods of time. All such experiments were carried out under complete surgical anesthesia, and recovery observations were so planned as to require but a small number of dogs. I

[*]Read before the General Session, Annual Meeting, April 26, 1944 in Tulsa.

may say, however, that our expectation of necessarily causing painful distress in dogs severely burned under anesthesia and treated immediately by closed-plaster dressings before permitting recovery was happily unrealized. It was as surprising to me as it would be to any of you to find that the foot of a dog could be immersed 45 seconds in boiling water and, if promptly encased in plaster, the dog gave no evidence of pain when he recovered from the anesthetic, indeed had to be confined rather closely in order to prevent injury to the dressing from active use of the burned part.

When Dr. Glenn and I began work, I believed that clotting of the exudate in inflamed, swollen tissues, such as would result from severe scalds, must have a good deal to do with the problem of local healing, since all such exudate must disappear before healing could be complete. It is imperative that exudation from blood vessels should occur in inflamed tissues. Highly active metabolic processes must go on in such regions in order to accomplish removal of dead cells and production of new. Inflamed tissue means tissue supplied with a maximum amount of oxygen through wide dilation of the smallest blood vessels from the blood due to abnormal leakage through the walls of many of the capillaries in the area. The exudate in a region of severe inflammation is practically blood plasma. It contains serum albumin, serum globulin, fibrinogen, and prothrombin. The last two are concerned with clotting. The reaction of coagulation takes place when, in the presence of calcium salts, injured tissues provide thromboplastic material. Some years ago, Menkin[1] (1931) showed that fibrin formation in and about foci of inflammation hinders absorption of toxic substances and bacteria by blocking lymphatic drainage. This is true to a certain extent and tends to isolate harmful agents and processes. But the exudate in and from severely injured parts and severe burns forms a good example of a productive sort of injury. It is often far greater in amount and more continuous than can be helpful. It is axiomatic that the size, or better, the volume of any solid part of the body is as definitely set as is the chemical composition of the body fluids. If injury occurs and the part is enlarged temporarily, it does not recover completely unless it returns to the original size, and the presence of unduly large exudation not only promotes infection and deformity, but always delays healing. While recognizing that clotting of exudate was necessary to control hemorrhage and that it might help to isolate infectious processes, it was my feeling that the extensive laying down of clotted plasma through inflamed tissue could not accomplish real good and that swelling, of itself, was a factor accompanying injury which should be considered as something to be prevented or treated, not as the inevitable accompaniment of injury or inflammation which would disappear with time or with control of the cause.

In this direction Glenn, Peterson and I[2] (1942) burned one front paw of an anesthetized dog by two minutes' immersion in boiling water. After several hours, when swelling was maximum, the animal was given a large intravenous injection of heparin so that coagulation was no longer possible. The companion foot was then burned to the same level in the same way. Comparatively slight local swelling occurred, only that due to accumulation of free fluid in the part, in contrast to the fluid imprisoned in the gelatinous coagulum which spread slowly through the first foot. While these experiments were in progress it had become clear that burns were one of the most frequent lessons of this War, and as a member of the Committee on Aviation Medicine, the first National Research Council group selected to attack the medical problems of the War, I had begun to hear a great deal about crippling burns of the hands in aviators. The efforts of our laboratory were turned at once toward exploration of burn problems, making use of techniques and experience in the study of the lymph and blood circulation we had developed over a number of years.

WHAT IS A BURN?

Intelligent attack upon any medical problem must be based upon the most thorough knowledge possible if all that is directly involved in the lesion, the complications promoted by it, and the ways in which methods of treatment combat the situations encountered. A burn is a lesion due to heat in which living cells are killed and neighboring cells injured in every degree. Blood capillaries, arteriovenous anastomotic channels, and the finest arteries and veins are dilated and somewhat increased in permeability as the initial normal physiological reaction to painful irritation, but in addition the heat injury may kill the walls of certain vessels and hemolyze the red cells in them. From this extreme effect upon the endothelium all graduations of damage to capillary walls will be present and it is possible to assert that in a severe superficial burn the capillaries most injured by the heat, but living and capable of recovering, may require a week to become normal in the sense of not leaking plasma excessively if subjected to ordinary pressures of the capillary blood. Abnormal leakage from the capillaries is the dominant continuing characteristic of the burn lesion. It causes loss of plasma into the part and through the part for surface escape. Local accumulation of exudate makes an excellent medium for the growth of micro-organisms, and frequently plasma loss is so great as to require plasma infusion to combat serious general effects.

There are further physiological matters of fundamental importance for the understanding of burns which are not properly appreciated. They are as follows:

1. The vascular dilatation which gives the redness, the heat, and part of the swelling in all painful inflammatory lesions is caused at first through what is called an axone reflex operating as indicated in the diagram, Figure 1. A sensory impulse interpreted as pain in the brain, branches to arterioles, capillaries, and arteriovenous connections in the adjacent tissue and dilatation results. Dilatation alone does not mean increased leakage through the walls of blood vessels until it has been pushed so far that stretching takes place. Wide dilatation and opening of all the vessels in a local area at once results in a maximum supply of oxygenated blood to the injured tissues. This widening of the vascular bed may last for a week or even more in infected lesions. Though initiated nervously, it is sustained by a variety of chemical agents formed in the burned tissue. In this connection it is well to refer to the shock-like state which is often thought to be due to the absorption of toxic substances from burns and from other severe wounds. These toxins absorbed from the lesions are considered responsible for lowered

blood volume by inducing capillary dilatation and some degree of abnormal leakage in the vessels of sound tissues. It may be the fact that something of the sort occurs, but as yet

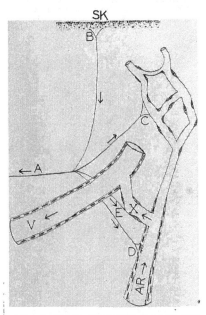

Figure 1. Diagram of the parts involved in the axone reflex which initiates the vascular dilatation in painful inflammatory lesions of which burns are prominent examples. A painful stimulus received at SK passes not only to the central nervous system to be recognized as pain, but to out-branching fibers to the smaller blood vessels which dilate as a result. SK, skin containing a pain ending; B, afferent nerve with A going to the spinal cord and branches, C, D, and E to a capillary, an arteriole, and an arteriovenous channel, X; V, a vein.

no one has detected such toxins in general distribution or even that capillaries in sound parts are abnormally affected after burns (Cope and Moore[3], 1944). One must, however, realize that even a very slight generalized increase in capillary permeability over the normal, especially if it continues for some time, might produce shock, particularly if added to a high degree of plasma loss by exudation in the actual burn. To my mind it is most satisfactory at the present time to consider that dilator and possibly permeability-increasing substances are formed in burns as an indispensable part of the inflammatory for the protection and healing of the

local situation in which they are formed. If the burned area is very large, some degree of absorption may occur, enough perhaps to act systemically where the effects are disastrous.

2. Recently, Muus and Hardenbergh[4] (1944) have shown that the lymph from a severely burned leg of a calf or dog increases the oxygen use of liver and muscle slices and that the serum of the burned animals shows traces of the same effect, the weaker stimulation to metabolism being due to the high dilution caused by the large volume of the blood. This observation is again important in that it indicates the presence in the burn exudate of something which stimulates the metabolism in an area where repair must go on as rapidly as possible. It is thus the fact that in such regions of inflammation there is local provision for dilatation of blood vessels and maximum oxygen supply and at the same time the production of something which increases oxygen use. With this arrangement, favorable locally, there goes the possibility of the overflow of metabolism increasing substance into the circulation with unfavorable general effects. We have found it necessary to guard constantly against rises in body temperature in severely burned animals. This fever is in no way related to infection. It comes within a few hours following the burn, and death from hyperpyrexia may result in the first 12 to 18 hours. Following the Cocoanut Grove disaster in Boston, hyperpyrexia was observed in several fatal cases. The use of heat for treating shock-like states is strongly ingrained in the profession, and warning against it have been given for surgical shock. External heat has but one purpose: to raise the body temperature to normal. Anything more than this is unfavorable in the treatment of shock, and for the collapse following severe burns even greater care must be exercised since, as these patients improve and the general circulation becomes normal, they will be in a position to absorb substances from the burn which will cause increased body temperature without the assistance of added external heat.

3. I have made a point of the fact that coagulation of burn exudate through the tissues has a serious part in the production of swelling which complicates healing. There is no doubt that coagulation of the exudate in burned tissue does occur, but if the burn is unaccompanied by crashing and mutilation of the tissue, coagulation is slow. At first this is possibly due to the fact that the dead cells in the lesion are simply heat coagulated bits of protein and do not give off thromboplastic material until they begin to disintegrate as a result of digestion. In addition to

this situation there is a further interesting fact which begins to be evident in the lymph collected from burned tissues soon after the burn takes place. Normal lymph clots just as does blood, but we soon noticed that lymph, in reality the burn exudate, begins to show delay and inefficiency in clotting quite soon. It will clot if allowed to pool in the tissues, but there is so much delay in this that a great deal of the swelling one expects from a burn can be prevented by elevation which allows the exudate to flow away through the tissues and lymphatics. It may be thought that preventing the accumulation of masses of coagulum around a burn is dangerous on account of allowing toxic absorption, but I do not think this possibility is important enough to overbalance the advantage to healing which arises through preventing the accumulation of undue amounts of coagulated exudate and consider the interference with coagulation, resulting locally in burns, of advantage toward healing of the lesion.

4. *The extent of destruction and fatal injury to the tissues involved in a burn is always less than is thought of the case upon first examination.* No one causing burns under laboratory conditions can fail to be surprised at the recovery which results from injuries treated promptly and properly. This lesson shows at once how much damage may be done by extensive debridement which destroys cells that may recover from mild degrees of injury and exposes sound cells to mutilation from contact with the dressing. Too much emphasis cannot be laid upon the harm resulting from enthusiastic scrubbing and debridement. Dirt in such injuries, unless deposited on the surface after the burn, has usually been subjected to high heat, and no amount of cleansing can keep such injuries from contamination by skin organisms from adjacent areas.

THE TREATMENT OF BURNS

The management of serious injuries of the extremities by enclosing them in plaster of paris dressings was not new when Orr[4] (1943), of Nebraska, began to advocate the method. It is, however, due to him and secondarily to the wide experience of Trueta[6] (1943) in the Spanish Revolution that we owe the great practical benefits which have resulted for the widespread war and civilian use of the method. Glenn, Gilbert, and I[7] (1943) examined the principles involved when the severely burned foot of a dog is encased in plaster immediately after burning. We dipped the foot of an anesthetized dog in

hot or boiling water for precise periods, and at once immersed the part in liquid plaster of paris which hardened in a few minutes and confined the injury in a rigid, indistensible dressing. The plaster cast included the entire foot and extended an inch to an inch and a half on to sound tissue above the upper

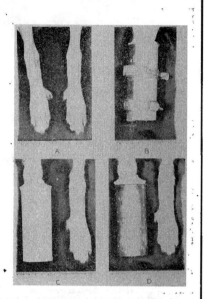

Figure 2. Application of a plaster cast to a burned paw.

A. Hind heel of an anesthetized dog, prior to burning. B. The right foot has been burned by immersion in hot water, and immediately after removal was thrust into a brass can containing liquid dental plaster. This can was in two halves, held tightly together by hose clamps. In the illustration, the plaster had hardened and one half of the can has been removed. C. The casted foot after removal of the can and ready for thorough drying by means of an electric fan. D. A perforated can to permit further evaporaton from the plaster has been cemented in place in order to protect the cast as the animal moves about, following recovery from anesthesia.   (From: W. W. L. Glenn, H. H. Gilbert, and C. K. Drinker. Jour Clin. Investigation, 1943, 22, 613.)

margin of hot water immersion. Beneath the plaster we used at most one or two layers of lightly vaselined gauze, not enough to leave room for swelling. This technique had the advantage of actually holding the part at the precise normal size. It met the physiological requirements of our experiment perfectly, since the foot was absolutely immobile in the rigid plaster and no matter what occurred, could not swell. Figure 2 shows the way in which casting of a burned foot was accomplished. The hind feet of a dog are shown in A. Immediately after burning the right foot by immersion in hot water, it was dried quickly, wrapped in a single layer of vaselined gauze or left uncovered, and then thrust into liquid plaster of paris in a brass container made in two parts and held together by hose clamps until the plaster solidified. In C

shown in Figure 3. Both hind feet of a dog were burned by simultaneous immersion to the cross lines in water at 100 degrees C. for 30 seconds. The right foot was at once cast as shown in Figure 2. The left was not treated. After 24 hours the cast was removed from the right foot and the photograph made. The casted foot is quite normal in appearance, and the uncasted left foot greatly swollen, with blisters between the toes from which serum drips.

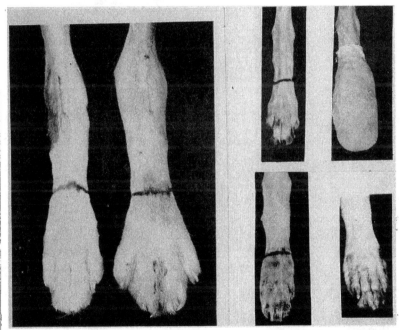

Figure 3
Figure 3. Both feet were burned for 30 seconds by simultaneous immersion in boiling water. The right foot was at once encased in plaster, and left untreated. Just before the photograph was made the cast on the right foot was removed. (Modified from: W. W. L. Glenn, H. H. Gilbert, and C. K. Drinker. Jour. Clin. Investigation, 1943, 22, 611.)

Figure 4
Figure 4. The upper left photograph is the hind foot of an anesthetized dog with a cross line to indicate the limit of burning. After immersion for 30 seconds in boiling water, it has been wrapped in one layer of gauze held lightly in place by gauze bandage and then covered with a plaster bandage extending well above the upper limit of the burn. The lower left photograph is the foot of another dog from which a similar plaster bandage has been removed 12 days after a 30 seconds' burn in boiling water. The final photograph shows recovery 86 days after this major injury.

the brass can has been removed and the plaster thoroughly dried. Then, in D, a second light can has been slipped over the casting and held in place with glue. This second can protects the plaster as the dog moves about. The manner in which this skin-tight method of applying plaster holds a foot so treated is

Before discussing the extraordinary way in which these skin-tight casts meet the physiological reactions of these burns, it is best to make the situation more practical, and this is possible by examination of Figure 4. In this case a burn due to 30 seconds' immersion in boiling water has been treated by an ordinary plaster bandage put on over a minimum amount of gauze covering. The left photograph of the lower pair shows the condition of such a foot on removal of the dressing 12 days after the burn, and the final illustration the same foot on the 86th day. Except for the fact that a small amount of hair is permanently destroyed, the foot is normal. There is no scar tissue; the epithelium is soft and smooth; there are no adhesions between the toes; and this recovery from a burn of major severity can be secured with mathematical regularity by simple closure in a plaster of paris dressing.

Why does the closed-plaster treatment work? I have devoted much time to examining the reasons why the closed-plaster treatment works so efficiently, since everything physicians have been taught runs counter to closing an infected or potentially infected part in a rigid dressing and then leaving it untouched for three weeks.

a. *The circulation.* Our first fear arises from a conviction that the close fitting, inelastic dressing will cut off the blood supply. I will not give the details of many different experiments, since all showed the circulation in an extremity cast in plaster or enclosed in the usual plaster bandage is unrestricted and wholly adequate. This will not be the case if the dressing is applied over a burn at the middle of an extremity and the lower part is not enclosed. It will swell promptly and can readily be made gangrenous if the dressing is left in place. There is but one course to take, namely the inclusion of the entire extremity in the dressing, and there can be no compromise with this.

b. *Edema and swelling.* I have said that abnormal leakage from the capillaries in a burned area is the major physiological derangement in the lesion. It requires very little thought to understand how plaster closure meets the problem of controlling capillary leakage. Unless the vessels are blocked by thrombi they will contain a current of blood when the plaster is applied. As soon as the dressing sets, it, in reality, becomes the wall of the capillaries, since even if they are highly permeable to water and solutes as a result of heat injury, the incompressible watery medium between the intravascular blood and the cast must bring about a situation in which, although the vessels are leaky, only minimal damage can occur. The restraint of seepage from seriously burned extremities will never be complete, and the plaster covering will always become stained with foul-smelling exudate, but the loss of

plasma may be so much lessened by prompt application of plaster dressings as to reduce the seriousness of the burn in terms of the extent of surface affected. It thus happens that a treatment which fits the local problem of healing by checking undue swelling, also improves the general condition of the patient.

c. *Absorption.* The closed-plaster treatment does not prevent direct absorption by the blood vessels, and in any burned region the activity of the curculation is so great as to make absorption steadily possible. This is a factor which cannot be controlled specifically by any method of management. If one collects lymph from the burned foot of a dog which is not confined in plaster and from the opposite foot encased in plaster and is prevented from swelling, it is apparent at once that the flow of lymph from the swollen foot is many times greater than from that held to normal size. This is due to the fact that though coagulation of exudate through the tissues and lymphatics of the swollen foot may restrain lymph flow to a slight degree, it does not counteract the promotion of lymphatic absorption which accompanies the wide opening of lymphatics always present in swollen tissues. It is the general impression that lymphatics are pressed shut in the presence of swelling. The opposite is true. The walls of the smallest lymphatics are completely permeable to burn exudates, and are attached on their outer surfaces to surrounding tissue so that swelling pulls them open and the permeability of their walls results in easy filling for eventual delivery to regions outside the burn.

d. *Pain.* I have referred to the apparent absence of pain in our experimental animals. The same experience is most striking in human burns. Our expectation would be the contrary. We think of mysterious pressure effects against the plaster covering, which would be excessively painful. But it is apparent that in a very short time after application, pressures under the dressing become equal in all directions and there is no fluctuant stretching of the tissues. Pain in burns, after the first effects of the heat wear off, is due to stretching of fine nerve fibrils from swelling or to mutilation of them in applying new dressings. The part in a closed-plaster case cannot swell beyond the state in which it existed when the dressing was applied. It always shrinks somewhat, and one may readily observe that if an extremity put up in plaster is allowed to hang down a day or two after the original dressing, pain will begin fairly promptly, and is relieved equally rapidly when the part is elevated and vascular turgescence removed. Another very real reason why the closed-plaster treatment saves the patient from pain resides in the fact that this dressing once in place is let alone for 21 days. It must contain no windows, and every impulse to open the dressing and ascertain the course of events must be resisted. If regional lymph nodes become inflamed and if fever and leucocytosis indicate an extending infection, it may be necessary to remove the cast; but these are not frequent complications, and in the ordinary case the plaster bandage may remain untouched for three weeks when its removal will not cause the slightest pain.

e. *Infection.* Experience has shown that local bacterial growth is, on the whole, less with closed treatment than when frequent dressings are used. At the outset the burned surfaces were dusted with one of the sulfa drugs, but the degree of absorption into the blood was unpredictable and the procedure was not continued. If medication by these drugs is thought necessary they are much better given in the usual way, since the increase capillary permeability in the burned area will mean thorough dosage where it is needed. Penicillin locally, because of its effect on staphylococci, has proved well worth while and should become in fairly wide use. There is little doubt that the complete degree of immobilization provided by the plaster dressing has part in the restraint of infection.

f. *Some special considerations.* In Figure 5 is shown a badly burned hand prior to treatment and after being enclosed in a plaster bandage. As a first covering one or two layers of dry gauze are now used. Grease of any kind has proved quite unnecessary to prevent sticking and may interfere with epithelialization. The fingers need not be wrapped separately. The dressing is applied so as to make a snug fit, but without pressure, the object being to hold the part at the volume existing when it is put in place, not to squeeze exudate out of it. Obviously the smaller the part when the dressing is applied the better. Consequently when a patient comes in for treatment the part should be elevated at once and kept so until the dressing is in place.

When our colleagues, Doctors Lund and Levenson at the Boston City Hospital, began to apply the methods and reasoning we had found satisfactory in our experiments upon dogs, it was believed the plaster bandage would not work well, since many patients could not be treated until some hours after the accident. It was found this was not the

case. They were more comfortable at once and they were easily cared for if closed-plaster dressings were used immediately. So far as I can see, the complete immobilization and absence of meddlesome redressings had most to do with this.

The use of rigid plaster instead of the

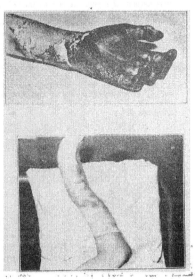

Figure 5. *Upper photograph,* appearance of hand before treatment. Note broken and unbroken blisters. Sooty appearance from electric flash. *Lower photograph,* after five days. Note medium position of fingers. Slight exudate stains the cast. (From: S. M. Levenson and C. C. Lund, Jour. A.M.A., 1943, 123, 273.)

more popular pressure dressing is still a matter of careful observation. In putting on a pressure dressing, the part is covered with layer after layer of elastic and absorbent material of the general nature of sterile cotton waste, and is finally enclosed in bandage which makes a relatively indistensible outside coat. Between the bandage and the skin there is a variable amount of elastic packing which is bound on so that some degree of pressure exists. How much this is or how much it ought to be no one can tell. From the physiological point of view the technique does not possess the clear-cut advantage of the closed-plaster dressing, but being a physiologist with a good deal of clinical experience, I have learned that the physiological point of view may readily be wrong. Certainly the use of plaster of paris is largely limited to burns of the extremities, and for those about the genitalia, trunk, neck, and head the pressure bandage must be employed in the majority of cases.

In conclusion, I regret that time does not permit me to discuss the eminently physiological problem of plasma and whole blood transfusions, the pernicious damage which may be done by intemperate administration of salt and glucose solutions, and the anemia and protein malnutrition following burns. I have confined my remarks to a discussion of the physiological nature of an extremely common sort of injury, and of the profit to be gained by treating the injury as a physiological problem. In simple terms, this means nothing more than *really thinking about* the medical job which confronts us, and thoughtful sagacious attacks on all jobs are the master words today.

BIBLIOGRAPHY

1. Menkin. V.: An aspect of Inflammation in Relation to Immunity. Arch. of Path., 12, 802. 1931. See also by the same author, Dynamics of Inflammation, An Inquiry into the Mechanism of Infectious Processes, The Macmillan Co., New York. 1940.

2. Glenn, W. W. L., Peterson, D. K., and Drinker, C. K.: The Flow of Lymph from Burned Tissue, with Particular Reference to the Effects of Fibrin Formation upon Lymph Drainage and Composition. Surgery, 12, 685. 1942.

3. Cope, O., and Moore, F.: A Study of Capillary Permeability in Experimental Burns and Burn Shock Using Radio-Active Dyes in Blood and Lymph. Jour. Clin. Investigation, 23, 241. 1944.

4. Muus, J., and Hardenbergh, E.: The Oxygen Consumption of Normal Rat Liver Slices in Serum and in Lymph Taken from the Legs Before and After Severe Burns. Jour. Biol. Chem., 152, 1. 1944.

5. Orr, H. W.: The Physiologic Factors Involved in Protecting the Patient Against Infection in the Healing of Fractures in Compound Wounds. Transactions and Studies, College of Physicians, Philadelphia, 10, 187. 1943. (This reference is a summary of Orr's work and goes back to 1923 when he began his advocacy on the closed-plaster method.

6. Trueta, J.: The Principles and Practices of War Surgery. C. V. Mosby Company, St. Louis. 1943.

7. Glenn, W. W. L., Gilbert, H. H., and Drinker, C. K.: The Treatment of Burns by the Closed-Plaster Method, with Certain Physiological Considerations Implicit in the Success of this Technique. Jour. Clin. Investigation, 22, 609. 1943

Public Health Aspects of Infantile Paralysis[*]

G. F. MATHEWS, M.D.

Commissioner of Health
Oklahoma State Health Department

OKLAHOMA CITY, OKLAHOMA

The epidemiological information on cases of infantile paralysis occurring in 1943 is not as complete as we should like to have. This is particularly true with respect to field investigations which would have included data on environmental sanitation. All field investigations which were made were carried out by individual county health officers and these were limited because of the shortage of personnel. The figures which are presented here were gathered for the most part from physicians' morbidity report cards supplemented by data from the Crippled Children's Commission on cases hospitalized but not reported. These records are fairly complete. Of the 594 known cases, 394 or 66 per cent were hospitalized , thus giving valuable statistical information of a clinical nature. We wish to recognize the splendid efforts on the part of our full-time county health officers in their assistance with the early recognition, diagnosis and isolation of cases.

*Presented to the Oklahoma State Medical Association, Tulsa, April 26, 1944.

DEFINITION

Infantile paralysis is an acute, generalized infection due to a filtrable virus, occurring both in epidemics and sporadically. From the standpoint of prevention, it is important to note that social and hygienic conditions apparently have no influence whatever in determining the infection. All classes are infected in about equal proportions.

HISTORICAL

Infantile parlysis has the ear-marks of a new infection, although some incidence of sudden paralysis in babies are found in the literature of antiquity. These might be assumed to be infantile paralysis.

The first outbreak described in the United States was reported by Caverly in 1894.

Wickman of Sweden, in 1905 and 1906, made the first systematic study of the disease from an epidemiological point of view. He directed special attention to several factors in the spread; namely, routes of travel, public gatherings of children, abortive and ambulant cases, and healthy intermediate carriers.

In 1909, the disease was transmitted to two monkeys by inoculating them from the spinal cord of a child who had died of infantile paralysis. Later in the year, Flexner and Lewis obtained the same results in further transmissions from monkey to monkey through an indefinite number of passages.

INCUBATION

The incubation period is commonly 7 to 14 days, with limits of 5 to 24 days. In making epidemiological studies, we consider happenings about two weeks prior to the onset of the disease.

The disease has gradually spread until it now exists in all countries of the world. The distribution, however, is quite unequal and irregular. From 1910 to 1914, inclusive, 18,800 cases were reported in the United States, and 31,500 cases were reported in the next two years. In 1916, an epidemic swept the United States involving numbers far in excess of anything recorded. There were 29,000 cases reported, and 6,000 deaths. This epidemic was the worst known in the history of the disease.

Cold countries having marked seasonal variations in temperature have been most affected. One of the many pecularities about infantile paralysis is that, while it

TABLE NO. 1

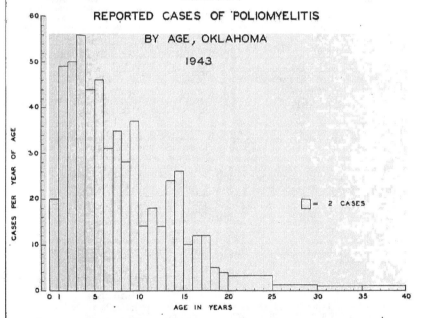

REPORTED CASES OF POLIOMYELITIS BY AGE, OKLAHOMA 1943

EPIDEMICS AND PREVALENCE

In the past, epidemics have been more severe in small towns and rural districts than in densely populated areas. However, there was an exception to this in the epidemic in 1916 which struck New York City with unusual force. But, in general, the incidence is lowest in metropolitan areas, and higher in small towns and villages of the country.

is a warm weather disease, it spares warm countries. A comparatively small number of cases have been reported from the tropics. The northern countries of Europe and the northern part of the United States have suffered most.

Infantile paralysis is strikingly a warm weather disease. It is true that during the winter, cases occur sporadically, but the number increases as the summer advances. The curve rises in July and reaches its peak in August or early September, and declines rapidly with the advent of cold weather. This seasonal periodicity repeats itself with marked regularity in epidemic regions of temperate zones. A community having an epidemic one year is usually spared the next.

SEX AND AGE

Rosenau states that about 56 per cent of all cases reported are males, and about 44 per cent females. In the past epidemics in the State of Oklahoma, 58 per cent of all cases reported were males, and 42 per cent females.

Infantile paralysis is primarily a disease of childhood, probably because the young are more susceptible to the infection. In the past epidemic in Oklahoma, 38 per cent of all cases reported were under five years of age, and 69 per cent of all cases reported were under ten years of age.

Note Age-Grouping Chart. (Table No. 1.)

Any age may be affected, however. Probably the most outstanding among adult cases is our President who was 39 years old when he contracted the disease.

CASE FATALITY

From 1894 to 1921, studies of 38 epidemics. totalling 20,568 cases were made and the case fatality rate ranged from 30 per cent to 5 per cent. The disease appeared to be more virulent in winter than in spring and in summer. Thus, the case fatality rate was 86 per cent in March and 20 per cent in August in 1921. There is a possibility of inaccuracy in these figures, due to the lack of recognition and incomplete reporting of mild cases during the off-season.

In the 1943 epidemic in Oklahoma, the case fatality rate was 5 per cent. The case fatality rate is lowest from one to five years of age. It is high under one year, and becomes proportionately higher as age advances. (Table No. 2.)

SPREAD IN FAMILIES

The disease as a rule does not spread in families; only about 4 per cent of the over 8,000 families attacked in New York City in 1916 had more than one case per family.

However, in the 1943 Oklahoma epidemic, we had one family with five cases and five families with three cases each, and eighteen families with two cases each. It is significant that when multiple cases do occur in a family, they usually come down together or within a short time of each other. The instance of five cases in one family occurred in Texas county and the onsets ranged from August 30 to September 12, 1943.

TABLE II
POLIOMYELITIS CASES, DEATHS, AND CASE FATALITY BY AGE, OKLAHOMA, 1943

Ages	Cases	Deaths	Case Fatality Per cent
All Ages	594	33	5.6
Under 1	20	7	35.0
1—4	199	7	3.5
5—9	177	7	4.0
10—14	96	5	5.2
15—19	43	1	2.3
20—29	24	1	4.2
30—39	9	2	22.2
40 and over	7	3	42.9
Age unstated	19	0	0.0

THE VIRUS

The virus is present in greatest virulence and concentration in the spinal cord and also in the brain of an infected person or animal. It has been found in other organs and tissues, such as the mucous membrane of the nose and pharynx. It has also been found in intestinal excretions.

Intestinal discharges should be disinfected in all cases until further knowledge of the source is at hand. It has been shown that ordinary chlorine treatment of sewage will not affect the virus. Trask has on numerous occasions detected the virus of poliomyelitis in urban sewage. It has not yet been possible to detect the virus in sewage during nonepidemic periods.

Infantile paralysis is not known to occur in nature in any other animal than man, although an animal reservoir is suspected. Only certain monkeys are susceptible. The old world monkeys have been found to be more suitable for experimental purposes. The disease in monkeys is a fairly accurate reproduction of infantile paralysis as seen in children. Monkeys have been infected by placing the virulent material upon the healthy mucous membrane of the nose, and by injecting the virus subcutaneously or into the peritoneal cavity. Also, by the introduction of the virus in the stomach. Lavan, in a talk in Oklahoma City last fall said that eight strains of the virus have been demonstrated.

IMMUNITY

One attack of infantile paralysis confers a high degree of immunity. Second attacks are almost unknown. Monkeys which have recovered from the infection show a high degree of immunity and their blood serum contains antibodies capable of rendering the virus harmless.

No racial immunity to the infection is known, although infantile paralysis has been for the most part confined to the white race. (No negro deaths, but 24 cases—4 per cent of total.) (Table No. 3.)

TABLE III
POLIOMYELITIS CASES BY SEX AND RACE
OKLAHOMA, 1943

Race	Total		Sex		
	No	Per Cent	Male	Female	Unstated
White	551	92.8	323	228	0
Negro	24	4.0	12	12	0
Indian	8	1.3	3	4	0
Unstated	11	1.9	1	2	8
TOTAL	594	100.0	339	247	8

MODES OF TRANSMISSION

(A) There is evidence to support the theory that the disease is directly transmissible from person to person. There is also a strong suspicion that healthy carriers play an important role in spreading the infection. There are epidemiological features of infantile paralysis that cannot be explained with the theory of contact infection; such as, the seasonal prevalence, rural incidence, lack of tendency to spread in families, and the disinclination to attack congested centers or to spread in hospitals, schools, or other crowded places.

(B) Insect-borne theory.
(C) Milk-borne theory.
(D) Other theories.

PREVENTION

No definite, effective system of prevention can be formulated until we are sure of the mode of transmission. We think that health authorities are entirely justified, in the meantime, in requiring cases to be reported, and isolated along the lines of preventive measures applied to typhoid fever; such as, disinfection, screening, guarding against insects, laying unnecessary dust, pasteurization of milk, closing of swimming pools, etc.

However, until we have something definite on the exact modes of transmission, all this resembles the old shot-gun prescription.

Both serums and vaccines have proved ineffective as prophylactic agents. Of course, no one can say that some kind of vaccine may not yet be realized.

Chemical phophylaxis will be of no definite value until the natural portal of entry is definitely known, and granting that it could be safely used.

Trask and Paul made the observation that infantile paralysis should be classed among the intestinal diseases rather than among the respiratory diseases. They further suggest that the principle of control may eventually turn out to be somewhat similar to those which have been used in typhoid fever. We are quite in the dark as to the control of any virus disease which is also an intestinal disease. And, in the control of poliomyelitis, our ignorance remains profound. Among other things, we still have to wait for more knowledge regarding the significance of insect vectors, and also regarding the existence of other possible extra-human carrier such as mammals or birds.

BIBLIOGRAPHY

1. Preventive Medicine and Hygiene—Rosenau, Chapter 5, "Infantile Paralysis."
2. Public Health Reports, Volume 58, Page 937.

The Significance of Abnormal Spinal Fluid Findings in the Diagnosis and Treatment of Neurosyphilis[*]

WILLIAM E. GRAHAM, SENIOR SURGEON

U. S. PUBLIC HEALTH SERVICE
U. S. Public Health Service Medical Center

HOT SPRINGS NATIONAL PARK, ARKANSAS

Most Public Health Officers and others interested in the control of syphilis have very properly concerned themselves chiefly with clinical and epidemiologic aspects of the early stages of this disease. This policy is based upon sound principles. Syphilis, except when congenitally acquired, is usually transmitted by persons in whom the disease is in the primary or secondary stage.

*Delivered before the Section on Public Health at the Annual State Meeting, April 26, 1944, in Tulsa.

If these individuals can be found, brought to treatment and kept under treatment until cured—or at least until rendered noninfectious, the chain of infection will be quickly broken, thereby preventing many new infections.

The most important single factor in syphilis control has been the availability of adequate treatment facilities regardless of the patients' ability to pay. It has been necessary, therefore, to set up more than three thousand free and part-pay clinics all over the country to care for indigent persons and those with a small income. These clinics and physicians treating patients privately have been doing such a good job that, despite wartime conditions, there has been no measurable increase in the amount of syphilis in this Country, and the last official reported rate in the armed forces is the lowest in history.

When a physician accepts a patient for treatment, he accepts the responsibility of treating that patient to the best of his ability. If he contents himself with giving injections of mapharsen and bismuth until the patient has had twenty of each and then discharges him or lets him lapse treatment, he has probably fulfilled his public health duty to the community but perhaps not his private duty to the individual. If the patient develops symptoms of neurosyphilis or some late manifestation of the disease fifteen or twenty years later and thereby becomes a public charge, the physician becomes partly responsible for the eventual physical breakdown of this individual and the consequent prolonged and expensive custodial care which he may require for the remainder of his life.

For the proper treatment of a patient who has syphilis, it is mandatory at some time or other during the course of his treatment that his spinal fluid be examined. About 10 per cent of infected persons who have been entirely untreated can be expected, eventually, to develop neurologic manifestations of the disease. It is difficult to estimate the percentage of persons who have received routine therapy with arsenic and bismuth who will become symptomatic, but it is certainly an appreciable percentage, especially when there has been a treatment lapse in early syphilis early in the treatment regime.

If the spinal fluid is ever to become positive, it nearly always does so very early after the infection has become established and, therefore, the fluid should be examined early. In early syphilis, when a patient is being treated on a conservative schedule of one injection per week, the spinal fluid may well be examined after about six months of treatment. If the tests are negative, the examination should be repeated at the completion of treatment. If intensive treatment is used, the fluid may be examined when the treatment has been completed. If the spinal fluid is negative at the completion of intensive treatment or after six months of routine treatment, there is slight chance that it will ever be positive. If it is still negative a year later, the test need never be repeated.

When a patient is seen in whom the in-

fection has occurred two or more years previously, a spinal fluid examination should be done at once in order to avoid wasting valuable time. If the test is negative, it will probably remain negative since immunity, if present, is usually well established after two years. If the test is positive, appropriate therapy should be instituted.

Until comparatively recently, very few registrants who had syphilis were accepted by the Selective Service Boards for induction into the armed forces. As was inevitable, this has all been changed and thousands of spinal fluid examinations are being made—many of them on persons who would otherwise never have received an examination of their spinal fluid. Many hitherto unsuspected cases of neurosyphilis are consequently being discovered. The finding of these cases present difficult problems to many a physician who has not had the training or the experience necessary to cope with it adequately. Very often he is not familiar with the significance of the various findings in the spinal fluid, and these findings are often misinterpreted. The practioner is perturbed when he discovers that the diagnosis and treatment of a symptomatic and clinical neurosyphilis fall short of being an exact science and that the problems which arise are often complex and confusing. He may be disappointed to find that the spinal fluid alone is not always a satisfactory guide to follow but that it is only an aid in the diagnosis and management of a patient with neurosyphilis. He discovers that false positive Wassermann tests are sometimes reported on spinal fluid specimens. He finds that laboratories vary widely in the types of tests which they perform and that they occasionally make conflicting reports. In short, all the familiar pitfalls found in the serologic diagnostic tests on blood are present and, in addition, there are many more occasioned by the greater complexity of spinal fluid tests and by the added gravity of that condition.

One should always remember that the sooner the presence of a syphilitic involvement of the nervous system is discovered, the more likely it is that that patient can be cured. This means that for best results the condition should be discovered during the fifteen to twenty-five years in which most neurosyphilis patients are asymptomatic. The earlier in this period the spinal fluid is found to be positive, the better.

Having concluded this somewhat lengthy preamble, it might be well to devote at least a paragraph or two to the subject under discussion, namely, "The Significance of Abnormal Spinal Fluid Findings in the Diagnosis and Treatment of Neurosyphilis."

There are, so far as we know, only three

changes in the spinal fluid that are of significance in the diagnosis of neurosyphilis. These are: the presence of reagin as manifested by a positive complement fixation or flocculation test, an increased number of cells, and changes in the spinal fluid protein.

Omitting the possibility of a false Wassermann test (w h i c h, incidentally, we shouldn't do), a positive complement fixation of flocculation test in the spinal fluid is pathognomonic of syphilitic involvement of the central nervous system. In fact, it is the only spinal fluid test that is pathognomonic. An abnormal cell count and an increased total protein or globulin content only indicate that meningeal irritation is present, and this may be caused by a variety of conditions. When the latter tests are positive in a person known to have syphilis, and when no other reason for them is apparent, a diagnosis of neurosyphilis should be made.

Eagle maintains that, for various technical reasons, precipitation tests on the spinal fluid are usually less satisfactory than an adequate complement fixation test. A quantitative test gives the maximum information. The titration should be carried downward as far as it will go. When a quantitative test has not been done, a fluid in which a 2 plus test has been obtained only in the first tube (E.G. containing 1 cc of fluid) is ordinarily reported as being "positive." The interpretation of this report may be much different from that made on a fluid reported as being strongly positive in four dilutions, that is, 4 4 4 4 0. Yet, without a quantitative test, the laboratory report on both tubes is identical.

Physicians are learning that a positive blood serologic test does not necessaarily indicate that a patient has syphilis. False positive Wassermahn reactions due to laboratory error or to some property of the serum producing biologic false positive reactions are by no means uncommon. The performance of serologic tests on blood has improved tremendously during the past few years. This improvement has been due to a very great extent to the introduction of the annual serologic evaluation study of state laboratories by the U. S. Public Health Service and, in turn, to similar intrastate evaluations conducted by the State Health Departments on laboratories within the states. Unfortunately, it does not seem practicable at this time to do similar surveys with spinal fluid specimens. Many physicians have the impression that false positive reactions are rarely obtained in the spinal fluid. This is not true. The average physician sees the results of only one spinal fluid examination on a given patient, and he—and the patient—are likely to stand or fall on the result of this single test. No reputable syphilologist will begin syphilis therapy on a patient with only the evidence of a single positive blood test. The implications of a false diagnosis of syphilis are too great to render such a policy tolerable. Consider the far greater implications to the patient of a false diagnosis of neurosyphilis which was based upon a single positive spinal fluid Wassermann test. All too often such patients are branded erroneously with the diagnosis of neurosyphilis, and then begins a tedious, prolonged, dangerous, and very expensive treatment regime involving perhaps artificial fever, Swift Ellis, and tryparsamide therapy. I am not advocating repeating all spinal fluid examinations which are reported positive immediately, but when the patient presents no symptoms of neurosyphilis and the spinal fluid Wassermann is positive with a normal cell count and a normal protein or globulin content, the suspicion of a false test should be entertained. Another spinal fluid specimen can then be obtained and sent to another laboratory or to several laboratories. Surely the additional information obtained by a repeated examination in such doubtful cases is well worth the added inconvenience to the patient—especially when the fluid is found to be normal.

When the spinal fluid Wassermann is found to be positive and all other tests are negative, it is likely, though not always certain, that there is not much "activity" in the neurosyphilitic process. This picture is sometimes found after a patient has had fever treatment. After such therapy the cell count usually drops to normal first, then the Wassermann test becomes negative (perhaps several years later) and finally, in favorable cases, the total protein drops to normal; but this order is by no means invariable. One must also keep in mind the possibility that the spinal fluid may remain "Wassermann fast" in the same manner so frequently seen in the blood of many patients with late syphilis.

The cell count is a procedure which is all too often neglected in examinations on the spinal fluid. To be satisfactorily performed, this test must be done on absolutely fresh fluid since sedimentation, clumping and autolysis may invalidate the results of such a test within a few hours. The test is easily performed and requires only a microscope and a leucocyte blood counting pipette and a counting chamber. It is customary to consider a cell count of 5 cells or less as normal and 5 to 10 cells as of doubtful significance. If more than 10 cells per cu. mm. of spinal fluid are found, some type of meningeal irritation is indicated. The intensity of the meningeal irritation is indicated by the number of cells present. In acute syphilitic meningitis, from 50 to 2,000 cells may be found. We may expect to find any number of cells up to 100 in late meningovascular syphilis and in tabes dorsalis, and up to 200 cells in general paresis. In a symptomatic neurosyphilis the cell count ranges from 0 to 200. A count of 150 or above presages the imminence of acute syphilitic meningitis and makes immediate intensive treatment mandatory.

Changes in the spinal fluid proteins are usually found when syphilis involves the central nervous system. The changes may consist of an increase in globulin, an increase in albumin, or an increase in varying ratios of both. A globulin increase can be determined by adding spinal fluid to an equal amount of saturated ammonia sulfate and grading the turbidity produced as one plus, two plus, three plus, and four plus. Normal spinal fluid contains too little globulin to be demonstrated by this test.

The well known Pandy test is not a test for globulin, but it is a test for total protein. In our experience the Pandy test has been somewhat disappointing. There is an increasing tendency to measure the amount of total protein present in the spinal fluid quantitatively. The total protein may be precipitated in a variety of ways and the amount of turbidity compared with standards in order to determine the number of mg. per cent of total protein. The amount present in normal fluid is generally considered to be from 15 to 40 mg. per cent though occasionally the content may be somewhat higher. This quantitative test is more informative than a qualitative test in much the same way that a quantitative Wasserman test is superior to a qualitative Wassermann in the diagnosis and management of neurosyphilis.

The best known colloidal tests are the gold, mastic, and benzoin. They are all fundamentally similar. They are entirely nonspecific and their diagnostic value has been greatly exaggerated. The type of cure obtained probably depends upon the absolute and relative concentrations of albumin and globulin in the fluid. The total protein determinations therefore actually give us more factual information than do the colloidal tests.

The idea that colloidal test zone curves are helpful in distinguishing between paresis, tabes, unclassified neurosyphilis, and infectious meningitis is fallacious. If the fluid contains a large excess of globulin as compared to albumin, it will give a paretic curve; and conversely, if it contains both albumin and globulin in large concentration, it will give a meningitic curve. Any type of curve may appear in any type of central

nervous system involvement, syphilitic or otherwise. It is truly illuminating to see, as we frequently do, three successive colloidal spinal fluid reports on the same patient six months apart, often from the same laboratory, indicating e. g. first a tabetic curve, second a meningitic curve, and finally a paretic curve. It would be truly weird to assume that such a patient had tabes first, then meningitis six months later, and finally paresis.

Unquestionably, one of the chief reasons for the popularity of the colloidal tests is that there is something exhilarating in a macabre sort of way in discovering that a patient has "numbers in his spinal fluid." It is more stimulating to see a report that says "colloidal mastic 5555543210" than one that says "total protein 75 mg. per cent." Undoubtedly, colloidal tests may be helpful to the physician in the evaluation of the status of the spinal fluid, but he should understand what a positive test means, and he should be cognizant of the limitations of the test. He should understand that, as is the case with an abnormally high cell count and an abnormally high protein content, a positive colloidal test indicates only meningeal irritation from some cause, not necessarily syphilis. He should consider the "zonal reactions" with suspicion, and he should remember that unless the degree of precipitaion exceeds two, the colloidal test should be considered normal. In other words, the colloidal curve 2222110000 is within normal limits.

A few general remarks on the treatment of asymptomatic neurosyphilis might not be amiss at this point. Routine treatment consisting of alternating courses of weekly injections of trivalent arsenic and bismuth for a total of forty to seventy injections usually is not adequate for the successful management of such a patient. When spinal fluid changes are minimal with a normal Wassermann test, usually a prolongation of six months to a year of the routine alternating courses of trivalent arsenic and bismuth will be adequate.

When moderate abnormalities are present in the spinal fluid including a positive Wasserman test, an intensified treatment routine should be used for at least six months to a year. The spinal fluid should be examined every six months. If the titre of the spinal fluid does not show signs of falling, fever or tryparsamide should be considered. In resistant cases fever should be used before treatment is stopped. The total duration of treatment in such patients will usually be two to two and one-half years.

When marked changes are present in the spinal fluid (paretic formula), routine treatment with trivalent arsenicals and bismuth is not sufficient to bring about a serologic reversal. Fever therapy is indicated on such patients, either as soon as the spinal fluid changes are discovered or as soon as is convenient for the patient. The total period of treatment for this type of patient should be at least three years.

Tryparsamide should never be used in any type of syphilis other than neurosyphilis, and it should never be used then unless adequate facilities for routine visual field examinations are available. Subdural therapy has been steadily losing ground, and we agree with Moore that its use should be entirely abandoned.

The fact that early treatment of asymptomatic neurosyphilis gives the best results cannot be overemphasized. After nerve tissue in the brain or spinal cord has been destroyed in patients with paresis and tabes dorsalis, little can be done with any type of therapy save possibly to prevent the process from advancing any further. Adequate therapy, including fever when indicated, long before actual neurologic damage has occurred is the proper prophylaxis against the development of asymptomatic neurosyphilis. It is indeed fortunate that the spinal fluid gives us a fairly accurate prophecy concerning what will happen perhaps years later. It is tragic that better use is not more frequently made of this device. The greater the extent of the spinal fluid abnormalities, the greater is the likelihood that, without proper treatment, paresis or tabes will be the eventual outcome.

It is hoped that this discussion may have been helpful in pointing out a few of the pitfalls that so frequently beset the practitioner in the management of patients who have syphilis. No apology is made for the fact that the methods of treatment of syphilis of the central nervous system have barely been touched. The routinized treatment schedules which are acceptable in early syphilis are impossible in neurosyphilis. Each patient requires individual treatment. As Moore says, "Success in therapy in this type of syphilis implies some things which no text can supply, namely, a basic knowledge of neurology, psychiatry and internal medicine, a working acquaintanceship with the art, as well as the science, of medicine, and experience. Lacking any one of these, the practitioner will secure better results with his patients if he carries out treatment procedures which have been advised for the particular individual patient by a consultant expert."

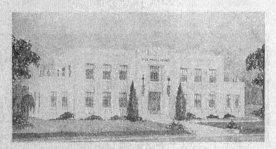

· THE PRESIDENT'S PAGE ·

This letter is to remind you to mail in your cards on the prepaid medical and surgical plan. This is one of the most important matters ever brought to the attention of the doctors of this State. We want each and every member of the Association to express himself on this proposition.

The action which the House of Delegates will take depends largely on the results of this survey. No doctor in this State is too busy to spend the very few moments it will require to fill out the card. If you are against it, say so. If you favor it, say so. If you have any constructive criticism to offer, send it in. But, for goodness sake, express yourself in some way in connection with this most important matter.

President.

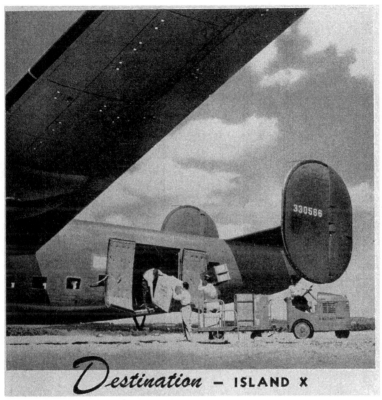
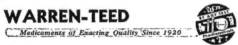

The JOURNAL Of The
OKLAHOMA STATE MEDICAL ASSOCIATION

EDITORIAL BOARD
L. J. MOORMAN, Oklahoma City, Editor-in-Chief
E. EUGENE RICE, Shawnee   BEN H. NICHOLSON, Oklahoma City
MR. PAUL H. FESLER, Oklahoma City, Business Manager

CONTRIBUTIONS: Articles accepted by this Journal for publication including those read at the annual meetings of the State Association are the sole property of this Journal.

The Editorial Department is not responsible for the opinions expressed in the original articles of contributors.

Manuscripts may be withdrawn by authors for publication elsewhere only upon the approval of the Editorial Board.

MANUSCRIPTS: Manuscripts should be typewritten, double-spaced, on white paper 8½ x 11 inches. The original copy, not the carbon copy, should be submitted.

Footnotes, bibliographies and legends for cuts should be typed on separate sheets in double space. Bibliography listing should follow this order: Name of author, title of article, name of periodical with volume, page and date of publication.

Manuscripts are accepted subject to the usual editorial revisions and with the understanding that they have not been published elsewhere.

NEWS: Local news of interest to the medical profession, changes of address, births, deaths and weddings will be gratefully received.

ADVERTISING: Advertising of articles, drugs or compounds unapproved by the Council on Pharmacy of the A.M.A. will not be accepted. Advertising rates will be supplied on application.

It is suggested that members of the State Association patronize our advertisers in preference to others.

SUBSCRIPTIONS: Failure to receive The Journal should call for immediate notification.

REPRINTS: Reprints of original articles will be supplied at actual cost provided request for them is attached to manuscripts or made in sufficient time before publication. Checks for reprints should be made payable to Industrial Printing Company, Oklahoma City.

Address all communications to THE JOURNAL OF THE OKLAHOMA STATE MEDICAL ASSOCIATION,
210 Plaza Court, Oklahoma City. (3)

OFFICIAL PUBLICATION OF THE OKLAHOMA STATE MEDICAL ASSOCIATION
Copyrighted August, 1944

· EDITORIALS

SHAME ON OKLAHOMA

According to fairly accurate estimates, less than half the members of the Oklahoma State Medical Association receive the Journal of The American Medical Association.

There is no point in belonging to the greatest medical association in the world if you are wholly ignorant of what this organization stands for; of the progress it sponsors, and the scientific knowledge it strives to disseminate.

Every doctor who belongs to the State Association should subscribe to the Journal of the American Medical Association. This much he owes to his patients, to his profession and to himself. There can be no economy in pocketing the subscription price. There is danger in procrastination, a patient may die for want of knowledge contained in the Journal.

Subscribe—scrutinize—lift your head and fraternlize—shell out and make the Journal of the American Medical Association your shiboleth.

YOUR COUNCIL

Under the guidance of the affable, capable new President, the Council in full attendance on Sunday, July 9, transacted the business of your State Association with a forthright sincerity and clarity of purpose calculated to warm the cockles of your heart with confidence and pride.

You may rest assured that the officers and the members of the Council are moving forward with the principles, purposes and the mandates of your House of Delegates. Are you doing what you can through your County Society, through your social and business contacts and through the care of your patients to put the profession of your State on the lasting pedestal of scientific accomplishments and laudable ambitions? Without your loyal cooperation, the work of your officers and the Council will be in vain. Wake up and make your own work your "master word."

BURNS

In this issue of the Journal appears Cecil K. Drinker's significant, logical discussion of experimental studies of burns and the clinical application of the principles established through the same.

On account of the War and increasing civilian hazards, this subject demands serious consideration by every doctor who may be called upon to treat burns. During the past two or three years medical literature has been loaded with articles on this subject. These reports and discussions, while revealing what may be accepted as a gradual accumulation of valuable knowledge, the careful reader has been disturbed by the want of uniformity; the absence of a dependable consensus of opinion by which the average doctor may be guided in the treatment of burns.

It is to be hoped that the work of Drinker and his associates may lead to a crystalization of principles and methods for the guidance of the physician with the greatest possible benefit to the patient. Every doctor who receives the Journal should read the Drinker article and all who anticipate the treatment of burns should re-read it with unction.

CHEMOTHERAPY IN TUBERCULOSIS

Internists with a special interest in diseases of the chest are being besieged by inquiries about Diasone, Promin and Promizole in the treatment of tuberculosis. No doubt the general practitioner has to meet the same inquiries.

For the information of those who have not had occasion to follow the progress of experimental work in this field and the clinical trial of certain chemical agents in the human being, it should be known that during the past year the American Trudeau Society (Medical Section of the National Tuberculosis Association) has had an active Committee on Therapy for the purpose of evaluating all therapeutic claims and advances in the treatment of pulmonary conditions.

The following report was published in the American Review of Tuberculosis, April, 1944:

"The Committee on Therapy of the American Trudeau Society (Medical Section of the National Tuberculosis Association), in session March 17 and 18, 1944, at Chicago and Waukegan, Illinois, has reviewed information so far made available to it on the effects of Promin, Diasone, Promizole, Diaminodiphenylsulfone and some related drugs upon previous established experimental tuberculosis in guinea pigs. It has also reviewed the very limited amount of roentgenological and clinical data from one institution so far made available regarding patients treated with one of the drugs, viz. Diasone. On the basis of these data the following statement has been authorized:

"Promin, Diasone, Promizole and certain related compounds appear to possess in varying degree the striking ability to restrain the development of experimental tuberculosis in guinea pigs offers many contrasts with clinical tuberculosis in human beings, even though the causative organism is the same.

"It is the opinion of the Committee that the clinical and roentgenological data so far made available to the Committee on the action of Diasone in human tuberculosis is as yet inadequate both quantitatively and qualitatively to permit, even tentatively, a positive evaluation of its curative effects upon tuberculosis in humans. The Committee believes that there is, at this time, no adequate basis for the optimistic implications of the magazine articles or of the releases to the press which are now so well known to both the profession and public. It is believed, on the contrary, that such implications are distinctly unwarranted and not in accord with the clinical evidence which has been reviewed by the Committee. The Committee regrets exceedingly that the magazine articles mentioned previously were published in spite of efforts on the part of both the Committee and the clinician quoted to stop their publication.

"Until controlled studies of adequate scope have been reported it is recommended that none of these drugs be used for treating tuberculosis patients except under conditions which will appreciably add to our knowledge of their clinical action, and in the presence of adequate facilities to protect patients effectively from their potentially serious toxic effects. Patients and physicians must also be reminded of the provisions of the federal regulations which prohibit the distribution of a drug in the experimental phase of development to other than reserve institutions to which the material is assigned by the manufacturer for either laboratory or clinical investigation. The Committee is informed that other clinical investigations are now in progress, and it is the expressed opinion of the Committee that such further controlled clinical investigation is distinctly desirable.

"Any use of chemotherapeutic agents, including Diasone, in the treatment of tuberculosis patients must, therefore, be regarded as purely a project in clinical investigation. It must be again emphasized that such use is not without hazard and that the roentgenological and clinical evidence reviewed by the Committee gives no justification at this time for any attitude concerning the value of these drugs in patients other than one of critical interest."

At the Annual Meeting of the National Tuberculosis Association and the American Trudeau Society in Chicago in May, this Committee presented a similar report. More recent studies and reports do not warrant any alterations in the above report.

The unfortunate publicity in lay periodicals has caused many people who are suffering from tuberculosis, to be unduly optimistic and their hopeful inquiries have brought a lot of trouble upon conscientious physicians. If premature babies were as virile as premature lay publicity, we could throw away our incubators.

The following paragraph is from a letter written by the Chairman of this Committee on July 20, 1944, in response to the author's inquiry about a newspaper story on sulfabenamide.

"The situation is just as you probably anticipated; namely that the newspapers are several jumps ahead of the investigators, and actually there is no evidence whatever that sulfabenamide is of benefit in pulmonary tuberculosis, nor has Doctor Gubner made any such claims directly or indirectly."

The following lines entitled "Fake Cures", written by a patient 28 years ago, serves as an example of what has been going on for many generations and expressive of the yearning for health and life always in the victim's heart. Let us hope for a genuine cure while we protect our patients from premature and false claims.

FAKE CURES

Some T. B.'s thought they had a cure
In Eckman's Alterative,—
   But they died.
Some others tried Tuberclecide
And thought it superlative,—
   And they died.

Some more poor dupes pinned all their faith
To the dope called Lung Germine,
Another bunch spent all their cash
For Virgin Oil of Pine,—
   Then they died.

Whittington's Specific is another fake cure name.
Oxomulsion is another and their results are just the same,—
   The suckers died.

Alpha Institute will cure (?) if you have the cash to pay,
The treatment is successful but the patients pass away,—
   They all died.

Miller's International is one that's somewhat new,
Lost forty-eight poor lungers of a possible sixty-two,—
   They just died.

Aicsol's another, made by a man named Lloyd,
And Nature's Creation is one more you must avoid,—
   Or you'll die.

There's a man in Jackson, Mich., by the name of Lawrence Hill,
Who'll guarantee to cure you if you will foot the bill,—
   And then die.

There's Wilson's cure and Roger's cure, Pulmonol and Sanosin,
Hydrocine and Oleozone and one called Sartolin,
All guaranteed to cure you 'till you're broke and near all in,—
   Then you die.

If you think you have consumption, don't waste time on a quack,
For he'll take all your money and you'll get nothing back.
Just go to some good doctor, and if he says you're right,
Follow his instructions and make a good stiff fight.—
   And you'll live.
    —E. E. Dunnigan, The Barlow Sanatorium, June 1, 1916.

What is Medical History?

This is the title of the third article in Sudhoff's "Skizzen" in the perusal of which the sincerely interested physician and surgeon will discover that he has entered a domain of science in which he may have thought he was hitherto quite well versed, to suddenly discover that he is passing through new territory with every step and has really not fully grasped what is meant under the term—medical history. It is not simply a record of medical events nor of the actions of eminent Ascelepiads nor of the discoveries of research workers. It is not a history of the revelation of other sciences bearing upon medicine. It is not a chronologic arrangement of years or dates in which important medical ideas originated or discoveries were made, it is not a record of various doctrines that were taught or of the different conceptions of anatomic, pathologic, physiologic, clinical, therapeutic and surgical endeavors that were conceived and executed. All these things, important though they are, constitute nothing but the material of Medical Historiography. As the surgeon would term it, it is the instrumentarium. What then is Medical History? It is the evolution and elucidation of the historic cultural and scientific developments, medical ideas, events, doctrines, etc., with regard to their inner connections. Medical history aims at a real understanding of the periods, their physicians and their manner of healing.—Master Minds in Medicine. John C. Hemmeter. Pages 14-15. New York Medical Life Press. 1927.

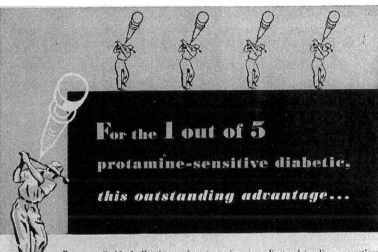

For the 1 out of 5 protamine-sensitive diabetic, this outstanding advantage...

Recent studies[1,2] of allergic reactions to various ingredients of insulin preparations demonstrate that approximately one out of five patients experiences skin reactions after intradermal injection of protamine. In the same study only two out of 81 diabetic patients exhibited sensitivity following the intradermal injection of globin.

Bauman,[1,3] and Duncan,[4] as well as others, have reported that patients who suffered from severe skin reactions following the use of protamine zinc insulin obtained immediate relief upon changing to globin insulin with zinc.

WITH 'WELLCOME' GLOBIN INSULIN WITH ZINC, these other advantages:

A single injection daily of 'Wellcome' Globin Insulin with Zinc will control many moderately severe and severe cases of diabetes, helping to reconcile patients who resent more frequent injections. Timed to achieve morning onset of action and then maximum effectiveness during the afternoon, 'Wellcome' Globin Insulin with Zinc provides control during peak eating and working hours. Diminishing action after 16 hours allays the dread of "night shock".

'Wellcome' Globin Insulin with Zinc, a new advance in insulin therapy, is a clear solution permitting a more uniform dosage. It was developed in the Wellcome Research Laboratories, Tuckahoe, New York. U. S. Pat. No. 2,161,198. Available in vials of 10 cc., 80 units in 1 cc.   'Wellcome' Trademark Reg.

(1) Page, R. C., and Bauman, L.: J.A.M.A. 124:704 (March 11) 1944. • (2) Bauman, L.: Bull. N. E. Med. Cen. V:17-21 (Feb.) 1943. • (3) Bauman, L.: Am. J. Med. Sc. 198:475 (Oct.) 1939, Ibid. 200:299, 1940. • (4) Duncan, G. G., Diseases of Metabolism, Phila., Saunders Co., 1942, p. 782.

'WELLCOME' GLOBIN INSULIN WITH ZINC

Literature on request

BURROUGHS WELLCOME & CO. (U.S.A.) INC. 9-11 E. 41st St., New York 17

ASSOCIATION ACTIVITIES

PREPAID MEDICAL AND SURGICAL PLAN GOES TO MEMBERS

The Prepaid Medical and Surgical Planning Committee met on July 9 preceding the Council Meeting. Most of the members were in attendance. It was decided to mail a revised plan to all members of the Association including those in the Armed Forces. A post card was to be included with the plan, for approval, disapproval or suggestions and criticisms.

The plans were carried out and approximately 300 replies have been received, a great majority of which are favorable to the Plan. Members inquired as to the inclusion of medical cases. The Committee has found that, in States where all services are included, the plans have not been successful and that it is best to start with those types of services which are mentioned in the printed plan and gradually extend the plan to include other types of services.

IT IS URGED THAT ALL MEMBERS RETURN THE POSTCARD IMMEDIATELY in order that the Committee will have the benefit of all suggestions before any final action is recommended to the Council and the House of Delegates.

ADVISORY COMMITTEE TO VOCATIONAL REHABILITATION DIVISION NAMED BY DR. ROUNTREE

As per action of the Council, Dr. C. R. Rountree, President, appointed the following Advisory Committee to the State Vocational Rehabilitation Division. In addition to these appointments there will be a dental representative appointed.

Clinton Gallaher, Shawnee, Chairman; Bert F. Keltz, Oklahoma City; James O. Asher, Clinton; Ennis M. Gullatt, Ada; and Harry D. Murdock, Tulsa. Mr. Bert Loy, Superintendent of Oklahoma City General Hospital was appointed on recommendation of the Oklahoma Hospital Association.

NEW STEPHENSON-TRAVERSE CLINIC OPENS IN ALVA

On Monday, June 19, patients were being received in the new Stephenson-Traverse Clinic in Alva. Dr. C. A. Traverse and Dr. I. F. Stephenson of Alva are to be complimented on this new addition to the medical facilities of the city.

Completely modern throughout, the tile brick building houses, besides the doctors' consultation and treatment rooms, an X-ray room, a laboratory, utility room, recovery rooms and a surgery room for minor operations. All rooms open off corridors and are heated and cooled by a single air-conditioning unit. A large, quietly-decorated reception room is at the front entrance of the building.

SPECIAL COURSE IN OTOLARYNGOLOGY ANNOUNCED

The University of Illinois College of Medicine announces that its fall didactic and clinical refresher course for specialists in otolaryngology will be held at the College from September 25 to 30 inclusive. The fee for the course is $50.00. Since registration is limited to twenty-five, applications should be filed as early as possible. Write for information to Department of Otolaryngology, University of Illinois College of Medicine, 1853 West Polk Street, Chicago 12, Ill.

CONGRESSMAN PAUL STEWART CONFERS AT EXECUTIVE OFFICE

Congressman Paul Stewart called at the Executive Office of the State Association on Tuesday, July 25, in regard to the legislation pending in Congress relative to the deferment of pre-medical students.

The War and Navy Departments and the Selective Service Board has issued regulations against the deferment of such students and the American Medical Association had their ruling appealed to the President who concurred. The officials of the A.M.A., the Oklahoma State Medical Association and Dean Tom Lowry of the Medical School have protested this ruling and have urged the Congressmen to support a bill which has been introduced in Congress providing for such deferment.

If pre-medical students are not deferred there will be a great shortage of doctors for both the Armed Forces and civilian needs by the year 1949. It is hoped that the doctors of the State will urge their Congressmen and Senators to support H.R. 5128, the details of which will be found in the Medicine at War page of this issue of the Journal.

REMODELING OF EXECTIVE OFFICES NEARING COMPLETION

The remodeling of the Council Room and Library of the Executive Offices in Oklahoma City is expected to be finished by the time this Journal reaches you. All members of the Association are invited to visit the offices when they are in Oklahoma City.

PAUL H. FESLER VISITS COUNTY SECRETARIES AND COUNCILORS

Mr. Paul H. Fesler, Executive Secretary of the State Association, has recently visited the Secretaries and Councilors in Choctaw, Bryan, Atoka, Pittsburg and Muskogee Counties.

Mr. Fesler has also surveyed the hospital facilities in McAlester and Muskogee in order to ascertain whether or not these hospitals could be utilized in connection with the training of men returning from the War. About one-half of the Oklahoma doctors in the service have indicated a desire for either internship, residency or postgraduate courses after the War.

MEETINGS OF COMMITTEES URGED

The Cancer, Prepaid Medical Plan, Public Policy and Public Health Committees have met since the Annual Meeting. It is hoped that all of the Committees will have meetings before the usual time of the Fall meetings of the local Medical Societies. The Societies will be kept informed so that these Committees may cooperate in matters affecting the entire Association.

NEW REQUIREMENTS OF AMERICAN BOARD OF OBSTETRICS AND GYNECOLOGY, INC.

A number of changes in Board regulations and requirements were put into effect at the Board's last annual meeting. These were designed to aid civilians as well as candidates in the Service. Among these is the waiver, temporarily, of the AMA requirement for men in the Army or Navy, especially for those who proceeded directly or almost so from hospital services into Army or Navy Service, upon a statement of intention to join promptly upon return to civilian practice. At this meeting the Board decided also to accept a period of

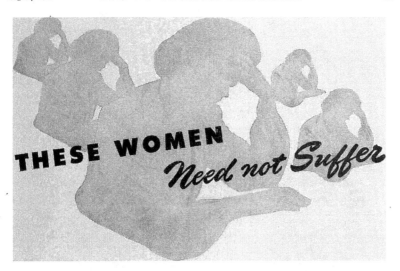
FOR SOME WOMEN the climacteric is practically uneventful except for the cessation of menstrual function. To others the cessation of ovarian activity becomes a crisis to themselves and their families.

One of the valued contributions of endocrinology was the discovery and isolation of potent estrogens and their usefulness in alleviating the distressing symptoms of the menopause.

Within the last five years the natural estrogens have decreased in cost while orally administered diethylstilbestrol costing only one or two cents a day has brought estrogenic therapy within the reach of every woman.

The Squibb Laboratories supply the *natural* estrogens Amniotin, in a variety of dosage forms for use orally, intravaginally or by hypodermic injection. The present price of Amniotin in Oil in capsules is the lowest in history; for injection, Amniotin in Oil in the vial packages makes the cost per dose relatively inexpensive and enables the physician to vary the dosage to fit the patient's requirements.

Diethylstilbestrol Squibb is available in a like variety of dosage forms except that for oral administration it is supplied in tablets rather than capsules. Reports in the literature indicate that, where excessive dosage is avoided, many patients acquire a tolerance to the drug and are able to take it without discomfort.

nine months as an academic year in satisfying our requirement for certain years of training. This is only for the duration and even men who are not eligible for military service but who are nevertheless in hospitals where the accelerated program is in effect have been allowed to submit to us this short-time period of training in lieu of our previous requirements.

Beginning with the next written examination, which is scheduled to be held the first Saturday afternoon in February, 1945, this Board will limit the written examination to a maximum period of three hours and in submitting case records at this time, all obstetrical reports which do not include measurements either by calipers and, as indicated, by acceptable x-ray pelvimetry, will be considered incomplete.

Prospective applicants or candidates in military service are urged to obtain from the Office of the Secretary a copy of the ''Record of Professional Assignments for Prospective Applicants for Certification by Specialty Boards'' which will be supplied upon request. This record was compiled by the Advisory Board for Medical Specialties and is approved by the Offices of the Surgeon-General, having been recommended to the Services in a circular letter, No. 76, from the War Department Army Service Record. These will enable prospective applicants and candidates to keep an accurate record of work done while in military service and should be submitted with the candidate's application, so that the Credentials Committee may have this information available in reviewing the application.

Applications and Bulletins of detailed information regarding the Board requirements will be sent upon request to the Secretary's Office, 1015 Highland Building, Pittsburg 6, Pennsylvania. Applications must be in the Office of the Secretary by November 15, 1944, ninety days in advance of the examination date. The time and place of the Spring 1945 (Part II) examination will be announced later.

Paul Titus, M.D., Secretary

W. T. Salmon, M.D.
1868-1944

Dr. William T. Salmon, Duncan, died on June 26 at his home. He had been in poor health for some time but had been seriously ill for only three weeks.

Dr. Salmon was born in Lynchburg, Tennessee. He graduated from the University of Tennessee and practiced in Cowan, Tennessee and Sherman, Texas before moving to Oklahoma City in 1898. After taking special work in New York in 1897, he confined his practice to eye, ear, nose and throat. In 1927 the family moved to Duncan where Dr. Salmon practiced until shortly before his death.

Dr. Salmon was past president of the Stephens County Medical Society and was active in medical legislation in Oklahoma during the early days of statehood.

Surviving are his wife, Mrs. W. T. Salmon, Duncan; a daughters, Miss Sue Salmon, Los Angeles; and two sisters, both of Nashville, Tennessee.

John R. Pollock, M.D.
1883-1944

Dr. John R. Pollock, Ardmore, died June 28 as a result of shock induced by the tragic drowning of his young granddaughter on June 27. Dr. Pollock was in ill health and was unable to sustain the impact of the tragedy of the child who fell into a lily pond at the Pollock residence.

Dr. Pollock graduated from the Chicago College of Medicine and Surgery in 1909 and shortly thereafter began practice in Ardmore where he carried on his profession many years. In the last few years he was handicapped by ill health. Dr. Pollock was a pioneer member of the Ardmore Rotary Club and was active in Boy Scout

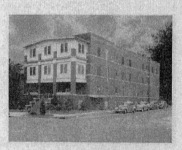
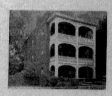

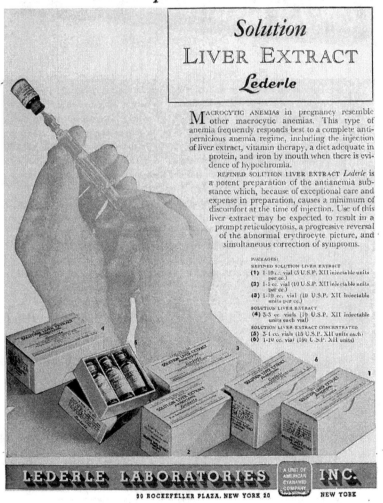

Why PENICILLIN-C.S.C.

Penicillin-C.S.C.—available as penicillin calcium as well as penicillin sodium—is packaged only in rubber-stoppered serum-type vials containing 100,000 Oxford Units. The vials are used in preference to sealed ampuls because they make for greater convenience in storing the solution and because they lessen the danger of contamination after the solution is made.

Only vials of 100,000 units are offered at present because experience designates them as the most advantageous size. If there IS a factor in therapy which may undermine or lessen the remarkable therapeutic efficacy of penicillin, it may be underdosage. Even if therapy is instituted late in the course of the disease, penicillin in many instances will prove effective if adequately high dosage is used for the proper length of time.

In the conditions so far explored and reported, effective dosage in some instances will be less than 100,000 units per day; in many instances it may have to be several times this amount Hence in a large percentage cf cases the Penicillin-C.S.C. vial of 100,000 units will prove most advantageous.

The convenience of the vial will be readily appreciated. After removal of the tear-off portion of the aluminum seal, sterilize the exposed surface of the rubber stopper

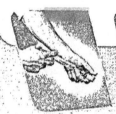
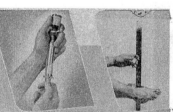

For the usual concentration (5000 Oxford Units per cc.) inject 20 cc. of physiologic salt solution into the vial in the usual aseptic procedure.

Invert the vial and syringe (with needle in vial), and withdraw the amount of penicillin solution required for the first injection.

Store vial with remainder of solution in refrigerator. Solution is ready for subsequent injections during the next 24 hours.

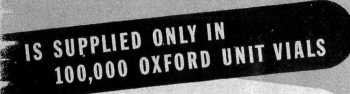
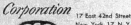

work. He was a member of the Carter County Medical Society, the Oklahoma State Medical Association and the American Medical Association.

Dr. Pollock is survived by his wife, Mrs. John R. Pollock and daughter Mrs. John Sullivan, both of Ardmore.

J. B. Gilbert. M.D.
1889-1944

Dr. J. B. Gilbert, Tulsa, died July 4 following a short illness. He had practiced medicine in Tulsa since 1909 when he moved there from Meridian, Mississippi. Dr. Gilbert became county physician in 1929 and served for a number of years in that office. He was a graduate of the University of Mississippi and Tulane University at New Orleans.

He was formerly on the staff of the Morningside Hospital and at the time of his death was on the staff at Hillcrest Memorial Hospital and the assistant staff of St. John's. He was a member of the American College of Surgeons, the State and County Medical Associations and the American Medical Association.

Surviving Dr. Gilbert are his wife, Mrs. Edna Gilbert; one son, Dr. J. B. Gilbert, Crippled Children's hospital in Oklahoma City; three sisters and three brothers.

Resolution

WHEREAS, Death has removed from our society its honorary member and most distinguished member in the person of Dr. G. P. Cherry of Mangum, and

WHEREAS, His personal and professional life was always an inspiration to the other members of the society, and

WHEREAS, His high conception of his professional duty to both his patients and to his fellow practitioners, was ever a source of pride to the members of this society, and

WHEREAS, Every member of the Greer County County Medical Society feels a personal loss in his going, but feel that his advice and council, his upright gentlemanly conduct and devotion to duty, has left us a heritage of which we can be proud to emulate.

THEREFORE BE IT RESOLVED, That this testimonial of love and high esteem of his colleagues of the Society be made a record in the minutes of the Society, and that copies of this resolution be given to his family, the local press and the Journal of the Oklahoma State Medical Association.

J. B. Hollis, M.D., Secretary
Greer County Medical Society

Classified Advertisements

News From The State Health Department

Dental Caries in Oklahoma

Selective Service data has revealed that dental condition of selectees from the Southwest is much better than the national average. This corroborates findings of public health studies made in the school populations of Oklahoma. One of these studies consisted in dental inspections of children in the 12-13 and 14 year age group, and was reported in "Public Health Bulletin" No. 226.

The dental caries attack rate was computed by combining these factors, namely: decayed permanent teeth; extracted (because of caries) permanent teeth; filled permanent teeth.

Some typical rates in Oklahoma per 100 children are as follows:

County	Caries Attack Rate
Comanche	199.2
Grady	152.3
Muskogee	258.3
Oklahoma	224.1
Tulsa	275.5

Contrasting these relatively low rates are some selected at random from the same bulletin. These rates are again for 100 children in the 12, 13, and 14 year age groups:

Town or County	Caries Attack Rate
Lake County, Indiana	513.5
Davenport, Iowa	657.5
South Portland, Maine	970.0
Queen Annes County, Maryland	649.0
Milwaukee, Wisconsin	917.0

These are significant differences which are not yet fully explained. Suggested explanations have been variations in climate, dietary habits, racial susceptibility, and water supplies.

The most promising of these possibilities for purposes of mass control is that of water. A definite correlation exists between dental caries rates and the type of water consumed. One of the first studies to establish this correlation was a dental survey made in the schools of Quincy and Galesburg, Illinois, some eight years ago In this study variables other than the community water supplies were, to all practical purposes, neutralized. The caries attack rate per 100 children in Galesburg was 201, whereas in Quincy the rate was 633. Similarly controlled surveys in other areas have had like results. Just what element or combination of elements in water has the inhibitory effect has not been determined. Fluorine seems to be one constant in water associated with low caries rates. However, fluorine bearing waters are usually heavily mineralized and the dental effect of these minerals should be considered. The pH of water is another factor which is deserving of close scrutiny.

Until the inhibitory factor in water is clearly established, control through this medium is obviously by pure chance, and whether water is exclusively responsible for low state-wide caries rates is also difficult of proof. However, the fact remains that dental caries, although a problem of major proportions here, does not have so heavy an impact on the child population as in many other sections of the country.

Oklahoma State Health Department

IMPORTANT

The following letter was received from the Federal Security Agency of the U. S. Public Health Service, Washington, D. C.

June 30, 1944

Dr. G. F. Mathews
State Health Commissioner
Oklahoma City, Oklahoma.
Dear Dr. Mathews:

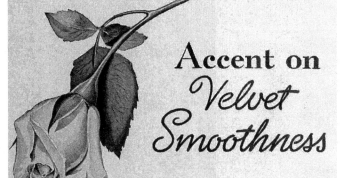

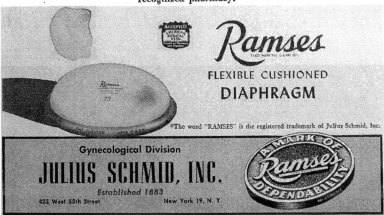

This is to advise that the program for the relocation of physicians and dentists under Public Law 216 which became operative December 23, 1943, has been terminated by Congress, effective June 30, 1944. It will therefore be impossible to arrange any further relocations under the benefits of this program.

For those communities in your state which have contributed their share of relocation expense and for which physicians or dentists have been contracted, the arrangement will be carried out according to the terms of the contract, from funds obligated for this purpose.

Those communities which have submitted their checks for $300.00 and for which it has been impossible as yet to locate a physician or dentist, will have their monies refunded promptly.

We deeply appreciate your cooperation and assistance in this program which, in the short time it has been in operation, has effected the relocation of a number of physicians and dentists in needy areas.

Sincerely yours,
(signed) L. H. THOMPSON
Assistant Surgeon General

SUMMER-TIME HEALTH

Summertime can be dangerous to the health, or it can be a time to store up extra vitality for winter, the Bureau of Publicity of the Indiana State Medical Association said in a recent bulletin.

"Food can be a dangerpoint for infection," the bulletin states. "Its source should be carefully watched. Grade A milk is a necessity. Vegetables should be fresh —preferably right from the garden—thoroughly washed, and kept cool. Bread, particularly whole wheat, should be kept in the refrigerator.

"Pies with cream fillings, cream puffs, eclairs, ham and hollandaise sauce are particularly susceptible to the staphylococcus germ which causes severe cases of food poisoning, and should be kept thoroughly chilled.

"Sunbathing should be taken in moderation, so should swimming. Swimmers should not go into the water right after meals or when completely exhausted. They should keep the nose free from water when it is submerged to avoid ear, nose and throat infections, and should not remain in the water too long, as thorough chilling of the body has the same effect in summer as in the winter.

"Flies and mosquitoes and other insects should be kept out of the house by strong screens, and quick exterminators are necessary. Breeding places of mosquitoes should be destroyed. Bird baths and pools should be drained and cleaned frequently. Water in which flowers stand in the house can be a breeding place too, and should be changed every day.

"Light, loose clothing without belts, tight armholes or tight sleeves lets the air reach the skin, allows ease of motion and makes one cooler," the bulletin continued. "Labor-saving devices are worth more in summer than at any other season. The wise housewife gets up early in the morning, uses her electric washer, her ironer, her vacum cleaner, her pressure cooker when the day is cool, finishes her work and is not pursued by chores all day long. She will do well to prepare her meals in the cool early morning hours too.

"Much heat will be kept out if houses are kept closed and darkened during the day. Fans should be placed on the floor to do the most good. Frequent showers, with cold water if you like, are recommended.

BOOK REVIEWS

TROPICAL NURSING. A. L. Gregg, M.A., M.D., M.Ch., B.A.O. (Dublin) D.T.M. & H. (London) L.M. (Rotunda Hospital). Member of Associate Staff of, and Lecturer to Nurses at the Hospital for Tropical Diseases, London, Lecturer on Tropical Diseases, Westminister Hospital Medical School. Philosophical Library, Inc., 15 E. 40th Street, New York, N. Y. 185 pages. 1944.

This text-book is the second edition of this timely topic. Timely, because tropical diseases are becoming increasingly important, due to the war which has taken our American soldiers and other personnel into the tropical areas, with the inevitable exposure to and acquisition of certain tropical diseases.

The book is divided into five sections—Personal Hygiene in the Tropics; Tropical diseases; Techniques; Care of the Eyes; and a Glossary.

Stress is given to the principal variants in relation to personal hygiene, such as the climate, the food, and the living conditions, because the body's adjustment to the climatic conditions depends upon adjusted habits of life. In the discussion of each disease the essential points on the causative agents, clinical condition, clinical course of the disease, complications, prophylaxis, medica and surgical treatment are emphasized. Each subject is given position and space in proportion to its relative importance, the malarias, dysenteries, and filiaries receive the most attention. Other diseases of an infectious nature which are discussed are: typhus, yellow, undulant, dengue, blackwater, relapsing, and sandfly fevers; the bubonic, pneumonic, and septicemia forms of plague; cholera, leprosy, yaws, bubo, rabies and sprue. Tropical skin infections and ulcers caused by mites or fungus. Two noncommunicable diseases, beri-beri and pellagra, are included. Space is given to heat exhaustion, sunstroke; snake, scorpion and spider bites.

The section on the care of the eyes is most interesting. Stress is placed on the protection of the eyes from glare, burns, and insects. The common eye diseases are: styes, conjunctivitis, corneal ulcers, glaucomia, and epidemic ophthalmia. A small amount of space is given to nursing technique which are quite in keeping with our present general and communicable disease nursing care. The same may be said of the medications and treatments prescribed.

The public health and sociological aspects of tropical diseases are not discussed. However, mention is made of the importance of screening, the use of mosquito netting, avoidance of uncooked foods, and the purification of water for drinking and bathing purposes.

This text-book should be in the library of every graduate nurse. It should be of special value to the nurses in government services who are now or expect to have a tour of duty in the tropics. They should be fortified with the information contained therein. The book is of small dimensions, measuring 7 x 5 x 1, which makes it ideal to pack in a nurse's kit for ready reference.—Golda B. Slief, A. B., R. N., Medical Social Service, Oklahoma County Health Association, Inc., Variety Club Health Center, Oklahoma City.

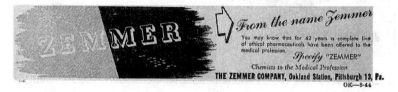

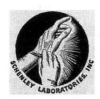

MEDICINE AT WAR

TIME NOW TO PROTEST AGAINST GOVERNMENT'S THREAT TO MEDICAL EDUCATION

Journal Says Present Policies of the Armed Forces and Selective Service Will Result in an Annual Deficit of 2,000 Doctors

Declaring that medical educators and the medical profession of the country refuse to accept the responsibility for the acute shortage of medical care which will threaten this country within a few years if current regulations and policies persist, The Journal of the A.M.A. for July 8 points out that the present situation will result in an annual and cumulative deficit of 2,000 physicians a year in face of new and increased demands for medical service. It advises the medical profession that now is the time to protest to the House and Senate Military Affairs Committees against this blind disregard for medical care in the future. The Journal says:

"In January 1944 it seemed that civilian and military needs for doctors would be met reasonably satisfactory by the arrangement in which the 55 per cent of entering medical school classes would be provided by the Army Specialized Training Program, 25 per cent by the Navy V-12 Program and 20 per cent from civilian sources. In the past six months this program has rapidly deteriorated. Today medical educators and the medical profession of the country refuse to accept the responsibilty for the acute shortage of medical care which will threaten this country within a few years if current regulations and policies persist. The responsibility must rest with the armed forces, the Selective Service System, the President and the Congress of the United States.

"In February the Army drastically curtailed the Army Specialized Training Program and has since renegotiated its contracts with medical schools to provide 28 per cent of the 1945 entering classes instead of 55 per cent, increasing to 47 per cent the numbers medical schools must obtain from civilian sources.

"In April the Selective Service System abolished all further occupational deferments of premedical and medical students not enrolled in medical schools by July 1, 1944. As a consequence, it was estimated that the entering classes of 1945 would be reduced 25 to 30 per cent.

"The threat to medical care entailed in these policies was pointed out to General Hershey, the Secretaries of War and the Navy, the President and others with the suggestions that the situation be met by (a) reinstitution of the inactive reserves by the Army and Navy, which functioned well for a year, and/or (b) an appropriate Selective Service adjustment, which was definitely a second best arrangement.

"The Army and Navy rejected the first alternative as an evasion of the Selective Service law, and the Selective Service System rejected the alternate proposal because of the acute need of the Army for young men. The needs for medical care were considered to be subordinate to the needs of the fighting forces.

"Alarmed at these developments, the House of Delegates of the American Medical Association, on 'the' recommendation of the Council on Medical Education and Hospitals of the American Medical Association, passed the following resolution at its opening session, June 12:

"WHEREAS, The present policy of the Army and the Selective Service System in preventing the enrollment of a sufficient number of qualified medical students will inevitably result in an overall shortage of qualified physicians, with imminent danger to the health and well being of our citizens; therefore be it

"RESOLVED, That it is imperative that immediate action be taken by the President or the Congress of the United States to correct the current drastic regulations, which result in a restriction of the number of students qualified to enter the courses of medical instruction in approved medical schools.

"This resolution was sent to the President, the Secretaries of War and the Navy, the Selective Service System and all members of the House and Senate Military Affairs committees.

"The latest measure still further jeopardizing medical education and medical care was the passage of the Army appropriation bill by Congress June 21. This bill includes the following provision:

"Provided that no appropriation contained in this Act shall be available for any expense incident to education of persons in medicine (including veterinary) or dentistry if any expense on account of this education in such subjects was not being defrayed out of appropriations for the military establishment for the fiscal year 1944 prior to June 7, 1944. . . .

"This provision would seem to eliminate from 1946 entering medical classes the 28 per cent of places contracted for by the Army. Even if the Navy increases its quota from 25 per cent to 31 per cent, schools will be obliged to obtain 69 per cent of their students from women and physically disqualified males. Nothing even approaching this number of qualified civilian students is available. Classes will probably be half filled in the country at large.

"Should an adjustment not be made to correct the present alarming situation, a tremendous reduction of graduates after the war will ensue. Although schools will continue the accelerated program, they will admit classes only once annually instead of every nine months. This of itself will reduce the number of graduates from the present annual average of 7,000 to 5,000. If classes can be only half filled, this number will be reduced to 2,500 graduates per year. Since 3,300 to 3,500 physicians die each year, there will result an annual and cumulative deficit of 2,000 doctors a year.

"Still further reductions in graduates and permanent damage to the 'plant' of medical education will result from some schools being forced to close their doors because of drastically curtailed enrollments. An unknown number of war casualties among medical officers will also reduce the supply of physicians.

"These reductions in medical graduates will occur in the face of new and increased demands for medical services, mainly from the civilian population, the standing army and navy, the Veterans Administration and the liberated countries of Europe.

"Full support should be forthcoming from the medical profession for the Miller bill (H.R. 5128), with modifications, which reads:

"Be it enacted by the Senate and House of Representatives of the United States of America in Congress assembled, That section 5 of the Selective Training and Service Act of 1940, as amended by inserting at the end thereof a new subsection reading as follows:

" '(n) There shall be deferred from training and service under this Act in the land and naval forces of the United States, as necessary to the maintenance of the national health, safety, and interest, in each calendar year not less than six thousand medical students and not less than four thousand dental students. As used in this subsection the term 'medical or dental student' means (1) a person who is enrolled in, and who is pursuing a course of instruction prescribed for the degree of doctor of medicine at an accredited medical col-

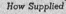

logs; and a person who is enrolled in, and who is pursuing a course of instruction prescribed for the degree of doctor of dentistry at an accredited dental college; or (2) a person who is pursuing a regular course of instruction at an accredited college or university (satisfactory completion of which will make such person eligible for enrolment in an accredited medical or dental college) with the bona fide intention of entering an accredited medical or dental college and pursuing and completing the course of instruction prescribed for the degree of doctor of medicine or for the degree of doctor of dentistry.''

''Protests against the blind disregard for medical care in the future should be addressed to the Senate (Senator Robert R. Reynolds, Chairman) and House (Representative Andrey J. May, Chairman) Committees on Military Affairs, the Senate Committee on Education and Labor (Senator Elbert D. Thomas, Chairman) and the House Committee on Education (Representative Graham A. Barden, Chairman). Every state medical society, medical school and scientific society should express itself in no uncertain terms on these developments.

The Forum

Notice to First Aid Workers and Others in the Immediate Handling of Burned Patients

It is high time that a warning is sounded against indiscriminate removal of burned clothing from a burned patient until he is removed to a hospital or to an environment where he can be attended under aseptic precautions. The clothing must not be removed if we are to accept and practice the teachings of authorities, such as the Surgeon General's Staff; that all burned areas must be considered and treated as an open wound. When some well-meaning layman tears or cuts off the burned clothing and exposes the area to contamination, it may mean the sacrifice of the victim's life. To smear on a lot of contaminated greases and oils only adds to the danger.

Do not remove any clothing. If any burned areas are exposed, cover with dry gauze if available. If not available use clean sheets or towels over the burned areas. Whether the face is burned or not the burned person should be masked during transportation and during aseptic care of the burn. As soon as the fire of the clothing is out, place the victim on a clean sheet, if available without disturbing any garment, wrap the sheet about him and if necessary in inclement weather, use blankets on top of the sheets. When he arrives at the hospital he is treated for shock. As soon as this is sufficiently controlled, he is removed to an operating room. The attendants are gowned, masked and gloved and under sterile precautions all burned clothing is then removed. The burned areas should then be very gently cleansed with sterile mild soap and water using every precaution as in any surgical operation.

It is not the object of this article to give details. This is written as an appeal to First Aid Workers in Industry, Red Cross Members and other laymen against the improper handling of the victims before they are seen by a surgeon. Do not destroy what may be the victim's only chance for recovery.

—A. Ray Wiley, M.D.

It is true that Society itself is an effect, but the great personality can neither produce nor prevent this effect. It can only modify it and give direction to it after it has been brought into existence. It is perfectly hopeless to contrast Society and the great individual as antagonistic agents. In fact this way of looking upon their mutual relations has already produced a great deal of harm. They mutually interact with and interpenetrate each other and each is incomplete without the other.— Master Minds in Medicine. John C. Hemmeter. Page vii. New York Medical Life Press. 1927.

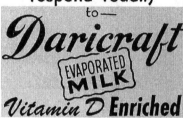
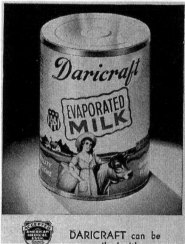

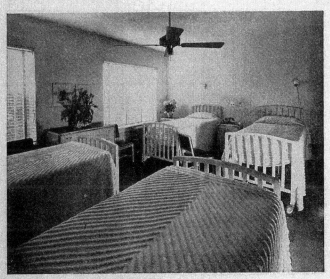

Medical School Notes

Dr. L. Everard Napier, Director of the Calcutta (India) School of Tropical Medicine, under the John and Mary R. Markle Foundation to the National Research Council, recently visited the School of Medicine. On July 7 Dr. Napier gave a general lecture on "The Tropical Diseases of India" and on July 8 he lectured on "Plague."

Other lectures will be delivered from time to time under the auspices of the National Research Council in co-operation with the Department of Preventive Medicine and Public Health. Announcement of such lectures will be made well in advance and a cordial invitation is extended to all those interested particularly to the Visiting and House Staff of hospitals.

Miss Elizabeth Hall, Instructor in Bacteriology, has resigned her position effective July 1 to do graduate work at the University of Washington, Seattle.

Dr. G. N. Barry, Medical Director of the hospitals, attended a postgraduate course in Cardiology in Boston during the month of July.

Seventy-two candidates took the Basic Science Examinations held at the Medical School on July 3. It is understood that the results will be available in August.

The Oklahoma State Dental Board also held its examinations at the school the latter part of June.

Dr. Charles Allen Winter has recently joined the Faculty of the School of Medicine as Assistant Professor of Physiology. Dr. Winter received the A. B. degree from Southwestern College, Winfield, Kansas, in 1926, attended the Johns Hopkins University, and was granted the Ph .D. Degree from the University of Buffalo in 1935. Prior to his coming to Oklahoma, Dr. Winter was on the Faculty of the University of Iowa. He is a member of the American Association of University Professors, the American Association for the Advancement of Science, the Society for Experimental Biology and Medicine, the American Physiological Society, and Sigma XI.

Dr. Noble F. Wynn, Instructor in Pharmacology, has recently resigned his position with the medical school to enter the United States Navy.

The Kiwanis Club was recently entertained with an Open House at the Crippled Children's Hospital. Mr. Jim Griffin, Secretary of the Club, presented to the School for Crippled Children a beautiful twelve volume set of Encyclopedia Britannica Junior. This set of books is a decided addition to the School Library and is a source of information and joy to the young patients confined to the hospital.

The following Residents of the University and Crippled Children's Hospitals have completed their contracts with these institutions:

Dr. J. D. Ashley, Jr., Resident in Medicine; Dr. Willard C. McClure, Resident in Eye, Ear, Nose and Throat, and Dr. John B. Jarrott, Resident in Ortho-

pedics, all of whom have entered the United States Army and have reported to Carlisle Barracks, Pennsylvania. Dr. Paul B. Rice, Resident in Surgery, is now doing private practive in Corpus Christi. Dr. J. Paul Shively, Resident in Obstetrics and Gynecology, is now connected with the Chicago Lying-In Hospital.

Two interns have reported for duty from the University of Texas School of Medicine, namely; Dr. Robert Lee Mathis and Dr. Henry K. May.

Dr. John F. Hackler, Professor of Preventive Medicine and Public Health, returned July 1 from New York where, for a period of eight weeks, he participated in the teaching at the De Lamar Institute, Columbia University College of Physicians and Surgeons and observed the teaching of courses at the medical schools of Cornell, New York University and Long Island College.

Dr. Hackler's visit was made possible through a grant from the Commonwealth Fund which, with the State Health Department, has assisted the Oklahoma State Medical Association in a rather extensive program of post-graduate medical education.

The Library has now added the following journals to its subscription list: American Review of Soviet Medicine; Annals of Allergy; Digest of Treatment; Industrial Medicine; Journal of Neurosurgery; Quarterly Review of Medicine.

New books from the summer book order are being received. The following are available at the present time: Association for Research in Nervous and Mental Disease—Pain, 1943: Modern Management of Colitis— Bargen, 1943: Human Constitution in Clinical Medicine —Draper, Dupertuis and Caughey, 1944: Medical Radiographic Technic—General Electric X-Ray Corporation, 1943: Office Endocrinology—Greenblatt, 1944: Facts for Childless Couples — Hamblin, 1942: Pathology and Therapy of Rheumatic Fever—Lichtwitz, 1944: Geriatric Medicine—Stieglitz, 1943: Fractures and Joint Injuries, Third Edition—Watson, Jones, 1943: Clinical Lectures on the Gallbladder and Bile Ducts—Weiss, 1944.

Miss J. Marie Melgaard, Director, Dietary Department of the University Hospital, has been selected as one of three candidates representing the hospital field for the Nominating Committee of the American Dietic Association for 1944-1945.

"Care and Food Service Equipment" has been published by the Burgess Publishing Company, Minneapolis, and reviewed in The Journal of the American Dietetic Association, Vol. 20, No. 7, Page 472, July-August, 1944. This paper was prepared by a Committee of the Administration Section of the American Dietetic Association of which Miss Melgaard is Chairman. The review states, "As to the form in which it is presented, it is outstanding as an example of organization and condensation which might well be emulated by others attempting to present similar material for publication."

According to Miss Melgaard, three student dietitians were admitted to the University Hospitals for a year of training beginning July 1, namely; Frances Gentile of Mount Mary College; Marjory McCollom of Kansas State College; and Elizabeth Wall of the Louisiana State University.

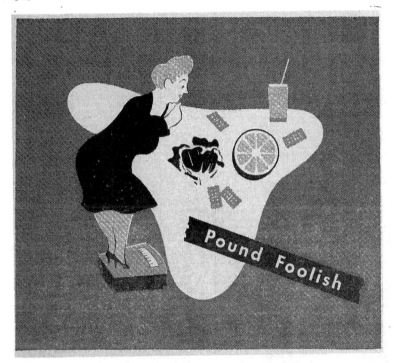

In treating those who recklessly "eat on" extra pounds, the physician may recommend a low calory diet which fails to achieve vitamin balance and thus afflicts the patient with a more serious condition than obesity. While chastening these patients on grapefruit and lettuce, the doctor can supplement their daily diet with one of Upjohn's small, easy-to-take vitamin preparations and provide an indispensable minimum of protective vitamins without the material addition of calories. Upjohn's penny-wise vitamins, small in size, high in potency, ensure safe reducing diets for the pound-foolish.

UPJOHN VITAMINS

DO MORE THAN BEFORE— KEEP ON BUYING WAR BONDS

★ FIGHTIN' TALK ★

The following have been called to active duty: LT. (jg) NOBLE FRANKLIN WYNN, Oklahoma City; LT. JOHN 'HOWARD BAKER, JR., Eufaula; LT. CHARLES S. NEER, Vinita; LT. JAMES GARTRELLE PHILLIPS, Oklahoma City.

The following have been promoted recently from lieutenant to captain: RICHARD HUFFMAN GRAHAM, Oklahoma City; CHESTER RANDALL SEBA, Oklahoma City; JOHN ENGENE HIGHLAND, Oklahoma City; CLAUDE WILLIAMS, Anadarko; John GEORGE MATT, Tulsa: From captain to major; E. B. LEY, Perry.

As will be noted in the above list of promotions, the Executive Secretary (on leave of absence) of the Oklahoma State Medical Association, DICK GRAHAM, is now a Captain. Dick is stationed in Washington at the Surgeon General's office.

The office recently received a picture of the young heir of the Graham's and it was the unanimous opinion that he is 'quite a boy.' Mrs. Graham and Richard, Jr., are with Dick in Washington.

The Evacuation Hospital in Italy, to which CAPTAIN WILLIAM R. TURNBOW, Tulsa, is attached, has been commended for its heroic work on the Anzio beachhead by General Mark Clark. Captain Turnbow is an anesthetist on the staff of the hospital, which was under daily artillery fire for over ten weeks at Anzio. The Hospital was activated at Fort Sam Houston, Texas in April, 1942 and went overseas a year later. It was stationed at Bizerte before going to Italy.

Oklahoma Doctor Awarded D. S. C.

CAPTAIN DONOVAN TOOL, Edmond, with the Fifth Army at Salerno, has been awarded the Distinquished Service Cross with the following citation:

"Charles D. Tool, Captain, Medical Corps, United States Army. For extraordinary heroism in action, on March 18, 1944, in the vicinity of Cassino, Italy. An urgent call for aid was received from a battery that was suffering many casualties during a heavy enemy counter-battery barrage. Captain Tool drove his ambulance into a position in the midst of the shelling in order to attend to the wounded. After treating some of the more seriously wounded who had been moved to a stone culvert for protection, he made his way through flying shell fragments to care for men in a gun pit where many hits were being sustained. Finding a survivor who was seriously wounded, he immediately set to work to save him, oblivious to the crash of incoming rounds. Fragments from a shell bursting nearby struck Captain Tool and pierced his spine. Captain Tool calmly continued working to save the wounded men and only when certain that all casualties had received treatment did he allow his own wound to be dressed. By his courageous performance under fire, Captain Tool saved the lives of eleven men. His fearless calm gave comfort to the wounded and contributed to the high morale of the troops under fire. Entered military service from Edmond, Oklahoma."

(Signed) Mark W. Clark
Lt. General, U. S. Army
Commanding.

Captain Tool was born in Edmond, Oklahoma and received his pre-medic work at East Central. After graduation from the University of Oklahoma School of Medicine and his internship, he returned, in 1932, to Edmond to take up his practice. At the time he enlisted, in 1942, he was serving on the staff of the University of Oklahoma School of Medicine.

After training at Carlisle Barracks, he was sent to Africa in February, 1943. He was placed in a division of one of the first troops to set foot on European soil at Salerno.

Captain Tool is now at Bushnell General Hospital in Birgham City, Utah, where he was flown from Charleston, S. C. after his ship docked there. He will be in the United States for at least a year to recover from the wounds he received at the battle front.

LT. STANLEY DRENNAN, Oklahoma City, has just returned from two years service in the South Pacific. Lt. Drennan's wife, Lt. Aloha Drennan, an army nurse, left for duty in the South Pacific just eight days after Lt. Drennan's arrival in the States.

Lt. Drennan has not fully recovered from a siege of malaria and is now stationed in Memphis, Tennessee, after spending some time with his parents in Oklahoma City.

He was based on several islands during his overseas service and the LST of which he was "both junior and senior medical officer" made 26 beachhead landings on Jap-held islands.

During one of the trips, Lt. Drennan was informed that a private, who had walked twelve miles through the jungle in severe pain, was having an acute attack of appendicitis. Having no adequate equipment at hand, Lt. Drennan, using a table in the washroom, operated. He states that bent spoons were used to hold back the muscle tissue. "I knew instantly that what I had been so long in life preparing for was now at hand," said Lt. Drennan.

CAPTAIN WELDON A. MURPHY, Mangum, has returned to the States after seven months in India. While in India, after a crash landing, Captain Murphy became lost from his command and spent 11 days dodging Japs in the jungles, living on weeds and herbs.

CAPTAIN L. C. McGEE, Newkirk, has recently been transferred from Chungking, China, to another point in China.

Lawton Physician Missing in Action

CAPTAIN WOODROW L. PICKHARDT, Lawton, paratrooper medical officer, has been reported missing in action in France since June 7. No further word has been received from the War Department.

Captain Pickhardt, raised in Seminole, attended the University of Oklahoma School of Medicine, graduating in 1917. He then served a two year internship at the University Hospital and one year at Lying-In Hospital in Chicago. He had served two years as director of the Creek County Health Department when he entered the armed forces August 11, 1942. In September 1942, he was transferred from San Antonio, Texas to Fort Sill. In January, 1943, he was sent to Ann Arbor, Michigan, for a special school, then in April was ordered to Trinidad in the Caribbean Area. Captain Pickhardt returned in November and volunteered for paratroop service, being sent to Fort Benning. He received his wings there on January 7, 1944, and was sent to England.

COMDR. RAYMOND G. JACOBS, Enid, returned from the South Pacific in March and is now at Mayo Clinic, Rochester, taking a three month course in plastic surgery.

MAJOR HERVEY A. FOESTER, Oklahoma City, now serving in England, writes that he has been recently elected a Fellow of the Royal Society of Medicine. The Society, has, as its patron, H.M. the King, and is located at 1, Wimpole St., London, England.

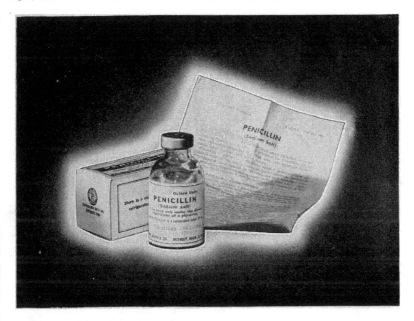

LT. COLONEL ONIS G. HAZEL, Oklahoma City, has recently been promoted from Major. Col. Hazel is Chief of Preventive Medicine and Consultant in Skin Diseases in the Office of the Surgeon, Headquarters Third Air Force, Tampa, Florida.

LT. WEBBER MERRELL, Oklahoma City, is reported critically ill in an English Hospital as a result of injuries received on D-Day.

While a resident of Guthrie, Lt. Merrell made his home with Lt. Col. and Mrs. Louis H. Ritzhaupt. He was graduated from the University of Oklahoma School of Medicine and interned at Wesley Hospital in Oklahoma City before he received his commission. He was stationed at Camp Gruber before going overseas in April of this year.

The following word has been received from CAPTAIN JOHN F. DALY, Pawhuska:

"After three and a half years duty with the medical service of the 45th Division, we'd reached the Anzio Beachhead in Italy. One morning I absorbed a load of scrap metal from a German bomb and since then I've been learning at first hand about the quality of army medical care. A month's stay in Naples and another in North Africa was followed by a splendid trip home on a hospital ship, landing in Charleston, S. C. I was soon transferred to the hospital at Framingham, Mass., where I'm awaiting various repairs."

MAJOR R. E. ROBERTS, Stillwater, recently reported that he had operated on his first German prisoner who was a 23-year old boy who had lived just outside of Berlin. Major Roberts states that the prisoner did more than his share of the groaning when shell fragments were removed from his chest. The shell fragments are being saved by Major Roberts to bring home to his two sons who live in Stillwater.

LT. COL. S. E. STRADER, Oklahoma City, is home for a rest after several months in the South Pacific. Col. Strader was called to duty in June, 1942, having served in France during the last war.

Col. Strader, in his statement to the Daily Oklahoman, lauded the performance of the American troops, the C-47 cargo ships and the Mitchell B-25 bomber. Following are excerps of his statement.

"It was surprising how quickly the Americans became expert jungle fighters, meeting the Japs on their own terms. Fighting in New Guinea isn't anything like trench or moble warfare. You are sniped at continually. You can't see your enemy. It's rough and tumble fighting, with knives, bayonets and whatever you've got in your hand, or even your bare hands if you're caught off guard.

"The average temperature, day and night, is 93 degrees, and the humidity is awful. But in spite of that heat, there are snow covered mountains there. I almost froze flying over them once.

"We couldn't have gotten anywhere without the C-47. And those kids who are flying them are doing a grand job moving our supplies in and out. Those pilots don't give a hoot, they just get in there and fly 'em, rain or shine.

"Those ships (B-25) get shot to pieces, but believe me they are tops. I recall one job they did that played havoc with a Jap air base. There were four strips for the takeoffs and landings. Our Liberators went in with P-38 escort and took out two of the strips. That done, the bombers and fighters high-tailed for home, leaving the Japs free to use the other strips and take off in pursuit. And they did that. Off in the haze, however, our Mitchells were waiting, and when those 95 Jap Zeros came back from the chase, they got the surprise of their lives. After all the Zeros had landed the Mitchells sailed over and not only knocked out the remaining strips, but blew all the Zeros to kingdom come. It was a great show."

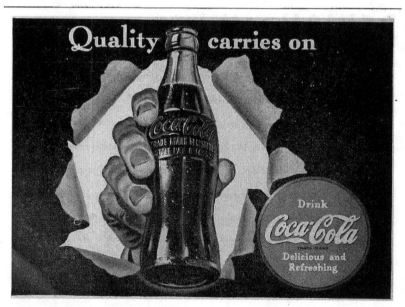

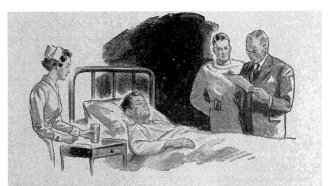

Proteins...Vitamins...Minerals

AS SOON AS LIQUIDS ARE RETAINED

The insult of anesthesia, tissue manipulation, unavoidable trauma, and enforced starvation sharply raise the nutritional requirements of the postoperative patient. Hence feeding must be started as early as possible to prevent too great a nutritional imbalance. Also, recovery is hastened and strength is gained more quickly when postoperative metabolic needs are supplied adequately.

Usually tolerated as early as liquids are retained, Ovaltine as a beverage provides a simple yet highly effective means of improving the nutritional state of the postsurgical patient. Its essential nutrients, well balanced and generously supplied, are in easily assimilated form. Thus the digestive burden is materially reduced. The delicious taste of this food drink proves appealing to all patients, young and old, making Ovaltine acceptable when many other foods are refused.

THE WANDER COMPANY, 360 North Michigan Avenue, Chicago 1, Illinois

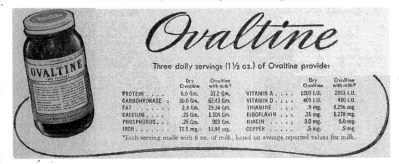

Ovaltine

Three daily servings (1½ oz.) of Ovaltine provide:

	Dry Ovaltine	Ovaltine with milk*		Dry Ovaltine	Ovaltine with milk*
PROTEIN	6.0 Gm.	31.2 Gm.	VITAMIN A	1500 I.U.	2953 I.U.
CARBOHYDRATE	30.0 Gm.	62.43 Gm.	VITAMIN D	405 I.U.	480 I.U.
FAT	2.8 Gm.	29.34 Gm.	THIAMINE	.9 mg.	1.296 mg.
CALCIUM	.25 Gm.	1.104 Gm.	RIBOFLAVIN	.25 mg.	1.278 mg.
PHOSPHORUS	.25 Gm.	.903 Gm.	NIACIN	3.0 mg.	5.0 mg.
IRON	10.5 mg.	11.94 mg.	COPPER	.5 mg.	.5 mg.

*Each serving made with 8 oz. of milk; based on average reported values for milk.

MEDICAL ABSTRACTS

"A NEW AID IN REMOVAL OF FOREIGN BODIES OF THE CORNEA." D. F. Gillette. Archives of Ophthalmology. Vol . 31, pages 129-133. February, 1944.

The author describes a new method of removal of foreign bodies from the superficial epithelium of the cornea. It is applicable to all foreign particles but especially to foreign bodies with an iron content encountered in industry. Most ophthalmologists demand that the foreign body, burn and stain be carefully and completely removed as soon after the injury as possible. A minority, however, prefer to leave the stain of rusty iron particle, and at times even the foreign body and burn, to slough out rather than risk the added trauma of removal. This sloughing out requires a variable length of time and usually results in infection, with painful and disabling complications. The method described anticipates the localized softening of the epithelium and aids in the immediate, safe and complete removal of the foreign body, burn and stain.

A one per cent solution of silver nitrate is topically applied to the foreign body and the surrounding epithelium by a small thread of cotton spun on the sharpened end of a round wooden toothpick. The silver nitrate produces a reaction which is a faint gray swelling of the superficial epithelium. This swelling elevates the foreign body slightly above the level of the surrounding epithelium.

Experimental investigation of the author proved to be so successful that he applied the method to clinical cases with very good results. The patient was tilted back in a dressing chair, which supported his head in a firm position. The injured eye was carefully anesthetized, and then inspected with a binocular loupe. The slit lamp was used to locate the minute foreign particles that could not be satisfactorily seen without the loupe. The conjunctival sac was irrigated with 5 or 6 drops of a mild solution of mercury oxycyanate. The one per cent solution of silver nitrate was then applied to the foreign body. The reaction which developed in one minute was sufficient. Removal of the foreign body was then attempted with a sterile, pointed wooden applicator, tightly wound with cotton. The author also used the sharpened end of a round toothpick. This method aided the complete removal of the foreign body, burn and stain when the patient was treated soon after the injury. When, however, the stain did not come away readily, the point of the cystotome was used gently to lift it out. When the patient was seen later, the foreign body and burn were easily removed, but the stain, having further penetrated the tissues, was not always dislodged with the applicator.

In such cases the point of the cystotome was used carefully to free and lift out the stain. The use of the cystotome is better than that of the curet or of the dental burr. Injury to Bowman's membrane was avoided, and if this membrane was injured, the silver nitrate procedure was not used, for it allowed the solution to spread into the deep interspaces and produce unwanted stain.

Sulfathiazole ointment, 5 per cent, was immediately instilled after the removal of the foreign body and stain. When possible the eye was protected with a sterile eye patch, held in space with a Scotch tape. The patient was instructed to instill some of the ointment if the eye became uncomfortable. The use of sulfathiazole powder and ointment gave also good results in cases of corneal ulcers. The use of tincture of iodine for corneal ulcers was discounted by the author. Sulfathiazole was used also in cases with signs of infection, in combination with the use of hot compresses and instillation of a weal solution of mercury oxycyanate at regular intervals.—M. D. II., M.D.

"FRESH FRACTURES OF THE CARPAL SCAPHOID." Benjamin Obletz. Surg. Gyn. & Obst., LXXVIII. 83. January, 1944.

This report is based on a study of forty-five consecutive fractures of the carpal scaphoid in an infantry training camp. During the same period, only ten typical Colles's fractures occurred. This was explained by the fact that the jarring impact of injury did not hyperextend the wrist, because it was rightly fixed by the soldier's strong forearm muscles. This impact cracked the scaphoid bone at its mechanically weak point, the waist.

In an anatomical study, 13 per cent of the carpal scaphoids had no arterial foramina proximal to the waist. On the basis of the variations in blood supply, the forty-five fractured scaphoids were divided into two groups: Type I, fractures without interruption of blood supply to either fragment: Type II, fractures with interruptions of the blood supply to the proximal fragment. Thirty-seven cases fell into Type I and eight into Type II. This classification was made possible by serial roentgenograms taken three to four weeks apart. In Type II cases, the roentgenograms at the end of three or four weeks showed generalized decalcification in all of the bones except the proximal fragment of the fractured scaphoid. At sixteen to twenty weeks, the densities of the two fragments seemed to blend and the fracture line was obliterated. In the early weeks, the proximal fragment retained its normal calcium, because of a temporary avascularity, which should not be confused with aseptic necrosis, as the latter would appear in the roentgenogram as an irregular mottled density with partial collapse. The clinical importance of this differentiation is to maintain immobilization long enough to allow revascularization of the proximal fragment. In the Type I cases, eight and three-tenths weeks was the average time required for healing, as opposed to 19 weeks for Type I fractures.—E. D. M., M.D.

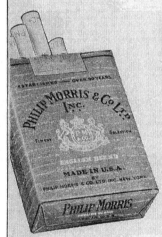

"THE RELATIONSHIP OF OPHTHALMOLOGY AND RHINOLOGY. V. E. Negus. The British Journal of Ophthalmology. Vol. 27, pages 554-557. December, 1943.

The two specialties have far too few opportunities for discussion and mutual criticism. There are, however, many interesting correlations. If a penetrating injury involves maxillary antrum or ethmoid, the removal of any loose fragments of bone, or foreign bodies is advised. Sulfonamide powder should be applied to such wounds. It must not be forgotten that there is close connection between the nasal sinuses and the cranial cavity; unnecesary interference may easily give rise to meningitis. Blood in sinuses is usually absorbed. Gross injuries to the antrum are best approached through the sublabial route.

The lacrimal gland rarely enters into the sphere of a rhinologist. The author noted cessation of lacrimation when the geniculate ganglion of the facial was affected by herpes. Sometimes it may be necessary to inject Meckl's ganglion in cases of excessive lacrimation. The habit of injecting the ganglion through the orbital fissure is a bad one. The route through the posterior palatine canal or sphenopalatine foramen is not as easy as through the pterygomaxillary fossa. No case should be submitted to injection unless the application of cocaine paste behind the posterior end of the middle turbinal has previously shown that lacrimation can be stopped by blocking the ganglion.

The lacrimal sac should not be forgotten when operating on frontal or ethmoidal sinuses through the external route. The usual incision does not involve the sac, except when an incision is made below the orbit. Chronic dacryocystitis is a condition met with by ophthalmologists and rhinologists alike. Excision of the sac may sometimes be necessary, but the reconstitution of the passages is a more physiological ideal. In the past West's operation of opening the sac through the nose was employed. The operation seems to be superseded now by the external operation of Toti, or better the modern modification of Dupuy-Dutemps. Nobody should perform the operation without having had training in its special technique.

Orbital cellulitis is a misnomer. It is really a case of frontal sinusitis and acute ethmoiditis with obital edema. Usually they should be treated by lavage of the maxillary sinus, which is always also infected and by an ephedrine spray. External incision is very rarely necessary or advisable. Some cases of orbital cellulitis in children are due to osteomyelitis of the maxilla or molar bone.

There are many cases of ethmoidal and sphenoidal suppuration in which the optic nerve is not affected. Conversely the cases of papilledema and retrobubar neuritis generally do not seem to associate with nasal sepsis. In cases of iridocyclitis one may look for a focus of infection. According to the author's experience the focus is seldom in the nasal sinuses, more often in the tonsils.

Osteomas of the orbit usually have a soft basis and are not difficult to deal with. Certain nasopharyngeal fibromas may cause proptosis, and are first seen by the ophthalmologist. Some of these tumors are radiosensitive. Indiscriminate irradiation, however, is not recommended; the author has seen intractable bone necrosis result. The eyes are sometimes displaced by a carcinoma of the antrum, or by mucocele of the frontal sinus or ethmoid. Antral carcinoma should be attacked by the sublabial rather than by the external route.—M. D. H., M.D.

"DIVISION OF THE FLEXOR TENDONS WITHIN THE DIGITAL SHEATH." Sumner L. Koch. Surg., Gyn. & Obst. LXXVIII. 9. January, 1944.

Despite the pessimistic attitude sometimes expressed concerning the possibility of successful repair of flexor tendons divided within the digital sheath, good results can be secured, if conditions are favorable, and if the surgeon is willing to use sufficient time and patience. The conditions essential for success are:

1. Fingers with an adequate blood supply and free from excessive scar-tissue formation.

2. Sufficient tendon with a smooth uninjured synovial covering.

3. A retentive mechanism to hold the tendon in contact with the volar surface of the finger when tension is put upon it.

4. Normal mobility at the interphalangeal and metacarpophalangel joints.

The author elaborates on each of these points, stressing the following: It is hopeless to expect free movement if both tendon surface and tendon sheath are injured. At least one-half of the normal gliding mechanism which nature has provided must be present, if free movement is to result. The advice sometimes given the surgeon to anchor a divided tendon to the surrounding tissues, so as to prevent retraction and facilitate subsequent repair, is ill-conceived, because it leads to dense scar formation. A tendon which has retracted into the palm may be brought distalward through an intact sheath. If the available tendon is irreparably damaged, one must provide a tendon graft, which is perferably taken from the sublimis tendon or the long extensor tendons to the dorsum of the foot. If a retentive mechanism is necessary, a new annular ligament is formed by passing a slip of normal tendon around the finger and suturing the ends at a point away from the gliding mechanism. At all times it is important to preserve all of the fibrous tendon sheath possible.

For the details of tendon suture, reformation of the fibrous sheath, closure of the finger incision, suture of the proximal end of the graft to the proximal segment of the tendon, the reader is referred to the original article.

Early active movement is not necessary to prevent adhesions. The hands are immobilized in optimum flexion for six to seven days. The dressing is left undisturbed during this period. Active movement, without permitting relaxation of the flexed finger and hand, is begun at the end of the third week. Some support is provided in a partially relaxed position until the end of the fifth or sixth week.

The author reports forty-one cases of secondary repair, of which a tendon graft was necessary in twenty-seven. Primary union took place in all but three cases. —E. D. M., M.D.

KEY TO ABSTRACTORS

M. D. H., M.D. ....Marvin D. Henley
E. D. M., M.D. ....Earl D. McBride

---

In the continuous world process, medical science has developed from prehistoric beginnings to its present status for the purpose of preserving the human race. Objectively considered, everything that medical men do or have done in the never ceasing changes of this process has aimed to produce results that were intended to be of enduring utility and value. All such results can be designated as conforming to the purpose of medicine and it is not always necessary that the medical workers and thinkers that are tending toward this purpose shall have the consciousness of purposeful action in their minds, but it is absolutely necessary that such workers should be mindful of the contemporary and preceding status and course of the medical changes which they desire to influence. This is another characteristic in which medical history and general history differ, for in general history great changes are often effected by persons who appear to act instinctively, unconsciously, without a knowledge of the inner connection of their action with the needs and intentions of their period.—Master Minds in Medicine. John C. Hemmeter. Page 104. New York Medical Life Press. 1927.

THE JOURNAL

OF THE

OKLAHOMA STATE MEDICAL ASSOCIATION

| VOLUME XXXVII | OKLAHOMA CITY, OKLAHOMA, SEPTEMBER, 1944 | NUMBER 9 |

Modern Concepts in the Treatment of Syphilis*

CHARLES B. TAYLOR, M.D.

OKLAHOMA CITY, OKLAHOMA

When in 1530 Hieronymus Fracastor described and named the disease called syphilis, he originated the first rapid treatment. He used crude mercury. This was used by inhalation, by mouth and by inuncation. He pushed his treatment to the point of extreme salivation and bloody diarrhea. All of his patients who did not die of the treatment, lost all of their teeth. Over fifty per cent of them died. He probably cured many of them in a short period of time. This rapid treatment was no doubt successful in a limited number of cases. Mercury remained the sheet anchor in the treatment of syphilis until 1909. For nearly four hundred years no other drug of importance was discovered, although many refinements of mercurial preparations came into use.

Ehrlich, in 1909 perfected the next drug to be used for rapid treatment. Ehrilich's edict set forth at the time he made his announcement of the discovery of salvarsan, was that one dose would cure syphilis. He called it "Therpia Sterilisans Magna," one large sterilizing dose. It didn't take long to prove that his rapid treatment was not a rapid cure at all, but an important adjunct in the treatment. Now, four hundred years after the first recognition of the disease, we are experimenting again with a rapid cure. The rationale of the present experiment is more logical than the other attempts and gives promise of being a success. Several methods are being used, each giving rather startling results. They all, however, must stand the test of time. When these treatments are evaluated, consideration must be

*Read before Annual Meeting April 25, 1944, in Tulsa.

given to the results obtained by previous methods. It is perhaps true, that fifty per cent of people with syphilis never complete what is considered a maximum period of treatment. This leaves us an astonishing number of people with latent syphilis who are a danger to no one but themselves. It is quite possible that those who undergo the present rapid treatments, are at least in as good condition as those who discontinued the older methods too soon.

The new modern rapid treatment of syphilis does not introduce any new drug other than penicillin which is at the present time purely experimental. The latest arsenical, mapharsen, at present, is the drug used almost exclusively. It differs only from our previous, long drawn out routine treatments, in that larger doses are given in a shorter period of time. In some methods, other adjuncts are added, particularly heat therapy.

It is not my intention in this paper to treat of various methods, dosage, or time. I am concerned especially now with the amount of drug given, benefits derived, the danger to the patient and the probability of complete cure. Regardless of the method used, the danger inherent in the treatment is concerned with the vital functions of the various organs. Interference with the functions may produce complications which render the treatment hazardous. It is essential, therefore, that certain specific routine examinations must be carried out prior to beginning the treatment. These examinations consist of:

(1) Liver function test.

(2) Determination of icteric index.

(3) Kidney function test.

(4) Estimation of N.P.N. and urea nitrogen in the blood.

(5) Total and differential blood and platelet counts.

On the third day of intensive treatment, blood chemistry, liver function test and determination of icteric index should be done and repeated at the end of treatment. Serious complications, which should be looked for carefully, are hemorrhagic encephalitis, failure of hepatic and renal function.

It is obvious that, since so many precautions must be taken to insure the safety of the patient, hospitilization is necessary. Since the majority of people who acquire syphilis are in the lower age bracket, and have not reached the point of economic security, the monetary requirements incident to institutional care are often prohibitive. If rapid treatment were available to all who have early syphilis, it would be justified, even though it proved later not be a permanent cure. Rendering individuals with early syphilis non-infectious in a period of a few days, would cut down the incidence of new infections tremendously. Time alone can tell whether or not we are to have these people who took a rapid treatment developing late manifestations, either of central nervous origin or the many systemic involvements. I feel that the rapid, massive therapy of syphilis must be considered still in the experimental stage. While brilliant results are seemingly being obtained many years must elapse before definite conclusions can be reached. When the risks attached to this method are eliminated it will probably be hailed as the greatest advance yet made in the treatment of syphilis.

DISCUSSION

ARDELL B. COLYAR, ASSISTANT SURGEON (R), U.S.P.H.S.

RUSH SPRINGS, OKLAHOMA

Ehrilich's attempts to cure syphilis with one dose of arsphenamine were the result of a very feasible conclusion, on which we are basing our attempts to cure syphilis. We do not expect to develop "one large sterilizing dose," but we do hope to develop a method of shortest possible duration, of maximum safety and greatest therapeutic efficiency. Syphilis, in its early stage, is an acute infectious disease, for which we have a specific drug. Though one dose won't cure, we know that five doses in five days will cure a certain number of cases. Ehrilich's idea was not so far afield as he thought.

No one will claim that the old method extending over one and one-half years is the ideal treatment. It may offer the most effective cure for those who complete it. We do not know. There are failures even among those who complete the maximum period of treatment. We may expect failures under the ideal method when we find that. But when we consider the fact that fifty to seventy per cent of patients on routine treatment do not receive enough injections to render them permanently non-infectious, we cannot fail to conclude that the old-fashioned method is inadequate. Ninety to one hundred per cent of patients started on intensive plans may complete treatment, barring reactions which necessitate discontinuing treatment.

This fifty to seventy per cent who do not complete treatment are dangerous, not only to themselves, but to their wives, husbands, children, and other contacts. They are potentially infectious. Ten per cent will have clinical relapse with infectious lesions. Thirty-five per cent may have other types of relapse if treatment is irregular. This represents more than one-fourth of all patients started on the old method. Certainly we can hope for better results by an intensive plan. I do not believe any of these plans have shown a twenty-five per cent relapse during the period of observation.

We cannot attempt to prove by statistics, at this date, which method is the best. We can only be stimulated by the "figures" to search for a better way to cure syphilis. We cannot do this by clinging to the "old-fashioned" nor by adopting too quickly the new.

There are many "plans" that may be called intensive—ranging from one day to three months. Dosage varies from 150 milligrams of Mapharsen to 2100 milligrams. The dangers to the patient, likewise, vary from one death in each two hundred fifty to little more than that involved in the routine method. The probability of cure promises to equal that of any other plan.

We have had some experience with three different plans of intensive treatment. The five-day has been used in Des Moines since 1939.

The indications for this treatment are:

1. Recent infection—less than 2 years.

2. No previous treatment or not more than 3 arsenicals.

Contraindications are:

1. Active tuberculosis.

2. Impaired kidney or liver function.

3. Certain blood dyscrasias.

4. Previous treatment.

Routine on admission was:

1. Physical examination.
2. Chest X-ray.
3. Electrocardiogram.
4. Complete blood count.
5. Complete urinalysis.
6. Bromsulfthalein liver function test.
7. P.S.P.
8. Icterus index.

Complete blood count and urinalysis was given daily. The Bromsulfthalein liver function test was given on the third and last days of treatment. Electrocardiogram was repeated in this clinic on the first, third, and last days of treatment for experimental purposes. We found changes in the complexes almost identical to that following completion of treatment.

Two thousand cc's of normal saline solution in 5 per cent glucose containing 240 mg. of Mapharsen are given intravenously daily over an 8-hour period. The flow of solution is kept at a constant rate, approximately 4 cc per hour. The needle is inserted into a vein in the lower forearm or hand to allow the patient to move about in bed. A nurse is in constant attendance. She may watch from ten to twelve patients. Very little sedation is given, none that might mask presenting signs of a cerebral reaction. Codeine, aspirin, or an ice bag may be used, if necessary, for pain and restlessness. The patient may be up and about when not on the intravenous, the Upjohn, or the bottle, as this method of treatment has been variously named by patients in different centers. Only one serious reaction occurred; a toxic hepatitis, from which the patient recovered. Other reactions include:

1. Pain in the arm due to spasm of the veins. This is relieved by speeding up the rate of intravenous drip for five or ten minutes.
2. Nausea and vomiting, usually relieved with large doses of Vitamin C, intravenously.
3. Elevation of temperature, and chills, sometimes considered an intravenous reaction. If temperature rises to about 102 degrees and is persistent, the treatment is interrupted until temperature becomes normal.
4. Headache, if persistent, calls for interruption of treatment and a careful search for any additional signs of a beginning encephalopathy.
5. C o n f u s i o n and other personality changes, which might indicate an hemorraghic encephalitis.
6. Accentuation of secondary lesions, usually occurring at the end of the first day or beginning of the second day's treatment.
7. Edema. This occurred when glucose in normal saline was given as previously indicated. We changed the solution to glucose in distilled water and had no further difficulty with retention of fluids.

Spirochetes disappear from lesions in from three to five hours. Primary lesions begin to heal the second day. Secondary lesions begin to fade the third day. The serologic reversal to negative may occur from one to ten months following treatment, depending on the duration of infection and the original level of the reagin titer. Early primaries may never have a positive Wassermann or Kahn. Sero-positive primaries reverse in from one to two months. Sero-positive secondaries reverse in from three to four months. Early latent infections (from 8 to 9 months duration) reverse in from five to ten months.

Here, I wish to emphasize an important point, and one which is not clearly understood by many physicians who see patients following intensive treatment. A positive Wassermann does not mean syphilis has not been cured. It does not call for more treatment. Follow-up on intensive treatment cases is of little value if additional treatment is given when not indicated. We are not treating "blood tests." A very definite plan of follow-up is desired. A serologic test for syphilis at frequent intervals includes a standard Wassermann and a Kahn quantitative determination of the reagin titer. A great deal depends on the quantitative test. It is expressed in Kahn units. In secondary syphilis, the time required for the serology to become negative depends on the original height of the titer, as well as the duration of infection. The blood test remains positive longer in a patient whose original titer is 1260 Kahn units than in one whose titer, for example, is 180 Kahn units. Therefore, it is not necessary to give additional arsenic to a patient following intensive treatment until it is shown that he has relapsed. The relapse is proved by the quantitative determinations of positivity and/or clinically infectious lesions.

Another short course is a six-week plan, which provides for five Mapharsen and one Bismuth injection a week. The amount of Mapharsen is based on the Eagle-Hogan dosage: 25 milligrams per kilogram body weight. This dosage divided into 30 injections constitutes the arsenical treatment. This scheme combines safety and brevity perhaps better than most of the other plans in use. The Mapharsen is given so as to provide two rest days a week, to prevent excessive accumulation of arsenic in the tissues.

The third plan is a 12-week plan, using three Mapharsen and one Bismuth injection a week. This is the method employed at Rush Springs. It is a modification of Eagle's treatment. On January 15, 1944, treatment had been completed on 290 patients. To date, there have been no deaths, one re-treated by a private physician, eleven sero-logic relapses, representing 3.79 per cent. Eight reactions necessitating discontinuation of treatment, or 2.37 per cent. These figures are not at all accurate, and when we have worked our statistics better, we may find an altogether different picture.

Intensive treatment is experimental. There is no ideal plan. Witness the one-day, five-day, twenty-day, twenty-one day, seven and one-half day with penicillin, the six-week, eight-week, ten-week, and the twelve-week. Ten schemes, and this is not all. There are at least two variations of each. But what an intense activity they indicate! We are on our way to the development of an ideal treatment for syphilis. If social management of venereal diseases can keep pace with the scientific progress, we will have the battle against syphilis won in a few years.

Ruptured Intervertebral Disc*

ARNOLD H. UNGERMAN, M.D.

TULSA, OKLAHOMA

No subject has received more attention or aroused more controversy than that of "low back and sciatic pain." To those suffering such pain finally appeared a ray of hope through the introduction of a new clinical-pathological entity, the Ruptured Interverte-bral Disc. Only through intimate coopera-tion between the Neuro-Surgeon and the Or-thopedic Surgeon, has this latest chapter in the etiologic diagnosis of sciatic pain been written.

Mixter and Barr in 1934 demonstrated that root compression, as the result of patho-logy in the Intervertebral Disc, was a com-mon cause of severe sciatic pain. Prior to this important contribution, the diagnosis of Ruptured Intervertebral Disc was made only at operation and then, usually, the lesion was mistaken for a neoplasm. In the typical clinical case of Ruptured Intervertebral Disc, a large part of the tumor mass is usually composed of the nucleus pulposus. The pre-sence of portions of the annulus fibrosus in this mass does not alter the fact that the presence of nucleus pulposus is the funda-mental consideration. The proper name for this entity is rupture of the annulus fibrosus with posteriolateral or posterior herniation of the nucleus pulposus. In order to under-stand more clearly this pathological process, a brief summary of the anatomy and physio-logy of the adult vertebral column should be reviewed.

The elements that we are most interested in are: 1. Intervertebral Discs; 2. Nucleus Pulposus; 3. Annulus Fibrosus; 4. nerve roots; 5. their relationship to the surround-ing bony portions of each vertebra. Between each vertebra there is an intervertebral disc. From the second cervical to the first sacral there are 23 of these discs. Each is cemented to the intervertebral surfaces of the verte-bral bodies above and below by a thin layer of calcifiied cartilage. On the interverte-bral face of each cartilage plate and intimate-ly blended with it is a fibrocartilaginous lay-er. This layer separates the nucleus pulposus from actual contact with the hyalin cartilage. The annulus fibrosus is a strong but some-what elastic membrane binding the adjacent vertebral bodies firmly. The fiber bundle ar-rangement contributes to the elasticity of this membrane.

In the adult the nuceleus pulposus is con-tained in a fibro-cartilage envelope, not a distinct layer, but merges with the annulus fiibrosus which in turn encloses the nucleus pulposus peripherally.

The nucleus pulposus consists of cartilage cells suspended in a gelatinous matrix in-terlaced by fine fibers from the fibro-cartilage envelope. It is composed of moderately tough tissue, but very plastic, resembling moist

*Presented to Section on Neurology, Psychiatry and Endocrin-ology, Annual State Meeting, April 26, 1944, Tulsa, Oklahoma.

fascia. Due to the structural nature of this tissue, it's function obeys the physical laws of an incompressible fluid. Studies upon the H_2O contents of the nucleus pulposus indicates dehydration with advancing age, as well as, a decreased pliability; resulting in additional wear and stress on the annulus fibrosus. Another factor which must be mentioned is the avascularity of the mature intervertebral disc. This adds to it's early decadence and feeble reparative efforts.

The nerve roots extrude from the dural envelope of the spinal cord and pass posteriorly through their respective foraminae. The vertebral canal, though sufficiently large to accommodate the cord and roots and to allow for normal freedom of movement, can easily be encroached upon by a rupture of the annulus fiibrosus with extrusion posteriorly of the nucleus pulposus, resulting in the syndrome under discussion. This composite structure of the vertebral column, if born in mind, will readily explain the signs and symptoms of this condition.

Normally when a sudden force is put upon the vertebral column it is transmitted to the Intervertebral Disc, with subsequent compression of the nucleus pulposus and a distension of the elastic annulus fibrosus, resulting in typical shock-absorber action. Besides this function, it equalizes the pressure over the entire intervertebral surface of each vertebra, following the physical laws of a fluid media. In summary, the fluid nucleus pulposus serves to distribute the force evenly over the intervertebral surfaces of the vertebra in whatever position, within limits, the spine is transmitting that force. In the intact disc, the annulus fibrosus is subjected only to forces tending to stretch it, forces which it normally withstands. If the nucleus pulposus herniates or loses it's fluidity, the annulus fibrosus is subjected to compression forces which are alien to it. The result is further damage to the disc and the vertebral surfaces.

The clinical examination is comparatively simple. There are but a few points in the history and physical examination of this group of patients, which would not be included in the complete routine examination.

The history of pain is always the incapacitating symptom of Rupture of the Intervertebral Disc. The sciatic pain so characteristic is limited to the course of the sciatic nerve and the structures innervated by it. The Gluteal, Hamstring, and leg muscles are frequently painful. The pain is, usually, exaggerated by coughing, straining or sneezing. Most cases give a history of mild trauma with or without the back pain following directly. The sciatic pain may be absent for weeks or months or years after the initial injury. Recurring attacks of lumbago occupy the interim. Many individuals give no history of injury but have occupations which produce constant wear and tear upon the lumbo- sacral spine. These must be considered as important an etiologic factor as frank trauma. This pain is worse upon activity. They find it easier to stand than to sit and complain more upon bending the back and straightening up afterward. Their's are attacks of recurrent sciatic pain.

Thirty five per cent of the cases are in the fourth decade. Seventy-five per cent of the cases are males. The most common single type of injury is the lifting of heavy objects in a bent-forward position, but, such minor trauma as an irregular swing or stepping off a curb can initiate this syndrome.

The sciatic pain is usually present along the entire course of the sciatic nerve, but points of maximum pain are often present in the gluteal region, the upper posterior thigh, the back of the knee, and lateral aspect of the leg and ankle. Coughing, sneezing, and straining intensifies the pain most often in the gluteal region.

Sixty per cent of the patients with herniated nucleus pulposus show straightening of the lumbar curve with listing away from the side of the lesion. Manipulation of the lower two lumbar spinous processes is painful and pressure applied just lateral to these processes reveals tenderness in many patients; this is quite significant if it reproduces the radicular pain. Las'gue test is positive in every case. This test consists of flexing the thigh to right angles with the trunk, then, extending the leg upon the thigh until pain begins in the gluteal or hamstring region, without further movement of the leg or thigh, the foot is dosoflexed, thus effecting a marked pull on the tibial (hence the sciatic) nerve. The jugular compression test has been found positive in over 75 per cent of the cases. This test is performed with the patient erect, and the jugular compression is maintained for two minutes before recording as negative. The venous return may be impeded either by digital compression or by the cuff of a spygnomanometer applied about the neck with the pressure maintained at 40 mm Hg.

Alteration in the sensations are of a common occurrence. Burning, stinging, prickling, tingling and the feeling of electrical shocks are symptoms frequently described. Objectively, hyperesthetic areas are found in approximately 75 per cent of the cases. If the hyperesthesia is more anterior on the lateral aspect of the leg, including the great toe, the herniation is probably at the fourth lumbar disc. If it is more posterior on the lateral aspect of the leg, including the lateral aspect of the foot, the herniation is probably at the lumbo-sacral disc. Diminution or absence of the ankle jerk on the affected side occurs in 80 per cent of the cases of lumbo-sacral herniation and in 25 per cent of the fourth lumbar herniation. Foot drop and peroneal paralysis do occur in the more severe cases. I might merely mention a few conditions which come to mind in the differential diagnosis of herniated nucleus pulposus: prostatis, rectal, abdominal, and pelvic neoplasm: cauda equina tumors: old spinal injuries with old adhesions in the arachnoid: neoplasms of spine, primary and metastatic: scar formations about nerve roots: spinal anomaly—congenital 5th lumbar: spondylolisthesis: hypertrophy of the ligamentum flavum: injury of the sciatic nerve: syphilis: abscess: neurofibrosus: peripheral tumors: herpes zoster: gluteal injections: hypertrophic arthritis: aneurysm of the iliac or popliteal artery: vascular disease: polyneuritis: psychoneurosis.

The diagnosis of a ruptured disc can be made solely from the patient's story of low back ache plus sciatica occurring in attacks, usually, after a relatively trivial injury, such as a lift, bend, or strain; and usually, during the acute stages, the pain in the back and the sciatica are intensified by coughing and sneezing. There may or may not be a sensory and motor loss from local pressure on the nerve. The only really valuable objective finding is a diminution or loss of the Achilles reflex and this occurs only in one half the cases. If this sign is present, the disc is ruptured at the fifth lumbar. The subjective story, therefore, is all important and the negative objective findings should not discourage the diagnosis. In Dandy's recent resume of this disease, consisting of the some 350 cases operated, the diagnosis failed only one time; a spinal cord tumor being the causative lesion. Ninety-five per cent of the cases with such symptoms have a ruptured Intervertebral Disc. Three conditions account for the other five per cent, namely, spondylolisthesis, 2 per cent; congenitally defective fifth lumbar, 2 per cent; and tumors of the cauda-equina, 1 per cent. An x-ray of the lumbar spine will diagnose or eliminate the first two. Therefore, tumors of the cauda-equina present the only problem. Though the symptoms may not differ from those of a ruptured disc, the backache is usually higher and there is frequently a diminution or loss of the patellar reflex. Should a tumor be present a lumbar puncture will usually show Xanthochrome fluid. The question of the intraspinal use of contrast media has been a source of controversy, but, there is no doubt that iodized oil is not only unnecessary but contra-indicated. Many men have used oxygen, as a

contrast medium introduced intraspinally in diagnosing ruptured discs other than the fourth and fifth. Dandy does not advocate this at all, and states, that if relied upon alone, two thirds of the total number will be missed. Particularly, the concealed disc.

There are two types of Ruptured Discs; protruding and concealed (very slightly protruding or not protruding at all.) It has been the disclosure of the latter by Dandy, that has cleared up the entire subject of those cases that are diagnosed, then operated and missed. Dandy devised two very simple tests at operation: the finding of the nerve root adherent to the underlying disc and the sense of fluctuation to forceps obtained by pressure upon the thinned ligament overlying the disc: horizontal or downward pressure on the spinous processes will reveal increased mobility over the affected disc. About 20 per cent of all the patients with ruptured discs have two, one at the fourth and the other at the fifth. The very unusual case of a disc at the second and third is localized by pain in the front of the thigh or pain in the back of the leg.

At operation, one sees that the affected discs really consist of two components; the necrotic interior; and the part that protrudes or attaches itself to the nerve. According to Dandy, the former causes the backache and the latter the sciatica. The realization of this one point accounts for the cure.

The treatment consists in removing the protruding disc, and curetting the necrotic interior. The disc is removed through a partial lamenectomy, or no bone at all need be removed, in some cases. It seems that there is no indication for either spinal fusion or for any stabilization of the lateral joint. It adds nothing except the severe ordeal of one to two months in a plaster cast. When the necrotic center of the disc is curetted, there remains a large area for natural fusion. The patient is out of the hospital in two weeks.

SUMMARY

1. Ruptured Intervertebral Disc is a comparatively new clinical-pathological entity and its recognition has brought relief to countless sufferers of "Sciatic Rheumatism" and low back pain.

2. The diagnosis can be made solely upon the signs and symptoms and X-rays of the lumbar spine. The use of intraspinal injections are of no significant help, except in the rare case of Ruptured Disc higher than the fourth and fifth lumbar; this occurs in less than two per cent of the total number of cases. Air can be used, but iodized oil is contraindicated. Two discs are ruptured in about 20 per cent of the cases.

3. There are two components of a Ruptured Disc: the necrotic interior of the disc, causing backache; the protruding portion causing sciatica. The small non-protruding or concealed discs are two times as frequent as the protruding one, and are, frequently, missed at operation. This accounts for recurrence and persistence of symptoms in some cases.

4. Cure is effected by removal of the disc and thorough curettment of the entire necrotic center, usually approached through a unilateral exposure and between the laminae without removal of any bone (Love's operation) or by the removal of a small bite of laminae.

5. Fusion operations after removal of the disc are contraindicted, as fixation of the opposing vertebral surfaces occur following through curettment.

6. Spontaneous cures must be rare, although temporary remissions are the rule.

Rheumatic Fever*

CLARK H. HALL, M.D.,

OKLAHOMA CITY, OKLAHOMA

Rheumatic fever is receiving an increasing amount of attention. It has been recognized as a serious disease but too often only after the heart has suffered serious damage. Comparatively little attention is given to the acute phases except to give relief of symptoms. After this has passed, the disease is often forgotten until another acute phase occurs or until the child has clinical evidence of considerable heart damage. In the United States for the year 1941 the Bureau of the Census reports that there were 26,235 deaths reported due to chronic rheumatic disease of the heart and 1,640 deaths due to acute rheumatic fever. In our own state there were 316 deaths due to chronic rheumatic disease of the heart and 32 reported due to acute rheumatic fever. The death rate per 100,000 population in 1941 for chronic rheumatic disease of the heart in the United States was 19.8 and in Oklahoma 13.5, for acute rheumatic fever in the United States 1.2 and for Oklahoma 1.4. These figures, of course, tell us nothing of the children and adults who have to live more or less modified lives due to the effects of the disease. Among industrial policy holders of the Metropolitian Life Insurance Company between the ages of 5 and 24, the death rate from rheumatic fever and chronic heart disease (about 90 per cent of which is rheumatic in origin during these years) was 9.7 per 100,000 as compared with 32.3 in 1917-1918. Thus, in the interval between the world wars, the mortality from rheumatic fever among young people has declined about 70 per cent.

*Presented at Annual State Meeting, April 25, Tulsa.

The navy is reporting rheumatic fever as a real problem. Conditions peculiar to naval training and military service in general may bring about recrudescences. Masters is of the opinion that the disease should be a cause for rejection as it is a continuous condition which usually starts in childhood. Levy et al., found in re-examination of men disqualified for general military service because of the diagnosis of cardio-vascular defects, that the chief cause for rejection was rheumatic heart disease found in 2,476 men or 50 per cent of the total of 4,994. Mitral valvular disease without aortic valvular disease was diagnosed in the majority of these rheumatic heart cases.

ETIOLOGY

The etiology of rheumatic fever is not a closed question. Usually there is an upper respiratory infection or even scarlet fever preceding a rheumatic fever episode. A number of investigators have demonstrated the beta-hemolytic streptococci of Group A.

SYMPTOMS

The rheumatic infection is a systemic one. The clear cut case is not difficult to recognize but often the history is not clear and may be confusing. It affects various tissues of the body in varying degrees. The heart is probably involved from the onset although the pathologic change may be difficult to demonstrate. Fever usually ranges from 100 to 102, occasionally higher. This may continue for a few days or a number of weeks and then return to normal. The child may have only one attack but usually there are repeated attacks at different intervals. These are more common during the late winter months and early spring. The pulse rate is increased. If there is an increase out of proportion to the temperature, a varying amount of heart involvement is indicated, especially of the myocardium.

The joint symptoms may be vague and often overlooked or disregarded by the parents and may be considered of little or no significance. Any child having joint pains deserves a careful investigation as to the cause. In younger children there may be little evidence of redness, swelling and fever, but more of stiffness which is not severe and disappears from time to time. In older children we are more likely to find the acutely involved joints. One or more may be affected. Usually we find several involved successively. The joints usually involved are the knees, ankles and wrists. Any of the joints may be effected including the smaller ones of the hands and feet. We have been impressed with the frequency of shoulder pain in older children.

Epistaxis is frequently encountered in rheumatic children. It may occur at any time but is quite often severe during a frank recurrence.

The leucocyte count is usually moderately increased during the acute phase, the average in a group of Wilson's cases being around 13,200. In chorea the count is lower, averaging 10,700. This increase is present during the period of activity and normal or below during quisence. It appears to be higher in patients with considerable heart involvement. There is generally an increase in the neutrophils.

The skin symptoms vary from time to time. Sweating is quite common and may be very troublesome. This may be present at any time including convalescence. The rheumatic nodules are not a common finding in our cases, in fact we have been impressed with their infrequency. Other skin manifestations may be present during the period of activity.

Chorea is frequently encountered. It may be the first known manifestation of rheumatic fever but many times is just another phase of the infection. Some of our cases give no history of joint pains, etc., but on physical examination very definite evidence of heart involvement is found.

The general condition of the patient, the involvement of the joints and chorea cause considerable worry but we know that all of this will clear up eventually. The really disturbing feature is the heart damage. Even in mild cases heart damage is evident sooner or later. It varies in degree and if there are repeated attacks, and there usually are, it progresses. Often the patient will complain of heart symptoms and the parents are not aware of a rheumatic infection because of its mildness. The younger the patient the greater the probability of serious heart damage. There may be pain in the precardium during the acute phase. The myocardium is involved in every case. The heart rate is out of proportion to the fever present. This increased rate may persist for some time after the acute infection seems to have subsided. The first sound at the apex is muffled and a soft systolic murmur may develop as a result of dilation of the mitral ring. A blowing systolic murmur heard over the base of the heart or along the sternum indicates involvement of the aortic valve.

In the early cases and those with only slight involvement, the X-Ray is not of great value. The fluoroscope and the flat plate are of aid when there is enlargement. The electrocardiogram changes, in the opinion of Levine, are the increased conduction time or P-R interval and alterations in the R-T complex.

Hemolytic anemia develops in proportion to the acuteness of the rheumatic infection. During convalescence this improves somewhat with the general condition of the patient. The sedimentation rate is increased when the rheumatic infection is active.

Abdominal pain is not an uncommon symptom in children with rheumatic fever. Freidberg and Goss have reported cases of abdominal rheumatism. They state that when acute abdominal symptoms are present in a patient suffering from rheumatic fever, complicating periarteritis nodosa should be considered. This complication is offered as an organic base for some instances of abdominal pain. There are times when the symptoms indicate appendicitis and it is wise to explore the abdomen. Referred pain in the abdomen is sometimes due to acute carditis, especially pericarditis.

PROGNOSIS

Not many deaths occur during the early acute phase. The younger the patient at the onset the more serious the prognosis. Recurrences are common and each time cardiac involvement usually progresses. There is a higher death rate in those who suffer marked cardia involvement early in the disease. Mitral stenosis and aortic insufficiency are more common in those cases that have continued for sometime. Levine has been impressed with the findings in older people that had chorea when children and no other evidence of rheumatic infection. At 30 or 40 they have mitral stenosis. The prognosis in chorea as to heart involvement is not as good as formerly believed; these cases must be followed for years.

DIAGNOSIS

This is not difficult in the case with a typical history of involvement of several joints, large or small, in succession, fever, increased white count and sedimentation rate. Usually there is a history of an upper respiratory infection from one to three weeks previously. Sometimes there is a rheumatic family history. In the vague cases the history of epistaxis, low grade fever at times, fatigue, sweating, and indefinite joint pains should make us suspect rheumatic fever. It may be necessary to follow the child for a time before a definite diagnosis can be made, especially if there is no laboratory evidence of infection at the time. It is wise not to be hasty in these cases. Many times the reaction to salicylates is of diagnostic significance since they usually relieve the rheumatic pains. .

TREATMENT

There is no specific treatment for the disease. It is entirely symptomatic. Full bed rest is the first order. Salicyates are given for the relief of pain and reduction of fever. If there is restlessness, sedation is given and at times it may be necessary to give codeine or morphine for relief of pain. The affected joints are supported and much comfort is obtained with heat either as hot packs or the light cradle. The ice cap often relieves precordial pain. It must be applied properly and kept in place. The skin must not be neglected as the sweating often causes irritation. Digitalis is not of value in the acute case but is given for heart failure. Swift has shown that sulfanilamide should not be given the patient with acute rheumatic fever as it may do harm. It is wise to keep the patient in bed until evidence of infection has disappeared for several weeks. This means no symptoms, normal temperature, pulse, white count and sedimentation rate. It has been our experience that the sedimentation rate is usually the last to return to normal. The child is allowed to sit up in accordance to his reaction to this activity. There is a big difference in children and there can be no set procedure; each case should have individual consideration. Nutrition is important. The child must be encouraged to eat a well balanced diet and if possible gain weight. The vitamins must be adequate, especially "C" as a deficiency is thought to have a bearing on the rheumatic infection by some workers. Iron is usually indicated because of the anemia.

CONVALESCENCE

This is a phase so often overlooked. The case must be kept under medical supervision. It is our procedure to send the rheumatic fever patient to the convalescent home after the acute infection has subsided, where his general condition and activities may be supervised. If he is from a good home, convalescence may continue there. All members of the family must be informed as to the situation so that cooperation may be obtained from every member of the household. This is especially true if there is considerable heart damage.

As soon as the patient's condition will permit all sources of chronic infection must be removed if possible. If the tonsils are the source of trouble and affect the general health, they should be removed. This should not be done just because the patient has a rheumatic infection.

There is considerable interest in the use of the sulfonamides as a means of preventing streptococcus infections and recurrent episodes of rheumatic fever. There has been a number of encouraging reports and among them one by Thomas who points out "that prophylactic sulfanilamide is effective in preventing rheumatic recrudescences, that it is relatively safe, and if the routine is stripped to essentials, the cost is far less than the cost of caring for the cardiac invalids these rheumatic subjects would eventually become. It is our practice to use it in patients who can be watched carefully. After the drug is started it is continued throughout the year. The blood concentration does not need to be high to be effective. In our limited number of cases on sulfonamide we are encouraged with the results so far. Change of climate is not practical.

A very perplexing problem in many instances is that of education. It is important, as these patients need all the training they can get so that they can earn their livelihood comfortably. As far as we know, this problem has not been completely solved by anyone. Some children are not able to attend school at all, while others are handicapped by not being able to attend regularly.

SUMMARY

Rheumatic infections are serious even though the individual attacks may not appear to be dangerous. In some instances the real damage may not become apparent until years later. It is important that it be recognized as early as possible and followed carefully. Every effort should be made to see that the convalescence is supervised and supplemented by an attempt to prevent infections that may lead to recurrent fever.

DISCUSSION

BEN H. NICHOLSON, M.D.,
OKLAHOMA CITY, OKLAHOMA

As Attendant of the Out-Patient Service at the Crippled Children's Hospital, I have

worked with Dr. Hall on the State rheumatic fever program.

Unfortunately, we have not had the time
or the help to evaluate the work to date but
I have gained the following impressions.

The most effective part of the program,
from my viewpoint has been an educational
one, teaching the parents what the disease
is, what we mean by recurrences and when
recurrences are apt to come, the meaning
of an adequate diet, and the meaning of restriction of activity. I have not been able to
bring myself to give any of the sulfonamide
drugs continuously since our patients come
from all over the State and are not under
close observation, but I have been giving
each child from 15 to 22 grains a day for
five days with each respiratory infection in
the hope of preventing invasion of the respiratory tract with the hemolytic streptococcus.

Our recurrences have been reduced in
number but to what extent I cannot as yet
say. Dr. Hall and I are not exactly in agreement on the question of activity. I feel that
just as soon as an active infection is pretty
much on the wane, the youngster should begin his activity and that it can be increased

as rapidly as it does not produce fatigue or
cause an untoward increase in pulse rate.
For these children school is more important
than for normal children because they must
eventually make their living with their heads
rather than their hands. It is a tremendous
disturbance of an individual child's morale
to be too far behind chilldren of his own age
in school.

I think, as a whole, the program headed
by Dr. Hall has been well worth the effort
and eventually I hope we can give an accurate evaluation of it.

BIBLIOGRAPHY

1. Bureau of the Census. Vital Statistics. Special Reports, Vol 17, No. 31. August 18, 1943.
2. Friedberg, C. K. and Goss, L.: Arch. Int. Med., Vol.
54, pp. 170-198. August, 1934.
3. Levine: Clinical Heart Disease, pp. 20 and 29. W.
B. Saunders & Co.
4. Levy, Robert L., et al.: Report of Re-examination of
4,994 Men Disqualified for Gen. Military Service. J.A.M.A.,
Vol. 123, No. 16. Dec. 18, 1943.
5. Master, A. M.: Rheumatic Fever in the Navy. Med.
Bull. Vol. 41, pp. 1019-1021. July, 1943.
6. Metropolitan Life Ins. Co.: Bull. Vol. 24, No. 9. Sept.
1943.
7. Swift, Moen and Hirst: The Action of Sulfanilamide in
Rheumatic Fever. J.A.M.A. Vol. 110, page 426. 1938.
8. Thomas, Caroline B.: The Prophylactic Treatment of
Rheumatic Fever by Sulfanilamide. Bull. of New York Academy of Med., Vol. 18, No. 8, pp. 508-526. August, 1942.
9. Wilson, May G.: Rheumatic Fever. Commonwealth
Fund. Page 133.

Some Laboratory Phases of Clinical Diagnosis*

I. H. NELSON, M.D.,

TULSA, OKLAHOMA

Strictly speaking, this subject might well
include roentgenology, electro-cardiography,
ophthalmoscopy, and many other specialties.
In a broad sense, even the stethoscope and
sphygmomanometer can be considered laboratory aids in clinical diagnosis. However,
to narrow the range of discussion we shall
consider here only those phases which can
be grouped under the general term 'Clinical
Pathology.'

In the earlier days of laboratory medicine
the clinician examined the urine, blood, sputum or other body materials at the bedside.
The facts learned from these tests, together
with those gained by inspection, percussion,
and auscultation, were fitted to the history
to arrive at a diagnosis. As the numbers
of tests increased and their complexity became greater it was found essential that
some physicians become full time clinical

*Read at Annual Meeting. Section on General Medicine, April
25, at Tulsa.

pathologists and that the specimens for examination be taken to a central location
where a wider collection of apparatus and
chemicals could bring about a saving of time
and enhance the accuracy of the determinations. This divorce of laboratory examinations from the bedside did not, or should not,
change the basic principle involved, namely,
that the laboratory findings are not an end
in themselves, but are simply aids to the
clinician.

The past 70 to 80 years might well be
called the Golden Age of Medicine. In no
branch of Medicine is this more true than
in that of Clinical Pathology. The knowledge gained in hematology, bacteriology, immunology, serology, biochemistry, mycology,
parasitology and other allied subjects is so
vast that any one individual can hope only
to learn some basic principles in each of
them and the numerous specific examina-

tions which may be found necessary in any of them. For the next few minutes we shall attempt to discuss briefly some of these special fields and mention some of the ways by which the clinician can get the most cooperation from the laboratory in his effort to attain the greatest degree of accuracy in diagnosis.

Hematology is the study of the blood and the blood forming organs. We believe that more erroneous findings are reported here than in any other branch of clinical medicine. Perhaps the greatest cause for these errors lies in the common belief that "anybody can make a blood count." As a matter of fact, even with the best of technique and the utmost care, there is a five per cent error which cannot be avoided. This error can easily become 40 per cent, even up to 100 per cent, in the hands of a poorly trained or careless worker. The only remedy possible is constant supervision on the part of the clinician or laboratory director, as well as the insistence on well trained technologists. The leukemias in the early stage may easily be overlooked unless the technologist is alert to the presence of a few abnormal leucocytes and calls them to the attention of the clinician or clinical pathologist.

Bacteriology has made great strides in the 70 years elapsing since the days of Pasteur and Koch. The clinician, with the aid of the clinical pathologist, must be able to isolate or identify scores of different strains of bacteria. Identification may involve the use of various kinds of culture media, and usually this is left to the technologist. This problem of identification will be greater in the future, as we will probably be called upon to determine the virulence or non-virulence of the many strains of streptococci, just to cite one example. The clinician has a great responsibility in deciding the proper time or methods used in obtaining material for bacteriological examination. It is astonishing to notice how many times a blood culture is requested long after the optimum time has passed in the course of the infection, or how often we are asked to examine slides obtained after the eye, for example, has been carefully washed and a therapeutic agent instilled.

Immunology and serology we shall consider together, principally because most of the laboratory tests are run on blood serum. In these fields the responsibility of the internist as to the proper time to run the tests is of the utmost importance because of timing, economics, and the conservation of the time of the technologist. A negative agglutination early in the course of typhoid fever is of no value usually, and may give a false sense of security. The same is true of the Wasserman test if it be taken the pri-

mary stage of syphilis. The patient has to pay for services which are of no benefit to him. The over-worked technologist wastes time and energy which is no small item these days when there is a shortage of competent workers. Another source of error or waste of time and material which crops up too frequently is caused by the use of syringes or needles which are wet either with alcohol or water.

In the field of biochemistry it is particularly necessary that the specimens be taken at the proper time (usually on a fasting stomach), and that the tests be done as soon as possible. The value of glucose, for example, usually drops rapidly after the specimen is obtained. Functional tests, such as the Phenolsulphathalein, Bromsulphalein, and other similar tests will probably assume a larger place in diagnosis as the clinician learns by experience the value of each of them. While discussing biochemistry it is well to mention the rapid advances in chemotherapy in the past ten years which have thrown added burdens on the laboratory because of the need during the time you are becoming familiar with the drug, to determine the blood level of the agent being administered. This is a field in which we all anticipate still further progress and perhaps most of the new drugs discovered will require blood level determinations, in their early use, at least.

Parasitology is a subject which should take on new interest in the minds of all of us in the very near future. The clinical pathologist has to learn with you. The return of our servicemen from overseas should bring to us cases of parasitic infestation which in normal times we would never encounter. We mention only leishmaniasis and filariasis. We may also see many relapses of malaria or dysentery, with or without complications, some of which may require the utmost ingenuity and cooperation between the clinical pathologist and clinician.

We shall mention briefly only one more subject before closing, and that is the examination of tissues. The utmost care should be taken by the clinician to obtain a representative specimen, and one that is large enough. It should be placed in fixing solution quickly so that cellular details will be well preserved, and it should be labeled properly.

In conclusion we should like to stress again three points: first, that the clinician use proper consultation and care in procuring the specimen for the clinical pathologist; second, that the accuracy of the determination cannot be any greater than the skill and care exercised by the technologist; third, that the findings must be properly interpreted.

DISCUSSION

ELIZABETH M. CHAMBERLIN, M.D.,
BARTLESVILLE, OKLAHOMA

It has been interesting to me in preparing a discussion of Dr. Nelson's excellent and timely paper, to learn that the problems of the younger pathologist in relation to the clinician are identical with those which the older generation has faced for many years. However, the pathologist of the immediate future has economic problems confronting him, which either did not exist for my generation or which we have either evaded or ignored. Also the clinician is face to face with some of the facts of professional life which have haunted the pathologist since the very beginning of clinical pathology. I refer to the threatened control of all forms of medical practice by non-professional agencies. This threat should work toward a better understanding among us all.

Dr. Nelson quotes the saying that "any one can make a blood count," and alas for the patient, almost anyone is likely to try it. Fortunately, in the routine examination in the doctor's office the majority of blood counts are normal, or very nearly so, consequently the poorly trained worker has the law of averages in his favor. I believe that more consultations are held in the field of hematology between the clinician and the pathologist than in any other branch.

In addition to what Dr. Nelson said of bacteriology, I would add that often we are asked to identify organisms after sulfa drugs have been given, sometimes for long periods. This obscures and renders impossible an accurate identification.

It is indeed an annoyance to receive a hemolysed specimen of blood due chiefly to a wet syringe, and it is equally maddening to have an oxlated specimen sent in, improperly mixed and full of small clots. In such cases it is better to have the patient sent to the laboratory.

In the field of parasitology, I am as ignorant as anyone could be who has never worked in the tropics, indeed we shall have to learn together.

I am glad that the day is gone when the pathologist was expected to be a magician, and produce a diagnosis with poorly prepared material and meager clinical data. Today more is expected of us, and we in turn expect ample data and properly prepared material, in order that the best results may be obtained. I should like to quote a sentence which often comes to my mind, a saying of the late Dr. Richard Jaffe, when asked about the advisability of giving an opinion as to the so-called "pre-cancerous" nature of any tumor. He replied, "We are pathologists, we are not prophets."

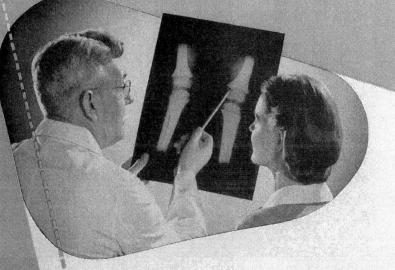

· THE PRESIDENT'S PAGE ·

Each month your Association publishes a Journal for the benefit and enlightenment of the membership. Besides the scientific articles, which are of a high quality and well worth reading, it contains many other items of interest and some excellent editorials.

I wonder how many of you realize what an enormous amount of work is required of your Editorial Board and the Editor - in - Chief month after month and year after year in order to compile this material for publication. By actual comparison, our Journal ranks very favorably with the best state medical journals in the country. We are most fortunate in having an Editorial Board composed of outstanding and capable men. The work of Mrs. Jane Tucker, the Editorial Assistant, is most praiseworthy. The Editor-in-Chief is nationally known for his literary as well as his scientific skill.

I wonder how many of us *read* the Journal and appreciate its worth? I am certain if these men knew that their labor is not in vain it would be a source of great inspiration and stimulate them to greater effort. If you have not been in the habit of reading the Journal, make it a point to do so. Failure to do this will cause you to lose contact with your Association at a time when some vital issues are at stake. We also urge you to send in news items and matters of interest to the Editorial Board. Remember, this is YOUR Journal and YOUR Association.

President.

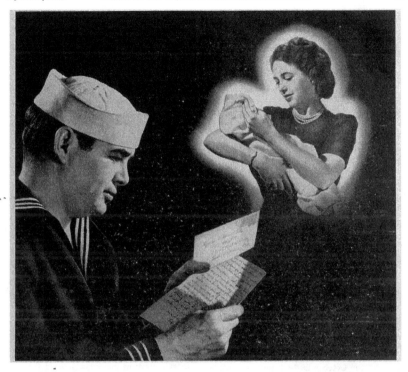

"Dear Jim... JUDY AND I ARE VERY WELL"

Thrilling words for a father at sea. They fortify a man with courage and breed new hope in an uncertain future.

That all our fighting men may be blessed with this confidence . . . home-front physicians and pharmacists are doing more than their share to safeguard the health of American families.

Warren-Teed representatives give constant thought to conserving the time of these busy wartime physicians and pharmacists.

WARREN-TEED
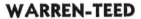

Medicaments of Exacting Quality Since 1920

THE WARREN-TEED PRODUCTS COMPANY, COLUMBUS 8, OHIO

The JOURNAL Of The
OKLAHOMA STATE MEDICAL ASSOCIATION

L. J. MOORMAN, Oklahoma City, Editor-in-Chief

E. EUGENE RICE, Shawnee   BEN H. NICHOLSON, Oklahoma City

MR. PAUL H. FESLER, Oklahoma City, Business Manager

JANE FIRRELL TUCKER, Editorial Assistant

CONTRIBUTIONS: Articles accepted by this Journal for publication including those read at the annual meetings of the State Association are the sole property of this Journal.

The Editorial Department is not responsible for the opinions expressed in the original articles of contributors.

Manuscripts may be withdrawn by authors for publication elsewhere only upon the approval of the Editorial Board.

MANUSCRIPTS: Manuscripts should be typewritten, double-spaced, on white paper 8½ x 11 inches. The original copy, not the carbon copy, should be submitted.

Footnotes, bibliographies and legends for cuts should be typed on separate sheets in double space. Bibliography listing should follow this order: Name of author, title of article, name of periodical with volume, page and date of publication.

Manuscripts are accepted subject to the usual editorial revisions and with the understanding that they have not been published elsewhere.

NEWS: Local news of interest to the medical profession, changes of address, births, deaths and weddings will be gratefully received.

ADVERTISING: Advertising of articles, drugs or compounds unapproved by the Council on Pharmacy of the A.M.A. will not be accepted. Advertising rates will be supplied on application.

It is suggested that members of the State Association patronize our advertisers in preference to others.

SUBSCRIPTIONS: Failure to receive The Journal should call for immediate notification.

REPRINTS: Reprints of original articles will be supplied at actual cost provided request for them is attached to manuscripts or made in sufficient time before publication. Checks for reprints should be made payable to Industrial Printing Company, Oklahoma City.

Address all communications to THE JOURNAL OF THE OKLAHOMA STATE MEDICAL ASSOCIATION, 210 Plaza Court, Oklahoma City. (3)

OFFICIAL PUBLICATION OF THE OKLAHOMA STATE MEDICAL ASSOCIATION
Copyrighted September, 1944

EDITORIALS

MARK YOUR CALENDAR

Now is the time to look ahead and "clear the deck" for October 23-26 inclusive. Put a ring around these dates for the Oklahoma City Clinical Society Meeting. This meeting has been planned for the benefit of the hardworked doctor. All the frills have been put aside and the program has been shaken down and packed full of practical facts for busy practitioners.

The War has made it necessary for the family doctor to work with skill and dispatch. The acquisition of knowledge is imperative. Opportunity is knocking at your door. On another page in this issue of the Journal will be found a list of the distinguished speakers for this meeting. Look this list over and make your plans.

Through the Oklahoma City Clinical Society the best and most up-to-date knowledge in diagnosis and therapy is being made available to the doctors of Oklahoma virtually without cost.

THE MOTHERS' MILK BANK

In the August, 1943 issue of the Journal a brief history of our knowledge of the nutritional and therapeutic value of milk appeared under the appropriate title, "The Milky Way." Supplementary to this discussion, attention is called to the important development of The Mothers' Milk Bank.

Since Dr. Fritz B. Talbot of Boston, in 1910, initiated interest in this field, the lives of many babies have been saved by mothers' milk made available through the methods of collection, preservation and distribution, gradually developed through the influence of Dr. Talbot's process, passing through various stages including difficult and expensive drying methods up to the present quick freezing now satisfactorily employed.

The following, quoted from a recent issue of Hygeia, shows the present status of Milk Banks and discusses the present difficulties and the need of wider coverage. "Today there are twenty-two milk bureaus in the United States and foreign countries. Two are in Canada, one at Toronto, the other at Montreal. London, England, has a center, and there is one in Lima, Peru.

"Many mothers who are now contributing their surplus milk are probably not giving as much as they might because they are anxious and worried about the war and other problems and uncertainties of the day. Some cannot come to centers to express their milk because they cannot provide care for their children while they are away, and others flatly refuse when they learn that they must have a physical examination. It is thus becoming increasingly harder to get breast milk for infants who require it. A hospital for children in Toronto is having trouble collecting milk because of restrictions on transportation. Since many hospitals still do not preserve mothers' milk, there is a definite need t o d a y for establishing more milk banks."

We are glad to announce to the doctors of Oklahoma that, through the generosity of Mr. and Mrs. Charles A. Vose whose own son was saved by frozen mothers' milk flown from Milwaukee, Oklahoma now has one of the few Mothers' Milk Banks in the world with frozen milk now available, when the need is established, for otherwise helpless babies.

"Oklahoma's mothers' milk bank has storage space for 800 to 1,000 ounces of frozen milk, when the happy day arrives when the supply exceeds the demand, and arrangements have been made for commercial cold storage space as needed. It is Miss Dryer's (Graduate Nurse in charge) dream to be able to have a supply on hand to be ready to answer the cry of sick infants throughout Oklahoma and Texas."

Every doctor who can find the time should visit the Oklahoma City Bank at the Oklahoma County Health Association, Variety Club Health Center, Oklahoma City. The management is efficient, the set-up emaculate and the routine most interesting to physicians and nurses who understand the meticulous care and technique required to collect and preserve milk with the exceptionally low bacterial count reported by the Oklahoma City Bank. All doctors are urged to help supply donors to make use of this life saving boon to unfortunate babies.

TOBACCO ROAD

It seems the irony of Fate that tobacco should be brought under the searching scrutiny of science. We are loath to decry the "holy herb," the "celestial manna", the "diving weed," the solace of savage and saint, the friend in solitude, silent, vital, warm and brave and mortal, yet reaching far beyond our verified experiences. For the doctor who loves the art of medicine and knows the comfort tobacco has given the priest, the peasant, the poet, the philosopher, the physician and his patients, it seems almost "folly to be wise."

Though the history of tobacco reveals much discussion and some controversy as to its original habitat, reliable botanists agree that it belongs to America. Tobacco was among the gifts the Indians presented to Christopher Columbus as peace offerings. Obviously the habit of smoking was well established in the new world and "the adventurers met people who apparently drank smoke in order to enjoy it." In this weed with its social and commercial potentialities, they had discovered the treasure of the Indies unawares. The American Indians held tobacco in high esteem, they believed in its divine origin and they gave expression to their belief in their primitive rituals. Apparently they knew little of its therapeutic application, which received such wide acclaim from the time of its introduction into European countries to the beginning of the 18th Century. It was used internally and externally and the scope of its therapeutic application ranged from the reduction of fatigue to the induction of abortion.

In the latter part of the 16th and the first part of the 17th Centuries, smoking had become so popular in England, especially among the "elite," there was a growing alarm and James the First (1556-1625) expressed his disapproval in no uncertain terms. Apparently he thought his smoking aristocracy was going to the dogs. But he hated Raleigh, who had been credited with the introduction of tobacco into England and it is well to attribute a part of his antipathy toward smoking to jealousy and envy. He branded the use of the "outlandish weed" as "A custome lothsome to the eye, hateful to the nose, harmfull to the braine, daungerous to the lungs, and in the blacke stinking fume thereof, neerest resembling the horrible Stigian smoke of the pit that is bottomlesse."[1]

Many, more liberal, English writers considered tobacco good for therapeutic use but bad when employed for pleasure. The controversy raged in prose and poetry while smoking thrived among the rich and the poor, the high and the low. The question was debated at Oxford and Robert Burton no doubt a student or, perhaps, at that time, Vicar at Oxford, had his say, "Tobacco, divine, rare, superexcellent tobacco, which goes far beyond all the panaceas, potable gold, and philosophers' stones, a sovereign remedy to all diseases. A good vomit, I confess, a virtuous herb, if it be well qualified, opportunely taken, and medicinally used; but as it is commonly abused by most men, which take it as tinkers do ale, 'tis a plague, a mischief, a violent purger of goods, lands, health; hellish, devilish, and damned tobacco, the ruin and overthrow of body and soul."[2]

It is not necessary to chart the subsequent course of the controversy which has continued to this day. Suffice it to say we are glad the American Indian had his glamorous past with his nicotinic pow-wow and his pipe of peace, and that the good old backwoods grandmother could dip her clay pipe in the hot coals for a light and smoke at the chimneyside with impunity while basting her rheumatism. Where ignorance is such bliss it seems a shame that science must sound the inexorable warning. Historically it is interesting to note that in 1671 Francisco Redi, one of the great scientists of his time, wrote a letter to Athanasius Kircher which Castiglioni discusses as follows: "In this letter he refers to experiments on various natural objects, and particularly on some which were brought from the Indies. His judgment is very objective and impartial. Speaking of the action of tobacco he says that it is one of the most virulent and toxic agents for injection into animals."[3]

Though its therapeutic claims were gradually relinquished, it was not until after the middle of the 19th Century that the scientific study of tobacco was well under way. In spite of increasing knowledge which proved its medicinal virtues had been greatly exaggerated and which led to organized opposition to smoking, the habit has gradually. grown to sush proportions that it literally covers the world.

Early in the 19th Century in Boston, someone looked in upon the Saturday Club and found the scientist Agassiz' with a lighted cigar in each hand, entertaining his fellow clubmen, Longfellow, Lowell, Whittier, Holmes, Sumner, Hedge, Prescott and others. Henry Thoreau looked in and said it was all cigar smoke. The scientific studies cannot be reported in detail but it may be said that they reveal definite effects upon the nervous system, manifested chiefly through circulatory changes with elevation of blood pressure and acceleration of the pulse, perhaps varying in significance with individual susceptibility. These scientific investigations dealing with the vasoconstrictor action of tobacco smoke were initiated by Bruce and his associates.[4] The history of progress in this field is briefly reviewed by Roth, McDonald and Sheard, with their own observations, in The Journal of the American Medical Association under the following title, "The Effect of Smoking Cigarets—and of intravenous administration of nicotine on the electrocardiogram, basal metabolic rate, cutaneous temperature, blood pressure and pulse rate of normal persons."[4] After a very interesting discus-

sion the authors reach the following conclusions: "After our subjects had smoked standard cigarets it was found that the blood pressure and pulse rate and the electrocardiogram returned to normal within five to fifteen minutes. However, the peripheral vascular constriction indicated by the cutaneous temperatures of the extremities persisted from half an hour to an hour and in some cases much longer. These observations make us conclude, as did Maddock and Coller, that the smoking of standard cigarets should be avoided in the presence of peripheral vascular disease. As Pratt has suggested, the habit of giving an injured soldier a cigaret is not advisable if arterial injury has occurred, as segmental spasm of the artery is common in such trauma and the vasoconstriction in a person sensitive to tobacco may cause irreparable damage."[5]

The above paragraph is followed by this significant Summary:

"Observations on six normal subjects yielded the following results:

"1. When the subjects were resting in a supine position after smoking two standard cigarets or French ashless cigaret paper with standard tobacco or standard cigarets in the British cigaret filter holder the cutaneous temperatures of the extremities of all the subjects decreased. In contrast, when two corn silk cigarets were smoked there was little if any change of the cutaneous temperatures of the extremities.

"2. When fully clothed normal subjects were sitting or engaged in slow walking, the temperatures of the extremities also decreased to the same degree after the smoking of two standard cigarets as while the subjects were in a resting, supine position.

"3. An increase of the basal metabolic rate occurred after the smoking of two standard cigarets, whereas the rate decreased after the smoking of two corn silk cigarets.

"4. Consistent changes of the electrocardiographic tracing developed after the smoking of two standard cigarets. The changes consisted in an increase of heart rate and a lowering of the amplitude of the T wave. Such changes were negligible after the smoking of corn silk cigarets.

"5. When saline solution was given intravenously previous to the intravenous injection of nicotine there was at first a slight drop of the cutaneous temperatures of the extremities, but when nicotine was added to the solution the decrease was rapid and pronounced. After the injection of nicotine the electrocardiographic t r a c i n g demonstrated a definite increase of heart rate and a lowering of the T waves even greater than that seen after the subjects had smoked two standard cigarets.

"6. There was an increase of blood pressure and pulse rate after either the smoking of two standard cigarets or the intravenous injection of 2 mg. of nicotine. After the smoking of two corn silk cigarets there was little or no change of blood pressure and pulse rate.

"7. While some subjects may show a parallelism between hyper-reaction to the cold pressor test and hyper-sensitiveness to tobacco, many other persons may hyper-react to one or the other alone."[6]

The following story not only serves as a striking illustration but coming from a great clinician and a renowned surgeon, it is of special medical interest. Soon after the death of Harvey Cushing the author was informed by Llwellys F. Barker of Johns Hopkins that Cushing requested him to come up to Yale to see him. When Barker arrived, Cushing said, "Barker, these surgeons want to amputate my foot. I am not going to let them do it. I will quit smoking." Barker said that Cushing gave up cigarets and got so much better, the amputation was unnecessary and he lived to die later of coronary occlusion. If patients could stop smoking as easily as Joe Lewis stopped Schmelling, our problem would be solved.

BIBLIOGRAPHY

1. Castiglioni, Arturo: Tobacco in Europe. Ciba Symposia, Vol. 4, Nos. 11 and 12, page 1443. February, March, 1943.
2. Burton, Robert: The Anatomy of Melancholy. Vol. 2, page, 228, 1932.
3. Castiglioni, Arturo: Tobacco in Europe. Ciba Symposia, Vol. 4, Nos. 11 and 12, page 1449. February, March, 1943.
4. Roth, Grace M.; McDonald, John B.; Sheard, Charles: The Effect of Smoking Cigarets. J.A.M.A., Vol. 125, No. 11, page 761. July 15, 1944.
5. Roth, Grace M.; McDonald, John B.; Sheard, Charles: The Effect of Smoking Cigarets. J.A.M.A., Vol. 125, No. 11, page 767. July 15, 1944.
6. Roth, Grace M.; McDonald, John B.; Sheard, Charles: The Effect of Smoking Cigarets. J.A.M.A., Vol. 125, No. 11, page 767. July 15, 1944.

THE POETRY OF TOBACCO
PRO AND CON
Savory Seasoning for Science

Little tube of mighty power,
Charmer of an idle hour.
    —Issac H. Browne

O thou weed,
Who art so lovely fair, and smell'st so sweet,
That the sense aches at thee, would thou hadst ne-er
    been born!
    —Shakespeare.—Othello, Act 4, 2
    (not so applied by Shakespeare.)

Yes, social friend, I love thee well,
    In learned doctor's spite;
Thy clouds all other clouds dispel,
    And lap me in delight.
        —C. Sprague—Tony Cigar.

Sweet, when the morn is gray,
Sweet, when they've cleared away
Lunch; and at close of day
Possibly sweetest.
    —C. S. Calverley—Ode to Tobacco.

Sublime tobacco! which, from east to west,
Cheers the tar's labour or the Turk man's rest.
    —Byron—The Island, 2, 19.

Like other charmers, wooing the caress
More dazzlingly when daring in full dress;
Yet thy true lovers more admire by far
Thy naked beauties—give me a cigar.
    Byron—Ib.

You abuse snuff! Perhaps it is the final cause of the
    human nose.
        Coleridge—Table Talk (Jan. 4, 1823.)

For thy sake, tobacco, I
Would do anything but die.
        —Lamb—Farewell to Tobacco

Ods me! I marvel what pleasure of felicity they have in taking their roguish tobacco. It is good for nothing but to choke a man, and fill him full of smoke and embers.
    —Ben Johnson—Every Man in his Humour, Act 3,3

James the First was a knave, a tyrant, a fool, a liar, a coward; but I love him, I worship him, because he slit the throat of that blackguard Raleigh, who invented this filthy smoking.
    —Swinburne—Spoken in the Arts Club

Pernicious weed! whose scent the fair annoys,
Unfriendly to society's chief joys,
Thy worst effect is banishing for hours,
The sex whose presence civilises ours.
        Cowper—Conversation

Tobacco is a filthy weed—
    I like it!
It satisfies no normal need—
    I like it!
It makes you grow both thin and lean,
It takes the hair right off your bean,
It's the worst darned stuff I've ever seen.
    I like it!
    —Anon.—American College Magazine, 1919

NED R. SMITH

On August 18, Dr. Ned R. Smith of Tulsa passed over the shining horizon. His obituary, which appears in this issue of the Journal sets forth his sterling qualities and highlights his professional and social career.

For a period of approximately four years he was a member of the Editorial Board where he served with distinction, giving of his time and talent for the benefit of the State Medical Association without remuneration. Because of his broad knowledge, sound judgment and wise council, his services were of great value to the Editorial Board and to the common cause for which the Journal stands.

Every doctor in the State is indebted to this departed champion of a great profession.

ASSOCIATION ACTIVITIES

ADVISORY COMMITTEE TO VOCATIONAL AND REHABILITATION DIVISION MEETS

The Advisory Committee to the Vocational and Rehabilitation Division met in the Executive Office of the Association on Sunday, August 13. The Committee is composed of the following: Clinton Gallaher, Shawnee, Chairman; Bert F. Keltz, Oklahoma City; James O. Asher, Clinton; Ennis M. Gullatt, Ada; Harry D. Murdock, Tulsa; Mr. Bert Loy, Oklahoma City.

This was the Committee's first meeting and Dr. Gallaher, Chairman, outlined the purposes after which Mr. Scurlock, Director of the Rehabilitation, and Miss Carr, Medical Social Worker, presented the various problems to be considered. A brochure was presented to all members of the Committee. It was decided that the Committee was to meet monthly either in the Office of the Department of Rehabilitation or the Oklahoma State Medical Association Office. The next meeting is to be called on September 3.

EXECUTIVE SECRETARY OF ASSOCIATION VISITS COUNTY SOCIETIES

Mr. Paul H. Fesler, Executive Secretary of the Association, has recently visited the Secretaries of the Medical Societies at Enid, Ponca City, Stillwater, Tulsa and Bartlesville.

Mr. Fesler surveyed the hospital facilities in these cities for the Post-War Planning Committee.

At a meeting of the Washington-Nowata County Society the following problems were discussed: Prepaid Medical Plan, Post-War Planning, Post-graduate courses after the War and other pertinent problems.

NEW COUNCIL ROOM AND LIBRARY COMPLETED

All members of the Association are cordially invited to visit the Council Room and Library at the Executive Office, 210 Plaza Court, Oklahoma City, Oklahoma.

The Oklahoma Hospital Association used the new room for a meeting on August 25.

HENRY H. TURNER RECEIVES HONORARY APPOINTMENT

In recognition of a series of lectures in endocrinology given in the Medical School and Academy of Medicine in Mexico City last April, Dr. Henry Turner, Oklahoma City, has been honored with the appointment as "Professor Extraordinario" of the National University of Mexico.

Dr. Turner also has received an invitation to participate in the Eighth Medical Week in Monterey, Mexico, September 3-9.

Captain Charles Donovan Tool (Class of 1931) has been awarded the Distinguished Service Cross "for extraordinary heroism in action on March 18, 1944, in the vicinity of Cassino, Italy." He has been returned to the States and is now assigned to the Bushnell General Hospital, Brigham City, Utah, recovering from wounds received in the battle of Cassino.

Captain Tool is a member of the Faculty of the Medical school and served in the capacity of Assistant in medicine before entering the Service.

TO AID THE WAR EFFORT, AMERICAN COLLEGE OF SURGEONS CANCELS 1944 CLINICAL CONGRESS

The American College of Surgeons, upon action of its Board of Regents, has cancelled its Annual Clinical Congress because of the acute war situation that has developed, involving greater demands than at any time in the past upon our transportation systems for the carrying of wounded military personnel, troops, and war material. The Congress was to have been held in Chicago, October 24 to 27.

Dr. Irvin Abell of Louisville, Chairman of the Board of Regents, in making the announcement, said that this action was taken after consultation with officials in Washington. Some of the replies which were received from these officials read in part as follows:

From Major General T. Kirk, Surgeon General, United States Army:

"Naturally, we all like these meetings to be held and to attend them. However, from an official standpoint I must say we are needing more and more railroad transportation to move our battle casualties from the ports to our hospitals. And there are still many troops in the United States who require railroad transportation to ports in order to get them overseas. In addition, difficulty is being experienced in obtaining the necessary material to continue the battle. This means transportation for the raw materials that go into munitions and the shipping of these munitions to the ports after they are fabricated. Each month the need for this material overseas is increasing rather than diminishing.

"The war is far from won and I think we should all consider the war effort rather than the satisfaction of our individual desires. That should give us the answer. After seeing the bomb craters and destroyed homes, factories and transportation facilities in Europe, I am not surprised that this nation feels it is far removed from war and that the war is about over. It isn't."

From R. H. Clare, Assistant Director, Passenger Section, Division of Traffic Movement, Office of Defense Transportation:

"This office cannot attempt to evaluate the importance or the essentiality of any particular meeting. We have attempted to clearly portray the present critical transportation situation. The transportation requirements of the armed forces are not at present being entirely satisfied. At the same time, soldiers and sailors on leave from duty overseas are unable to secure Pullman accomodations to their homes and frequently have to stand in coaches for considerable distances. The responsibility, therefore, rests upon the officers of your organization to determine if, in the light of these conditions, you should go through with your Chicago meeting.

"I believe you will agree that the Office of Defense Transportation cannot attempt to make this decision for you. We assure you that there is an urgent need for the curtailment of convention travel in order to clear the transportation channels of the country for the movement of military and essential civilian travel. We, therefore, ask you for your serious consideration of our appeal in the light of this situation."

Feeling that the many factors in favor of holding the Clinical Congress, however important, are less vital than the assurance of adequate transportation so far as possible for the conveying of troops and war material, the Ameri-

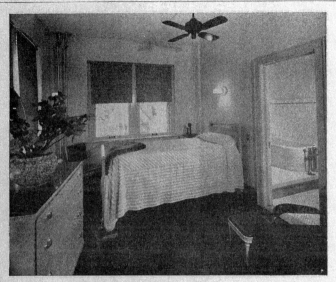

can College of Surgeons willingly cancels, for the third successive years, its annual meeting, in order to aid the war effort. The Regents recognize that there is a great burden on the members of the surgical profession in their local communities as the result of the large proportion of the profession which is serving with the armed forces. They also take cognizance of the desire of the profession to do nothing which would interfere with the successful prosecution of the war program, such as would be caused by the temporary absence of its members from duties during the period of Congress. More than three thousand surgeons and some two thousand hospital representatives usually attend the Clinical Congress.

At the annual meeting of the Board of Regents which will be held later in the year, fellowship in the College will be conferred *in absentia* on the class of initiates of 1944, as there will be no Convocation exercises. At the same time the list of hospitals, cancer clinics, medical services in industry, hospitals conducting programs of graduate training in surgery, and medical motion pictures, that meet the College standards, will be approved and later published.

All present Officers, Regents, Governors, and Standing Committees will continue in office.

War conditions permitting, the Clinical Congress will be held in the fall of 1945.

22nd ANNUAL FALL CLINICAL CONFERENCE OF THE KANSAS CITY SOUTHWEST CLINICAL SOCIETY

The Kansas City Southwest Clinical Society announces its Annual Conference, October 2, 3, 4, 1944, Municipal Auditorium, Kansas City, Missouri.

A list of distinguished guest speakers will be found elsewhere in this issue of the Journal. Their scientific presentations will be made before the general assemblies.

Symposia on the following systems will be presented by members of the society; gastrointestinal, obstetrics, pediatrics, cardiovascular, urogenital, headache and backache.

The meeting will open Monday morning with a Round Table Discussion on the Newer Things in Medicine as portrayed by the participating guest speakers.

A copy of the Kansas City Medical Journal, carrying the entire program will be mailed you upon request—208 Shukert Bldg., Kansas City 6, Mo.

One of the most ennobling attributes of greatness in medical men is their amazing unselfishness. Medical genius never seeks its own. Schopenhauer states: ''The ordinary men have their own interests in mind and as a rule know how to advance them, because they adapt themselves to their own times, ready to serve the requirements and notions of contemporaries. For this reason they generally live in happy circumstances, but the genius sacrifices his personal welfare to a great objective purpose. He cannot do otherwise because his heart and soul are embodied in this purpose. The great mass does otherwise. That's why they are small, but the genius is altruistic, that's why he is great.—Master Minds in Medicine. John C. Hemmeter. Pages 130-131. New York Life Press. 1927.

Medical School Notes

Miss Kathlyn Krammes, Superintendent of Nurses and Director of the School of Nursing, has been granted a leave of absence beginning August 1, 1944, for the purpose of taking graduate work leading to the Master's Degree at the University of Washington, Seattle. Miss Krammes has been awarded a Federal Scholarship under the Bolton Act.

Mrs. Clara Wolfe Jones, Educational Director of the School of Nursing, will serve as Director of the School and Superintendent of Nurses during the absence of Miss Krammes.

The Women Commandos, Radio Program of WKY under the sponsorship of Julie Bennell, have given $25.00 to the Crippled Children's Hospital for birthday parties. The Women Commandos furnish the money for gifts and refreshments for the birthday parties each month at the Crippled Children's Hospital, and expect to make this a permanent custom. This is the second check that has been donated this year.

Dr. Howard C. Hopps has been appointed Professor of Pathology and Chairman of the Department effective September 1, 1944. Dr. Hopps received the M.D. degree from the University of Oklahoma School of Medicine in 1937, interned at Evanston Hospital, Evanston, Illinois, and subsequently became connected with the Department of Pathology of the University of Chicago as Assistant Professor of Pathology.

Dr. Louis Alvin Turley after many years of faithful service to the medical school has been made Professor Emeritus of Pathology effective September 1, 1944. Dr. Turley will continue his connection with the School of Medicine doing research and other work.

Miss Mary Leidigh has been serving as Administrative Dietitian, University Hospital, since July 24, 1944. Miss Leidigh received the degree of Bachelor of Science from Texas Technological College, Lubbock, Texas, and the Masters' Degree from the University of Texas. She has served as Dietitian of Texas Technological College Dormitory System, as head of the Home Economics Department of Panhandle A. & M. College, Goodwell, Oklahoma, and as Area Supervisor with the Community School Lunch Program with headquarters at Ft. Worth.

Miss Ruby Wortham, Instructor in Histology, has resigned her position to go to the University of Washington, Seattle. Miss Wortham has been with the School of Medicine since 1939.

Lt. N. F. Vander Barkett, Class of 1939, has just been released from active duty with the United States Army after having served fourteen months in the Medical

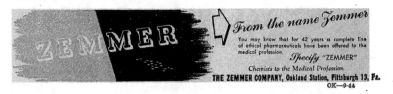

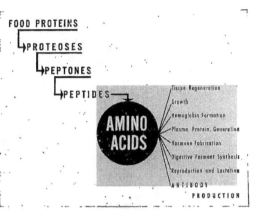

Corps. For the past year Lt. Barkett has been on the Surgical Staff of the Finney General Hospital, Thomasville, Georgia.

Lt. and Mrs. Barkett and their young son are establishing a home in Oklahoma City and he will practice in this vicinity.

Commencement Exercises for the School of Medicine and the School of Nursing will be held in the Auditorium of Oklahoma City University, Friday, September 15, at 8 P.M. Fifty-six medical students expect to receive the degree of Doctor of Medicine and 23 young women the Diploma of Graduate Nurse.

The medical profession is cordially invited to be present at these exercises.

• OBITUARIES •

Ned R. Smith, M.D.
1884-1944

Dr. Ned R. Smith, Tulsa, died on August 18 at St. John's Hospital in Tulsa. Death was attributed to a heart ailment from which he suffered about a year ago. He had been in the hospital since June 25, although a previous illness had sent him to the hospital last year. However, in recent months, Dr. Smith has been able to carry on his duties at the hospital.

Dr. Smith, a native of Bethany, Missouri, received his education at the University of Michigan where he held five degrees, a record for that institution. He came to Tulsa in 1928 from Halstead, Kansas, where he had been in charge of neurology and psychiatry at the Dr. Hertzler Clinic. He established an office at 703 Medical Arts Bldg. where he carried on his practice until the time of his death. In 1931 he turned the former Oklahoma Hospital into a sanitarium and two years later took over the Oakwood Sanitarium.

Within the past week, Dr. Smith was re-elected President of the City Board of Health. For a year he served as psychiatrist at the Tulsa Induction Center. He was on the staff at St. John's and Hillcrest Memorial Hospitals and taught neurology and psychiatry for ten years. Dr. Smith was on the Editorial Board of the Journal of the Oklahoma State Medical Association. He was a member of the Kiwanis Club, the American Medical Association, the American Psychiatric Association, Southern Medical Association, Tulsa County Medical Society, of which he was a past president and trustee, a 32nd degree Mason and Shriner and a member of the Chamber of Commerce.

Surviving are the widow, Mrs. Pluma Delore Smith of the home at Sand Springs, a daughter Mrs. Rawlins E. Haber, Tulsa and two sons, Lt. Col. William T. Smith, stationed in Alaska and Lt. Edward R. Smith, stationed in France.

Services were held on August 22 at the First Christian Church with Rev. J. Edgar Wright officiating. The body was shipped to Kansas City for cremation.

W. J. Mason. M.D.
1866-1944

Dr. W. J. Mason, Lawton, died on July 13 at his home after having been ill since the middle of January and bedfast for the past month.

Dr. Mason was born July 6, 1866 at Gasconade County Missouri and was educated at the St. Louis University, St. Louis. In 1918, he moved to Lawton where he remained until 1937 when he retired from active practice and moved to Springdale Arkansas. After living there four years, he and his family returned to Lawton where he re-established his practice.

Dr. Mason was a member of the Oklahoma State Medical Association, the American Medical Association and various civic organizations.

Surviving are three daughters Mrs. Edith Liles, Pocasset; Mrs. Blanche Needham, San Miguel, California and Mrs. Louise Mason, Oklahoma City; a stepson, Ed Blazier, Wichita, Kansas and two step daughters Mrs. R. F. Brown, Enid and Mrs. Janette LaGrone, Minneapolis, Minn.

Classified Advertisements

In judging the role and function of great men, particularly great men of science, we can reach a degree of clearness in understanding by holding in mind three perspectives: First, the degree in which the work, labors, and endeavors of the great men have met the hitherto uncontrolled forces of nature subservient to man. Secondly, the extent to which the work of the great man has advanced human culture. Thirdly, the extent to which the work of the great man has advanced human civilization.—Master Minds in Medicine. John C. Hemmeter. Page 212. New York Medical Life Press. 1927.

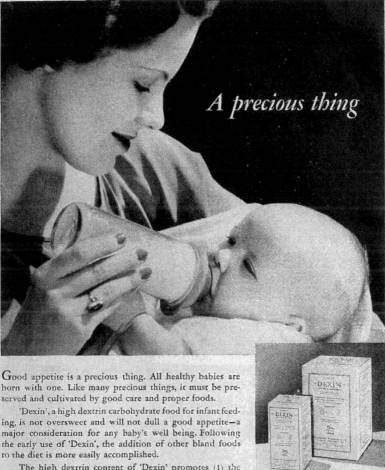

A precious thing

Good appetite is a precious thing. All healthy babies are born with one. Like many precious things, it must be preserved and cultivated by good care and proper foods.

'Dexin', a high dextrin carbohydrate food for infant feeding, is not oversweet and will not dull a good appetite—a major consideration for any baby's well being. Following the early use of 'Dexin', the addition of other bland foods to the diet is more easily accomplished.

The high dextrin content of 'Dexin' promotes (1) the formation of soft, flocculent, easily digested curds, and (2) diminishes intestinal fermentation and the tendency to colic and diarrhea. 'Dexin' is readily soluble in hot or cold milk.

'Dexin' Reg. U. S. Patent Office

'Dexin' does make a difference

| COMPOSITION | Dextrins | . . . . . | 75% | Mineral Ash | . | 0.25% |
| | Maltose | . . . . . | 24% | Moisture | . . | 0.75% |

Available carbohydrate 99%   115 calories per ounce
6 level packed tablespoonfuls equal 1 ounce

'DEXIN'
HIGH DEXTRIN CARBOHYDRATE

Literature on request

BURROUGHS WELLCOME & CO. (U.S.A. INC.) 9-11 E. 41st St., New York 17, N. Y.

STATE HEALTH DEPARTMENT

All physicians and hospitals in the State of Oklahoma whose practice includes obstetrics or pediatrics have had some experience with the Federal Emergency Maternity and Infant Care Program. Many practitioners undoubtedly wonder why the Oklahoma State Health Department has undertaken to administer this program. Many will probably also question some of the stringent rules and regulations concerned with this program. We quote some pertinent excerpts from the Emergency Act of the U. S. Congress of March 18, 1943 which will answer some of the questions which naturally involve some experiences with this program:

"For Grants to States to provide medical, nursing and hospital maternity and infant care for the wives and infants of enlisted men in the armed forces of the fourth, fifth, sixth and seventh grades under allotments by the Secretary of Labor and plans developed and administered by the State Health Departments and approved by the Chief of the Children's Bureau of the U. S. Department of Labor." We further quote pertinent excerpts from regulations and administrative rules of the U. S. Children's Bureau: "Services may be authorized when at the time of application the individual is the wife or an infant under one year, of an enlisted man in the fourth, fifth, sixth, or seventh pay grade. Service is without financial investigation and without cost to the patient or family the attending physician has agreed to accept payment only from the State Health Department for services authorized, the hospital has agreed to accept payment only from the State Health Department at the per diem rate or the established rate paid by the State Health Department and when it is understood that the patient or family cannot be required by a physician or hospital to pay for any part of either medical or hospital care to be authorized."

Since the beginning of this program in Oklahoma, May 6, 1943, and with the exception of two months during which the program was discontinued, the Oklahoma State Health Department has authorized under this act approximately 13,000 cases for maternity care. Our records show that 91 per cent of these cases are hospitalized, 3 per cent are delivered by practitioners other than doctors of medicine. Average cost per case is approximately $83.00 Nine per cent of deliveries occur in the home. The approximate annual expenditures for these services to physicians and hospitals in the State of Oklahoma is $1,000,000.00. The Children's Bureau Regulations provide that the expenditures of these funds must be in accordance with the State Laws. This means that the individual or organization providing any services under this Act must file claims in duplicate, duly notarized and sworn to in accordance with State Laws and filed with the State Health Department. The present procedure for processing these claims under the State Law requires at the minimum approximately thirty days. Approximately 2,500 claims are handled monthly by the Oklahoma State Health Department. (Approximately 1,250 to physicians and 1,250 to hospitals.)

"The administration of the 'EMIC' program is governed by the law and the funds available, and these factors are responsible for the difficulties and misunderstandings in part, but not entirely. The State Board of Health has had to call entirely upon its own limited resources to build up a large clerical and accounting staff when all types of personnel are at a premium, and to establish an administrative set-up without precedence in public health services. Every worker involved has felt duty bound to strive unstintingly, and all have put in many hours uncompensated overtime; but even with such a mighty effort, it has been difficult to keep up with a seemingly tidal wave of applications, queries, and correspondence. This, also, has undoubtedly added a measure to the confusion. Nevertheless, progress has been made, and all concerned have been sustained by the knowledge that they are working hand in hand with the physicians, nurses, and hospitals in a program to sustain the morale of the armed forces."

The physicians of our State, in particular, have contributed their skill generously and in return for only moderately recompense, to this wartime program for the families of our fighting men.

Oklahoma State Health Department.

Certain views have found wide acceptance to the effect that the collective effort of the masses has been of decisive influence in science as well as to progress in general. The collective energy is regarded as the decisive impulse in the development of medicine. Let us attack with sober historical method such doctrinaire constructive philosophizing which befuddles "modern" thinking. It will then become apparent that the assumption of a progress distilled from the instinct of the masses is a mere fiction. Real medical scientific progress cannot be produced by "communis opinio" or mass suggestions. Such progress demands intense effort of specially trained individuals, who obtain their guiding ideas from the intuitive genius of creative leaders.—Karl Sudhoff. Master Minds in Medicine. John C. Hemmeter. Page xxv-xxvi. New York Medical Life Press. 1927.

Great men are comparable to the gyroscope, because of their marvellous sense of orientation concerning specific scientific tendencies. Whenever the mass or even the professor deviates and errs from its correct direction, the great man undertakes to bring them back to the right road. This is not only true of science, but also of religion and philosophy. It is not necessary for great men to produce a great discovery, originate a doctrine, write great books to become great. Some of the greatest medical men are those who have left no such records.—Master Minds in Medicine. John C. Hemmeter. Page 131. New York Medical Life Press. 1927.

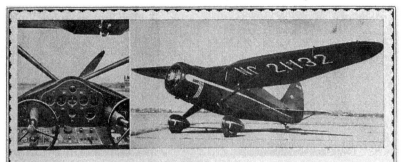
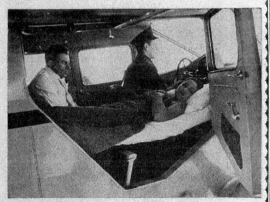
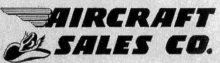

..and Morale

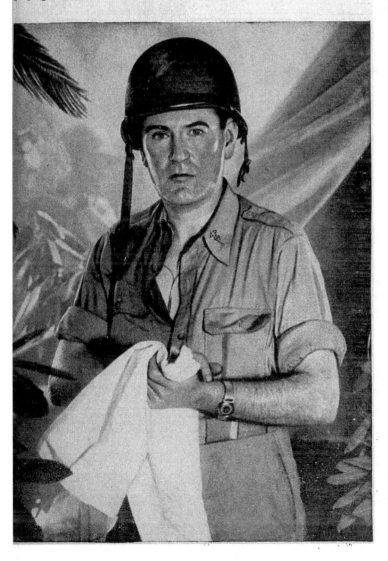

★ FIGHTIN' TALK ★

(*Note: Have been writing this column for some time and each month the number of letters received is smaller. Have had no letters for several weeks and it is becoming difficult to maintain the column—don't you want it anymore? If you do, please let's have some news.*)

Captain Woodrow L. Pickhardt found to be German Prisoner

In the August issue of the Journal, CAPTAIN WOODROW L. PICKHARDT, Lawton, was reported as missing in action. On August 16, the following wire was received by Mrs. Pickhardt, Lawton: "A report just received through the International Red Cross states that your husband Captain Woodrow L. Pickhardt, is a prisoner of war of the German government."

Captain Pickhardt was reported missing June 7, the day after the Western Front Invasion. His wife had received no word since the War Department message of June 30.

LT. JOHN H. BAKER, JR., Eufaula, has been ordered to active duty. He expects to leave soon and will report to an army hospital in Pennsylvania.

Captain Felix Adams, Vinita, Released by Nazis

One of the miracles of warfare was the capture, release and survival of CAPTAIN FELIX ADAMS, Vinita, by the Germans. Captain Adams survived the fire of the Germans as his parachute descended on French soil. He was shuttled around by the Nazis as they retreated under deadly American artillery shelling and is still active after the German refusal to yield to the Allied demands resulting in the intense blasting of Cherbourg from the air while Captain Adams was performing operations on wounded soldiers.

After being captured, Captain Adams was forced to care for the German wounded. After his release he was sent to a hospital in England to receive treatment for an injured knee and for flak wounds in his hand.

COLONEL DANIEL L. PERRY, Cushing, former member of the 45th Division, now with the Medical Corps in the Pacific, has recently been promoted from the rank of Lt. Colonel. He is commanding officer of an Evacuation Hospital "somewhere in New Guinea."

Colonel Perry practiced in Cushing prior to entering the Army. He, with Colonel Davidson, helped to organize the original Company A of the Oklahoma National Guards in the Cushing area.

CAPTAIN EDWIN C. YEARY, Oklahoma City, was on the first glider which landed on D-Day with a surgical team aboard. Their job was to establish a clearing station for battle casualties. Captain Yeary states that establishing the clearing station had to wait for a few hours as there were American wounded to be taken care of on the field where the gliders had landed. Enemy patrols were active and snipers were plentiful.

Captain Yeary received his medical degree from the University of Oklahoma in 1939 and served his internship at the University Hospital, Iowa City, Iowa, being called to active service on June 15, 1941.

Major Clinton S. Maupin Reported Japanese Prisoner

MAJOR CLINTON S. MAUPIN, Waurika, has been a prisoner of war in Japanese prison Camp No. 1, Cabanatuan, Phillippines, since he was captured on Bataan. Major Maupin sent a card in which he said that he

is in excellent health and is looking forward to seeing his family again soon.

Major Maupin graduated from the University of Oklahoma School of Medicine in 1934.

Captain H. Myles Johnson Receives Citation

CAPTAIN H. MYLES JOHNSON, Fort Supply, is attached to the famous Seagrave Hospital Unit headed by Lt. Col. Gordon S. Seagrave, author of the book, "Burma Surgeon." The Unit is with General Stilwell's forces who are clearing northern Burma so that American Engineers can extend the Ledo road to the Burma road. Captain Johnson is credited with helping to save the lives of 2,000 Chinese soldiers on the battlefields. He has been in China, Burma, India Theater of War for 26 months. Soon after the Myitkyina Airfield was captured by American and Chinese troops, the Seagrave Unit moved in and Captain Johnson was one of the first doctors on hand to take care of the wounded.

He received a special citation from Brig. Gen. W. L. Boatner on May 29, 1944, which reads as follows: "During this period he was under constant enemy fire, making his way over the most difficult of jungle terrain and, with utter disregard for personal safety, administered to the medical needs of both Chinese and American patients. The splendid performance of duty and disregard for personal safety reflects credit on his organization and the espirit de corps of the United States Army."

Captain Johnson attended school at Fort Supply and was graduated from the University of Oklahoma School of Medicine in 1940. He served his internship in Denver, Colorado and enlisted in the Army before Pearl Harbor in 1941. He sailed in March, 1942, and has never seen his daughter who was born in July, 1942. Captain Johnson's father, H. L. Johnson, is Assistant Superintendent of the Western Oklahoma Hospital at Fort Supply.

Major Ralph W. Hubbard Writes From Jap Prison Camp

MAJOR RALPH W. HUBBARD, Oklahoma City, had not been heard from since December, 1943, until the following card which was received by Mrs. Hubbard in August: "Health good. My love to you, the boys and entire family. One radiogram was inspiration. Do not worry this is only temporary. Am well and will soon be with you."

Major Hubbard was taken prisoner at the fall of Bataan where he was attached to a base hospital. His brother, Captain William E. Hubbard, a flight surgeon stationed with a bomber group in Australia, was recently awarded the Soldier's Medal for heroism. His father, Major John C. Hubbard is stationed at Fort Sill and another brother, Major John R. Hubbard is serving in India.

The following excerpt is taken from a letter received in the Executive Office from MAJOR C. G. STUARD, Tulsa:

"After being on duty with the Army for over three years and with many doctors from all sections of the country, one can safely say that no apologies are needed for the training that men from Oklahoma receive. The Army, like politics, makes strange bed fellows but I have yet to see a man from Oklahoma who could not make the proper adjustment and meet the situation.

"This is a processing station for overseas troops both for officers and enlisted men. I have been hoping that some of the Oklahoma M.D.'s in the A.A.F. who

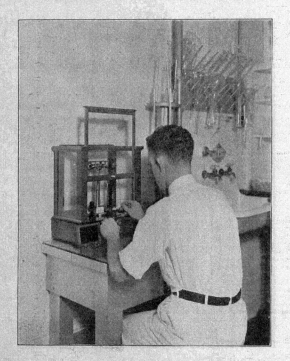

are preparing for overseas might come through and look me up.''

CAPTAIN WILLIAM E. HUBBARD, Oklahoma City, a flight surgeon now stationed with a bomber group in Australia, has been awarded the Soldier's Medal for heroism. He described the incident to his mother as follows:

''It was in January that I was up for an early morning takeoff for a combat mission. This airplane had taken off. Captain Glass and I were standing around shooting the breeze as usual, waiting for them to come over the field in formation as is our custom in case something happens.

''We noticed this airplane at the end of the strip flying for a crash landing. He came in for a landing without landing gear or flaps and all props turning but accidentally struck some parked aircraft at the end of the strip.

''While the fire was immense, full load of gasoline, and the ammunition was exploding, my boys and I made a search close to the fire for anyone who might be alive, although we considered the possibility very slight. We did find two boys still breathing but burned seriously and with multiple injuries. We dragged them out and headed for the hospital. Neither of them lived very long.

''Probably all of this will be censored, but it was so long ago now, I think it migh go through. I wanted my two enlisted men to have the medal, but for myself I wasn't very eager. The only thing I want to wear is to again have the privilege of wearing a blue suit and a red tie.''

Institute of Neuropsychiatry Announces New Offices

The Institute for Neuropsychiatry, formerly the Coyne Campbell Clinic, announces the removal of its offices from 131 N. E. 4th St., Oklahoma, Oklahoma (the Coyne-Campbell Sanitarium) to Suite 1212 Medical Arts Bldg., Oklahoma City. Office hours by appointment.

Journal Explains There is no Such Disease As 'Jungle Rot'

Apparently there is no such disease as ''jungle rot,'' *The Journal of the American Medical Association* for August 26 advises in answer to a query.

''The United States Army Medical Department,'' *The Journal* says, ''has no information concerning the disease called 'jungle rot.' Perhaps the term applies to a condition known as 'Bareco rot,' which is a synoym for 'desert sore' or 'veld sore.' . . .

''From Panama comes information that the terms 'jungle rot' and 'tropical rot' are used by laymen to describe any sort of sore developing on the body, usually a severe form of . . . fungus, mold or yeast infection.''

Journal Points to Increasing Danger of Rabies

''Throughout the country the reported increase of rabies in dogs is a cause of mounting concern.'' *The Journal of the American Medical Association* for August 26 says. ''Control measures have been instituted in many areas, including parts of southern California, eighteen Michigan counties, St. Louis, the environs of Baltimore and Newport, Ky. Reports from indiana and the Bronx indicate an increase in the number of rabid dogs and of persons bitten by rabid dogs. If still more serious outbreaks are to be forestalled, such well known preventive measures as muzzling, incarceration and destruction of stray animals, and restraining of all awned dogs by leash, will doubtless have to be undertaken in many other communities.''

They weren't trained so well for the civil war. That is why the casualty reports so often read: ''Died of exhaustion.''

Hitler beside himself in a double suicide pact would be a Wagnerian finish.

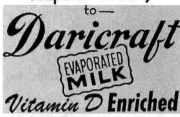
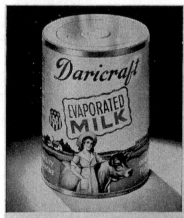

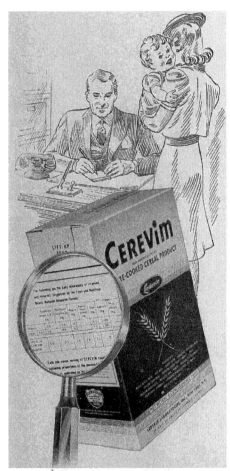
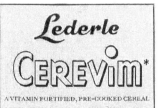
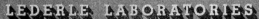

POINTS TO NEED OF AUGMENTING OUR REHABILITATION SERVICES

Doctor Says Health Resorts can be Utilized in Rehabilitation of Industrial and Other Civilian As Well as Military Casualties

Civilian hospitals as well as military hospitals must augment their rehabilitation services greatly and our American health resorts can be utilized to advantage for the rehabilitation of industrial and other civilian as well as military casualties. Frank H. Krusen, M.D., Rochester, Minn., declares in the Journal of the American Medical Association for July 29.

"It is undoubtedly a fact," Dr. Krusen says, "that we are now facing the most stupendous problem in rehabilitation which has ever existed in the history of the world.

"The number of war injuries sustained in the Army and Navy and also in industrial and other civilian pursuits will be the largest our country has ever known. Adequate utilization of our national health resorts will assist materially in solving our rehabilitation problems.

He points out that steps to meet this problem already have been taken by both the Army and Navy and also that civilian hospitals are beginning to consider plans for the rehabilitation of injured industrial workers and civilians in other fields. The importance of rehabilitation centers of the health resort type is emphasized by the British experience in this field, Dr. Krusen says. He tells of the care of an air gunner "who remained in a civilian orthopedic hospital for treatment of a torn and displaced semilunar cartilage (of the knee) for ten months and who was still totally incapacitated even though the diagnosis had been correct, a skillful operation had been performed, there had been no surgical complication and he was receiving daily massage. He limped, he did not cooperate, and he was depressed. He had been told that 'the nerve to his knee had been cut.' Then he was transferred to one of the orthopedic rehabilitation centers of the Royal Air Force medical service.

"Watson Jones (in a recent issue of the British Medical Journal) described subsequent events as follows: 'He saw the sky, the sea, the open spaces. For many months he had seen only the stone walls of many corridors. His new surroundings were different: there was a lounge and a writing room, tasteful decorations and flowers, a menu which was varied and excellent, an atmosphere of well being and contentment. After a few days he smiled. There was sometimes a sparkle in his eye. Within a week he sensed the spirit of optimism. It grew upon him and he was reassured. His difficulties were explained and he was taught special exercises. He learned to walk, then to run. He became an enthusiast and worked hard. He worked in the gym, played on the fields, swam in the pool, cycled on the track. Time raced past, for he was busy. He attended lectures, played billiards and went to concerts. He became bronzed and fit. He laughed and was full of the joy of life. In seven weeks he reurned to his unit and to full duty. He forgot about the 'nerve in his knee.'

" 'Ten months—total incapacity; seven weeks—full recovery.'

"What better argument could one present for the importance of the health resort in rehabilitation of the disabled? Watson Jones has stressed the fact that this is not an isolated case but is 'typical of the experience of many victims of bone and joint injury."

Dr. Krusen describes some of the work that is being done, at several of the rehabilitation hospitals of the Army and the Navy. The effectiveness of the program is illustrated by his comments on the program at the Army's Fitzsimmons General Hospital, Denver.

"Convalescent care of these patients,' he says, "includes drill, calisthenics and gymnastic sports such as volley ball, basketball and football signal practice. The convalescent patients who require physical therapy report regularly to the physical therapy clinic for treat-

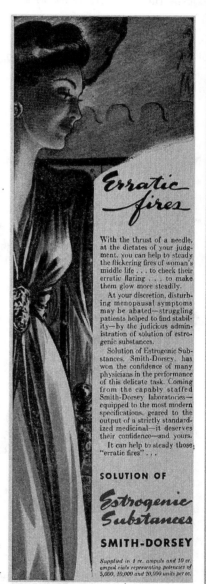

Insulin action *timed* to the needs of the day

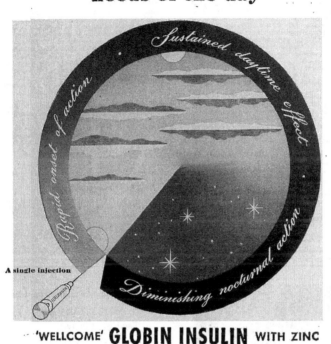

A single injection

'WELLCOME' GLOBIN INSULIN WITH ZINC

● As the diabetic goes through the day, his insulin requirements vary. 'Wellcome' Globin Insulin with Zinc provides an action timed to meet these changing needs. An injection in the morning is followed by rapid onset of action which is sustained for continued blood sugar control as the day wears on. Finally by night insulin action begins to wane, minimizing the occurrence of nocturnal reactions.

Many moderately severe and severe cases of diabetes may be controlled with only a single, daily injection of 'Wellcome' Globin Insulin with Zinc. This new long acting insulin is a clear solution of uniform potency. In its freedom from allergenic skin reaction, it is comparable to regular insulin. This advance in diabetic control was developed in the Wellcome Research Laboratories, Tuckahoe, N.Y. U.S. Pat. 2,161,198.

Vials of 10 cc.   80 units in 1 cc.

Literature on request

'Wellcome' Trademark Registered

BURROUGHS WELLCOME & CO. (U.S.A.) Inc. 9-11 E. 41st St., New York 17, N. Y.

ment. The therapeutic program is coordinated so that patients are kept busy most of the day.

"When patients are assigned to the convalescent ward program they are no longer under liberal hospital regulations but under strict military discipline. Surprisingly they prefer this strict supervision of regimentation to the liberal and somewhat relaxed discipline of the ordinary hospital ward. Most of the patients were in the surgical service and their morale improved materially when they were transferred to the convalescent-ward program. Interestingly, the patients on this program have exhibited a decided increase in the rate of progress toward recovery over the rate achieved when they were receiving only physical therapy. It is proposed to coordinate this convalescent ward plan with occupational therapy and work therapy. This is the type of program which undoubtedly will tend to improve morale and speed recovery. . . . "

Dr. Krusen says that the growing recognition of the rehabilitation problem by civilian hospitals is reflected in the fact that the Michael Reese Hospital in Chicago is contemplating an elaborate convalescent center which can serve this purpose.

He says that "Obviously a rehabilitation plan which is conducted at a health resort such as White Sulphur Springs (West Virginia, operated by the Army) of Glenwood Springs (Colorado, operated by the Navy) will tend to appeal to an injured man more than one conducted in less pleasant surroundings, and surely a well organized, properly administered scheme of treatment will be more likely to gain his cooperation than would the ordinary hospital routine.

"We can assume, therefore, that well developed rehabilitation programs at certain health resorts will have very definite places in treatment for injuries. The program is just beginning to take form, and it is to be hoped that it will continue to expand and grow.

"As the pattern becomes clearer and clearer, one can already catch glimpses of an almost ideal reconstruction regimen. All of us must strive to bring this program into sharp focus, giving to it our best health resorts, our most skillful rehabilitation workers and some of our finest executives. A lesser effort for the care of the injured defenders of our way of life cannot possibly be considered acceptable."

The progress of medicine is the history of the work of individuals and that is the principal reason why I have devoted this work to a description of a few selected master minds in medicine, in order to make it clearer to us by which mental operations and at what cost and effort our present knowledge of medicine has been attained.—Master Minds in Medicine. John C. Hemmeter. Page 10. New York Medical Life Press. 1927.

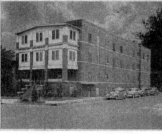
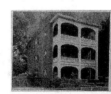

THE HOSPITALIZATION PROGRAM FOR VETERANS

At the end of the last war no provision had been made for the medical care of veterans returning from the service, and within a very short time it became evident that many of them had to be hospitalized. The only place available in Oklahoma was the University Hospital, and with the assistance of the American Legion and others a large number of beds was set aside for this purpose. Later, the Legislature provided for an administration building for the hospital, thereby releasing space for about 100 patients. This filled the gap until the Veterans Hospital at Muskogee was completed and even after most of the patients were transferred to Muskogee, it was necessary to set aside a ward at the University Hospital for 25 or 30 beds for the care of such patients. After 25 years, this ward is still in use at the expense of the State.

The same problem developed in connection with patients with mental conditions and tuberculosis. Special buildings were erected by the State at Norman for mental patients, and a special hospital was built at Sulphur for tuberculosis patients.

This same condition was true in other states, and because of the bad administration of the Veterans Bureau at that time some of the states were not reimbursed for the expenses involved.

There were 90,000 men from Oklahoma in the other war, whereby there are 250,000 in this war.

The men are now being discharged at the rate of 12 per hour, according to an editorial in the Los Angeles Examiner, and many of them because of physical disabilities, many of which are minor at present, but if not properly cared for may develop into serious conditions. In order that the men will have the best of care, many of them could and should be cared for in local hospitals or in special hospitals located in their home states. They should also be cared for by a physician of their choice.

In order that the men with physical disabilities may be properly classified, there should be a diagnostic center in states where the medical profession is organized to conduct such a center.

In most of the states, the medical profession is thoroughly competent to care for the average patient. The complicated cases should be kept in the Army, Navy, or Veterans Hospitals for care, but most of them could be transferred to facilities nearer home. These men and women want to get home, and while the government hospitals may be more elaborate and in some instances more efficient, those with experience know that if the patient is not satisfied, he will not respond as well as he will where he can be near his relatives and friends. The expense involved for relatives to visit the veterans in distant hospitals should also be considered.

In 1931 and 1932, the Veterans Administration was urged by the leaders in the medical and hospital professions to use local hospitals for acute conditions and to use the Veterans Hospitals for tuberculosis and mental conditions. If this policy had been followed, many of those with tuberculosis would be alive today, and many of those now occupying mental hospitals would be useful self-supporting members of society.

The best place for a sick man is as near home as possible where he can be cared for by those who know him best and are interested in him as an individual and not just as another patient.

In order to avoid the confusion following the last war, a resolution was passed by the American Legion Convention appealing to the Veterans' Administration to set up diagnostic facilities in Oklahoma. This is not a post war plan. The need is now present as men are being discharged at the rate of 2,000 per week, and more than 600,000 had been discharged on December 1 of last year.

The Oklahoma men have been active on all fronts, and we must see that not a single man in need of intelligent medical care is neglected.

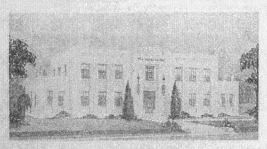

OL' DOC WAGONER

(Reprint)

Ol' Doc Wagoner has a prescription he wants to try out on you. It's Senate Bill No. 1161 to set up a government doctoring and hospital bureaucracy that would just about finish off the private doctor—and also the American's right to pick his own physician or to provide his own pills.

We have received several warnings against Ol' Doc's new concoction. It's no good for man or beast, for chills, fits or falling hair, we are told by a good many doctors.

Ol' Doc Wagoner's principal patients up to now have been labor unions. He prescribed for many baby unions and some of these bottle-fed infants grew up to be giants, flabby maybe, but fat. The labor press in its review of labor's status on last Labor Day, however didn't carry many testimonials for the Ol' Doc's sovereign remedy, the Wagoner Law. It seems the Ol' Doc's tonic pepped up the appetite all right, but what good is an appetite with OPA and WLB hanging 'round.

The Ol' Doc's new Golden Prescription calls for a bigger "social security" bite out of the worker's pay check so that the Surgeon General of the Public Health Service can spend $3,000,000,000 a year buying hospitals and hiring doctors.

The pay check is getting so frayed on the edges with withholding taxes and other "deducts" that a few more dog-ears won't leave enough space for the dollar mark.

Our guess is that the American people will never write a "Before and after Taking" testimonial for Ol' Doc Wagoner's socialized medicine. There just isn't going to be any taking.

Oh, yes, the Ol' Doc is an M.D. all right—Doctor of Meddling.

The reciprocal relation between the great master minds which the human race has produced and Society at large, has not received the concentrated study which this great problem deserves.—Master Minds in Medicine. John C. Hemmeter, Page vii. New York Medical Life Press. 1927.

The medical man and the natural scientist of today, more particularly the biologist in every process of thinking, in all research, is under the influence of the evolutionary idea—that is History. And if we make clear to ourselves that biologic processes can only be grasped adequately in their evolution, a slight deviation from the narrow path of the specialist's method of investigation will lead us to recognize that science itself, is a living entity of an intellectual nature and has its life in evolution. Thus it comes about that the most approved natural scientist of today brings with him a considerable mental equipment for historic contemplation and perception of his subject, his special discipline; in truth this has risen out of his work of investigation itself.

In order to be able to enter intelligently into the inherent life of science, one must be in constant contact with the present status of one's specialty, whatever it may be, down to its latest developments. The scientist of today possesses qualifications for the understanding of the historic past of his specialty and in consequence, of all earlier developments of the same; this the scientist or physician who is trained only historically has to obtain by earnest application and laborious study while the contemporaneous scientist almost industively, with unerring precision, grasps the truth. It happens that the historian who is not likewise a scientfic specialist at times misses the mark.—Karl Sudhoff. Master Minds in Medicine. John C. Hemmeter. Page xxiv. New York Medical Life Press. 1927.

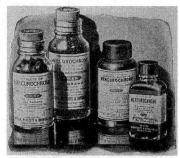

MEDICAL ABSTRACTS

"GANGRENE COMPLICATING FRACTURES ABOUT THE KNEE." Joseph M. King and Bruce J. Brewer. Surgery, Gynecology and Obstetrics. LXXVIII. 29. January, 1944.

The authors found, in reviewing the literature from 1840 to 1941, inclusive, that forty-seven cases of gangrene following fractures about the knee had been reported. They added four cases which had come under their direct treatment during the preceding twelve months.

Certain factors which tended to enhance the occurrence of vascular complications in fractures about the knee were demonstrated by anatomical dissection, namely, the proximity of the artery to the bone, and the fact that the artery is restrained or "locked in place" by the muscles and fascia. Either of these factors allows the artery to be easily traumatized, or even lacerated, by jagged fragments, or minimum displacement of fragments. It was emphasized that it is essential to make an early differential diagnosis between a laceration and a thrombosis of the main artery. This can be made from the clinical picture, usually within a few hours. In the presence of a laceration of the main artery, early exploration is imperative to prevent a sequence of events that may result in death to the patient. The therapy instituted for a thrombosis of the main vessel is not early surgery. Rather, the therapy should be directed toward the support of the ischaemic tissue by enhancing the collateral circulation. The latter can be accomplished by immediate alignment of the fragments and immobilization, plus relief of the vasomotor spasm in the obliterated segment, which almost invariably occurs. Chemical lumbar sympathectomy with novocain should be performed as soon as diagnosis is made, and should be repeated as often thereafter as the clinical response indicates. In the early states of occlusion, the collateral circulation may be enhanced by a moderate application of heat. If the circulation is not restored to normal or nearly normal at that time, then the extremity should be treated as anaemic tissue and the metabolism should be retarded by refrigeration. Finally, in those cases in which therapy fails to re-establish an adequate circulation, amputation should be performed as soon as there is a definite line of demarcation between the normal and gangrenous tissue.—E. D. M., M.D.

"ELIMINATION OF INTRANASAL PACK BY THE TOPICAL USE OF THROMBIN." H. N. Stevenson. The Annals of Otology, Rhinology, and Laryngology. Vol. 53, pages 159-162. March, 1944.

The use of thrombin as an aid in operative surgery has been recorded by various authors since 1943. It is valuable in controlling bleeding surfaces in plastic surgery and brain surgery. The author recommends its use for postoperative treatment after intranasal surgery for drainage of the accessory nasal sinuses. He obtained the thrombin as a dry powder prepared from bovine serum. Ten thousand Iowa units of the powder was dissolved in 10 cc of saline. It was applied in the following manner:

At the termination of the operation the field was well covered with tampons soaked in ephedrine-adrenaline solution to bring about vasoconstriction. After the removal of these tampons the field was thoroughly suctioned and the thrombin solution was then sprayed freely over the area. After the oozing was controlled in this way the external nares were closed with plugs covered with petrolatum to prevent the passage of air and so insure against disturbance of the operative field. Twenty

four hours later the external nares plugs were removed and the nasal chamber and exposed sinuses irrigated with 1/20,000 tyrothricin solution. Similar irrigations were done daily.

The results obtained were quite satisfactory. The postoperative bleeding was less than is usually seen in this type of operation. The patient was able to breath moderately through each side of the nose as soon as the external nares plugs were removed and he never entirely lost his airway. The postoperative swelling of the nasal membranes was decidedly less than usually seen.—M. D. H., M.D.

"RELATIONSHIP OF POLIOMYELITIS AND TONSILLECTOMY." R. E. Howard. The Annals of Otology, Rhinology, and Laryngology. Vol. 53, pages 15-34. March, 1944.

As early as 1910 Sheppard and Boyd mentioned that tonsillectomy should be done with caution during the season of a poliomyelitis epidemic. The warning was repeated later, and cases of bulbar poliomyelitis were described following tonsillectomy and adenoidectomy. The percentage of poliomyelitis infection in tonsillectomized children cannot be determined with exactness. Looking over the statistics of seven years of Cincinnati hospitals, the author finds that the approximate ratio of poliomyelitis to tonsillectomies performed in summer and autumn is 1 to 2,000, and to the total number of cases of poliomyelitis during these months 1 to 40. The possibility of poliomyelitis during July, August, September and October in non-epidemic years following tonsillectomy and adenoidectomy is minimal, but when it does occur, it is serious and most often bulbar in type. The possibility of poliomyelitis following tonsillectomy and adenoidectomy in the other eight months is nil, except in Texas and California where the poliomyelitis season is extended from June to November and sometimes includes December.

The organism causing poliomyelitis is a filtrable virus and may be present on any surface of the gastro-intestinal tract from the lips to the lower bowel of persons afflicted with the disease, convalescent or associating with carriers. The virus is widely distributed among normal people and manifests itself only in those who are susceptible. The infection may be transferred by the hands, handerchiefs, towels, and other recently handled articles of so-called carriers. It may also spread by coughing, sneezing, loud talking or laughing. There may be also indirect methods of spread. During months of epidemics of poliomyelitis, operations on the nose and throat should be avoided.—M. D. H., M.D.

"THE PLASTIC REPAIR OF SCAR CONTRACTURES." Paul W. Greeley. Surgery XV. 224, February, 1944.

In this article, Greeley has described several methods of repair of deformities or defects produced by scar contractures. He has not concerned himself merely with the treatment, but has outlined some of the steps which could be taken in the prevention of scar contractures. Cutaneous defects following third-degree burns should be covered early with properly selected skin grafts, as the best method of preventing severe scar contractures. It is not possible to prevent contractures from scars merely by traction or splinting, unless the offending scar itself is eliminated.

The treatment of healed scar contractures consists first, of the most careful excision tracting scar tissue, and second, of the filling in of the cutaneous defect. The use of the Z or multiple Z plastic incisions, with rotation of flaps, has been widely and successfully used by Greely. Case reports are presented, showing the marked disability resulting from scar contractures which limit ranges of motion of extremities or immobilize the head by fixing the chin to the chest, and the successful relief of this condition is described and illustrated. Contractures in growing children should be corrected as soon as possible after they develop. If they are permittd to continue through the growing period, permanent deformities of the bones and joints may result.—E. D. M., M.D.

"PRESENT STATUS · OF MEDICAL AND SURGICAL THERAPY FOR THE DEAFENED." Samuel J. Kopetzky. Laryngoscope. Vol. 54, pages 217-228. May, 1944.

Therapy for the deafened is still for the most part an empirical procedure. Exact diagnosis of the lesions causing progressive deafness is possible only in a small number of patients. The surgical approach has failed in approximately 50 per cent of the cases. The acceptance of a surgical operation by the patient still entails a gamble on his part as to the final success. A more exact differential diagnosis as to the cause of deafness may finally result in proper selection of surgical cases.

The basic foundations for surgical therapy were developed by Holmgren and Sourdille. The essence of surgical therapy is the fenestration of the horizontal semicircular canal, and the maintenance of the fenestra. The methods of approach are different in the hands of different surgeons. One may ascribe success to the procedure if permanently improved hearing of practical value results from the surgery. It should be realized, however, that normal hearing is not obtained by fenestration of the semicircular canal. Only a practical gain is attainable. Providing the loss of hearing has not fallen below the 40 decibel level prior to operation.

No case should be subjected to surgery until it has been under observation and medical treatment has been tried for a considerable length of time, preferably for at least six months. Before surgery is suggested to the patient, a properly fitted hearing aid should be used for a period of time, the results of its use as to social and business adjustments awaited. The very use of a hearing aid has therapeutic value. Surgery should be reserved for those cases which present an evident rapid deterioration of hearing in spite of medical treatment and for cases where hearing impairment is below the level of practical hearing; namely, 40 decibel loss and no improvement is obtainable by medical means.

The medical treatment must consist in handling allergies and of water imbalance by suitable medication and diets. Deafness in children is often caused by hypertrophy of lymphatic tissue around the Eustachian tube; this type of deafness can be cured by radium application in the area of the pharyngeal orifice of the Eustachian tube. Deafness is sometimes improved by removing the accompanying tinnitus; bezyl cinnamate injections may be tried for this aim.

Of all the drugs and bichemicals tried by the author the administration of carotine-in-oil (Caritol) in doses of 25,000 units a day, with yeast concentrate (B complex) in doses of 4 gr., given three times a day, has given him the best results. Anterior pituitary extract has also beneficial effects. Dietary habits, the interdiction of the use of mineral oils in food salads or as purges is necessary. Mineral oils will result in a loss of vitamin absorption. By vitamin therapy, hearing may be held at its existing point both in chronically suppurating ears and in cases in which there is a family history of deafness. This type of mediation may also result in improvement of hearing.—M. D. H., M.D.

"WAR SURGERY OF THE EYE: AN ANALYSIS OF 102 CASES OF INTRAOCULAR FOREIGN BODIES." H. B.

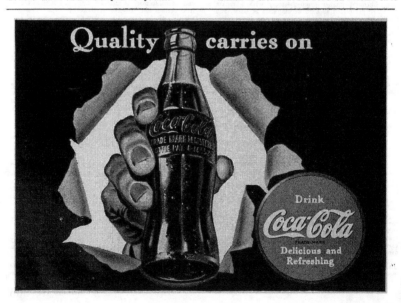

The Development of
PENICILLIN *Schenley*

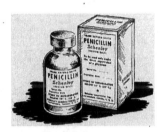

ONE of the most important phases of Schenley enterprise has long been extensive research on mycology and fermentation processes.

With this background, it was a natural step for Schenley to apply its entire research effort to devising a large-scale penicillin production method. A procedure was perfected which earned Schenley's inclusion among the 21 firms designated to produce penicillin.

Non-toxicity in therapeutic dosage is one of the most valuable features of penicillin. It is most important, of course, that the finished drug be uniformly free of pyrogens. PENICILLIN *Schenley* is produced under precautions for sterility more rigid than those taken in the most modern surgical operating rooms, and each lot is biologically tested before release.

•

Stallard. The British Journal of Ophthalmology, Vol. 28, pages 105-135. March, 1944.

In the present war, penetrating injuries of the eye were chiefly caused by fragments of shell, hand grenades and land mines. There were all types of injuries at various sites of the eye. The foreign body could be seen occasionally by the ophthalmoscope. Most often, x-ray apparatus had to be used. Movement of the foreign body is the essential feature in diagnosis. Intraocular foreign bodies due to fragmentation of war missiles are generally low-magnetic or possess no magnetic properties at all. The fragments are irregular in shape, have ragged edges and a rough granular surface. The posterior route is the method of choice in extracting war missiles.

After extraction, the patient is placed in a position in which there is the minimum pressure of intraocular contents into the wound. Aspirin is given immediately after the patient is settled in bed. Some postoperative pain begins one hour after operation and continues one to two hours. The dressing is removed 48 hours after operation. The lid margins are swabbed with warm normal saline. A drop of warm sterile atropine 1 per cent is instilled. No pad is placed over the eye but a strip of gamgee is laid along the infra-orbital margin to absorb any tears and the eye covered with a shield. On the third day the conjunctival stitch is removed under cocaine or pantocain surface anesthesia. The patient is allowed to sit up in a chair on the eighth day. The scleral stitch is left buried beneath the conjunctiva and Tenon's capsule and in no case has it given rise to any trouble.

In the majority of cases the scleral entry wound is closed by the time a soldier reaches the base hospital. If the wound is under 3 mm., has not prolapsed uveal tissue and is apparently closed and well shut off by surrounding fibrous tissue it can be left alone. In some cases surface diathermy is applied around the edge of the wound and causes it to contract. The associated retinal detachment with a ragged tear through which the foreign body had passed may necessitate the application of surface diathermy so as to include the edges of the tear.

According to the author's statistics, in 23 cases vision improved; in 47 cases vision remained the same; in some cases vision became worse. Evisceration had to be done in seven cases. Five developed panophthalmitis; the eyes began to shrink. It is probable that some surgeons fearing the danger of sympathetic ophthalmia excised eyes unnecessarily; but the decision is a difficult problem in which courage, worry and possible folly may become intermingled. Unfortunately there is no infallible test to show whether an eye is liable to sympathetic ophthalmia.

Sulfonamides have been used, but under such conditions that their value could not be determined. In some cases sulfonamide seemed to have no effect; subsidence of inflammatory signs was slow. In one case sulfonamide administered eight days after wounding did not check the process of endophthalmitis and excision was necessary. Generally it was not until the patient had reached the hospital that regularized sulfonamide therapy could be given.

"REPAIR OF THE BURNED HAND." George Warren Pierce, E. H. Klabunde, and D. Emerson. Surgery, XV. 153. January, 1944.

These authors have again brought into sharp profile the problem of repair of the burned hand. The intricate mechanism of the hand, from the point of view of its multiple small joints, muscles, tendons, and nerves, and their interrelationships, requires a covering which is both strong and flexible, as nearly as possible resembling that of the normal skin, in order that the best possible function may be obtained. In this paper, the study has

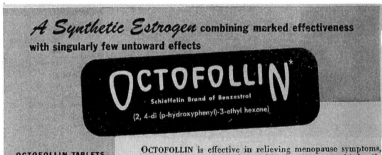

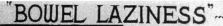

been confined to repair after the acute stage has passed.

Since the hand is most often uncovered and hence unprotected, it is burned more frequently than any other single part of the body, with the possible exception of the face. The tendency to protect the hand by closing it results in more frequent and more severe burns of the dorsum than of the palm.

The authors have emphasized the fact that restoration of function and of appearance of the burned hand demands a most thorough knowledge of the anatomy and physiology of the part. The amount of tissue loss and tissue damage must be carefully determined before planning the repair. The earlier the diagnosis is made and the treatment begun, the better the opportunity of the surgeon for obtaining a good result.—E. D. M., M.D.

"THE EUSTACHIAN TUBE: A REVIEW OF ITS DE-SCRIPTIVE, MICROSCOPIC, TOPOGRAPHIC AND CLINICAL ANATOMY." Graves, Grant O., Edwards, Linden F., Columbus, Ohio. Archives of Otolaryngology, Vol. 39, page 359-397, May, 1944.

The entire tube varies in length from 31 to 38 mm; the cartilaginous portion measures 24 or 25 mm, and the osseous portion 11 or 12 mm. The tube passes laterally from a sagital plane through the pharyngeal orifice, at an angle of about 45 degrees. The course of the tube is that of an inverted S. The pharyngeal orifice is a vertical slit when at rest, which becomes triangular only during the act of swallowing or during the act of raising the soft palate. The boundaries of the orifice consist of folds anteriorly and posteriorly and elevations superiorly and inferiorly.

The cartilaginous portion of the eustachian tube is composed of mucous membrane supported partly by cartilage and partly by a connective tissue layer. Near the pharyngeal ostium the shape of the lumen as seen on cross-sections is irregularly triangular with its apex directed superiorly. Traced posterolaterally toward the isthmus, the lumen assumes an elliptic shape; it gradually becomes reduced to a narrow vertical fissure.

The osseous portion of the tube is situated within the petrous portion of the temporal bone, where it occupies a semicanal which is directed laterally, superiorly and posteriorly to the tympanic ostium. The osseous portion lies on a more horizontal plane than the cartilaginous, the two forming an obtuse angle of about 160 degrees opening outward at their junction. This junction is called the isthmus, and it is in the region of the spheno-petrosal fissure at the level of the medical surface of the angular spine of the sphenoid bone.

Three muscles are intimately associated with the eustachian tube; the tensor palati, the levator palati and the salpingopharyngeus. The blood supply of the tube is derived from several arteries: the ascending palatine artery from below, the tubal branch of the internal maxillary artery from above, the tubal branch of the artery of the pterygoid canal from above, and other branches coming from the ascending pharyngeal and the middle meningeal arteries.

The pharyngeal end of the tube is richly supplied with lymph vessels. This fact substantiates the clinical findings of a greater frequency of lymphoid inflammation, acute inflammation, ulcerations, tuberculosis, adhesions and scars in the pharyngeal end of the tube, in contrast to the prevalence of ostetis, caries and necrosis with formation of granulation tissue in the osseous portion of the tube.

Little is known of the abnormal development of the tube. The osseous portion may be deficient, or there may be other defects in the tube. A few cases of tumors were also described. They can be diagnosed mostly by x-rays. Deafness seems to be the initial symptom, with tinnitus frequently complained of, occasionally full feeling in the ear or intermittent pain referred to the depths of the ear. A malignant tumor may cause metastases in the cervical nodes. If it infiltrates the tube,

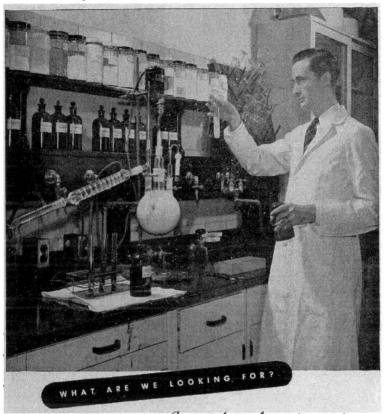

WHAT ARE WE LOOKING FOR?

In arsenical research we are seeking compounds which offer promise of greater effectiveness against the spirochete of syphilis with less toxicity to the patient . . . a syphilis therapy that will be even better than the dramatically successful Mapharsen* treatment of today. But that is not all we are looking for... we are making an exhaustive study of arsenic compounds, searching for the one that may bring amebic dysentery and other diseases of protozoan origin under control, and open up new fields of effective therapeutics.

*Trade-mark Reg. U. S. Pat. Off.

PARKE, DAVIS & COMPANY DETROIT 32, MICHIGAN

various symptoms may develop such as reduced visual acuity, diplopia and paralysis of the ocular muscles.

If foreign bodies are lodged in the tube, they can be removed by two approaches from the pharyngeal or from the tympanic end of the tube.

The eustachian tube gained in importance by the development of aviation. On level ground or in level flying the slight variations of pressure within and without the middle ear are adequately adjusted by the normal swallowing rates of man and the resultant contractions of the tensor palati muscles to open the tubes. An adult usually swallows once a minute while awake and once in five minutes while asleep. This rate is accelerated to one swallow every one to thirty seconds while chewing.

On ascending into the air from the take-off, the decreasing pressure of the atmosphere allows a slight sense of fullness in the ears when the distance from the earth is 100 feet (3 to 5 mm. of mercury differential), provided no swallowing has taken place. When the ascent has been made to 500 feet without swallowing, the hearing becomes distant and of less intensity and is then suddenly relieved as the increased air pressure in the middle ear forces an automatic opening of the tube with its attendant click. Thus on continued ascent the increased air pressure within the middle ear forces successive openings of the tube relatively decreasing frequencies. All of these openings are entirely independent of the openings produced by normal swallowing. With these two mechanisms working simultaneously to open the tube, little difficulty is experienced by aviators in ascent, provided infection or previous trauma does not preclude opening of the tube.

If, for some reason, the tube remains closed until there has been an ascent of 1,000 feet, tinnitus develops with sensations of hissing, roaring, snapping and crackling sounds in the ears, also vertigo, and sometimes pain.

Descents from altitude almost require some conscious maneuver to ventilate the middle ear in order to equalize the pressure there with the increasing barometric pressure. Swallowing, yawning, sneezing are the natural movements opening the tubes. Tensing and relaxing the tensor muscles by moving the mandible will often suffice; others have to close their nostrils and exerting enough pressure in the pharynx to initiate opening either by swallowing or by contracting the abdominal muscles. In the rapid descent of dive bombing the continuous yell or the continuous swallowing maneuver is used. Here the tube probably remains open while considerable gas enters the middle ear.

Passengers in commercial air liners often complain that the pressure will not equalize for several hours after descent. This is because the 21 per cent of oxygen of the air must be absorbed down to 12 per cent to 15 per cent in the capillaries. If they would inflate their ears at the end of expiration following moderate breath-holding, the period of recovery will be very much shortened.

Inefficiency of the eustachian tubes in opening has brought on a whole series of symptoms and signs, which have acquired in the recent past more accurate anatomic and physiologic explanations. The outstanding single symptom of the "blocked eustachian tube" is deafness of the conductive type for low tones, and it lasts the longest among the symptoms, sometimes for 16 days. Pain occurs in 61 per cent; tinnitus in 5 per cent; vertigo in 3 per cent. Similar symptoms may be seen in caisson workers and in submarine personnel, including divers. Warm, soothing oil in the external ear gives as much relief as attempts to equalize air pressure by means of the eustachian catheter or the politzer bag.—M. D. H., M.D.

KEY TO ABSTRACTORS

M. D. H., M.D. ....Marvin D. Henley
E. D. M., M.D. ....Earl D. McBride

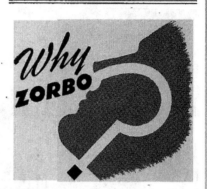
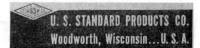

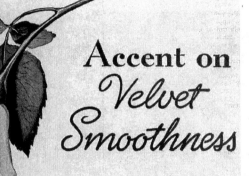

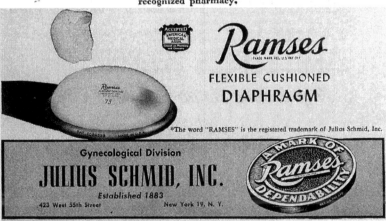

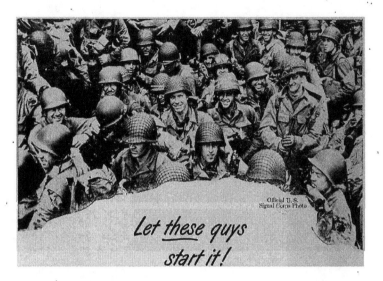

Official U. S.
Signal Corps Photo

Let these guys start it!

There's a day coming when the enemy will be licked, beaten, whipped to a fare-thee-well—every last vestige of fight knocked out of him.

And there's a day coming when every mother's son of us will want to stand up and yell, to cheer ourselves hoarse over the greatest victory in history.

But let's not start the cheering yet.
In fact, let's not start it at all—over here. Let's leave it to the fellows who are *doing* the job—the only fellows who will *know* when it's done—to begin the celebrating.

Our leaders have told us, over and over again, that the smashing of the Axis will be a slow job, a dangerous job, a bloody job.

And they've told us what our own common sense confirms: that, if we at home start throwing our hats in the air and easing up before the job's completely done, it will be slower, more dangerous, bloodier.

Right now, it's still up to us to buy War Bonds—and to *keep on* buying War Bonds until this war is completely won. That doesn't mean victory over the Nazis *alone*. It means bringing the Japs to their knees, too.

Let's keep bearing down till we get the news of final victory from the only place such news can come: the battle-line.

If we do that, we'll have the *right* to join the cheering when the time comes.

Keep backing 'em up with War Bonds

Oklahoma State Medical Association

OFFICERS OF COUNTY SOCIETIES, 1944

★

COUNTY	PRESIDENT	SECRETARY	MEETING TIME
Alfalfa	H. E. Huston, Cherokee	L. T. Lancaster, Cherokee	Last Tues. each Second Month
Atoka-Coal	R. C. Henry, Coalgate	J. S. Fulton, Atoka	
Beckham	G. H. Stagner, Erick	O. C. Standifer, Elk City	Second Tuesday
Blaine	L. R. Kirby, Okeene	W. F. Griffin, Watonga	
Bryan	John T. Wharton, Durant	W. K. Haynie, Durant	Second Tuesday
Caddo	F. L. Patterson, Carnegie	C. B. Sullivan, Carnegie	
Canadian	P. F. Herod, El Reno	A. L. Johnson, El Reno	Subject to call
Carter	J. R. Pollock, Ardmore	H. A. Higgins, Ardmore	
Cherokee	P. H. Medearis, Tahlequah	W. M. Wood, Tahlequah	First Tuesday
Choctaw		E. A. Johnson, Hugo	
Cleveland	F. T. Gastineau, Norman	Iva S. Merritt, Norman	Thursday nights
Comanche	George L. Berry, Lawton	Howard Angus, Lawton	
Cotton	A. B. Holstead, Temple	Mollie F. Scism, Walters	Third Friday
Craig	Lloyd H. McPike, Vinita	J. M. McMillan, Vinita	
Creek	J. E. Hollis, Bristow	F. H. Sisler, Bristow	
Custer	F. R. Vieregg, Clinton	C. J. Alexander, Clinton	Third Thursday
Garfield	Julian Feild, Enid	John R. Walker, Enid	Fourth Thursday
Garvin	T. F. Gross, Lindsay	John R. Callaway, Pauls Valley	Wednesday before Third Thursday
Grady	Walter J. Baze, Chickasha	Roy E. Emanuel, Chickasha	Third Thursday
Grant	I. V. Hardy, Medford		
Greer	R. W. Lewis, Granite	J. B. Hollis, Mangum	
Harmon	W. G. Husband, Hollis	R. H. Lynch, Hollis	First Wednesday
Haskell	William Carson, Keota	N. K. Williams, McCurtain	
Hughes	Wm. L. Taylor, Holdenville	Imogene Mayfield, Holdenville	First Friday
Jackson	C. G. Spears, Altus	E. A. Abernethy, Altus	Last Monday
Jefferson	F. M. Edwards, Ringling		Second Monday
Kay	J. Holland Howe, Ponca City	G. H. Yeary, Newkirk	Second Thursday
Kingfisher	A. O. Meredith, Kingfisher	H. Violet Sturgeon, Hennessey	
Kiowa	J. William Finch, Hobart	William Bernell, Hobart	
LeFlore	Neeson Rolle, Poteau	Rush L. Wright, Poteau	
Lincoln	W. B. Davis, Stroud	Carl H. Bailey, Stroud	First Wednesday
Logan	William C. Miller, Guthrie	J. L. LeHew, Jr., Guthrie	Last Tuesday
Marshall	J. L. Holland, Madill	J. F. York, Madill	
Mayes	Ralph V. Smith, Pryor	Paul B. Cameron, Pryor	
McClain	W. C. McCurdy, Sr., Purcell	W. C. McCurdy, Jr., Purcell	
McCurtain	A. W. Clarkson, Valliant	N. L. Barker, Broken Bow	Fourth Tuesday
McIntosh	Luster I. Jacobs, Hanna	Wm. A. Tolleson, Eufaula	First Thursday
Murray	P. V. Annadown, Sulphur	J. A. Wrenn, Sulphur	Second Tuesday
Muskogee-Sequoyah			
Wagoner	H. A. Scott, Muskogee	D. Evelyn Miller, Muskogee	First Monday
Noble	C. H. Cooke, Perry	J. W. Francis, Jerry	
Okfuskee	C. M. Cochran, Okemah	M. L. Whitney, Okemah	Second Monday
Oklahoma	W. E. Eastland, Oklahoma City	E. R. Musick, Oklahoma City	Fourth Tuesday
Okmulgee	S. B. Leslie, Okmulgee	J. C. Matheney, Okmulgee	Second Monday
Osage	C. R. Weirich, Pawhuska	George K. Hemphill, Pawhuska	Second Monday
Ottawa	Walter Kerr, Picher	B. W. Shelton, Miami	Third Thursday
Pawnee	E. T. Robinson, Cleveland	R. L. Browning, Pawnee	
Payne	H. C. Manning, Cushing	J. W. Martin, Cushing	Third Thursday
Pittsburg	P. T. Powell, McAlester	W. H. Kaeiser, McAlester	Third Friday
Pontotoc	A. R. Sugg, Ada	R. H. Mayes, Ada	First Wednesday
Pottawatomie	E. Eugene Rice, Shawnee	Clinton Gallaher, Shawnee	First and Third Saturday
Pushmataha	John S. Lawson, Clayton	B. M. Huckabay, Antlers	
Rogers	R. C. Meloy, Claremore	Chas. L. Caldwell, Chelsea	First Monday
Seminole	J. T. Price, Seminole	Mack I. Shanholtz, Wewoka	Third Wednesday
Stephens	W. K. Walker, Marlow	Wallis S. Ivy, Duncan	
Texas	R. G. Obermiller, Texhoma	Morris Smith, Guymon	
Tillman	C. C. Allen, Frederick	O. G. Bacon Frederick	
Tulsa	Ralph A. McGill, Tulsa	E. O. Johnson, Tulsa	Second and Fourth Monday
Washington-Nowata	K. D. Davis, Nowata	J. V. Athey, Bartlesville	Second Wednesday
Washita	A. S. Neal, Cordell	James F. McMurry, Sentinel	
Woods	Ishmael F. Stephenson, Alva	Oscar E. Templin, Alva	Last Tuesday Odd Months
Woodward	H. Walker, Buffalo	C. W. Tedrowe, Woodward	Second Thursday

(Serving in Armed Forces)

THE JOURNAL

OF THE

OKLAHOMA STATE MEDICAL ASSOCIATION

| VOLUME XXXVII | OKLAHOMA CITY, OKLAHOMA, OCTOBER, 1944 | NUMBER 10 |

The Clinical Diagnosis of Malignancies*

HUGH JETER, M.D.

OKLAHOMA CITY, OKLAHOMA

No practitioner of medicine can escape the problem of malignancy and we need only to be reminded of its frequency to realize the necessity of constant review of the subject. Recent public health reports indicate that one of every 250 persons have cancer. Twenty-five per cent more women than men have cancer. This would mean we have in Oklahoma, roughly, 10,000 cases of malignancy. There are 475,000 to 500,000 under treatment at any given time in the United States and about 300,000 new cases diagnosed for the first time each year. In addition to this, there are cases which have been treated and cured and, of course, an unlimited number which have been undiagnosed. Something like one out of each six of us, if we may assume that we are in the cancer age, are doomed to develop cancer if we have not already. This is an alarming figure if we give it serious thought. The percentage of morbidity and mortality corresponds closely with the percentage of deaths and casualties of our boys in the armed forces. Demobilization of the boys in the service may be expected, but with our present knowledge we have no reason to look forward to the demobilization of the various factors which go to cause and perpetuate malignancies, except through the efforts of physicians.

Physicians are prone to ask themselves, "Why should we make great effort to diagnose malignancies when we have no specific treatment?" Experience through recent decades has lowered the mortality rate in many forms of cancer and we have reason to be

optimistic about the future in this respect, even though we know certain forms of cancer are incurable. Dr. James Ewing, a few years before his death, remarked, "Cancer is the most curable of major causes of death." Other major causes of death being referred to are heart disease, which heads the list, intracranial vascular lesions, and accidents.

Furthermore, cure is by no means the only goal which we wish to attain. Palliation, relief of pain, euthanasia in general and, in short, general management of these cases is most important. No doctor can spend his time more profitably than in prescribing proper treatment and care for relief of the suffering, miserable and helpless case of malignancy. No people are more grateful to the physician than the relatives, friends and attendants of these unfortunates.

The question as to the actual increase in the incidence of malignancies would appear from statistics to be a mathematical fact. However, credit must be given the physicians for having actually developed great improvement in their diagnostic acumen along with more accurate knowledge of the behavior of the disease and better equipment to aid in the discovery of hidden forms. Physicians are also credited with the fact that there are many more people today who survive other diseases and live to the age which we know is the cancer age and will, therefore, be more subject to cancer. The average age given by one large series of malignancies was 53.9 years. We must, therefore, accept the fact that we have an increasingly large number of cases of malignancies and every practitioner, regard-

*Presented before Section on General Medicine, Annual Meeting, April 25, 1944, Tulsa.

less of his specialty, must anticipate that he is sure to see such cases and be on the alert for an early diagnosis.

Mortality rates have been substantially reduced, particularly in malignancies of the skin, breast and uterus, and early diagnosis is the greatest factor in this accomplishment.

Histopathological examinations, surgical pathology, necropsies, research, and pathology in general, have contributed much, if not more than any other department of medicine, to the present knowledge of malignancy. My own interest in the subject is, admittedly, largely the result of study in these departments. However, in this report it seems apropos to give fundamental clinical facts helpful in the diagnosis, rather than detailed pathological findings. Eighteen years of experience and the privilege of having aided in some capacity in the diagnosis of a large number of malignancies have impressed upon me at least one particular fact that seems worthy of emphasis, namely, that malignancies tend to behave in a more or less characteristic manner and knowledge of this behavior is most important in diagnosis. The expression, more or less characteristic behavior, has been used advisedly because although tumors, both benign and malignant, do have a characteristic behavior, as we will attempt to point out in connection with the specific instances, yet in hardly any instance should the term 'always' be used. It is perhaps this very subject that has made the old adage of, "Never say always and never say never," a favorite among pathologists.

Great difficulty has been encountered in this attempt to present the subject in such a brief period of time and the following review is only proposed as one which will hit the high points, or the most characteristic and useable facts. Details will necessarily be omitted.

Benign tumors offer many very interesting examples of specific behavior, but these will also have to be omitted, except as generalities apply to them.

Statistics, or probabilities based upon statistics, which are to be given in the following are not given as a result of my own experience, but from those of authentic reports or large series of cases. References are attached.

BRAIN TUMORS

Neuroepitheliomas, or t u m o r s arising strictly from brain substance, or the cells which go to make up brain tissue, namely, the glioma, spongioblastoma, astrocytoma, medullablastoma, oligodendroglioma, ependymoma, occur in young people, ordinarily from very early childhood to about 35 years of age and rarely occur in individuals over 70 years of age. These tumors, although malignant in their histological structure, are nonencapsulated and behave malignant in that they invade and destroy brain tissue, do not give metastases. This is perhaps because of the special and different type of lymphatic drainage in the brain. These tumors do not give bone destruction. If an x-ray of the skull shows destruction of bone, it may be concluded that if it is primary of the brain it is likely a meningioma of some type. It has been a curious thought to me that meningiomas give bone destruction and yet they are the least malignant and most curable of the tumors of the central nervous system.

OCULAR TUMORS

Glioma of the retina (neuroepithelioma, or retinoblastoma). Characteristic clinical behavior and peculiar structure render this tumor one of the most striking examples of specific tumor process. Twenty-three per cent are bilateral and ninety-four per cent occur under 4 years of age. The tendency to sudden hemorrhage into the tumor is striking. It is the second commonest tumor of the eye, malignant melanoma being the commonest. It displays a remarkable and tragic familial tendency. Ten children out of sixteen in one family have been known to die of this tumor.

In connection with tumors of children in general, there is an interesting behavior characteristic, well expressed by Roger Williams, "One noteworthy feature about the tumors of infancy and early life is, that the localities whence they are prone to originate, are very different than those whence malignant tumors commonly arise at later periods of life."

What about the question of heredity? So-called cancer families have been reported and are seemingly known to most of us. Napoleon Bonaparte, his father, his brother Lucien, and two of his sisters, Pauline and Caroline, all died of cancer of the stomach. A less illustrious family is that reported by Broca, the family of Madame Z, which had sixteen people out of twenty-six die of cancer of the breast, liver, or uterus. However, it may be said that from a practical point of view, in so far as diagnosis is concerned, the history in regards to heredity can not be used to any certain degree of accuracy.

PRIMARY SULCUS TUMOR

This tumor was described in 1932 by Pancoast, who had 8 cases. It originates in the region of the pleura of the superior sulcus of the chest, extends outward by direct contiguity destroying ribs and clavicle, invading the brachial plexus, has little tendency to metastasize, and forms a diffuse rather than nodular swelling of the lower cervical region. Involvement of the sympathetic nerves gives Horner's syndrome. They occur ordinarily in young adult males. Although carcinomatous in appearance, the specific type of cell origin is controversial. It has been suggested and seems highly plausible that it arises from an extrapulmonary rest, perhaps in the cervical sympathetics. Two such cases have come to my attention. X-ray serves to confirm the diagnosis. A snap diagnosis can be made—Horner's syndrome with inequality of pupils, perspiration excessive on one side in comparison to the opposite, and a tumorous bulging in the neck.

NEUROCYTOMA OF THE ADRENAL GLAND

This is another malignancy arising from nerve cells, some say the neuron, (Bailey—sympatheticoblastoma). It has a distinct behavior in that it invariably occurs in children under 8 years of age, gives generalized subperiosteal bony metastasis leading to hemorrhage. Post orbital bony involvement causes exophthalmus or proptosis. X-ray of the skull is ordinarily diagnostic. Dr. Dean Lewis of Johns Hopkins several years ago looked at the film of one of these cases in an exhibit and pronounced the diagnosis with no hesitancy and said, "Nothing else gives such a picture in a child of that age."

X-ray examination is confirmatory, if not of itself completely diagnostic, in many types of malignancy, neurosarcoma, myeloma, osteogenic sarcoma, chondrosarcoma, Ewing's sarcoma (endothelial myeloma), and a large group of tumors which give metastatic lesions, such as breast carcinoma, prostate carcinoma, thyriod carcinoma, hypernephroma, and others.

OSTEOSARCOMA

This tumor arises primarily from the osteocyte, has a remarkably characteristic behavior in that it occurs in an average age of 16 years, is more common in boys than girls. Of 13 cases which we have reported, all occurred at the metaphysis, 86 per cent at the knee, five of the upper end of the tibia, seven of the lower end of the femur, one the upper end of the fibula and two the upper humerus. The average period from onset to demonstrate metastasis was 7.6 months. Eight cases amputated gave demonstrable metastasis in an average of 4.5 months following operation. They uniformly gave metastasis to the lungs without local recurrence or lymph gland involvement. The mortality is 95 per cent regardless whether the leg is amputated or not.

Since this report we have seen 15 more cases, the statistics of which are remarkably similar.

The question of trauma has repeatedly been studied in connection with the cause of bone tumors and no definite connection has been proven.

Martland found a much higher incidence of osteogenic sarcoma resulting from the industrial exposure of radio-active substances in connection with the luminous paint in a watch manufacturing establishment.

This brings up the great question—the cause of cancer. Generally speaking, no specific cause is yet known. However, the following chemicals in industry have proven to be more or less specific factors and must be given consideration in connection with diagnosis:

1. X-ray exposure, such as physicians and x-ray technicians have experienced.
2. Cancer of the scrotum has proven to be common among chimney sweepers in England.
3. Coal tar products are carcinogenic in connection with tar distillation, coal gas manufacturing, etc.
4. Cancer of the bladder has occurred in aniline dye industry.
5. Skin cancer is caused by the long continued use of arsenic, such as Fowler's solution.

MULTIPLE MYELOMA

A malignant tumor arising within the bones of the trunk, primarily the spine, giving metastasis generally to the ribs and skull, with an x-ray picture much like that of neuroblastoma, but occurring not in young people, the average age being 42 years, and 72 per cent in males. About 65 to 80 per cent give a characteristic form of protein in the urine (Bence-Jones). Death occurs as a result of nephritis.

WILM'S TUMOR

Adenomyosarcoma of the kidney

An emboynal malignancy, males and females are equally represented, the average age is 3 years. The tumor is slow to give distant metastasis. Age is of utmost importance in connection with diagnosis of all tumors, such as is vividly illustrated by these cases. If a child, male or female, birth to 4 years of age, has a large abdominal mass, the chances are 9 to 1 that it is a Wilm's tumor.

It may be said that in infancy (birth to 10 months of age), Wilm's tumor and ocular glioma are of equal frequency. In childhood up to the 7th or 8th year, glioma is the most common, but Wilm's tumor frequently is found. From the 8th year to the presexual period of 13 or 14 years, it is unusual to find any type of malignant tumor. At the Memorial Hospital, out of 19,129 patients, there were no malignant tumors during this period of life. In our experience, brain tumors and one case of adenocarcinoma of the colon have been the only exceptions. During the pubital period, or from about 14 to

24 years, the tumors especially frequent are endothelial myelomas, thymomas, gliomas, osteogenic sarcomas and sarcomas of the testis.

Maturity in the male extends to sexual decline, which is an indefinite terminal, and in the female terminates at the menopause. A great host of malignant tumors occur at this period and the early part of the succeeding period.

Senescence may be said to begin with the menopause in the female and the sexual climacteric in the male and terminates in death. The cancers of salient interest in this epoch are the basal cell epitheliomas of the skin, the squamous cell carcinomas of the skin, lip, buccal mucosa, floor of the mouth, and vulva, and the carcinomas of the prostate gland.

In any discussion concerning the age occurrence of malignancies, it is to be emphasized that the anatomical and physiological age of the subject, as well as that of the particular organ under question, is of more importance than the chronological age of the individual. Cancers developing in such organs as the breast, thymus, uterus and prostate, all of which undergo physiological atrophy in definite periods of life, have specific relationships to age.

CARCINOMA OF THE STOMACH

This is the most frequent malignancy of the male, with the exception of skin cancer. Sixty to 70 per cent of all stomach cancers occur in males. Cancer of the alimentary tract has been reported four times as frequent in men as in women.

One curious form described by Krukenberg occurs in both ovaries and the stomach and the exact origin, whether ovaries or other portions of the gastrointestinal tract, has not been definitely decided.

MELANOSARCOMA OR MELANOEPITHELIOMA

This malignancy is known to "misbehave." It is one of the most malignant, occurs at any age, arises from skin, retina, arachnoid, or any pigmented area. Metastasis may be delayed. Biopsy of a suspected primary lesion ordinarily does not give sufficient positive information whereby it can be predicted, whether it has been, is, or will be malignant.

Much could be said of the value of biopsies as a means of diagnosis. It can probably be said that biopsy properly selected will lead to a positive and definite diagnosis, at least in so far as whether or not a tumorous lesion is malignant or benign in 95 per cent or more cases. Melanosarcoma is, therefore, mentioned because it is strikingly exceptional in this respect.

Ferguson discovered a substance called Intermedin (intermediate portion of the pituitary gland), which has a particular relation to chromophores and is excessive in the blood in case of melanoma, and reports that they are using a certain type of fish, Elritza, which will change the color of its spots if the urine from a case of melanoma is injected, thereby giving a test of the blood which is helpful in the diagnosis of melanoma. This brings up the question of tests for malignancy.

Serological tests, as applies to specific antigens, may be summarized by the report of the Brussels Congress, "A vast amount of work has been devoted to this subject and widely employed, but with no case with results of practical value."

MALIGNANT TUMORS OF THE SEX GLANDS

These tumors in both the male and female, particularly those arising from the placenta, or those of a teratomatous nature from testicles or ovaries give a positive aschheim-Zondek or Friedmann test in a high per cent of the cases. This affords one test which can be used in a specific way to make a diagnosis of malignancy.

Colloid carcinoma arises from certain mucus producing cells, ordinarily from the gastrointestinal tract, gives metastasis by direct extension and by transplantation to the peritoneal surface. Ovaries, not infrequently, are the primary site. Fluid in the peritoneal cavity develops sooner or later. The fluid is ordinarily lumpy, thick and of such character that the mere gross appearance is diagnostic.

Histological examination of paracentetic fluids, particularly those of the peritoneal cavity and the pleural cavities, have been found by us to yield positive diagnosis in 85 per cent of the cases, if the fluid is properly concentrated and handles. Carcinoma of the lung is, unfortunately, too many times not suspected until fluid develops in the cavity. Carcinoma of the ovary gives the highest percentage of positive fluid examinations in connection with the paracentetic fluids of the abdomen.

Cancer of the breast affords a single example in which its behavior is outstanding, namely, that it occurs practically altogether in the female, only 1 per cent in the male. It is extremely important because of its frequency, 30 per cent of all malignancies of the female occur in the breast, the average age is 51 years.

Any solitary nodule in the breast at any age must be suspected to be cancer until pathological proof of some other disease is obtained.

Transillumination gives positive findings only in hemangiomas.

Cancer of the uterus: Welch collected from the literature over 131,000 cases of cancer, of which 29.5 per cent were of the uterus. About 10 per cent of uterine cancers arise from the corpus and the remainder at about the junction of the cervical epithelium with thte cervical mucosa. The average of at least one large series was 48 years.

FUNCTIONAL TUMORS

Tumors of the endocrine glands: Although most of these tumors are not malignant, it seems fitting to make mention of them here because no discussion of the diagnosis of malignancies or tumors would be complete without the mention of advances in connection with these more or less recent discoveries. A clinical picture may lead to a diagnosis of tumors in such cases where the tumor itself can in no way be demonstrated.

The masculinizing tumors are pituitary. 1. Basophilic adenoma—usually in females. 2. Pineal—in males only. 3. Adrenal cortical tumors and hyperplasias. 4. Ovarian arrhenoblastoma—hypernephroma or adrenal cell tumor of the ovary. 5. Testicular interstitial cell—adrenal cell type.

Feminizing tumors: 1. Adrenal cortical tumors and hyperplasias—in adult males only. 2. Ovarian granulosa cell tumor—and thecoma.

Parathyroid adenoma causes a cystic disease of bone—osteitis fibrosa cystica, giving a remarkably characteristic roentgenological and clinical picture. Spectacular cures can be made by parathyroidectomy.

Hyperinsulinism may lead to a definite diagnosis of adenoma of the pancreas.

SUMMARY

Tumors tend to behave in a more or less characteristic manner, especially as regards age, sex, anatomical location, anatomical distribution and the progress of the disease. Adequate knowledge of these more or less specific tendencies is of utmost importance in connection with the suspicion of the existence and consequent diagnosis.

Early diagnosis is the most important single factor in the cure of malignancies and diagnosis at any stage is mandatory for the proper treatment and satisfactory management of the case.

Numerous additional examples illustrating interesting and practical facts about malignancies have necessarily been omitted.

DISCUSSION

PAUL B. CHAMPLIN, M.D.
ENID, OKLAHOMA

Doctor Jeter has given you as complete a resume of all the different forms and locations of cancer as it is possible to do in a short paper of this kind.

There has been a great deal of pessimism in the past in regard to the treatment of malignant diseases so I want to again call your attention to the statement of Doctor Ewing's which Doctor Jeter quoted, that "Cancer is the most curable of the major causes of death." This is true if all types of malignant diseases are included because great strides have been made in curing the malignancies of the skin, breast, uterus and intra-oral cancers; but the extensive campaign of public education on early signs of cancer have produced little result with the inaccessible forms of the disease, such as lesions of the gastro-intestinal tract with the possible exception of the rectum.

Considerable progress has been made in regard to carinoma of the lung, its early recognition and treatment. There is no question but what the incidence of carcinoma of the lung is increasing. Ochsner reports that in 1938 among 825 necropsies performed in the Charity Hospital in New Orleans there were 17 primary carcinomas of the lung and only 16 carcinomas of the stomach. This is a rather startling statement inasmuch as carcinoma of the stomach is supposed to be a rather common disease and carcinoma of the lung a rather rare one. If this is true then we have been overlooking a large number of carcinomas of the lung which have been diagnosed as either a pulmonary or a cardiac condition.

We are looking forward to the time when some universal test of malignant diseases will be at our disposal, and to the time when some definite causitive etiological factor will be found. So far there is no scientific data which leads us to hope for any early solution of this problem. We must rely altogether on early diagnosis and early treatment so eternal vigilance is our only hope at the present time.

BIBLIOGRAPHY

1. 1942 Summary of Vital Statistics, Published by the Bureau of the Census, Washington, D. C., Vol. 20, No. 2 of Vital Statistics Special Report.
2. Dorn, Harold F.: Public Health Reports.
3. Lewis, Dean: Department of Surgery, Johns Hopkins University. Personal interview.
4. Williams, W. Roger: The Natural History of Cancer.
5. Boyd, William: Text Book of Pathology, Third Edition
6. Ewing, James: Neoplastic Diseases, Fourth Edition.
7. Pack, George T., and LeFevre, Robert G.: The Age and Sex Distribution and Incidence of Neoplastic Diseases at the Memorial Hospital, New York City.
8. Martland, Harrison S.: Occurrence of Malignancy in Radio-active Persons, Am. J. Cancer 15: 2535, 1931.
9. Cancer. A Manual for Practitioners. American Society For the Control of Cancer, 1940.

Tantalum has assisted surgeons to return to active life many cases which in the last war would have been disfigured and incapacitated for life. Lost portions of the skull, ears, noses and other parts of the face are being replaced with tantalum. On veteran has a tantalum "belly wall." Nerves which control motion in arms and legs are stitched with tantalum thread and protected while healing with tantalum cuffs. Facial paralysis is relieved by small saddle-shaped pieces of tantalum and wire used to pull the corners of the mouth to a normal position. This stops the unpleasant drooling and facial distortion which go with the condition. Cleft plates also are being corrected.

A Physician Looks at Public Health Education*

Clinton Gallaher, M.D.

SHAWNEE, OKLAHOMA

By way of introduction may I review the meaning of the democratic principle and may I insist that it be applied to the problems of health education. There are two tenets which characterize a democracy. The first is the conviction that all men will eventually do what is right. It implies an appeal to reason. Deny this and all teaching is wasted. For a time men may be coerced by necessity, or threats, or violence, but they at length begin to distinguish truth and deception, and they voluntarily do what is right, because it is right, and because it is the only way to get along with people. A certain amount of faith in this concept of human relations is indispensable in a democracy.

One should not fail to observe that health can never be safeguarded by legislation alone. Health education must prepare the way for public health legislation. To be effective, law must represent public opinion, its enforcement must be in tune with majority convictions. Obviously, good public health laws should proceed from the people, and it is the job of those interested in health education to teach the value of public health measures and to give the people an intelligent grasp of existing and anticipated health legislation.

The second tenet of democracy is the recognition of the value and the intregity of men as individuals, the concept that each man has certain rights which must be respected and preserved, even against the State. This idea gets very close to religion, any religion. It is implicit in the teaching of the great religious leaders, Confucious, Buddah, and the Christ. Some of our misery may be due to the fact that the teachings of these great leaders have been forgotten or neglected. Health education may be truly considered a part of a great movement which has a specific aim: the relief of suffering, particularly as it is related to disease. In a broad sense, health educators are contributing to the concerted effort of a great people to make the world a better place in which to live. Their chief function consists in dissemination of knowledge including an understanding of the agencies employed in the prevention of disease and the preservation of health.

*Read at the Annual State Meeting April 26, 1944, Tulsa, Oklahoma.

Throughout the ages we know that people have spent much time at war. But in war and peace there has been a less obvious but never ending battle between man and the scourges of poverty, ignorance and disease. Their toll of human suffering and death is greater than that brought about by all man-made violence combined. In the face of the present World War it is imperative that the people have every possible protection. This is also a time wherein the principles of democracy are on trial, and our way of doing things is being questioned by men and groups of men all over the world. Our way of living is challenged not only on the battle fields, but by many people who have honestly, though misguidedly, lost much of their faith in humanity and in democracy.

We cannot directly cure the ills of poverty. That is accomplished by the productive wealth of our people, by those who are productively engaged in agriculture, transportation, processing, manufacturing, and distributing. Therein lies the true measure of wealth in any nation. It must not be confused with the amount of money that people have. It is of course a trite observation that no wealth is possible without reasonable good health, and in attempting to improve health through education it is in our province to advance the common cause of men.

The need for proper adult health education is based on three assumptions: (1) That a great many people are eager for information about matters having to do with personal and public health. (2) That the medical and public health agencies are the best and most logical channels for the dissemination of such information. (3) That if these proper agencies do not assume their full responsibility, less worthy groups will usurp the field and hamper the cause through inadequate or false teaching.

The interest in medicine as such, in hygiene, eugenics, diet, and kindred subjects is more obvious than ever before. Health educators should be sure they have the right answers, according to available knowledge. The public should be taught that medical science is not static and that principles and practices change with increasing knowledge. Established fundamentals should be taught and controversial questions avoided. What is known should be taught with dignity and authority. If this is done there will be no time for controversial problems.

Of all things, however, which will tend to unite and strengthen the efforts of those who are working for the improvement of health conditions, it seems to me there is nothing which can be so beneficial as the free assembly of groups large and small. Small groups are better, I think, wherein the problems are discussed openly and frankly. When we were in school we heard lectures by scholarly men, a fine thing for youngsters, but bull sessions in the evening got a lot of good ideas across to minds that would otherwise have been in the dark, more or less to this day. Those sessions also taught us to know each other better and to become more friendly.

This orderly dissemination of knowledge concerning the factors related to physical welfare, which we call Health Education, must be planned upon a basis of long term effort. It must be recognized that all educational influences are brought about slowly, and often results are remote. This very time element predicates the deliberation which is necessary for orderly and proper development. It tends toward building a stability of thought and process which, in the long run, will be most effective. Those who are interested in Health Education cannot limit their activities to merely telling the old story of preventive medicine, nutrition, hygiene, prenatal care and venereal disease control. A full Public Health Education program must include an organized effort to bring about a practical application of a number of factors, which must include: A survey of need and a proper evaluation of relative needs of communities; a co-ordinated understanding of all social and medical agencies and agents, a realization of their proper abilities and spheres of usefulness, and a mutual understanding and confidence; a specific program adapted to possibilities of accomplishment, and the ideals desired; a presentation which will tend to popularize Health Education through the facility of participation.

Do not seek a standard pattern which is to be used in formulating a community organization. Community problems and resources are never identical, but they do hold certain regard for basic principles which may apply in any community. They are as follows:

1. The objectives should represent real and definite needs worthy of the best possible efforts.
2. The program should have community interest and approval or it is unlikely to survive.
3. The program should include participation by all people concerned.
4. The plans should be developed under the guidance of a central representative planning group.
5. The program should relate itself acceptably to all other existing community program organizations and agencies.
6. The community should have a report of conditions and of progress at regular intervals.

The people of Oklahoma who are now most interested in Public Health Education have thus far advanced their programs along well considered channels. They are people of understanding and personal integrity. Their activities have already meant much to the welfare of the people of this State. Although my acquaintance with Health Education as such, is somewhat limited, I cannot help feeling a selfish pride in the accomplishment.

In closing may I insist that all groups who are interested in Public Health Education must work together toward the development of programs, which are thoroughly understood, and which, according to mutual agreement, represent the best possible direction for efforts. Please assume that local physicians will be glad to co-operate with any program that merits their support. At times some of you may question this statement, but when and if you do, I believe sober consideration will convince you the difficulty is one of lack of understanding and not a willful obstruction. When purposes of Health Education are well defined, most differences of opinion merely represent poor acquaintance either with the subject or with the individuals or groups involved.

DISCUSSION

CHARLES W. HAYGOOD, M.D.

I am confident that we all agree that the so-called "rambling thoughts" of the essayist have been most provocative and worthwhile. In fact, Dr. Gallaher succeeded in "throwing his words and phrases together" in such a fine manner that it has been difficult for me to decide just which of his many points of emphasis should be discussed in my allotted five minutes.

To my mind Dr. Gallaher struck an important note when he referred to the first tenet characteristic of democracy; namely, the conviction that all men will eventually do what is right. May we as a profession never lose faith in that concept.

As we look back over the years to the public health movement in its early stages, all of us can appreciate how and why the law enforcement of early days has given away to the educational approach. As Dr. Gallaher stated, "men may be persuaded for a time by necessity, or threats, or violence, but they at length begin to distinguish truth and deception." He further stated that legislation as such does not (and may I add never will) safeguard the health of the people unless it is the conviction of the people that such legislation is good, necessary and adequate.

During the early years of public health the health officer was considered primarily a law-enforcing officer. No doubt many of us have had that same experience even in 1944, indicating that this concept still lags in the minds of some of our people. As the public health program began to grow and health authorities realized that they could not depend on force, they turned to education.

The n e c e s s i t y for motivation toward sounder health practices becomes apparent when we consider the scope and breadth of the public health programs of today. How much public favor and support would we maintain and secure if our programs of prevention and control of communicable diseases, nutrition, sanitation, etc., were entirely dependent on law enforcement as a means of administration?

Certainly, another keynote of the foregoing paper was that the medical and public health agencies are the logical agencies for the disseminataion of health information to the people.

In this phase of his discussion Dr. Gallaher pointed to one of the primary purposes of health education; namely, as Dr. Hiscock has said, "To close the wide gap between scientific knowledge and the application of this knowledge to daily life."

All of us believe that preservation of health belongs primarily in the medical field, but the reality of health preservation will remain only a dream if the public at large is not awakened to its necessary and important role of cooperation. Therefore, in order to "bridge the gap" and to develop toward s o u n d e r personal and community health practices, we become dependent on public cooperation and understanding.

I was particularly pleased to hear Dr. Gallaher suggest to us that we assume that local physicians will be glad to cooperate with any program that merits their support. Leaders of note in public health have consistently stressed, and wisely so, that the practicing physicians and dentists in any community are the stanchions in the battle for better health. We need and must have the active support of the medical profession if we are to expect that our health education emphasis to the public, to seek and to use

proven scientific knowledge, is to result in the application of the health knowledge gained.

I hope that this brief discussion on my part has helped to re-emphasize a few of the basic considerations we should bear in mind.

As Health Director and associate of Dr. Gallaher in Pottawatomie County, I wish to express my personal appreciation to him for his excellent paper.

DISCUSSION

A. HELEN MARTIKAINEN, M.D.

I appreciate having this opportunity to discuss a few of the many aspects of health education, Dr. Gallaher has called to our attention so very ably this morning.

Early in his presentation Dr. Gallaher indicated that it behooves medical, public health, and allied leaders to encourage the active participation of our citizens in public health education programs. Pioneers in the growing health education movement have repeatedly demonstrated that in community programs of health education the principle of "learning by doing" is a very vital force in promoting and sustaining citizen interest in health education activities. Real credit should be given here to the many non-official agencies, as for example, the tuberculosis associations all over the country. These associations for some years now have continued to develop effective tools and methods of health education, and have above all consistently recognized the strength and influence of their citizenry well armed with the known facts of the prevention and control of tuberculosis.

We recognize the fact that health education is an activity that permeates the whole health field. Docotors, dentists, staff members of the state and county health departments, and allied workers have opportunities daily in person to person contact with patients and families to instruct people in particular health matters. The spoken word, radio and newspaper publcity, motion pictures on health, and other educational media are influencing people to become more health conscious and health curious.

There still exists the need for more thorough going health education in order that all classes of persons may be reached. Dr. Gallaher has outlined to us a number of principles basic to the development of an organized community health education program. I believe if we think through again and again the recommendations he has made and analyze them in our own local terms we can visualize the deficiencies and gaps in our own health education endeavors.

Surveys made by not able leaders in health education have disclosed that when official, non-official, and other community agencies have carried on independent programs of health education, the programs have been guided by special interests with overemphasis, duplication, and incompleteness the net result. A study in one urban area indicated that "health literature had been distributed to those who could not read, and those groups with the highest morbidity and mortality rates were not being reached."

May I hasten to add here that the principles of health education as outlined by Dr. Gallaher are as applicable to the building of school health education programs as to the general population.

Dictation of a preconceived plan of study of health administered in a super-imposed manner will, and rightly so, meet with indifference, apathy, and ridicule. Parents, teachers, students, and community workers alike will be far more in favor of developing any health education program if they are given an opportunity to have a part in it. As stated earlier, the principle of "learning by doing" is growth provoking and more endurable than simply being a passive onlooker on the side lines.

I was pleased to hear Dr. Gallaher stress the fact that enlisting community interest in the study of health problems and promoting active participation should be regarded in terms of a long range effort before all classes of people may be reached. There are however, a variety of intermediate steps in which a variety of experiences may be provided for the general public under proper guidance. I would like to specify a few of

them: serving on planning committees, health councils, assisting with conduct of various health surveys, sponsoring food handlers' courses, mothers' classes, sanitation programs, radio programs, visual aid projects, community film and health reference libraries, health legislation programs, volunteer assistance at clinics, summer-round up conferences, organizing nutrition and home nursing classes, interpreting various study programs to friends and organizations, interpreting local health problems and additional facilities needed. These mentioned are only a few of the many educational experiences which adults and students alike may have for real satisfaction in community service ventures with support of authorative and trained leaders for guidance.

Dr. Gallaher pointed out that there is no standard pattern for enlisting community wide participation in an organized manner. Whatever the nature or scope of the community plan providing for closer cooperation, we have within our power the opportunity to give a greater impetus to individual programs of health education and to make the total program of health study and concerted action the ever growing concern of everyone.

BIBLIOGRAPHY

1. Shephard, Wm. P.: Metropolitan Life Insurance Company.
2. Wriston, Henry M.: Challenge to Freedom. Harper.
3. Health Education: National Health Education Association of the U. S.
4. Committee Report from Public Health Association: Community Organization for Health Education.
5. Hiscock, Ira V.: Ways to Community Health Education. Commonwealth Fund; Oxford University Press.

Diabetes and Pregnancy

PAUL B. CAMERON, M.D.

PRYOR, OKLAHOMA

In the average general practice, the diabetic patient is not accorded the attention that the disease deserves. There are not many physicians who have made any great effort to familiarize themselves with any but the superficial principles of this rather common condition, and equally few who can calculate a diet with any facility. This is unfortunate for the average diabetic, who, with few exceptions, observes his or her diet with no great care, mainly because the physician has not impressed the patient with the fundamentals of the ailment. We are prone to order diets vaguely, or to hand the patient a sterotyped diet list. This is poor discip-

line for the diabetic. This manner of prescribing a diet is perhaps a tolerable compromise between the direction "do not eat any sugar," and the elaborate instructions possible in the large clinics where a staff of dieticians is available. It takes many hours to impart adequate knowledge to the diabetic patient and at the present time very few doctors have those hours to spare.

Perhaps the reason why more patients do not come to harm because of inadequate care is that most diabetic patients seen are overweight, middle-aged persons whose diabetes is comparatively benign, and which can be controlled merely by restricting the total food intake, by causing gradual weight reduction, or by elimination of the inflammatory lesion which made them seek medical advice. There is likewise a feeling on the part of many, in which I concur to some extent, that hyperglycemia and glycosuria do not, *in the absence of ketosis*, bring the patient to harm. I know of no final word in this debate, which will not be settled until large control groups are seen and studied for many years.

The mild type of diabetes, however, is seldom seen in the patient of childbearing age, which belongs to the group we are presently concerned with. These are more severe cases, requiring strict dietary supervision, and in most instances, rather substantial insulin doses to keep them under partial control. Only one in five diabetics over 50 years of age in a series we have studied, required insulin.

How shall we advise these younger people when they consult us, about marriage and rearing a family? We must first point out that they have an incurable disease, one which will always require vigilance on their part. The trained diabetic will do this as a matter of habit, but remember again, that few diabetics are well educated in their disease. The disease will interfere to an extent with their daily lives, and certainly hamper their domestic and social pursuits. There are certain positions not open to them for gainful occupation. They are not insurable for the most part, and those who are acceptable to an insurance company must pay large excess premiums, a factor preventing adequate protection for the dependents. Both parties should be equally well informed on matters diabetic. The families of each spouse should be surveyed for traces of diabetes, for if the non-diabetic spouse carried a diabetic tendency the mathematical probabilities of a diabetic offspring increases almost to a certainty. The young couple must be aware of the constant need for medical attention, either from the private physician, or in a clinic devoted to that disease which can be found only in the large centers. Both parties, it is needless to say, should be endowed with a reasonable amount of intelligence. If all conditions satisfy the physician, he may give his approval to a marriage. Some patients may abide by his decision.

In the question of raising a family, the writer feels that many sides appear in this discussion. We shall not dwell on the sociological aspects of childless marriages or a large family, but confine the discussion to the maternal and fetal considerations. We shall also draw observations and conclusions, not from the methods possible and workable in the large clinics, but from the manner in which the average doctor is able to conduct his private practice in these days.

Not all diabetics are fertile. Many have a poor general development, and exhibit added endocrine disturbances. Some will show persistent infantilism, and menstrual irregularities. We cannot predict, even after gynecologic survey, which patient can become pregnant. Such a diagnosis is not safe in any patient who menstruates. I believe we can tell the diabetic that most of them will show alterations in the diabetic state during the last half of pregnancy, if not earlier. They will require larger insulin doses, and careful dietary management to offset the loss of tolerance usually appearing at this time. Although animal experimentation indicates that the surgically diabetic dog gains tolerance during gestation through the added fetal supply of insulin, this does not seem to hold true in clinical observation. Most of our cases have become worse in pregnancy. This loss of tolerance is not necessarily permanent.

We must warn the prospective diabetic mother that if there is nausea of pregnancy in the earlier weeks of gestation, vomiting will derange the food intake to an annoying degree. She must be prepared to remain in the hospital for rather prolonged periods, to adequately control the ketosis which follows persistent vomiting. This appears rather easily even in the non-diabetic. Although the acidosis is controllable with intravenous replacements of dextrose and fluids, the diabetic is much closer to the danger line of hepatic damage, and there may appear a loss of tolerance in one who can ill afford it.

The toxemias of pregnancy appear with greater frequency in the diabetic. Careful watch must be kept for visual changes (difficult to evaluate in the insulin-taking patient) excessive weight gain (hence the desirability of being able to calculate a diet closely), edema, albuminuria and headaches. Hydramnios is relatively common in diabetics, presumably related to the rapid fluid shifts which come with changing insulin doses and salt intake.

The prospective diabetic mother does not run a greatly increased chance of losing her life, over that of her non-diabetic sister. Her hazards lie in uncontrolled toxemias, and in whatever aggravation of her diabetic state takes place in the last few months of pregnancy. Neither of these should be fatal.

In marked contrast to the maternal mortality, that of her fetus is high. The tendency to abortion, miscarriage,, and premature labor is great, and the number of premature deaths, and immediate postnatal deaths is excessive. Far less than half of the diabetic pregnancies come to a successful conclusion, with a living and healthy child.

Why these babies die prematurely in utero, and are delivered macerated, and why they survive the first few days of life is subject to much discussion, and there seems to be no reason for the question. The babies which reach full term are large, weights of over ten pounds not being rare. They are not postmature, but are fat, flabby, with poor tissue tone, and few are vigorous.

I do not believe that the severity of the maternal diabetic, or the excellence of her diabetic care has a great deal to do with the fetal mortality. We have seen macerated fetuses born of mild diabetics, and apparently well developed and healthy children from women who had persistent glycosuria during the entire pregnancy, with bouts of ketosis and even one, who in the seventh month, spent thirty hours in deep coma associated with lobar pneumonia. Indeed, in our case records there are numerous examples of stillbirth, and premature labor, with reports of babies who weighed much over the normal many years before diabetes was clinically discovered. We are beginning to view with suspicion the report of lactosuria in the latter monhs of pregnancy, in the belief that there is little we can state about its sole existence, and whether there is an additional factor or not controlling to its passage.

The feticidal factor must not be entirely a diabetic one. The pituitary gland can be involved, inasmuch as it seems to be concerned with all glandular activity. Experimental evidence is at hand showing that excessive production of gonadotropins is associated with overgrowth of animal fetuses, and the same has been determined with the human diabetic. Undeniably good results have been claimed by the employment of large doses of estrogens and progesterone in the latter months of the pregnancy, to nullify this excessive gonadotropic effect on the fetus.

Assuming that the baby is living at birth, there is still the hazard of the first few days to overcome. There is a possibility of fetal hypoglycemia and hyperinsulinism which may be fatal. Administration of weak glucose feedings is therefore desirable, and even pareateral glucose solutions may be used. It should be used routinely in these babies, until the danger zone of the first two days is passed. Some of the babies are born with radiologically enlarged hearts; some enlarged livers and spleens; some intracranial hemorrhages; some with excess nucleated red cells in the circulating blood, and some, after careful necropsies, show nothing at all to account for death. I do not know of any

thymus-caused deaths; this condition after all may be one of the misconceptions of medicine handed down the medical generations.

In the management of the pregnant diabetic, our duties are many. We must see that she does not gain much over 20 pounds, that her diet is calculated and changed at suitable intervals to insure this. No ketosis must go without immediate attention, no matter how mild. She, of course must be familiar with urine testing, both with Benedicts solution, and with an acetone test. We prefer the Rotheras test with ammonium sulfate-sodium nitroferricyanide and ammonia, in the belief that it is far more sensitive than the ferric chloride test. She should receive no salicylates, as they vitiate the acetone tests. She is to report all abnormalities at once. This is not so much to protect the baby, as we have said previously that the degree of diabetic control is not the principal factor in the babies survival, but to protect the mother's tolerance.

It would seem justifiable to administer large doses of stilbestrol in the latter months, although we have had no personal experience with this drug. This apparently is of equal value with the much more expensive glandular preparations.

I feel that, clinically, we can tell so little about the fetus and its chances of survival, we should make frequent observations on the fetal heart and activity in the last three weeks, and in the event of any weakening of either we should consider induction of labor, or Caesarian section. Low section under spinal anesthesia does not carry a high risk.

It is seriously to be doubted if we can advise the diabetic that childbearing is desirable. If their desire is great enough, after understanding the risk to themselves in view of the lowered probability of having a living child, they may wish to proceed. The writer is rather pessimistic about the situation as it stands. There is no question that this pessimism would be less if the patient were under the care of a clinic where she could receive the best of expert care, but under the condition of ordinary practice I feel that we should discourage child bearing. The average doctor finds himself burdened with more or less urgent cases these days, and he has little time to give to the more elective type of duties. If a diabetic comes under his care, already pregnant, he must do the best he can. I have little hesitation about suggesting a therapeutic abortion in a patient whose diabetes is severe, and in whose ability to cooperate most fully we cannot place confidence.

SUMMARY

1. The average diabetic does not receive

adequate care.

2. Diabetes in the woman of childbearing age is usually more severe.

3. The diabetic contemplating a child must be unusually well informed about her disease.

4. There are certain hazards in the pregnant diabetic, and she has greatly lessened chances of bearing a living child.

5. We are not optimistic about the whole problem, and feel that only selected diabetics should be permitted to have children.

6. In certain cases, therapeutic abortion is definitely feasible.

DISCUSSION

C. J. FISHMAN, M.D.,
OKLAHOMA CITY, OKLAHOMA

The statement by Dr. Cameron that diabetes most often occurs in older years and in the obese type of patients is exceedingly pertinent. In the old days, prior to the discovery of insulin, the average life of elderly patients with diabetes, even without any treatment whatever, was fifteen years while those that developed under 30 years of age had an average life of only two to four years, even with excellent dietetic management. It behooves us, therefore, to be on the alert to discover diabetes in pregnant women even though they are not usually in the generally accepted diabetic ages.

Dr. Cameron also wisely suggested prophylaxis in avoiding marriages among known diabetics. This is practical genetics which however is not as practical among human beings where sentiment plays such an important part in attraction, love, and marriage, that they can be deferred from their desires which are based upon sentiment rather than pure reason. I have tried in many instances to point out the evil possibilities of marriage among individuals who have hereditary diseases but have rarely succeeded.

Since it is estimated that there are 100,000 diabetic women of childbearing age in the United States the problem of pregnancy in diabetic women becomes important. Williams, at the Johns Hopkins Hospital, prior to the discovery of insulin, estimated that maternal mortality in diabetic pregnant women was from 25 per cent to 30 per cent. P. White of Boston, since the institution of insulin treatment, estimated the rate to be 3.8 per cent or six times that of non-diabetic patients, this in patients having superior care; while the infant mortality is more serious continuing from 20 per cent to 40 per cent of all pregnancies, almost as frequent as before the insulin era. Glycosuria in the early months of pregnancy is not due to lac-

tose but is always a true glycosuria and must be confirmed by a blood sugar, which, when over .120 per cent, means diabetes. The presence of glycosuria without increased blood sugar indicates a reduced renal threshold. Even though this is an explanation, the presence of sugar in the urine in a pregnant woman should not be considered lightly and the patient should be continuously under medical and laboratory guidance.

Acidosis which is the most serious complication, is aggravated by toxemia of pregnancy so that eclampsia is more than ten times as frequent in diabetics as in normal women and it has been repeatedly shown that there is an excess of placental prolan prior to the onset of toxemia. Another factor of importance is the nutritional deficiency and it is definitely established that the requirement for thiamine is increased three to five times in normal pregnant animals and there is further requirement in diabetics so that these extra factors are to be considered seriously during the presence of true diabetes or glycosuria in pregnant women.

Patients under satisfactory management with insulin require increased doses even in the early months of pregnancy based upon the extra metabolic requirements while in the later months of pregnancy less insulin may be required for the reason that the fetus reduces not only its necessary amount of insulin, but produces a sufficient added amount which is available to the diabetic mother. This has been confirmed repeatedly by many observers. After delivery this fetal insulin is no longer available and the mother again requires her usual dosage with at times, larger amounts.

During the later weeks of pregnancy lactose may be present in the urine which must be distinguished from glucose and if this is not done and insulin is increased, this would have no influence upon the lactosuria and even induce hypoglycemic reactions.

Stillbirths and congenital defects in a diabetic woman are more frequent than in normal women and in addition to this, the tendency to the development of large children has always been regarded as a probability even though these children were known to have been larger by reason of flabbiness and edema rather than because of actual increased growth. This may be explained upon the nutritional deficiency of the mother which is expected to be controlled by the better understanding and feeding and the substitutional use of vitamins particularly thiamine in pregnancies. If it is suspected that the child is large, premature delivery or Caesarian section is indicated. Futhermore the increased requirement of the mother for insulin, supplied by the fetus in the later months of pregnancy, seems to induce increased insulin supply in the child and immediately after birth the possibility of hyperinsulinism with hypoglycemic reactions in the child is sometimes seen so that the early feeding with sugar is indicated as soon as possible following birth,, as was pointed out by Dr. Cameron in his paper. Therefore, the necessity for increased quantities of insulin should be carefully guarded because the induction of hypoglycemia in the mother influences a hypoglycemic reaction on the part of the fetus with a possibility of hypoglycemic death.

It is obvious therefore, that in glycosuria during pregnancy, and certainly in a true diabetic, pregnancy becomes an important complicating factor which must be treated with utmost watchfulness and intelligence.

In almost all the counties of the United States there are local Chapters of The National Foundation for Infantile Paralysis prepared to help health officers, doctors, nurses, hospitals and patients in every way possible. These Chapters stand ready to assist the entire community. Know your Chapter—ask its help if needed—and volunteer to help your Chapter so that it will be able to render the necessary services.

The German who invented an edible paper had something. As the posse closes in, the high command can eat its plans for World war III.

An airplane pilot reports hitting a grasshopper at an altitute of 10,000 feet. One can only feel the time is here to mow the grass.

• OBITUARIES •

Resolution

WHEREAS, The Tulsa County Medical Society has sustained a great loss with the passing of Dr. Ned R. Smith on August 18, 1944, and

WHEREAS, Dr. Smith contributed greatly through his extreme foresight and high intelligence to the progress of the state and community in which he lived, to the health and well-being of its people, and to the advancement of professional and civic interests, and

WHEREAS, Dr. Smith served the Tulsa County Medical Society in the capacity of officer and trustee, and served many other civic and professional organizations in similiar capacities, acting in the interests of all,

NOW THEREFORE, BE IT RESOLVED: That the Tulsa County Medical Society commemorate the passing of Dr. Smith through this resolution, that it pay tribute to his achievements, and serve to express the heartfelt loss of the members in Dr. Smith's passing.

BE IT FURTHER RESOLVED: That this resolution convey the sympathy of the Tulsa County Medical Society to Dr. Smith's family and friends.

Approved this 11th day of September, 1944.

Average consumption of pharmaceuticals of men overseas is two pounds per man per month.

Pharmacists are serving in every branch of our armed forces. They are contributing much to the war effort on the home front by carrying on under discouraging handicaps of manpower shortages. They are helping the physicians carry their heavy loads under wartime conditions.

The people in every neighborhood should know these facts. This Upjohn display will tell them.

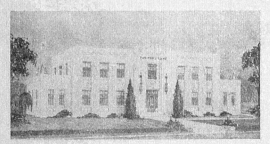

• *THE PRESIDENT'S PAGE* •

A Booth at the Oklahoma State Fair was maintained by the Oklahoma State Medical Association, the Oklahoma State Health Department, the American Society for the Control of Cancer and the Oklahoma State Tuberculosis Association. The title of the Booth was "Doctors at War" and movies were shown on War in the South Pacific, depicting surgeons at work with battle casualties. Also shown were movies on Cancer and on Tuberculosis.

Thousands of pieces of literature on Cancer were distributed by the American Federation of Women's Clubs through the cooperation of Mrs. E. Lee Ozbirn of the Cancer Committee. Representatives from the Federation were on duty at all times. The Oklahoma State Tuberculosis Society furnished interesting and educational literature on Tuberculosis which was distributed by their representative. In addition to the medical literature, thousands of Wagner-Murray cartoons were distributed.

The success of the Booth was apparent by the crowds which, at all times, were in attendance. Keen interest was shown in the moving pictures and the literature was well received. This medium presented a wonderful opportunity to educate the lay public in the early symptoms of cancer and tuberculosis and the necessity of consulting the physician at the first indications.

President.

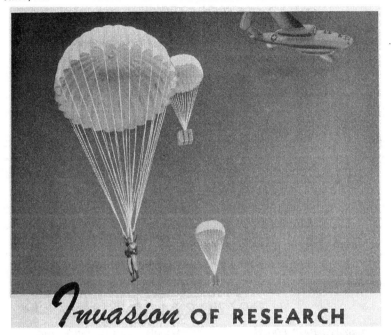

Invasion OF RESEARCH

Daily, a flight surgeon with complete medical supplies and equipment lands in a steaming jungle . . . To give lost infantry soldiers first aid and protection against infection . . . To relieve malaria victims . . . To prevent amputations . . . and save lives.

Today, the medical profession is doing a more important job than ever before.

Through careful manufacturing and efficient distribution of reliable Warren-Teed products, we are constantly endeavoring to save the time of physicians and pharmacists all over the world. Together, we shall speed the day of Victory.

WARREN-TEED

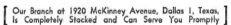

Medicaments of Exacting Quality Since 1920

THE WARREN-TEED PRODUCTS COMPANY, COLUMBUS 8, OHIO

[Our Branch at 1920 McKinney Avenue, Dallas 1, Texas, Is Completely Stocked and Can Serve You Promptly]

The JOURNAL Of The
OKLAHOMA STATE MEDICAL ASSOCIATION

EDITORIAL BOARD

L. J. MOORMAN, Oklahoma City, Editor-in-Chief

E. EUGENE RICE, Shawnee   BEN H. NICHOLSON, Oklahoma City

MR. PAUL H. FESLER, Oklahoma City, Business Manager

JANE FIRRELL TUCKER, Editorial Assistant

CONTRIBUTIONS: Articles accepted by this Journal for publication including those read at the annual meetings of the State Association are the sole property of this Journal.

The Editorial Department is not responsible for the opinions expressed in the original articles of contributors.

Manuscripts may be withdrawn by authors for publication elsewhere only upon the approval of the Editorial Board.

MANUSCRIPTS: Manuscripts should be typewritten, double-spaced, on white paper 8½ x 11 inches. The original copy, not the carbon copy, should be submitted.

Footnotes, bibliographies and legends for cuts should be typed on separate sheets in double space. Bibliography listing should follow this order: Name of author, title of article, name of periodical with volume, page and date of publication.

Manuscripts are accepted subject to the usual editorial revisions and with the understanding that they have not been published elsewhere.

NEWS: Local news of interest to the medical profession, changes of address, births, deaths and weddings will be gratefully received.

ADVERTISING: Advertising of articles, drugs or compounds unapproved by the Council on Pharmacy of the A.M.A. will not be accepted. Advertising rates will be supplied on application.

It is suggested that members of the State Association patronize our advertisers in preference to others.

SUBSCRIPTIONS: Failure to receive The Journal should call for immediate notification.

REPRINTS: Reprints of original articles will be supplied at actual cost provided request for them is attached to manuscripts or made in sufficient time before publication. Checks for reprints should be made payable to Industrial Printing Company, Oklahoma City.

Address all communications to THE JOURNAL OF THE OKLAHOMA STATE MEDICAL ASSOCIATION, 210 Plaza Court, Oklahoma City. (3)

OFFICIAL PUBLICATION OF THE OKLAHOMA STATE MEDICAL ASSOCIATION

Copyrighted October, 1944

EDITORIALS

STATE FAIR BOOTH

In keeping with the editorial policies of this Journal, the Oklahoma State Medical Association, the Oklahoma State Tuberculosis Association, the State Health Department and the American Society for the Control of Cancer, conducted an educational exhibit including pictures on cancer and tuberculosis and a War Film entitled "Life Line," showing the doctors at war, caring for casualties from the battle fields back to the hospitals. Suitable literature on cancer and tuberculosis and educational material on socialized medicine were distributed. Representatives from the above agencies were at all times present for the purpose of distributing the educational material and giving additional information.

Records show that thousands of people passed through this booth and manifested unusual interest in the exhibits, moving pictures and available literature, many returning to ask questions and express approval. This is a good way to counter-act the trend toward regimented medicine, since there is much truth in the adage that the American people are apt to be "down on what they are not up on."

We salute the participating agencies with the hope that they will never permit such an opportunity to pass without the effort to inform the people concerning the evolution of medicine, of present methods of practice and the danger of regimentation.

REGIONAL MEETING OF THE COLLEGE OF PHYSICIANS

On February 23 in Oklahoma City there will be a Regional Meeting of the American College of Physicians with Oklahoma, Missouri, Kansas and Nebraska participating. This meeting immediately follows the annual Washington Birthday Meeting of the Oklahoma Internists.

All of the members of the Oklahoma State Medical Association and all the doctors in military service are cordially invited to attend both meetings. No doubt, the Regional Meeting of the College will be of great significance for physicians who are holding the humble sectors on the home front. Please keep the date in mind.

LONG LIVE VIVISECTION

Since the days of Herophilus and Erasistratus in the 2nd Century, B.C., vivisection periodically has made important contributions to medical knowledge and has been instrumental in the saving of untold suffering and death.

The recent controversy before the Chicago City Council over the employment of dogs in experiments requiring vivisection is of momentous interest, not only to doctors but to the people at large. It shows how ignorance and prejudice cling to society with unrelenting tenacity.

The opposition of the anti-vivisectionists allegedly for humane purposes is essentially inhuman. Usually the opposition comes from women from mirrored and tiled bathrooms, clothed in furs and feathers and other wares processed from dead animals. They passionately plead for poodles versus people. If their husbands who provide their luxuries were to die of the plague, they would still have their poodles and pekinese and the potentiality of mange and fleas.

GERIATRICS AND SPECULATIVE GYMNASTICS

Increasing longevity is no mystery to physicians. It is the realization of a planned objective, but for some people, it is a great enigma. Medicine must ever strive to provide better health in order that people may find increasingly greater satisfaction in self expression over a longer period of time. Tallerand said, "Everybody wants to live long, but nobody wants to be old."

Certain politicians, while clammering for what they call better medical service become excited about the old age problem and unwittingly find themselves facing an embarrassing political paradox.

If, in the United States, the increase in the number of people reaching 65 years of age surpasses the alarming figure of two million in ten years, perhaps we should conclude the high quality of medical service is already over-taxing the ingenuity of lawmakers and administrators.

The time of senescence, in a given individual, is set by the germ plasma and not by the clock. The problem of the aging would not be so great if organized agencies would replace the fixed retirement age with a policy of common sense and critical judgment in keeping with biological facts, human genetics and constitutional potentialities. Allowing for reasonable variations, we know that within a period of nine months, a fertilized microscopic ovum will produce a full-fledged human being. But no one can accurately estimate the time between that period of

"mewling and puking in the nurses arms" and the "turning again toward childish treble." Certainly we should not hasten the "last scene of all" by a compulsory premature retirement from useful employment. In many cases a gradual transition may be possible. Certainly the psychological strain of sudden idleness should be avoided when possible. The aging individual dependent upon the decision of an employer or the rule of an organization may suffer serious mental strain in anticipation of the approaching hour when retirement is demanded. The judgement and experience of age should not be disregarded. It is remarkable how certain faculties, abilities and skills are retained in older people.

There is another sad paradox in the establishment of homes with expensive occupational schemes for aging people who otherwise might be individually and profitably employed with great personal satisfaction:

"Our nature here is not unlike our wine
Some sorts, when old, continue brisk and
      fine."

Old age, learning how to gradually leave off is no more dangerous to society than youth learning how to take on the duties of life. Regimentation is good only for prisoners of war and the mentally unsound. Growing old should not rest upon the arbitrary decision of a finite master, but as Amiel has said, it should be "the Master Work of Wisdom."

No matter how sad the lint and rags out of which a life is woven, nobody has a right to silence the shuttle, if hope is still alive with sufficient genes to finish the fabric. Without personal liberty we would be "no better than parsnips." Please let us grow frosty with frugality and, God willing, hoary with honor.

CULTURE AND MEDICAL SUPERIORITY

In the light of our editorial policy concerning the desirability of a broad scholastic foundation for the study of medicine and the continuance of the cultural graces in the practice of medicine, the following from Ralph Waldo Emerson's letters should be read with interest. It appears that his erudite, cantankerous Aunt Mary developed a "severe erysipelas." After being upbraided for his visit and his concern, Emerson writes his wife:

"We found Aunt Mary much better. Her disorder which on Friday night was such that Dr. Spofford believed she could not live until morning suddenly changed its character and she has rapidly mended. She says her head from the eyes upward is one lump of disease and she sits covered with burdock bandages down to the mouth, but so much of her face as is seen looks very well. . . . Dr. S. she says is as well pleased with his work as if he had built up an old wall, but she shall know better than ever to employ such a doctor again. She had dismissed her first physician because she wished to die in the presence of a superior and intelligent man, but that Dr. S. should have the assurance to cure her, was unlooked for."

MEDICINE AND MANPOWER

Approximately one-third of the doctors in the United States have volunteered for service in the Armed Forces. In spite of this great strain upon civilian medical services, the physicians left behind, regardless of age and physical fitness, have worked day and night in an effort to hold every sector on the home front. There have been no complaints about the increased working hours, no thought of strikes; only spontaneous individual effort to meet obvious needs, with no watching of clocks, no punching of time cards, no swinging of doors to mark the end of a day's work. The task must be done in order that the War may be won. Thus the physician sets the pattern of good citizenship through the prompt performance of patriotic duty unhampered by selfish motives.

In spite of the fact that we have given the best in our profession for medical service at the front and in military hospitals, it is significant that medical manpower has been sufficiently extended through voluntary effort to hold the health level, the morbidity and mortality rates remain virtually where they stood before Pearl Harbor. In spite of false accusations coming out of Washington over a period of ten years, physicians without demanding redress, without thought of extra pay for overtime or double pay for holidays, have held the line on the home front from the most humble sector up to the busy marts of war industry. Men belonging to labor unions who move only when the order comes from their leaders and racketeers cannot voluntarily extend the coverage of manpower. They are robbed of the fluidity and flexibility of life by a despicable form of slavery.

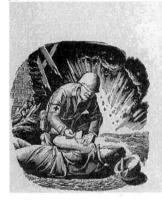
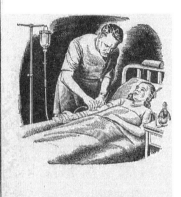

ASSOCIATION ACTIVITIES

KANSAS MEDICAL LEADER SPEAKS AT TULSA

Dr. Frank L. Feierabend, Kansas City medical leader, was guest speaker at the October 9 meeting of the Tulsa County Medical Society. Dr. Feierabend spoke on the subject "Medical Service Plans and the Doctor's Responsibility."

Slides from the National Physician's Committee relative to Prepaid Medical Plans were presented by Mr. Paul Fesler, Executive Secretary of the Oklahoma State Medical Association.

FIRST AWARD OF MARCUS PERRY SCHOLARSHIP MADE

Dr. John C. Perry, Tulsa, established the Marcus Perry Medic Scholarship to perpetuate the memory of his father, a pioneer Tulsa physician. The $250.00 Scholarship is awarded on the basis of past scholastic records, medical aptitude, character and financial need.

The award for the 1944-45 year was given to Clyde Goodnight, senior student at the University of Tulsa. Announcement of the awarding of the scholarship was made by Professor H. D. Chase, chairman of the premedic Committee.

PREPAID MEDICAL PLAN COMMITTEE MEETS

On Sunday, October 8, a meeting of the Prepaid Medical Plan Committee was held at the Skirvin Hotel in Oklahoma City. Final recommendations for an indemnity plan were adopted to be presented to the Council and the House of Delegates at the meeting on October 22.

NATIONAL TUBERCULOSIS ASSOCIATION EXECUTIVE COMMITTEE MEETS

On October 16, a meeting of the Executive Committee of the National Tuberculosis Association was held in New York City. Dr. Lewis J. Moorman, Oklahoma City, President of the Tuberculosis Association, attended the meeting. Dr. Moorman will go from the meeting in New York to New Jersey where, on October 17, the 40th anniversary of the New Jersey State Tuberculosis Association will be celebrated.

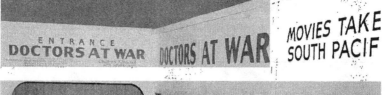

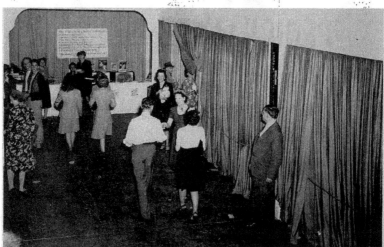

State Fair Booth, 1944

EXECUTIVE SECRETARY ATTENDS CLEVELAND MEETING

Mr. Paul Fesler, Executive Secretary, attended a meeting of the Planning Committee of the American Hospital Association in Cleveland on October 2. He also sat in with the Blue Cross and Medical Care Planning meetings.

PRESIDENT AND EXECUTIVE SECRETARY ATTEND GARFIELD COUNTY MEETING

Dr. C. R. Rountree, President and Mr. Paul Fesler, Executive Secretary, attended the meeting of the Garfield County Medical Society in Enid on September 28. Over thirty members were present and showed considerable interest in the slides furnished by the National Physician's Committee on Prepaid Medical Plans.

TIMELY MESSAGE GIVEN BY DR. KRETSCHMER ON RADIO

The following message was delivered by Dr. H. L. Kretschmer, President of the American Medical Association, on the radio program, "The Doctor Fights" which is sponsored by Schenley Laboratories, Inc.

"It is not a novel experience for American doctors to participate in war. The American Medical Association was organized in 1847 in the midst of war with Mexico. Since that time American doctors have taken part in the Civil War, the war with Spain, the Boxer Rebellion and World War I.

"Doctors serve voluntarily, you know—whether with the armed forces or on the home front. There is that within a man which leads him, yet impels him to enter this profession . . . and, having entered, to serve wherever and whenever his services are needed.

"I would pay my respect tonight especially to the older practitioners of medicine. All of them are doing more than double duty. Many who had retired from active practice re-entered the practice of medicine. Thousands of the older doctors who had retired gave up their leisure and are working harder than ever before.

"Despite the large number of doctors in the armed forces the people of this country have never enjoyed better health than now. The death rate is the lowest in our history except for a slight, not serious rise, last year. There have been no major epidemics like the influenza of the last War.

"The venereal diseases are almost completely controlled; and it is likely that the combined use of the sulfonamide drugs, of penicillin, of heat, and of new technics, may eliminate venereal diseases entirely within a few generations. Tuberculosis has now reached an all time low. During the past year more than three million babies were born in the United States with the lowest maternal and infant death rates in our history— and this in the midst of the War.

"Notwithstanding many exaggerated reports the fact is that the nutrition of our people is excellent. There are isolated areas where nutrition needs improving but we know how to control these conditions and we need only to apply the knowledge we have. People must be taught how to eat proper foods.

"Far too many people take vitamins without first getting professional guidance as to which—if any— vitamins they need. As a result of the wonderful achievements of medicine in reducing mortality, more people are reaching an advanced age where they are subject to degenerative diseases. Today nine per cent of our population are over 65 years of age. The new advances of medicine are going to increase that percentage and the care of the aged may well be one of the largest medical problems of the post war period."

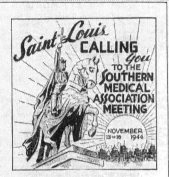

Saint Louis CALLING you TO THE SOUTHERN MEDICAL ASSOCIATION MEETING
NOVEMBER 13 to 16 1944

PHYSICIANS of the South have an urgent call to St. Louis for the annual meeting of the Southern Medical Association, Monday, Tuesday, Wednesday and Thursday, November 13-16 — a great wartime meeting. Medical meetings are essential, as essential in wartimes as in peace, even more so. Physicians, civilian and military, need medical meetings. At the St. Louis meeting, a streamlined essential wartime meeting, every phase of medicine and surgery will be covered in the general clinical sessions, the twenty sections, the four conjoint meetings, and the scientific and technical exhibits— the last word in modern, practical, scientific medicine and surgery. Addresses and papers will be given by distinguished physicians not only from the South but from other parts of the United States. Everything under one roof, the Municipal Auditorium.

REGARDLESS of what any physician may be interested in, regardless of how general or how limited his interest, there will be at St. Louis a program to challenge that interest and make it worth-while for him to attend.

ALL MEMBERS of State and County medical societies in the South are cordially invited to attend. And all members of state and county medical societies in the South should be and can be members of the Southern Medical Association. The annual dues of $4.00 include the Southern Medical Journal, a journal valuable to physicians of the South, one that each should have on his reading table.

SOUTHERN MEDICAL ASSOCIATION
Empire Building
BIRMINGHAM 3, ALABAMA

WAR FILM SHOWN AT WOODS COUNTY MEDICAL SOCIETY MEETING

At a meeting of the Woods County Medical Society on Tuesday, September 26, the feature of the evening was the colored film shown by Dr. J. H. Humphrey of the Mooreland hospital. Dr. Humphry is a former medical missionary to China and the films dipicted "China Before and After the Japanese Invasion."

WHO CAN MATCH RECORD OF DR. D. W. GRIFFIN?*

Near the town of Lenoir, N. C., a group of farm boys attending a country school were playing ball, among them a lad named David Griffin. As his brother threw the ball it struck a playmate who fell in an epileptic fit. Thoroughly alarmed, the boys believed their comrade was about to die. That was the beginning of a mental illness which became so acute that the sick boy's mother confined him in a log room some distance from her house. With other lads in the neighborhood David Griffin visited the log room, peering through cracks in the walls at their former playmate, chained in one corner.

"More than anything else, I believe, seeing that boy led to my study of mental illness," says Doctor D. W. Griffin, superintendent of the Central State Hospital at Norman who tomorrow completes 45 years of service to the people of Oklahoma.

Only 6 months after having been graduated from the medical college of North Carolina's State University, Doctor Griffin came to Norman. Had he possessed the price of a ticket back home he would have left immediately, so shocked was he by what he found. But how could he leave when his wordly goods consisted of $5.00, one suit of clothes, one pair of shoes, one suitcase and two shirts.

The hospital, privately owned, had been an old school building, and it had been run for profit. It housed 260 patients who slept on straw mattresses. The windows had no screens. To keep patients quiet, attendants gave them opiates and whisky. Realizing that if he undertook drastic reforms speedily he would incur the hostility of older men running the place, Doctor Griffin employed diplomacy to effect changes gradually.

It was in 1915 that Governor Robert L. Williams decided that the State should purchase the hospital. The price asked was $250,000.00 The governor continued bargaining with the owners until they agreed to accept $100,00.00. Then one morning he called Doctor Griffin, asking his to come to Oklahoma City.

"I've bought your hospital and I made a pretty good horse-trade. Now I want you to stay there and manage it." There he has remained, the faithful, hard-working, highly-efficient, kindly doctor, striving to maintain not only a hospital, but a home for his patients. No problem baffles him. When he no longer could hire men to mow the grounds he bought sheep and gave patients the job of shepherding them. Food-producting gardens are worked by patients who find healing in contact with the good earth, air and sunshine—they also work in kitchens, storerooms, and other places. Although he has not made money for the institution he managed to save a sum that, supplemented by a grant from the federal govern-

ment, he used in building a beautiful chapel where religious services and moving picture shows are held.

What other administrator of a state institution has carried on through 45 years—Doctor Griffin has been under every governor since Governor Cassius M. Barnes of territorial days and every governor has trusted him. So have the people of Oklahoma. Here is a man who knows his job thoroughly, a man of the highest integrity.

"The people of Oklahoma have been good to me," says Doctor Griffin. In any event, this is certain; Doctor Griffin has been good to them.

*Edith Johnson. Daily Oklahoman. October 6, 1944.

POSTGRADUATE COURSES BEING HELD BY AMERICAN COLLEGE OF PHYSICIANS

Courses on Cardiology, General Medicine, Internal Medicine and Allergy have been held by the American College of Physicians during the month of October. Still to be held are Courses on Internal Medicine and Special Medicine. These courses have been arranged through the generous cooperation of the directors and the institutions at which the courses will be given. The Advisory Committee on Postgraduate Courses will plan another course during the winter and spring of 1945.

The courses are organized especially for Fellows and Associates of the Colleges but where facilities are available, they will be open to non-members with adequate preliminary training preference to be given to non-members in the following order: (1) candidates for membership (2) medical officers in the armed forces (3) physicians preparing for examinations by their certifying boards (4) other non-members having adequate background for advanced work. By direction of the Board of Regents registrations from non-members of the College may not be accepted more than three weeks in advance of the opening of any course.

Course No. 5 (October 23—November 4) in Special Phases of Internal Medicine offers an unusual opportunity for physicians to familiarize themselves with recent developments in various fields of Internal Medicine. Among other outstanding physicians, Dr. Henry H. Turner, Oklahoma City, will speak on Endocrinology October 31, November 1 and November 3. The meeting place will be at Thorne Hall, Northwestern University in Chicago.

Course No. 6 (December 4—December 15) in Special Medicine allots for approximately one-half day to the consideration of each of several special fields of medicine. It offers a short but detailed resume in these several different specialties, and gives an opportunity to study under a selected faculty. The meeting place is the Philadelphia General Hospital of Philadelphia.

Continue To
BUY BONDS!

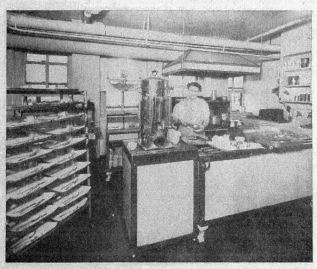

In Memoriam

Roy E. Baze, M.D.
1910-1944

Captain Roy Baze, Chickasha, was killed in action in France on August 24, 1944. Captain Baze participated in the invasion of Southern France, where he parachuted into occupied country.

Having served with the medical corps for three years, Captain Baze served in the African campaign before going to southern France. He attended high-school in Blanchard, was graduated from Wentworth military academy, Lexington, Missouri, Oklahoma City University and the University of Oklahoma School of Medicine, graduating with the Class of 1936. Before entering the armed forces he practiced in Chickasha with his uncle, Dr. W. J. Baze.

The following letter was received by Mrs. Baze just two days before the telegram that Captain Baze had been killed in action. The letter shows the wonderful work being carried on.

"Many things have happened since my last letter. . . . The stars were bright but no moon and I had bundles of food, medical supplies and gas mask distributed about the body requiring two men to help me into the plane. We are soon over water and lights show the correct way. An aircraft carrier with lights outlining it and a plane taking off from it were beautiful from above. Soon the fighters protecting us could be seen. They looked like black beetles with lights in their tails. The ships below looked like a swarm of water bugs. Later comes the order to stand up and hook up. Then go. It is a very beautiful scene; the wind perfectly calm. We go through a layer of clouds then we can see the ground beneath us. With my load I am wondering how hard I am going to hit. Fortunately I hit in a vineyard on a very soft spot of ground—a very easy landing. Soon discover that there are no Germans in the exact vicinity. The French are anxious to keep us so the Aid Station is put up in a French home. It is beginning to get daylight and the planes roar overhead. Noon and I have had very little business. Then a French ambulance comes saying there are several wounded in the hospital. We go to the hospital and operate with the help of a French surgeon. Cannot praise too highly the help that they gave us at the hospital. By 5 p.m. we were evacuating the wounded by American ambulances. Lot of business and am tired at bedtime, my first sleep in 36 hours.

"The following morning gather my equipment together and move to a hotel. Some of the men are getting a German truck with trailer body in shape so we can have portable surgery. A good night's sleep except an occasional sniper shooting somewhere in the town. The next morning the men have the truck running. Go to the square to see the leader of the French underground in this vicinity, who helped us so very much, receive the Silver Star from an American General. Got in the truck and drove 20 miles to the other part of our group. We get our truck equipped with equipment from a German hospital. Have lights inside the trailer so we work at nights. We have plasma, plaster, ether and surgical instruments, so we expect to do quite well."

Captain Baze is survived by his parents, his wife and one son, Frank Skirvin Baze. His wife and son live at LaBelle, Missouri with Mrs. Baze's parents.

In fitting tribute to a fine physician and a wonderful person, the following editorial appeared in the Chickasha Express of September 21.

"War is not a respecter of persons. It strikes down the bravest and best. Of the Son of Man it was said, 'He saved others, himself he could not save.' In the case of Chickasha's Dr. Roy Baze, it was literally true.

"As a member of the army medical corps, Captain Baze bound up the wounds of our fighting boys in North Africa and Italy. His last letter told a graphic story of parachuting down safely in France, with his surgical supplies. Next came the shocking news—killed in action, August 24.

"We haven't the least doubt that many boys coming home from the war will owe their lives to Dr. Baze. He did not die in vain. Making the supreme sacrifice, he gave to his country and to humanity the highest service of which any man is capable. The influence flowing from his unfinished life will live forever. It isn't how long we live but how well.

"Modest, genial Roy Baze had a heart of pure gold. Still quite a young man when he came to Chickasha to practice his profession, he soon had a host of friends. Blessed with civic spirit, it wasn't long before he became a useful member of the community. While he was city physician, the hour was never too late or the night too stormy to keep him from going to the aid of the needy and distressed.

> 'His life was gentle, and the elements
> 'So mixed in him that Nature might stand up
> 'And say to the world, This was a man.' "

A memorial service was held in Oklahoma City, the home of Captain Baze's parents Mr. and Mrs. G. T. Baze, on Sunday, October 8.

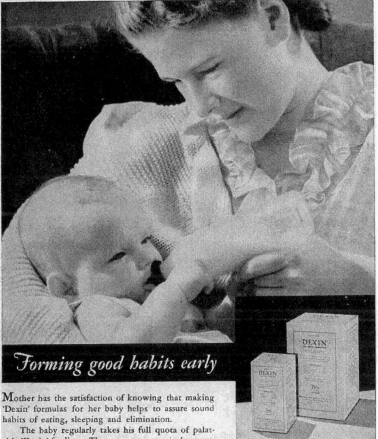

Forming good habits early

'Dexin' does make a difference

Mother has the satisfaction of knowing that making 'Dexin' formulas for her baby helps to assure sound habits of eating, sleeping and elimination.

The baby regularly takes his full quota of palatable 'Dexin' feedings. They are not excessively sweet, and do not dull the appetite. Adding bland foods to the diet is more easily accomplished.

A well-fed 'Dexin' baby is not awakened by unsatisfied hunger. 'Dexin' helps eliminate disturbances that might interrupt sleep. Its high dextrin content (1) reduces intestinal fermentation and the tendency to colic, diarrhea and constipation, (2) promotes the formation of soft, flocculent, easily digested curds. 'Dexin' Reg. U. S. Pat. Off

COMPOSITION

Dextrins	. . . . .75%	Mineral Ash	. 0.25%
Maltose	. . . . .24%	Moisture	. . 0.75%

Available carbohydrate 99% 115 calories per ounce
6 level packed tablespoonfuls equal 1 ounce

'DEXIN'

HIGH DEXTRIN CARBOHYDRATE

 Literature on request

BURROUGHS WELLCOME & CO. (U.S.A.)(INC.) 9-11 E. 41st St., New York 17, N. Y.

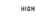

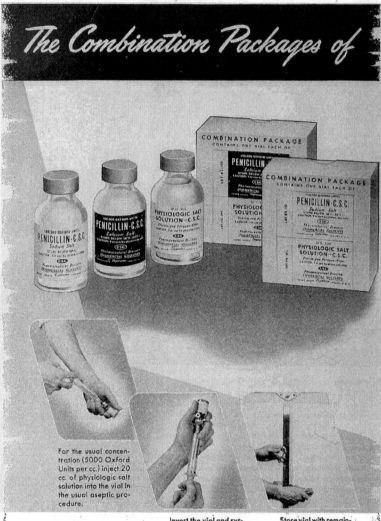

The Combination Packages of

For the usual concentration (5000 Oxford Units per cc.) inject 20 cc. of physiologic salt solution into the vial in the usual aseptic procedure.

Invert the vial and syringe (with needle in vial), and withdraw the amount of penicillin solution required for the first injection.

Store vial with remainder of solution in refrigerator. Solution is ready for subsequent injections during the next 24 hours.

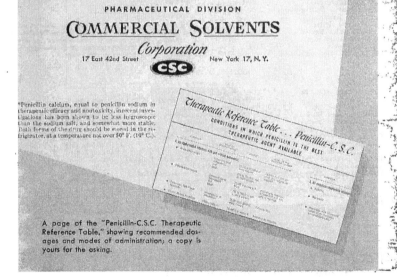

Medical School Notes

Commencement Exercises for the School of Medicine and the School of Nursing were held at 8:00 P.M., Friday, September 15, in the auditorium of Oklahoma City University. Dr. Chauncey D. Leake, Dean and Executive Vice-President of the University of Texas Medical Branch, and Principal Administrator of Hospitals, Galveston, Texas, delivered the Commencement Address.

Dr. G. L. Cross, President of the University of Oklahoma, conferred the Degree of Doctor of Medicine on 52 men and four women. Twenty-three nurses received the Diploma of Graduate Nurse.

Thirty young men were commissioned First Lieutenant, Medical Corps, Army of the United States; Nine were commissioned Lieutenant (jg), Medical Corps, U. S. Naval Reserve for Inactive Duty and nine for Active Duty.

Jack William Strode, son of Mr. V. C. Strode, Pawnee, served as Class Marshall of the medics. Miss Marie Elaine Blakely, daughter of Mrs. Amy Blakely, Stillwater served as Class Marshall of the Nurses. These students ranked highest scholastically in their respective classes.

GRADUATE NURSES

Geraldine Grimmett—President

Peggy Jo Wilson—Vice-President

Margaret Sue Hamburger—Secretary-Treasurer

Norean Eleanor Anne Anderson	Carnegie, Oklahoma
Eloise Virginia Baker	Hobart
Suzanne Sanders Bilger	Oklahoma City
Marie Elaine Blakely	Stillwater
Ruby Ivalee Blakely	Stillwater
Jessie Winiffed Bynum	Hulbert
Lorraine Louise Coble Combs	Seminole
Grace Ledbetter Cutler	Oklahoma City
Geraldine Lou Grimmett	Pauls Valley
Margaret Sue Hamburger	Weatherford
Rosemary Antoinette Piering Hardy	Duluth, Minn.
Margaret Ellen Harman	Elmore City
Virginia Charlene Hester	Oklahoma City
Ethel Estelle Smith Horner	Oklahoma City
Merilee Margaret Jennings	Kinta
Jennie Evalyn Lewis	Liberal, Kan.
Georgie Lorraine Price McCormick	Lone Wolf

Ethel Colena McKerracher	Peckham
Emma Bode Orman	Keota
Margaret Lillian Phillips	Norman
Mary Jane Kennedy Shackelford	Henryetta
Peggy Jo Wilson	Oklahoma City
Martha Agnes Zaleski	Harrah

Dr. Robert H. Bayley has recently been appointed Professor of Clinical Medicine and Vice Chairman of the Department of Medicine. Dr. Bayley received the Degree of Doctor of Medicine from Emory University in 1931. For the past several years he has served as Associate Professor of Medicine at the Lousiana State University School of Medicine.

Dr. Florene C. Kelly assumed the duties of Assistant Professor of Bacteriology on September 15. Dr. Kelly holds the Ph. D. degree from the University of Chicago and has been on the faculty of Simmons College for several years, serving in the capacity of Assistant Professor of Biology. She is a member of the Society of American Bacteriologists and the Massachusetts Public Health Association.

Miss Mary Leidgh has recently been employed as Assistant Administrative Dietitian at the hospitals. Miss Leidgh received the Bachelor of Science Degree from Texas Technilogical College, Lubbock, and the Master's Degree from the University of Texas. She has had extensive experience in dietetics work.

Dr. H. A. Shoemaker, Assistant Dean, and Mr. Jos. Smay, Director of the School of Architecture at the University, recently made a trip to inspect the University of Iowa and the University of Colorado College of Medicine and Hospitals for the purpose of obtaining ideas to be used in planning a building program for the School of Medicine and the University of Oklahoma Hospitals.

Miss Adeline Anne Johnson took up her duties as Research Assistant and Technician in the Department of Pathology on September 1. Miss Johnson has served as Technician in the Departments of Bacteriology and Pathology of the University of Chicago.

DOCTORS OF MEDICINE

NAME	INTERNSHIP	LOCATION
**Clifford Ward Allen, Jr.	U. S. Naval Hospital	
-Alex Barno	Jersey City Medical Center	Jersey City, N. J.
*Elmer Stanley Berger	University Hospital	Oklahoma City
Dorothy Frances Blackert	City-County Hospital	Ft. Worth, Texas
*George Randolph Booth	St. Francis Hospital	Wichita, Kansas
-Maurice Phillip Capehart	University Hospital	Oklahoma City
*Francis Patrick Cawley	Jersey City Medical Center	Jersey City, N. J.
-John Hatchett Clymer	University Hospital	Oklahoma City
-Leon Doyle Combs	St. Paul's Hospital	Dallas, Texas
Betty Louise Conrad	City of Detroit Receiving Hospital	Detroit, Mich.
*Evan Leonard Copeland	Wesley Hospital	Oklahoma City
*Robert Wendell Dixon	University of Michigan Hospital	Ann Harbor, Mich.
Julia Steele Eley	University Hospital	Oklahoma City
*Frederick Roscoe Ford	Grant Hospital	Chicago, Ill.
*Virgil Ray Forester	King County Hospital	Brooklyn, New York
*David Jackson Geigerman	St. Mary's Hospital	Cincinnati, Ohio
*Carl Holmes Guild, Jr.	University Hospital	Oklahoma City
**George Henry Guthrey	U. S. Naval Hospital	
*James Barnett Hampton	Good Samaritan Hospital	Portland, Oregon
**Samuel Isaac Hardy	U. S. Naval Hospital	
Minnie Marie Henson	Lutheran Hospital	Cleveland, Ohio
*James Fitton Hohl	State of Wisconsin General Hospital	Madison, Wisconsin
*Francis Willis Hollingsworth	Good Samaritan Hospital	Portland, Oregon
**Robert Ray Johnson	U. S. Naval Hospital	
Sidney Kaplan	Queens General Hospital	Long Island, New York

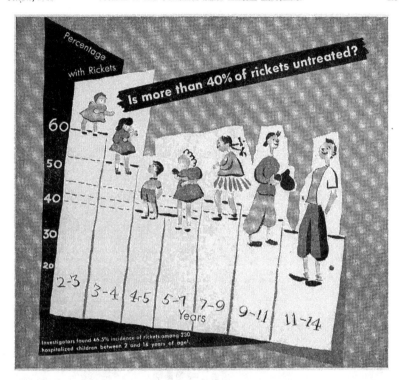

Percentage with Rickets

Is more than 40% of rickets untreated?

60
50
40
30
20

2-3 3-4 4-5 5-7 7-9 9-11 11-14
Years

Investigators found 46.5% incidence of rickets among 230 hospitalized children between 2 and 14 years of age[1].

It used to be thought that rickets is prevalent only in the first two years of life. This was when the roentgenological and clinical manifestations were accepted as the criteria for diagnosis. Recent studies suggest that perhaps as the result of this impression, as much as 40% of rickets has gone untreated.[1]

Microscopic examination of the long bones of children between the ages of 2 and 14 who died from various causes showed a startlingly high percentage of cases of rickets in older children. The highest incidence was found during the third year (57%). This suggests the need of continuing vitamin D supplementation beyond infancy. Evidently, as long as growth persists, and at least through the fourteenth year, administration of vitamin D should be made routine; because even in children who appear healthy, histologic bone studies show that disturbances in calcium-phosphate metabolism are fairly common.

Whether the vitamin supplements prescribed are for infants or for older children, Upjohn preparations may be given routinely with the assurance of dependable potency in pleasant, easy-to-take dosage forms.

1. Folki, R. H.; Jackson, D.; Eliot, M. M., and Park, E. A.: Am. Jrl. Dis. Child. 66:1 (July) 1943. Note: A reprint of this paper is being mailed to all physicians. Additional copies are available upon request.

Upjohn
KALAMAZOO, MICHIGAN

U P J O H N   V I T A M I N S

**Harry McGee	U. S. Naval Hospital	
*Willard Lyal McGraw	Wesley Hospital	Oklahoma City
*Floyd Fuller McSpadden	Grace Hospital	Detroit, Mich.
*Robert Jesse Morgan	St. Paul's Hospital	Dallas, Texas
*John Wildey Morrison	St. Anthony Hospital	Oklahoma City
*Marshall Opper	Mount Sinai Hospital	Chicago, Ill.
*William Nathan Oxley	Ohio State University Hospital	Columbus, Ohio
*Roy Gibson Parrish	Baltimore City Hospital	Baltimore, Md.
**James Coldren Peters	U. S. Naval Hospital	
-Robert Theodore Pfundt	Evangelical Deaconess Hospital	Detroit, Mich.
-Theodore Robert Pfundt	Hurley Hospital	Flint, Mich.
*John Phipps	Wesley Hospital	Oklahoma City
Pamela Richardson Prentice	Baltimore City Hospital	Baltimore, Md.
**James Hugh Rollins	U. S. Naval Hospital	
**Art Henry Rutledge	U. S. Naval Hospital	
*Ben Allen Rutledge	Gorgas Hospital	Panama Canal Zone
*Joseph Salamy	Methodist Hospital	Dallas, Texas
*Herbert Victor Louis Sapper, Jr.	Colorado General Hospital	Denver, Colorado
**Paul Olden Shackelford	U. S. Naval Hospital	
*Richard Floyd Shriner, Jr.	University Hospital	Oklahoma City
*Robert David Shuttee	Indiana University Medical Center	Indianapolis, Ind.
*Ralph Simon	St. Paul's Hospital	Dallas, Texas
James Ronald Smith	University Hospital	Oklahoma City
*William Thomas Snoddy	St. Josephs Hospital	St. Paul, Minn.
*Jack William Strode	Los Angeles County Hospital	Los Angeles, Cal.
-William Van Voorhis Thompson	University Hospitals, State U. of Iowa	Iowa City, Iowa
*Adolph Nathaniel Vammen	University Hospital	Oklahoma City
Glen Franklin Wade	St. Anthony Hospital	Oklahoma City
*Phillip Cook Waters	California Hospital	Los Angeles, Cal.
Jay Deane Wilson	St. Vincent's Hospital	Jacksonville, Florida
-Millington Oswald Young	Cleveland Clinic Foundation Hospital	Cleveland, Ohio

*Candidates for Commissions of First Lieutenant, Medical Corps, Army of the United States.

**Candidates for Commissions of Lieutenant (jg), Medical Corps, U. S. Naval Reserve for Active Duty.

-Candidates for Commissions of Lieutenant (jg), Medical Corps, U. S. Naval Reserve for Inactive Duty.

CLASSIFIED ADS

THREE GOOD CASTLE STERILIZERS FOR SALE: One 16 in. Chromium plated sterilizer, good as new, $35.00 (cost about $60.00); one old but serviceable 12 in. Chromium plated sterilizer, $15.00; one 8 in. syringe sterilizer, good as new, $20.00. Dr. A. C. Hirschfield, 407 Medical Arts Bldg., Oklahoma City 2, Okla.

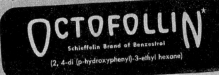

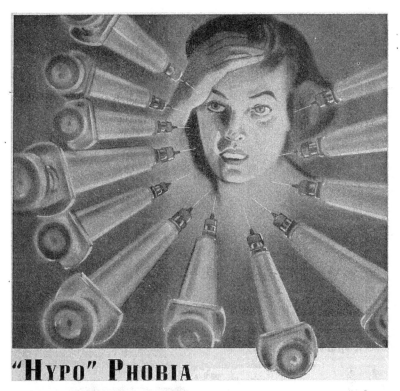

"HYPO" PHOBIA

● A single injection daily of 'Wellcome' Globin Insulin with Zinc will control most moderately severe and many severe cases of diabetes. Thus it helps diminish the "hypo" phobia which so often dominates the mental attitude of patients who have been receiving several injections daily.

'Wellcome' Globin Insulin with Zinc helps turn problem diabetics into better adjusted and more cooperative patients. 'Wellcome' Globin Insulin with Zinc is timed to the patient's needs. One injec-

tion provides a rapid onset of action in the morning and sustained daytime effect with the safety of diminishing activity during the night.

'Wellcome' Globin Insulin with Zinc is a clear solution and, in its freedom from allergenic reactions, is comparable to regular insulin. This new advance in insulin therapy was developed in the Wellcome Research Laboratories, Tuckahoe, New York. U. S. Patent No. 2,161,198. Available in vials of 10 cc., 80 units in 1 cc.   'Wellcome' Trademark Registered

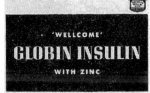

Medicine At War

DOCTOR SHORTAGE PAYS OFF

In the past, when great battles were fought, loss of life was multiplied tenfold because of lack of prompt and adequate medical care for the wounded. But in the present war the story has been different. Even yet the full account of the achievements of medicine on "D-Day" has not been impressed upon the country.

One correspondent reports that within 45 minutes after the first troops landed on the shores of France, a medical unit was on the beachhead picking up casualties, while in the background a landing craft had been converted into an operating theater.

During the first day, twenty-two major operations were performed by this single unit. From dawn on "D-Day" until four o'clock in the afternoon, the unit remained on the beach. Blood plasma had been landed and transfusions made from mobile equipment.

Fifty thousand American doctors are in the armed forces. Everyone of them is a trained expert at the business of saving lives. At least those civilians who have had to linger in crowded waiting rooms to secure the attention of the over-worked doctors on the home front, can see the reason for the inconvenience thrust upon them.—Chickasha Star 9-21-44.

Army Death Rate from Diseases Now at All-Time Low

The disease death rate among American soldiers of World War II is the lowest ever recorded for the U.S. Army and only one twentieth as high as that of World War I, thanks to an effective program of military preventive medicine, Brig. Gen. James S. Simmons, chief, Preventive Medicine Service, U. S. Army, reported in a nationwide broadcast Tuesday, August 29.

General Simmons, speaking as guest of Schenley Laboratories, pointed out that there have been no great epidemics among American soldiers in this war despite the fact that they have been exposed to every known disease under difficult field conditions. "U. S. troops," he said, "have experienced every kind of weather and climate and have lived among primitive peoples of the tropical world. In spite of all these handicaps, the sick rate has been comparatively low and the diseases mild."

The smashing through Axis defenses in France, England and the islands of the Pacific was credited by the speaker to the fact that "GI Joe is one of the healthest soldiers in the world."

"This is not just a matter of luck," General Simmons added. Owing to the effective program of military preventive medicine developed by the Surgeon General and carried out by the Medical Department of the Army, thousands of medical officers trained in disease prevention follow the soldier and guard his welfare from the moment of his induction until his return to civilian life, he pointed out.

Due to the vaccination of soldiers, he explained, smallpox, the typhoid and paratyphoid fevers, tetanus, yellow fever, plague, cholera and typhus "have been of no importance." Some meningities, pneumonia and mild influenza have occurred, General Simmons stated, but the

death rates have been insignificant, "Malaria, our No. 1 hazard overseas, has been controlled at home. Formerly, it caused much illness in certain tropical theaters but practically no deaths, and the disease has now been much reduced even in such regions," the medical officer disclosed.

"The Army's program of preventive medicine has paid enormous dividends by conserving our military manpower," he concluded. "Undoubtedly, it will also contribute richly to the future welfare of our country.

Medical Officers Needed

The Civil Service Commission has announced a new examination for Rotating Internship and Psychiatric Resident positions at St. Elizabeths Hospital, the Federal Institution for the treatment of mental disorders in Washington, D.C. The positions pay $2,433 a year, including overtime pay.

The Internship consists of 9 months of rotating service including medicine surgery, pediatrics (affiliation), obstetrics (affiliation), and as conditions permit, psychiatry and laboratory. Applicants must be third or fourth year students in an approved medical school.

Psychiatric Resident positions consist of 9 months in psychiatry. Applicants must have successfully completed their fourth year of study in a medical school and they must have the degree of B. M. or M.D. In addition they must have completed an accredited rotating internship of at least 9 months or be serving such internship at the time of making application. Persons who attain eligibility but who are still serving their internship may have their names submitted for appointment but they cannot enter on duty until they have completed their internship.

There are no age limits for this examination and no written test will be given. Applications will be accepted until the needs of the service have been met. Application forms may be secured at first and second class post offices, from the Commission's regional offices, or direct from the U. S. Civil Service Commission, Washington 25, D.C.

Appointments to Federal positions are made in accordance with War Manpower Commission policies and employment stabilization programs.

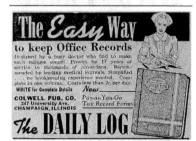

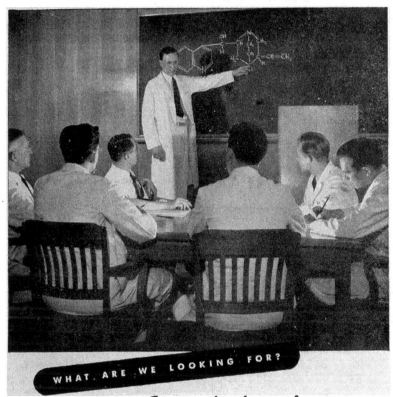

WHAT ARE WE LOOKING FOR?

In antimalarial research we are seeking the drug which will be not only more satisfactory than present synthetics, but will be superior to quinine also. In the laboratories of Parke, Davis & Company, and on research grants, new chemical compounds are being synthesized, studied for toxicity, and tested for effectiveness against malaria parasites. We are looking for a non-toxic, rapidly acting drug that will be an effective prophylactic and a permanent cure for this disease.

PARKE, DAVIS & COMPANY ➤ **DETROIT 32, MICHIGAN**

★ FIGHTIN' TALK ★

The following have been ordered to active duty: LT. ARMON M. MEIS, Enid; LT. HOMER VINCENT ARCHER, Oklahoma City; LT. DICK HOWARD P. HUFF, Norman; LT. JOSEPH PRICE BELL, Welch; LT. EDWIN CHARLES TURNER, Oklahoma City; LT. JACK BURGESS TOLBERT, Oklahoma City; LT. COMDR. LUVERN HAYS, Tulsa; LT. COMDR. H. B. JENKINS, Stillwater; LT. PAUL MACRORY, Bethany.

LT. COLONEL WARREN J. BARKER, Ponca City, has recently been promoted from Major. He was formerly connected with the Ponca City Clinic. For the past two years, Lt. Col. Barker has been overseas, serving in England, Africa, Sicily and in Italy. Suffering shrapnel wounds during the battle of Tunisia, he is the recipient of the Purple Heart. Lt. Col. Barker is now in command of a medical battalion.

CAPTAIN WILLIAM A. LOY, Norman, has recently been promoted from First Lieutenant.

State Doctor Captures Nazi Hospital and Staff Singlehanded

CAPTAIN JOHN Y. BATTENFIELD, Oklahoma City, certainly wins honors by the spectacular capture of a Nazi Hospital and Staff. Singlehanded and unarmed, Captain Battenfield effected the capture of several Nazi doctors, hospital attendants, equipment, vehicles and weapons. The following letter was received by MAJOR JOHN McDONALD, Ada, who is in the Surgeon General's office in Washington:

"I jumped in Southern France on D Day after a rather nervous but uneventful trip. I was very heavily loaded and fractured my left 6th rib when I landed in a vineyard but I was so excited that I didn't even know it was fractured until the next day. I was extremely busy for several hours taking care of just what you'd expect. I was not in any serious danger until later when I went ahead to treat some seriously wounded French civilians and I was trapped in a courtyard by German mortar fire. You must have been making some good luck medicine because I didn't get a scratch. Later I got lost and went into a German occupied town but again was not fired on. Later I went back to the same town looking for a place for wounded and walked up to a German hospital. You can imagine my surprise when I saw all the German soldiers carrying weapons including the doctors and a German sniper on the roof. I didn't know anything else to do except advance because I thought I'd get shot in the back if I turned around. The Germans must have seen the look on my face because they held their hands up and surrendeerd the entire hospital including all their vehicles and weapons to me. It was really a joke because I didn't have a weapon or any support. The German doctor in charge took me to another part of town and surrendered another hospital which was also empty. The Germans were still rather arrogant even though they surrendered and I had quite a bit of difficulty forcing them to feed me."

The following letter from CAPTAIN C. A. BISHOP, Picher, written from somewhere in New Guinea, was sent to the Executive Office by Dr. M. A. Connell:

"After several years of silence perhaps I should write a note of greeting. I haven't forgotten those ancient days before I joined the ranks of Uncle Sam's armed forces. However, that belongs as much to a distant past as my high school days.

"For a long time now I have lived an army life. For a good part of that time I have lived in the field where there are no cities or civilization. I have lived this time in jungles among mosquitoes and coconut palms. Atobrine is a delicious dessert which we have after breakfast. Coconut trees are beautiful in the moonlight—with bombs coming down, searchlights and ack ack fire—'Bogies' falling in flames, etc.

"I have enjoyed a Cook's Tour of the South and Southwest Pacific and frankly can't see any reason for fighting over these damn islands. I have seen a few beautiful spots but beauty alone isn't enough. Have you ever tried eating dehydrated and canned foods without fresh fruits or vegetables for periods of months? Try it and you'll understand what I mean.

"We've been away from home so long now that we would feel lost if we were to return. It would be like going to a strange country and meeting strange people. Civilians are a rare sight. I believe we would stare at real modern homes and buildings, good highways, civilian cars, etc. I have almost forgotten all of that.

"I'm still a captain, battalion surgeon, in a searchlight battalion. I hope that within another year or two I'll be able to return and begin all over again."

LT. (jg) E. EVANS CHAMBERS, Enid, has received the following citation of merit from Admiral C. W. Nimitz:

"The Commander in Chief, United States Pacific Fleet, takes pleasure in Commending Lt. (jg) Evander Evans Chambers, United States Naval Reserve, for service as set forth in the following Citation:

"For meritorious service in the line of his profession as Assisting Surgeon to the Senior Medical Officer on board a U. S. Navy transport during the invasion of Saipan Island 15-16 June, 1944. By his devotion to duty, untiring energy and professional skill, operating for over seventy-two hours without rest, he was instrumental in bringing relief to many of the wounded and undoubtedly saved the lives of many who would otherwise have perished. His conduct was at all times in keeping with the highest traditions of the naval service.

C. W. Nimitz,
Admiral, U. S. Navy."

CAPTAIN J. M. TAYLOR, Oklahoma City, has a new baby daughter, Nancy Virginia. Papa is serving with an evacuation hospital in the Southwest Pacific. Mrs. Taylor and young Nancy make their home in Oklahoma City.

CAPTAIN JAMES J. GABLE, graduate Class of '42, is serving in France. The following is taken from his letter to the Executive Office.

"I landed in France 8 June and we have been going after it since that time. My outfit is one of the best and I've had some exciting times. As you've read, that hedgerow fighting the first couple of months was rough as the proverbial cob, but now the going is much easier. So far I've had one swim, no baths, changed clothes twice; had a handful of hot meals but mostly cold K rations, lots of 'Jerry' souvenirs, French wine, flowers and kisses and probably adrenal insufficiency. I'm ready to come home to Mama and our two babies."

LT. COLONEL JOE C. RUDE, graduate Class of '30, writes from the European Theater of War that, after leaving Army X-Ray Technical School and after 23 months of service, he is overseas where they are trying to make a consultant out of him. He states that he would much prefer to stay in the practice of radiology than be a glorified personnel man who travels about and no one wishes to see.

CAPTAIN LAL DUNCAN THRELKELD, Oklahoma City, is quite pleased about his new daughter, Margaret Ann. Captain Threlkeld is serving in France while Mama and Margaret Ann wait in Oklahoma City.

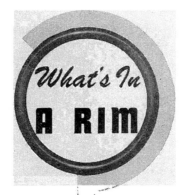
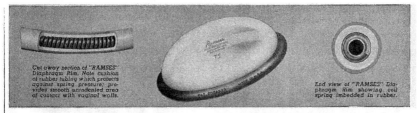

MAJOR JOHN R. HUBBARD, Oklahoma City, has been transferred from India to China. Major Hubbard is armed to the teeth with a carbine and a Chinese knife, also 45 pounds of personal luggage. The new equipment is standard Chinese officers' equipment as the major's new assignment transfers him from the American medical unit with which he was serving in India to a wholly Chinese division.

The following letter received in Cherokee from CAPTAIN JACK PARSONS who is now stationed at Pampa, tells a story of how the soldier feels about Post-War Planning:

"I am pleased to see the men and women of Cherokee are beginning to think about post-war planning for our town. As K. G. Braley says, 'Let's do it now.' I don't like to admit it but Alva has beat us to the draw on many things and I don't mean their prisoner of war camp either. I was happy to see the alfalfa mill come to town, also the corset factory. Let's make it interesting enough to keep them there. Your idea of a farmer's community house is great. Also we need a stadium and other things. I note that many good ideas were turned in to Paul Gray. I'll add one for him—I would like to see an annual celebration of the Cherokee Strip opening held at the logical place, namely, Cherokee. Enid sort of grabbed that one before we did and I have friends in Enid who wouldn't care to see us have the celebration. However, the Rose Bowl committee didn't like to see the other 'bowls' come into being either.

"The opening of the lake should help our town if we take advantage as we should. I have already completed plans for another office building twice as large as the one I left.

"I must close now but let me say again that we soldiers certainly appreciate seeing you folks at home taking such an interest in our future as expressed in your post-war planning drive."

After a long absence in the Southwest Pacific, COMDR. CLIFFORD C. FULTON, Oklahoma City, returned to his home. After his leave he will then report for duty at the naval air station in Corpus Christi, Texas. Comdr. Fulton is the son of Dr. J. S. Fulton, Atoka.

LT. PHIL DEVANNEY, Sayre, is now serving as chief surgeon of the Third Marine Division Hospital on Guam. Lt. Devanney entered the service two years ago and has served on Guadalcanal, Bougainville and Guam for the past year and a half. In an interview with a Marine corps correspondent, Lt. Devanney remarked "It's unhealthy to boast but so far haven't lost a case at this hospital—we realize a good deal of that is luck but we're thankful for it and hope it continues."

MAJOR FRED G. DORWART, Muskogee, has become quite an avid flower collector while spending his overseas stretch in the Aleutians. To most people the Aleutians are a vast frozen waste, but to Major Dorwart it is a wealth of odd flowers that have never been catalouged. The Alaskan University is interested in the collection of 78 species which Major Dorwart has collected in his spare time. He says that the land there has never before been inhabited but has been made liveable. The major is taking photos of the areas in which the various flowers are found for information when the pressed flowers are catalouged.

MAJOR O. H. COWART, Bristow, is stationed somewhere in France and has written that his brother, Major Edmond Cowart is also stationed at the same base but that he has not yet been able to meet him.

Oklahoma Doctor Visits Romanian King Recently

CAPTAIN JULIUS T. LEVINE, formerly of the Staff of the McAlester Clinic, was received recently in Romania by King Mihai and Queen Mother Helen who said, 'When I heard there were American doctors in the palace

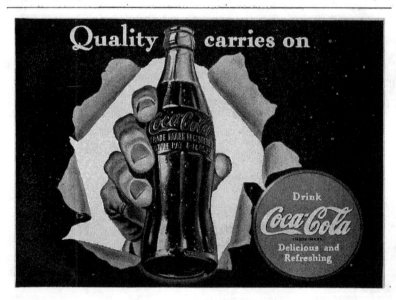

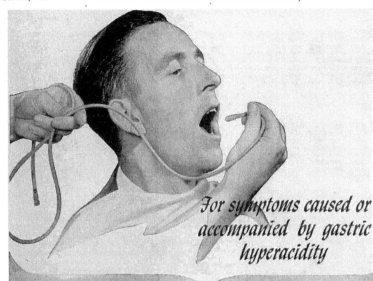

For symptoms caused or accompanied by gastric hyperacidity

Creamalin promptly reduces stomach hyperacidity by adsorption. The effect is persistent. It does not provoke a secondary rise in hydrochloric acid, such as is common after alkalies, nor does it disturb the acid-base balance of blood plasma. . . . Relief is promptly secured and maintained with safety. Hence the very extensive application of this highly useful agent in the management of peptic ulcer and symptoms caused by gastric hyperacidity.

•

Supplied in
8 oz., 12 oz. and 1 pint bottles.

★ ★ ★

CREAMALIN
Reg. U. S. Pat. Off.
Brand of ALUMINUM HYDROXIDE GEL
NON–ALKALINE ANTACID THERAPY

★ ★ ★

WINTHROP CHEMICAL COMPANY, INC.
Pharmaceuticals of merit for the physician
NEW YORK 13, N. Y.   WINDSOR, ONT.

grounds, I told them to lock the gates and not let them get away before I had seen them.'

Captain Levine and another flight surgeon assigned to the 15th Air Force went to Romania to care for wounded American Air Force members. They were called to the palace for consultation on the illness of the father of the king's private secretary. They wore regular work day clothes, the associated press reported.

MAJOR H. A. ZAMPETTI, Drumright, is stationed with a bombardment group in England. He is serving as flight surgeon.

MAJOR JESS D. HERRMANN, Oklahoma City, formerly associated with Dr. Harry Wilkins, has been awarded the Bronze Star for meritorious service. Major Herrmann is a member of the 21st Evacuation Hospital. The Star was awarded after Major Herrmann performed successfully a delicate and tiring brain operation on a soldier only six days after he was operated for appendicitis.

The following interesting excerpt is from a letter received from MAJOR HERVEY A. FOERSTER, Oklahoma City, now serving in England:

"I had occasion to visit a hospital recently and ran into MAJOR HARRY FORD, Oklahoma City, who is Chief of E. E. N. & T. and CAPTAIN JIMMY CURRY of Sapulpa, Oklahoma. Ford is keeping plenty busy, also Jim Curry with his big smile and wonderful personality is certainly cheering up the soldiers who have lost arms, legs and faces. I saw one soldier who had lost his entire nose, mouth and chin but he was still able to smoke by sucking on a cigarette with his hand clasped against what used to be his face. I saw several painfully writing out 'Dear Mother' with their left hand—since their right one was missing. I saw extensive burns and lots of graft work beautifully done. This war may be nearly over but there still is lots of reconstructive surgery to be done and I am afraid does will be kept in longer."

CAPTAIN RICHARD ROYS, Class of '39, company commander of a Medical unit on an island north of New Guinea, has been decorated with the Bronze Star for bravery in caring for the wounded under fire. Captain Roys already held the Silver Star, awarded for bravery in action in New Guinea last year.

MAJOR LLOYD W. TAYLOR, Class of '41, has been awarded the Legion of Merit by Major General James L. Frink, commanding general of the U. S. Army Services of Supply in the Southwest Pacific. The honor was bestowed upon Major Taylor for his work in late 1942 and early 1943 as supply officer of a Medical unit serving combat troops in New Guinea. Suffering from illness and fatigue, Major Taylor obtained badly needed medical supplies for American and Australian hospitals other than his own, in addition to doing his regular work caring for wounded men. He is now assigned to the Office of Chief Surgeon of the Southwest Pacific area, helping in the evacuation of patients from battle zones to Australia and the United States.

Johnson & Johnson Research Foundation Makes Announcement

Tantalum plates, foil, screws and wire to repair broken bones, nerves and skulls will shortly be available to civilian surgeons through a recent allocation of the War Production Board, according to an announcement made by Dr. Gustav S. Mathey, President of the Johnson & Johnson Research Foundation, New Brunswick, New Jersey.

The Johnson & Johnson Research Foundation is a non-profit organization, founded in 1940 to endow research in universities and hospitals and to disseminate summaries of findings to members of the medical profession. Dr. Mathey states that by an agreement between the Ethicon Suture Laboratories, Johnson & Johnson subsidiary, and the Fansteel Metallurgical Corporation of North Chicago, the availability of tantalum for civilian surgeons is assured at an early date.

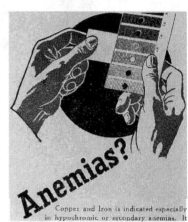

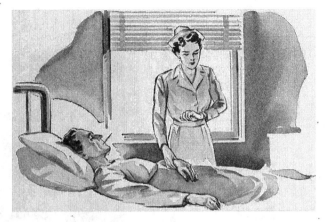

WHEN INCREASED METABOLISM
Increases Nutritional Needs

During periods of acute febrile disease, dietary adjustment must be made to satisfy the change in nutritional demands. Protein requirements are increased 50 to 100 per cent, caloric expenditure is raised because of increased heat production, and vitamin needs, especially those of the water-soluble groups, are greater. Only by fully meeting these altered requirements can recovery be hastened, can convalescence be shortened, and the usual state of lethargy reduced in severity.

Designed to supplement the diet during periods of increased metabolic activity, Ovaltine in milk is a powerful weapon in preventing nutritional insufficiency during these periods. The abundantly supplied nutrients of this palatable food drink are quickly assimilated and metabolized. Its delicious taste makes it appealing even to the seriously ill patient who usually presents a feeding problem. Because its curd tension is considerably lower than that of milk alone, it leaves the stomach promptly, rarely produces nausea or anorexia, and presents no undue digestive burden for the patient.

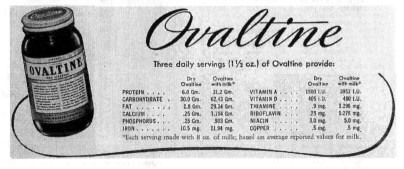

BOOK REVIEWS

MINOR SURGERY. Edited by Humphrey Rolleston and Alan Moncrieff. Philosophical Library, New York.. 1944. Price $5.00.

Eighteen British writers contribute to this volume of eighteen chapters. The chapters on hand infections and on childhood anaesthetia and analgesia are perhaps the most practical.

The arrangement is peculiar in that Amputations of the Cervix and Excisions of Bartholin's gland are included in Minor Surgery and in the Chapter on Genito-Urinary Disease. The Chapter on Gynecology adheres much more closely to minor procedures. Orthopedic conditions of minor significance are well and completely discussed.

Chapters on Minor wounds, mouth, nose and throat, ear, eye, ganglia, benign tumors and cysts, skin infections, rectum,-hernia, varicose veins, ulcers and phlebitis are included.—L. J. Starry, M.D.

PULLEN'S MEDICAL DIAGNOSIS. Twenty-seven authors. Edited by Roscoe L. Pullen, A.B., M.D., Instructor in Medicine, Tulane University of Louisiana School of Medicine; Assistant Clinical Director, Charity Hospital of Louisiana at New Orleans. 863 illustrations on 584 figures, 45 in colors. Published by W. B. Saunders. 1106 pages. Price $10.00.

This publication is quite a pretentious tome, with the collaborators all young men of distinction in various schools, both north and south. They represent surgery, orthopedy, pediatrics, pathology, obstetrics, gynecology, ophthalmology, otolaryngology, physiology, neurology, psychiatry, cardiology, etc. It especially stresses the matter of history taking, which gives us an insight into human frailties, "but this art is acquired only by experience and establishes a baseline from which further diagnostic and therapeutic procedures may be initiated." It is a bedside medical diagnosis aimed at making (rarus avis) clinicians. It has but little laboratory measures, and only a few x-ray illustrations.

It's physical diagnosis and electrocardiography are especially well handled in clear and understandable chapters. The use of the five senses is especially urged in estimating this. Normal conditions are expanded so as to be able to interpret the aberrations therefrom. Sydenham says to observe. Hence this necessity for understanding the anatomy, physiology and pathology, as manifested in various diseased conditions. It seeks to find out why the patient seeks the physician, and whether the ailment has a somatic or functional background, when he feels he has a just cause for his complaint. The anatomy and physiology may find the changes which ultimately cause the pathological conditions before the irreversible status to therapeutic measures is attained, and how much the symptoms are modified by psychic background.

Neurology and neuropsychiatric diagnosis are well handled in several chapters, and numerous illustrations, so as to illuminate the study of these conditions. The endocrine survey (covered by 50 odd pages) gives a lucid picture of this new phase of medicine. Peripheral vascular diseases, that new branch of cardiology, is given its place in the scheme of diagnosis.

This handy reference book should be for the medical students, active practitioners or one who has grown rusty during these strenuous years, when he is not able to study and do post-graduate work.—Lea A. Riley, M.D.

New Upjohn Display Features Pharmacy in the War

Pharmacists are performing herculean tasks in the armed services of our country and in civilian business. To pay tribute to these men, The Upjohn Company is featuring "Pharmacy in the War" in their new institutional window display.

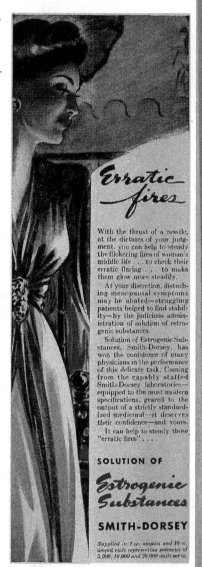

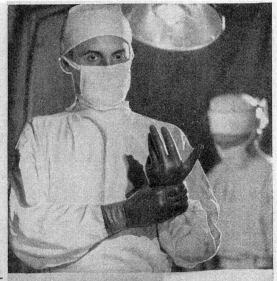

HEROES...Behind Masks

Bombs screaming down ... shells crashing ... the crazy clutter of strafing planes' machine guns ... they're the "background music" of the drama that's played on every fighting front every day by the surgeons of the field clearing-stations.

"Soldiers in white" ... heroes—behind masks.

Naturally we are proud that their choice of a cigarette—in those moments when there's a brief respite for a heartening smoke—is likely to be Camel. The milder, rich, full-flavored brand favored in the Armed Forces all over the world.

Camel is truly "the soldier's cigarette"!

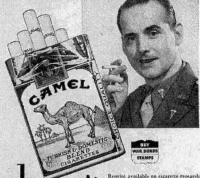

BUY WAR BONDS STAMPS

Reprint available on cigarette research—Archives of Otolaryngology, March, 1943, pp. 404-410. Camel Cigarettes, Medical Relations Division. One Pershing Square, New York 17, N. Y.

COSTLIER TOBACCOS **Camel**

Medical Abstracts

"DISCUSSION ON PAIN IN LARYNGOLOGY." Mollison. W. M., et al. The Journal of Laryngology and Otology. London. Vol. 58, pages 457-464. November. 1943.

In laryngology the position of pain is sometimes a guide to the affection of the underlying tissues but often it is not so, the pain being preferred remotely. The fifth nerve is very apt to refer pain from the deep structures. Reference may be made from one branch to another of the same division (as from lower teeth to the ear); from a branch of one division to a branch of another division, which is more common (carious lower canine gives rise to supra-orbital pain.) The commonest example is supra-orbital pain from antral infection; less recognized is the superorbital pain from acute tonsillitis or pharyngitis.

Pain due to affection of the sphenoidal sinus is frequently referred to remote parts of the head, e.g., to the occipital area, behind the ear and the top of the head.

The 9th nerve is also apt to refer pain remotely. The statement that a lump in the neck and a piece of wool in the ear is diagnostic of growth in the deep pharynx is as true as any sweeping generality. It is true that pain in the ear may be the only symptom of a carcinoma of the aryopiglottic fold. In the esophagus: the pain of a growth or impacted foreign body is often referred, either to the suprasternal notch or epgastrium even though the lesion is in the middle of the tube.

Frontal sinusitis is likely to be associated with pain referred along the supra-orbital nerve, with tenderness at the notch. External operations on this sinus may be followed by persistent supra-orbital pain and hyperesthesia, varying in severity. There is a pain around the eye and upper cheek and temple, often limited strictly to one side, lasting for a day or two days, sometimes only for an hour or two, or even shorter, so that six or more attacks may occur daily. This "migrainous neuralgia" is often thought to be the result of eyestrain, and glasses are prescribed; in many patients, turbinectomies, antral washouts, even exenteration of the ethmoid and antra, have been done without relief. Chronic neuralgia of the jaws is very difficult to relieve.

There are a number of remote diseases which may cause pain behind the eye; apical petrositis, antrum disease, frontal sinus diagnosis, sphenoidal sinusitis, enlargement of the shell of one middle turbinate. Pain around the eyes usually disappears after injection of the Gasserian ganglion.

Pain in the ear is commonly connected with the glossopharyngeal nerve and spasmodic pain occurring in the ear is strongly suggestive of this origin. It may be referred through Jacobson's nerve. There is a type of pain which may be called the "ice-cream complex." It refers to the side of the head after eating anything that is very cold. The reference is presumably up the bagus nerve and thence to the 5th nerve, and so to the various areas supplied by the 5th nerve.

A curious example of referred sensory disturbance is, that several patients complained for many months of the taste of iron or something rather bitter and unpleasant every time they ate after a tonsil operation.— M. D. H., M.D.

"LATENT MASTOIDITIS DURING TREATMENT WITH SULFA DRUGS." M. Aubry. La Presse Medicale, Paris. Vol. 52, page 124. April. 1944.

Latent mastoiditis in adults is a distinct pathological entity. Aside from the latent antritis in infants, which is of a special type, latent mastoiditis has been known for a long time. It may have various causes. It may be sometimes due to a special rare pathogenic bacterium (pneumococcus mucosus.) A distinct form of latent mastoiditis is the one which may develop during sulfonamide medication. The author calls attention to cases of mastoid osteitis the symptoms of which were masked by sulfonamide therapy. The first symptom of such masked mastoiditis cases usually developed, or became manifest, on the sixth week of illness: seemingly, the otitis media was cured, when suddenly paralysis of the facial nerve appeared, without any other sign of mastoid disease.

In other cases of latent mastoiditis, the first symptom may be general sepsis from thrombosis of the lateral sinus developing six to seven weeks in the course of a harmless looking otitis media. When the mastoid is opened in such cases, there may be a diffuse mastoid without pus, and the bone around the lateral sinus may seem to be healthy.

In otomastoiditis, a sulfa drug has triple action: (1) it acts upon the syndrome of infection by reducing the fever; (2) it acts upon the syndrome of otitis by drying up the discharge, and by causing indirectly the healing of the perforation in the eardrum; sometimes there remains a slight hyperemia at Shrapnell's membrane, and a certain thickness of the eardrum (Leroux-Robert); (3) it acts upon the mastoid syndrome by camouflaging the osteitis which, anatomically, may persist in a deceitful sleep while, clinically, all signs of mastoiditis, especially the spontaneous and provoked pain, may disappear.

In this form of latent mastoiditis there is only one single sign that remains for the clinician, and this is the radiographic picture. Even this sign may be misleading, if the radiogram is not technically perfect; or if there is no way to compare the radiogram of one mastoid with that of the opposite side (bilateral otitis, or previous otitis and mastoiditis of the opposite side); or if one forgot to take a radiogram of the mastoids at the beginning of otitis media. Only a comparison of the radiograms—one taken at the beginning of the disease and one taken at the time of suspected mastoiditis —will remain the only means for reaching a correct diagnosis.

The conclusion is that one should be extremely careful in prescribing sulfa drugs against otitis media. If it is a mild otitis, the best is to deal with it according to the old classical methods of treatment, without using sulfonamides. And this is the case for the majority of otitis patients. If mastoid complication is threatening, one should demand radiograms of both mastoids, and prescribe an intensive treatment with sulfonamides before surgical intervention is decided upon. During this treatment, successive radiograms have to be made in view of the camouflaging action of the drug. If the otitis is very severe, first thing to do is to make radiograms of the mastoids, and only then should sulfonamide be given. If this precaution is neglected, one may do much harm by continuing sulfonamide medication until suddenly a

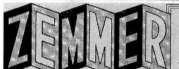

Bacillary dysentery—
a new conquest for

SULFADIAZINE
Lederle

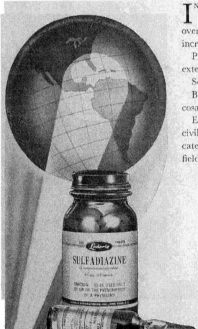

IN THE CONTROL of acute bacillary dysentery, SULFADIAZINE presents certain advantages over the other sulfonamides that have gained increasing recognition.

Prolonged high blood levels tend to prevent extension of the infection.

Secretions in the gut become bacteriostatic.

Bacterial growth within the intestinal mucosa tends to be inhibited.

Extensive clinical experience in military and civilian practice supports these views and indicates increasing use of SULFADIAZINE in this field.

REFERENCES:

HARDY, A. V., BURNS, W. and DE CAPITO, T.: Pub. Health Rep. 58: 689 (Apr. 30) 1943.
HARDY, A. V. and CUMMINS, S. D.: Pub. Health Rep. 58: 693 (Apr. 30) 1943.
HALL, W. W.: Am. Drug Mfgrs. Assoc. Annual Convention, Scientific Sec., Hot Springs, Va., May 1, 1944.
Annual Reports, U. S. Pub. Health Service, 1942-43, p. 122.

PACKAGES:

Sulfadiazine Tablets, 0.5 Gm. (7.7 grains) each (grooved) Bottles of 50, 100, 1000, 5000 and 10,000 tablets.
Solution Sodium Sulfadiazine (sodium 2-sulfanilamidopyrimidine) 25% w/v solution.
Packages of 6, 25, 100 ampuls, 10 cc. each.

Listen to the latest developments in research and practice—the new Lederle program, "THE DOCTORS TALK IT OVER" —on the blue network every Friday evening.

LEDERLE LABORATORIES INC.
30 ROCKEFELLER PLAZA, NEW YORK 20   NEW YORK

A UNIT OF AMERICAN CYANAMID COMPANY

serious complication develops, in which sulfa drugs would be very effective, but. meanwhile, the patient has been made resistant to sulfonamides by the previous long-continued, unwise medication.—M. D. H., M.D.

"COMMON EAR DISEASES IN CHILDREN AND THEIR TREATMENT." A. Furniss. The Prescriber. Vol. 38. pp. 82-83. June, 1944.

The vast majority of aural infections are secondary to bacterial invasion of the nasal and pharyngeal mucosa. It is obvious that to prevent such lesions we must provide and maintain a healthy upper respiratory tract, otherwise Eustachian catarrh may develop, rapidly leading to tympanic infection and suppuration, and other complications of otitis media. It is not sufficient to examine the tonsils and adenoids only, and then remove them; the doctor should also examine the nasal passages, teeth, sinuses, the neck for enlarged glands, and make careful inquiries into the general health, past illnesses, and so on. He will then be surprised to find how many cases of aural suppuration begin with sore throat; or what a large number of mastoid wounds will not heal because there is an undiscovered infected nasal sinus, or untreated diseased tooth.

Many writers have reported on the good results obtained by physical therapy in ear infections. In acute middle-ear disease, the action of lightrays on the affected structure and on adjacent structures arrest the inflammatory changes, limits the infective process, and in many instances prevents complications. For the treatment of acute otitis media the author recommends luminous heat irradiation with the Sollux lamp and localizer, as close as can be tolerated (about six inches is usual), 30 minutes exposure; the treatment should be repeated frequently, once to four times daily until the condition clears up.

Provided no definite surgical indications are present, ultra-violet therapy gives a good prospect of curative results also in chronic purulent otitis media. The ear is cleansed by suction and dry swabs. Mercurochrome solution (2.5 per cent) is instilled and allowed to remain in the meatal canal five to fifteen minutes. Then it is wiped out and the canal is irradiated using a Kromayer water-cooled mercury vapor lamp and a suitable applicator, gradually withdrawing so that a definite reaction results along its length. The reaction should be vigorous, but short of blister point. The irradiation is repeated every second day until the discharge ceases. Concomitant general tonic measures (light baths, etc.) are also indicated.

The common factor in the various and many remedies for otorrhea is cleanliness. Before the introduction of drops or the inflation of powder the ear must be thoroughly cleansed, mopped out or syringed. Cleansing is necessary also before light therapy, or before ionization. It may be that it is cleanliness that is mainly effective in bringing about the cessation of the discharge.

Far fewer radical operations are being done now than formerly. There are many cases of chronic otitis media, but just a few in which radical operation is really indicated. Some form of meato-mastoid operation gives better results than a simple Shwartze operation, as recurrences in the latter are not uncommon. Every case must be dealt with according to the pathological condition found at the operation. In some the attic wall will have to be removed, and in others the incus; in some no interference with the middle ear proper will be required, but in nearly all cases it will be found unnecessary to damage hearing. The majority of cases after a few months to discharge, with improved hearing.—M. D. H., M.D.

KEY TO ABSTRACTORS

M.D.H., M.D. ....Marvin D. Henley, M.D.

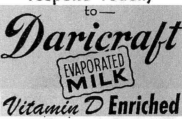
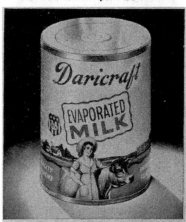

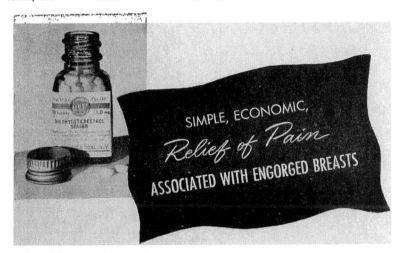

SIMPLE, ECONOMIC,
Relief of Pain
ASSOCIATED WITH ENGORGED BREASTS

IN WOMEN, in whom breast feeding is undesir-able or contraindicated, the early administration of Diethylstilbestrol provides an effective means of preventing the development and minimizing the intensity of breast pain. This simple proce-dure eliminates the use of breast binders, ice bags, restriction of foods and use of saline catharsis.

In large numbers of women the medication may consist of administration of 10 milligrams Diethylstilbestrol orally on the day of delivery or first day postpartum, and 5 milligrams at 24-hour intervals thereafter, for two or more days. Patients are not nauseated by Diethylstilbestrol thus administered, nor is there any vomiting or any other evidence of drug hypersensitivity.

Most physicians who have discovered the value of this hormonal treatment of engorged breasts find it most satisfactory.

Diethylstilbestrol Squibb is available in 5-mg.

tablets which are particularly useful for the treat-ment of this condition. The synthetic estrogen is available in a variety of other dosage forms for oral, intravaginal, or parenteral administration. Not the least among the advantages of Diethyl-stilbestrol is its low cost.

Given in doses of 0.5 mg. or less, it has made the cost of estrogen therapy relatively inexpen-sive to women of middle age whose distressing symptoms of the menopause require this form of alleviation.

The Squibb Laboratories also supply natural estrogens in the form of Amniotin—an extract of pregnant mares' urine. It, too, is available in a variety of dosage forms, for oral, intra-vaginal and parenteral use.

For literature address the Professional Service Dept., 745 Fifth Avenue, New York 22, N. Y.

E·R·SQUIBB & SONS, NEW YORK
MANUFACTURING CHEMISTS TO THE MEDICAL PROFESSION SINCE 1858

OFFICERS OF COUNTY SOCIETIES, 1944

★

COUNTY	PRESIDENT	SECRETARY	MEETING TIME
Alfalfa	H. E. Huston, Cherokee	L. T. Lancaster, Cherokee	Last Tues. each Second Month
Atoka-Coal	R. C. Henry, Coalgate	J. S. Fulton, Atoka	
Beckham	G. H. Stagner, Erick	O. C. Standifer, Elk City	Second Tuesday
Blaine	L. R. Kirby, Okeene	W. F. Griffin, Watonga	
Bryan	John T. Wharton, Durant	W. K. Haynie, Durant	Second Tuesday
Caddo	F. L. Patterson, Carnegie	C. B. Sullivan, Carnegie	
Canadian	P. F. Herod, El Reno	A. L. Johnson, El Reno	Subject to call
Carter	J. R. Pollock, Ardmore	H. A. Higgins, Ardmore	
Cherokee	P. H. Medcaris, Tahlequah	W. M. Wood, Tahlequah	First Tuesday
Choctaw		E. A. Johnson, Hugo	
Cleveland	F. T. Gastineau, Norman	Iva S. Merritt, Norman	Thursday nights
Comanche	George L. Berry, Lawton	Howard Angus, Lawton	
Cotton	A. B. Holstead, Temple	Mollie F. Scism, Walters	Third Friday
Craig	Lloyd H. McPike, Vinita	J. M. McMillan, Vinita	
Creek	J. E. Hollis, Bristow	F. H. Sisler, Bristow	
Custer	P. R. Vieregg, Clinton	C. J. Alexander, Clinton	Third Thursday
Garfield	Julian Feild, Enid	John R. Walker, Enid	Fourth Thursday
Garvin	T. F. Gross, Lindsay	John R. Callaway, Pauls Valley	Wednesday before Third Thursday
Grady	Walter J. Baze, Chickasha	Roy E. Emanuel, Chickasha	Third Thursday
Grant	L. V. Hardy, Medford		
Greer	R. W. Lewis, Granite	J. B. Hollis, Mangum	
Harmon	W. G. Husband, Hollis	R. H. Lynch, Hollis	First Wednesday
Haskell	William Carson, Keota	N. K. Williams, McCurtain	
Hughes	Wm. L. Taylor, Holdenville	Imogene Mayfield, Holdenville	First Friday
Jackson	C. G. Spears, Altus	E. A. Abernethy, Altus	Last Monday
Jefferson	F. M. Edwards, Ringling		Second Monday
Kay	J. Holland Howe, Ponca City	G. H. Yeary, Newkirk	Second Thursday
Kingfisher	**A. O. Meredith, Kingfisher**	**H. Violet Sturgeon, Hennessey**	
Kiowa	**J. William Finch, Hobart**	**William Bernell, Hobart**	
LeFlore	Neeson Rolfe, Poteau	Rush L. Wright, Poteau	
Lincoln	W. B. Davis, Stroud	Carl H. Bailey, Stroud	First Wednesday
Logan	William C. Miller, Guthrie	J. L. LeHew, Jr., Guthrie	Last Tuesday
Marshall	J. L. Holland, Madill	J. F. York, Madill	
Mayes	Ralph V. Smith, Pryor	Paul B. Cameron, Pryor	
McClain	W. C. McCurdy, Sr., Purcell	W. C. McCurdy, Jr., Purcell	
McCurtain	A. W. Clarkson, Valliant	N. L. Barker, Broken Bow	Fourth Tuesday
McIntosh	Lester I. Jacobs, Hanna	Wm. A. Tolleson, Eufaula	First Thursday
Murray	P. V. Annadown, Sulphur	J. A. Wrenn, Sulphur	Second Tuesday
Muskogee-Sequoyah			
Wagoner	H. A. Scott, Muskogee	D. Evelyn Miller, Muskogee	First Monday
Noble	C. H. Cooke, Perry	J. W. Francis, Perry	
Okfuskee	C. M. Cochran, Okemah	M. L. Whitney, Okemah	Second Monday
Oklahoma	W. E. Eastland, Oklahoma City	E. R. Musick, Oklahoma City	Fourth Tuesday
Okmulgee	S. B. Leslie, Okmulgee	J. C. Matheney, Okmulgee	Second Monday
Osage	C. R. Weirich, Pawhuska	George K. Hemphill, Pawhuska	Second Monday
Ottawa	Walter Kerr, Picher	B. W. Shelton, Miami	Third Thursday
Pawnee	E. T. Robinson, Cleveland	R. L. Browning, Pawnee	
Payne	H. C. Manning, Cushing	J. W. Martin, Cushing	Third Thursday
Pittsburg	P. T. Powell, McAlester	W. H. Kaeiser, McAlester	Third Friday
Pontotoc	A. R. Sugg, Ada	R. H. Mayes, Ada	First Wednesday
Pottawatomie	E. Eugene Rice, Shawnee	Clinton Gallaher, Shawnee	First and Third Saturday
Pushmataha	John S. Lawson, Clayton	B. M. Huckabay, Antlers	
Rogers	R. C. Meloy, Claremore	Chas. L. Caldwell, Chelsea	First Monday
Seminole	J. T. Price, Seminole	Mack I. Shanholtz, Wewoka	Third Wednesday
Stephens	W. K. Walker, Marlow	Wallis S. Ivy, Duncan	
Texas	R. G. Obermiller, Texhoma	Morris Smith, Guymon	
Tillman	C. C. Allen, Frederick	O. G. Bacon, Frederick	
Tulsa	Ralph A. McGill, Tulsa	E. O. Johnson, Tulsa	Second and Fourth Monday
Washington-Nowata	K. D. Davis, Nowata	J. V. Athey, Bartlesville	Second Wednesday
Washita	A. S. Neal, Cordell	James F. McMurry, Sentinel	
Woods	Ishmael F. Stephenson, Alva	Oscar E. Templin, Alva	Last Tuesday Odd Months
Woodward	H. Walker, Buffalo	C. W. Tedrowe, Woodward	Second Thursday

(Serving in Armed Forces)

THE JOURNAL

OF THE

OKLAHOMA STATE MEDICAL ASSOCIATION

| VOLUME XXXVII | OKLAHOMA CITY, OKLAHOMA, NOVEMBER, 1944 | NUMBER 11 |

Observations In "Thymus Disease"[*]

G. R. RUSSELL, M.D.

TULSA, OKLAHOMA

The age-old subject of thymus disease, or "the thymus problem" as the late Graeme Mitchell[1] has so aptly put it, is viewed by two diametrically opposite schools of thought. The first or affirmative side holds that excessive enlargement of the gland by pressure on the trachea, recurrent laryngeal nerve, great vessels and other mediastinal structures can and does at times produce spells of dyspnea, cyanosis and even death. The disciples of this school postulate that: 1. Bronchoscopic examinations and lateral roentgenograms demonstrate that tracheal compression may occur; 2. There is an apparent cessation of symptoms after radiological treatment of the gland; and 3. Occasionally, findings at necropsy suggest that compression had occurred during life. The second or negative side holds that: 1. It would be difficult for a soft organ such as the thymus to compress the cartilagenous trachea; 2. That great neoplastic enlargements may occur without symptoms of compression; 3. That there is no close correlation between the symptoms which might be attributed to pressure and the size of the roentgenographic shadow; and 4. That careful clinical study will show other causes for such symptoms as dyspnea and cyanosis in most cases.

It would seem reasonable to expect middle ground on which not all of the vague and ill-defined symptoms held by the affirmative side are due to this condition, but on which the odd case may occur with symptoms and signs which the negative side could not explain on any other basis. The writer has always held

to the latter or middle ground position, but after twenty years of practice in pediatrics, it would seem that the pot of gold at the foot of the diagnostic rainbow is as empty as ever.

The difficulties attendant upon the diagnosis of thymus disease are many. Since percussion of the para manubrial area seldom, if ever, gives reliable information as to the size of the gland, roentgenographic findings are the only available means of reaching a conclusion during the life of the individual. A comparison of roentgenographic impressions with post mortem findings shows frequent discrepancies in the diagnosis of hypertrophy. Boyd[2], in a large series of cases, has held that the gland on the average does not exceed 30 grams, while numerous instances at autopsy show an increase up to 50 grams (or 67 per cent increase) without any previous symptoms of thymus disease. The writer, in reviewing a series of hospital cases, has seen a roentgenographic diagnosis of hypertrophy made and the almost immediate subsequent autopsy report showing the gland to weigh 10 grams. Due consideration must be given to the phase of respiration in which the roentgenogram is taken as it must be remembered that in the phase of expiration the diaphragm is high and mediastinal structures are pushed together with the shadows appearing greatly wider than in the subsequent phase of inspection when, with the lowering of the diaphragm, these same structures are lengthened and stretched with an apparent, as well as real, narrowing of the shadows they cast. Many observers prefer, in addition to the conventional antero-

*Presented April 25, 1944, at the Annual State Meeting, Tulsa.

posterior view of the chest, additional right and left lateral and oblique exposures. However, regardless of the view taken, these same factors must be considered. Also, as the roentgenogram is merely a shadow, differentiation must be made from enlargement of regional lymph nodes, anomalies of the heart and great vessels changes in other mediastinal structures.

When the above criteria are met for a diagnosis of hypertrophy of the thymus gland and symptoms of dyspnea and cyanosis are present, there are still pitfalls on the path leading to the establishment of this hypertrophy as the cause of the symptoms produced.

The following two cases are given as examples of what might appear to satisfy the hypothesis, but which on critical analysis are proven to be otherwise:

CASE 1

Baby S., a female infant born at the end of the 9th month of gestation and with a birth weight of 7 pounds, 2 and one-half ounces. The child was Para I and was delivered following an episiotomy and a mid-low forceps application. It was slow to breath and cry and 0-2 and alpha lobelin were given. It was then sent to the nursery in good condition. About twelve hours later, it became cyanotic and apneic, requiring artificial respiration and 0-2 inhalations periodically. The respirations were improved following alpha lobelin. On the second day a radiological examination of the chest showed some enlargement of the thymus gland and a treatment was given. This was repeated 24 hours later. Immediately following each treatment, it was believed by some that the respirations became more normal. The periods of cyanosis still persisted and at times the extremities were rigid and an inability to suck were noted. Elixir Luminal in drams one-half to drams one doses were given and calcium gluconate intramuscularly.

About 72 hours after delivery, the child began to take small amounts of formula and water, but for the next 24 hours there were still periods of rigidity and cyanosis. From the fifth day on, the stay in the hospital was uneventful. The child gained regularly and was dismissed on the twelfth day.

Growth and development were average during the first six months of life. During the second six months of life, it was evident that muscular development was going to be delayed, and the child, by the age of one year was still unable to eat alone. The head growth had been average up to 11 months when it was slightly larger than normal and at one year was considerably larger. Some spacticity was also noticed at this time. An encephalogram, done at about this time, showed

definite evidence of both internal and external hydrocephalus.

Thus, while the first impression of this case may have been one of thymus disease, a critical analysis in retrospect calls attention to the fact that the cyanosis was not correlated with dyspnea as one should expect with upper respiratory obstruction as from pressure of an enlarged thymus on the trachea, but that the cyanosis was periodic and accompanied by periods of apnea which could only be central in nature. The rigidity of the extremities could be accounted for in the same way. The subsequent development made only one conclusion possible, namely a cerebral defect or injury.

CASE 2

Baby C., was the result of the fifth pregnancy which terminated in the eighth month of gestation. There had been three previous normal pregnancies and one miscarriage at six months following an electric shock which threw the mother into a bathtub. It was a male and weighted 5 pounds, 2 ounces. The delivery was spontaneous and respirations were immediate, but characterized by marked inspiratory difficulty. Suction was used and oxygen, but the respirations continued labored. An x-ray of the chest showed complete atelectasis of both lungs. The child died one hour and forty-five minutes after birth.

The post mortem examination, on opening the thorax, exposed a prominent thymus extending under the sternal notch. The thoracic contents were removed en block for a museum specimen, offering what was at first believed to be a very vivid example of tracheal obstruction caused by an enlarged thymus. This obstruction consisted in an enfolding of the soft non-cartilaginous portion of the wall which was made possible by the flabby soft cartilage deficiency of the anterior portion. Thus, the real pathology was not thymus disease, but really inability of the trachea to maintain a clear open air passage from the throat to the lungs.

It will be noted that the cases cited are both in the so-called newborn period. This is the period of life in which it would be most logical to expect thymus disease to occur since the gland normally undergoes involution with increasing age. In this connection, it is interesting to see what is going on in some of the large institutions of the country. Potter[3] in a recent article in the Journal of the American Medical Association has analyzed the causes of death in a series of approximately 1,000 autopsies at the Chicago Lying-In Hospital during the past ten years, and another series of approximately the same number from the New York Lying-In or Sloan Hospital. In not one single instance has thymic disease been given any significance as a cause of death. In the former institution no x-ray treatment to the thymus gland has been given in the past three years.

For those who are interested in the older infant as a possible source of thymic disease, the work going on in the Chicago area is noteworthy. In the past several years the Chicago Health Department lead by Dr. Bundesen and various obstetricians, pediatrists, and pathologists of the city have organized to carry out an extensive campaign to obtain autopsies on all infants dying under one year of age. The three main causes of death are listed as cerebral injury and anoxia, prematurity and infection. Efforts devoted to reducing these causative factors to a minimum have resulted in a definite reduction of infant mortality in this area. Death from thymic disease does not appear as a specific diagnosis in the records of the Chicago Health Department. The writer is told in a personal communication that the coroners use it on older infants only because they do not know what else to put down when they find an infant who has been previously well and suddenly dies.

For evidence that these sudden deaths do occur it is only necessary to examine the experience of the average physician. If he has not experienced such an occurrence personally he has a colleague, who has had an apparently perfectly healthy infant patient found dead in bed. A natural question follows, namely, if these infants, who are previously well and suddenly die, do not die of thymic disease then just what is the cause of their death?

A quick glance through the cumulative index shows numerous causes of sudden death in infants, paroxysmal ventricular tachycardia, spasmophialia, unrecognized diaphragmatic hernia, syphilitic aortitis, congenital heart disease, acute nondiphtheritic inflammatory edema of the larynx, laryngeal polyp and accidental mechanical suffocation. One very interesting series of autopsies shows a series of findings analagous to anaphylactic shock in the guinea pig with marked eosinophilic infiltration and ruptured alveoli of the lungs. With all these diagnoses possible as a cause of sudden death, it would seem unnecessary to place them all under the vague, indefinite diagnostic blanket of thymic disease.

No treatise on thymic disease is complete without at least the mention of status thymicolymphaticus. This is the condition usually given as the basis of sudden death in children who have died at the beginning of an anaesthetic or at the beginning of a minor operation such as a pleural puncture or a spinal puncture, or during a subcutaneous injection, or during the application of a fixed bandage or a cold pack, or immersion into water, or after sudden fright.

Stoeltzner[4] and others have called attention to the fact that the real pathology in these cases is a hypoplasia of the chromaffin system and of the vascular system with the thyms undergoing enlargement and changes present in the lymphatic system in general. In consequence they would apply the term status hypoplasticus as a term more inclusive of the pathology involved.

SUMMARY

1. The writer has presented a brief resume of some current opinions and findings in thymic disease and the usually related status thymicolymphaticus.

2. These findings has been seasoned by two typical cases chosen as examples of possible sources of confusion in the diagnosis of thymic disease.

3. The first type which primarily simulated thymic disease was finally and conclusively settled as a birth injury.

4. The second type case which at first even more met all the criteria for the diagnosis of thymic disease, was explained at autopsy by an insufficiency of the tracheal rings.

5. The term "Tracheal Insufficiency" is offered as another explanation of conditions which may simulate thymic disease.

BIBLIOGRAPHY

1. Mitchell, A. Graeme: Diseases of the Thymus Gland. Cecil's Medicine—6th Edition. Page 1244
2. Boyd, Edith: American Journal on Diseases of Children. Vol. 51; pp. 313-335. 1936.
3. Potter, Edith: Journal of the American Medical Association. Vol. 124, pp. 336-339. 1944.
4. Stoeltzner, Wilhelm translation Pfaundler and Schlossman: Diseases of Children (Peterman) pp. 322. 1935.

A Great Doctor

The following quotation has to do with Dr. Frances Adams who gave us the English translation of Hippocrates, originally published by the Syndenham Society.

"Dr. Adams's great work was the translation of Paulus Aeginetas, the Greek physician, whose teaching embodied all the earlier history of medicine. This translation was dedicated to Dr. Abercrombie of Edinburgh and Dr. Guthrie of London. In his preface he says: "I trust that I have been able to present the reader with a work from which he may, at one view, become familiar with the prevailing opinions of the profession upon all the most important points of medical practice during a period of more than fifteen centuries.' A herculean task, and faithfully discharged. A translation of Artæus followed, requiring research, a visit to the Bodleian Library at Oxford, and to great book collectors, who gave variety to his acquaintance, and introduced him to the literati of Britain.

"The contrast in Dr. Adams of the student burning the midnight oil, and the country surgeon sent for in hot haste at all hours of the day and night, makes his character all the more interesting. A writer says, with jaunty sarcasm: 'We well remember finding this great scholar at his careless jentaculum, diverting himself with doing an Ode of Horace into Greek verse; being then, and we daresay still, at the call of any shepherd's 'crying wife' up in the solitudes of Clochnaben.'"
—Aberdeen Doctors, At Home and Abroad, pp. 269-270. Ella Hill Burton Rodger. William Blackwood and Sons. Edinburgh and London. 1913.

Urological Pain With A Negative Urinalysis[*]

W F. LEWIS, M. D.

LAWTON, OKLAHOMA

During the first three years of my urological practice I saw a large number of patients who apparently had been neglected. They represented one of the most common of complaints—"pain in the kidney" or "pain across the kidneys." By far, the majority of these patients had a negative urinalysis and therefore, the kidneys were forgotten as a possible source of the pathology.

This paper will not include those cases that give a typical picture of ureteral colic due to calculus but those patients that have more of a chronic complaint or many acute exacerbations of a chronic condition.

Most of these patients have 'made the rounds.' That is to say, they have been here and there without relief of the backache that has partially disabled them for several years. I have found most of these patients to be in the third or fourth decade of life and about equally as common in the male as in the female. Very few of them admitted that they had had a back injury but many of them had consented to a series of joint adjustments. Some had had pelvic surgery or an appendectomy for chronic infections without relief of their original pain. Others received treatment for lumbago, muscle spasm, sprains, etc.

Too often, especially in these busy war times, these patients have not been given the attention they would like and for which they are willing to pay. Very few would object to a urological examination — including a series of x-rays. The most important procedure in the examination of these patients is the intravenous urogram. This can be done by any general practitioner. The patient is advised to take a cathartic, preferably epsom salts or castor oil, the night before the examination and to concentrate his body fluids by not taking any fluids or food after midnight. A preliminary film is usually taken, although it is not necessary in these patients. The intravenous dye is given and a ten minute film taken. In the majority of cases this will show the pathology, if present, but if delayed excretion is present, a twenty or thirty minute film is taken. A complete upright picture is taken, especially in the female, after the pa-

tient walks around for a while. This will show the excursion of the kidney and the emptying of the renal pelvis. Further examinations—such as retrograde urogram—may be necessary if the pathology is sufficient to prevent visulization of the dye. However, most of the cases are diagnosed by intravenous pyelograms.

The conditions which impede urinary flow or excretion of the intravenous contrast media are numerous. Any pathology which reduces the caliber of the ureteral lumen must be considered whether intrinsic or x-trinsic, temporary or permanent.

1. Intrinsic

   a. Stenosis of the ureter at any level.

   b. Hypertrophy of the ring muscles at the ureteropelvic junction.

   c. Congenital valves.

   d. Congenital pinpoint ureteral meatus.

2. Extrinsic

   a. Aberrant or accessory renal vessels.

   b. Fibrous bands around or across the ureter.

   c. Kinking of tthe ureter with or without ptosis of the kidney.

   d. Tumors pressing on the ureter.

Ureteral obstruction is much more common in persons with congenital anomalies of the kidneys such as: Ectopic kidney (unilateral, bilateral or crossed); Double kidneys; Fused kidneys ("horseshoe," "cake" or "sigmoid") ; d. Rotated kidney.

The outstanding complaint is a dull heavy costovertebral pain, usually varying from a vague sense of discomfort to a more severe constant type. It is generally in proportion to the rapidity with which the obstruction occurs rather than the size of the hydrocalyx or hydronephrosis. Frequently the pain is only temporary, as is the pain in a ptotic kidney, being present while ambulatory and being relieved by a few minutes rest in the recumbent position. The pain is usually more intense while the patient is walking, running or riding because the obstruction becomes more acute as the kidneys descend in their normal or abnormal excursion. Gastrointestinal manifestation with abdominal pain,

*Presented at the Annual State Meeting April 25, 1944, in Tulsa.

flatulence, nausea and vomiting may be the only symptoms.

The pathology found in the painful kidney is some degree of dilatation of the pelvis and calices. This, however, is not the most serious disturbance. The renal substance is subjected to back pressure which causes a pressure atrophy and is progressive in destroying the ability of the kidney to excrete the urinary by-products until in its later stages the excretions may contain only water and salt. If the obstruction is removed before advanced atrophy or infection results, normal function returns. We are urging the recognition of these cases before any appreciable damage is done.

The primary purpose of treatment is to relieve the obstruction of the urinary flow. The pathology in some cases can be relieved by ureteral dilation, but most cases require plastic surgery of the ureter or renal pelvis, nephropexy, or removal of obstructing extrinsic pressure.

In conclusion, I wish to emphasize the importance of recognizing these cases of urinary obstruction early before complications have developed. And also to remind you again that the type of pain is not always characteristic—being easily misconstrued, especially if the patient presents a normal urinalysis. Probably a large number of the x-rays will show normal urograms, but I'm sure none of the patients will be disappointed to know that the pain across his back is not due to his kidneys. Most of them will be pleased to see some concrete evidence whether it be positive or negative.

DISCUSSION
JOSEPH FULCHER, M.D.

First, I wish to compliment Dr. Lewis on his most excellent presentation of this complex problem. It is all too often that we find people with pain which is definitely urological, yet the urinalysis is negative. This, I think, he has proved very conclusively, especially with his most interesting urograms.

It is all very well that we urologists, have facilities and equipment to make these studies, but where these are not available, one can still have a great deal to rely upon. A case history means so very, very much and cannot be overemphasized. Often we find pains simulating a urological pain, which may be the result of an injury and not having any connection with the genito-urinary system.

Careful scrutiny of the patients contour may reveal some abnormality of the bony framework which will give rise to such symptoms. We should never forget that it is very important to use inspection, palpation, percussion and ausculation. In palpating for suspected renal pain have the patient comfortable, flat on his back with a pillow under his head, and thighs flexed. In palpating for the left kidney, first use one hand posteriorly in the casto-vertebral angle. This is done from the patient's right side. Then bi-manually palpate the left kidney for size, position and motility; this will bring out sensitivity, also. The right kidney should be palpated in the same manner, except with the examiner on the left side of the patient. Tenderness should be sought along the spine and the muscles of the back. Very often a neuritis of the ilioinguinal or iliohypogastric nerve, or the intercostal nerves may simulate pain from a urological condition. Foci of infection should never be forgotten, especially in connection with myositis, a neuritis, or an osteo-arthritis.

Percussion of the spinous processes may suggest that the trouble is in the spine.

Hyperesthesia of the skin is easy to elicit and is sometimes a deciding factor in ruling out the kidney as the cause of the existing pain.

In arriving at a conclusion as to whether or not a patient is suffering from a urological condition depends, first upon carefully eliciting and evaluating his symptoms and physical findings. These determinations can be made in many instances by using detailed principles of history taking and a careful physical examination. The more technical procedures will then follow suit.

Life
June 22

Fools and clowns and sots make the fringes of every one's tapestry of life, and give a certain reality to the picture. What could we do in Concord without Bigelow's and Wesson's Bar-rooms and their dependencies? What without such fixtures as Uncle Sol, and old Moore who sleeps in Doctor Hurd's barn, and the red charity house over the brook? Tragedy and comedy always go hand in hand. — *The Heart of Emerson's Journals, page* 200. *Houghton Mifflin Company. Boston and New York.*

John Hunter

John Hunter, the great anatomist, was the most distinguished medical man of the day. Scotland greatly reverenced him, for not only was he a famous surgeon and a profound anatomist, but he was a Scotsman. In invincible industry he was a grand example of that genius described as "an infinite capacity for taking pains," and putting anatomy on a sure foundation, he gave to the study of pathology its true place. It was said of him that he loved anatomy with all the fondness of a lover, and in his incessant industry laboured as if life was all too short for the work he had to do. He had a candid open nature, was entirely unreserved, despised artifice, was above all deceit, and hated to see it in others. His life was a sacrifice to science, and in his earnest aim and intense character he had much in common with students from the north, who, though they reverenced little, yet reverenced the best.—*Aberdeen Doctors, At Home and Abroad, pp.* 114-115. *William Blackwood and Sons. Edinburgh and London.* 1913.

The Science of Radiology*

W. S. Larrabee, M.D.
TULSA, OKLAHOMA

Some apology or explanation for your Chairman seems necessary as he is really the third choice of the general program committee. The first choice was forced to decline the honor about the middle of January. The second choice was unable to accept the appointment, therefore, in desperation he was drafted.

I could have chosen to search the literature, revamp several reams of statistics, compile many tables, and with a limited amount of plagarism, produced something you have already heard many times, something you could find elsewhere done much better by more able men.

After much cogitation, I decided to change the usual procedure and write something which, though not so scientific, may receive your interest and concern in your chosen speciality, this paper, therefore is titled "The Science of Radiology," and is sub-divided into several heads, namely: Conception, Birth, Infancy, Childhood, Adolescence, Graduation, Early Manhood, Courtship, Future Hopes and Dangers.

CONCEPTION

Remember that the apparatus, materials and knowledge used by Roentgen and the Curies represented the labor of many ingenious investigators, scientists, electricians, chemists and students, there can be little doubt that conception, the actual contact between the ovum and spermatazon, must have taken place somewhere in the three preceding centuries. Yes, "The Science of Radiology" had a long gestation.

BIRTH

To the mind of this essayist there is no doubt, that, on that October day in 1895 when William Roentgen, working with a Crook's tube and a Barium Platinum Cyanide screen, saw for the first time a 'faint flickering, greenish illumination on the bit of cardboard in a darkened room, "The Science of Radiology" was born.

INFANCY

From birth the "Infant Science" was a precocious child. At first a few men with very crude machines, worked with and learned about the new diagnostic and therapeutic agent. Soon some men were devoting all their

*Presented before the Annual State Meeting, April 25, 1944, Tulsa.

time and energy to this newest branch of the healing art. In a few years Radiology Societies were formed to acquire and disseminate accurate knowledge and to stimulate scientific research. Radiology was advancing more rapidly than any other branch of medicine and contributing something to almost every division of modern science. This baby, "The Science of Radiology" was indeed a promising infant.

CHILDHOOD

After some years, Radiology ceased to be an adjunct of medicine and became a part of specialized medicine. Workers began to interest and train other members of the medical profession. Courses in Radiology were organized in the medical schools. Electrical engineers developed and improved the methods of generating the ray. The hand-propelled static generator became the induction coil and then the mechanical rectifier. The gas tube became the hot anode or the Coolidge tube. Every conceivable gadget and device was developed and improved until at the time of the World War No. I, the child "The Science of Radiology" was ready for Junior High.

ADOLESCENCE

The necessities of war, as always happens with the increased need, brought marvelous changes and developments in the generation and application of the Roentgen Ray. A great many physicians were given fundamental training, and a lesser number, advanced training in Radiology through their army service.

GRADUATION

By the end of the War, "The Science of Radiology" had its commencement and received its diploma. Local organizations formed national organizations, and there followed, as the night the day, the international organization. The Congress of American Radiology made this the most glamourous, the most spectacular, the most convincing and the youngest speciality in medicine.

EARLY MANHOOD

At first, radiological equipment was very expensive and required a considerable amount of room for safe operation. The radiologist was found more often in the hospital, the clinic, or the group. The physician, following his internship, spent from six months to two years in advanced study to' become a radiologist. These comparatively few, highly trained, hard working students of science, developed "The Science of Radiology" to its present standards. The published results of their thought, experience and research became so voluminous and intricate that one had to be a mechanical engineer, a physicist and a physician to comprehend the subject. Meanwhile, the manufactures of x-ray equipment were not idle. They saw a vastly lucrative business awaiting them. The hot cathode tube, the single compact unit, the shock proof tube, the 30 ma., then the 100 ma., then the 500 ma. tubes, the rotating mode, etc., caused the radiologist to spend all he collected from January to November to purchase the newly advanced, more workable equipment. Thanks to a benevolent Government, we had no with-holding tax then.

COURTSHIP

The manufactures not only produced finer, safer and simpler equipment, but the price also dropped from about $10,000.00 to $500.00 for the small diagnostic units, while the therapy units ranged from $2.500.00 to $50,-000.00, depending upon the voltage and method of rectification.

The radiologist found fellow physicians purchasing a fluoroscope for the office or one of the small units to hasten their fracture work. Having seen a few stomachs at the radiologist's office, they thought it was a short step to lowering the fluoroscopic screen and giving the faithtful patient the benefit of knowing the progress of his ulcer, without the necessary loss of time and the added fee of the x-ray man. There followed the colleague's visit to the Roentgenologist's office with a film he was not quite sure about—consulta-tion without fee. Before long, there were many x-ray men and some Roentgenologists.

Not long could such a condition exist without being capitalized by "that throng of near respectability" who trade in the fantastic pretense of the many counterfeits that infest the outskirts of the medical profession, sheltered partly by the cloak of the thoughtless physician and partly by the ignorance and credulity of the general public. This throng lined their shelves with works on Radiology, equipped their offices with x-ray machines and attempted to appropriate, seize and confiscate "The Science of Radiology," adopting it as their own. The Radiologist found his science, his labors, his dreams, wedded against his will to the advertisers, the commercial laboratories and the cults.

FUTURE

Your essayist has no fear, but that the well trained, competent Radiologist will maintain "The Science of Radiology" on the high plane of its conception and that the general public is fast learning to sift the true from the false, for, "by their works ye shall know them."

You and I inherited the practice of medicine in a good healthy condition. It is our obligation to bequeath it alive and healthy, not morbid and dead to our posterity. Let us strive "to nobly save, not meanly lose this last great hope of medicine."

In conclusion let me remind you that the study of medicine and "The Science of Radiology" is never ended. Each day new facts and theories call for additional study. To keep abreast of the times, yours is a never ending task and let us always remember "that a little knowledge is a dangerous thing, drink deep or taste not of the Pierian Spring."

The Diagnosis and Medical Management of Poliomyelitis[*]

CARROLL M. POUNDERS, M.D.

OKLAHOMA CITY, OKLAHOMA

This paper is an attempt to review and clarify some of the most important points about the diagnosis of poliomyelitis and to briefly touch upon the medical management.

Until our present knowledge of the disease is improved upon, in all probability, there will always be a high per cent of cases undiagnosed and the reason for this will be brought out shortly.

*Presented before the Annual State Meeting, April 26, 1944, Tulsa.

The disease usually starts with mild general symptoms accompanied possibly by upper respiratory and digestive disturbances which last only 24 to 48 hours. Two or four days later there is some recurrence of the fever with signs of meningeal irritation and in another one to four days motor disturbances appear. The opinion is quite general that the disease may become arrested during any stage of this development and that a large proportion of all cases do stop short

of the development of the motor disturbances.

There naturally arises the question as to
whether or not, during an epidemic, there occur many cases which might be termed abortive and which go undiagnosed. During such
times it is not uncommon for us to see children who become sick with mild systemic disturbances including such symptoms as headache, sore throat and gastro-intestinal disturbances consisting of vomiting and constipation. The illness lasts only a day or two
and when spinal fluid examinations have
been made they have been normal. Observations have been made to the effect that these
children have not later contracted the disease
even after repeated exposures and their blood
serum has been found to contain antibodies
against the virus. It is felt that this type of
case is common and accounts for great numbers of people being immune to the disease.

With our present limitations we can actually make a diagnosis in only those cases
which show evidence of involvement of the
central nervous system. Whether or not the
preliminary stage of systemic involvement is
recognized, the onset of this recognizable
phase is apt to appear to be somewhat sudden
with fever, headache and vomiting being the
first complaints. The fever is usually around
102 degrees but it may occasionally go to 104
degrees and it generally lasts four or five
days but may last as long as ten days. Headache is not a common childhood complaint
but in this condition it is often severe and
may be general, occipital or frontal in type.
Vomiting is fairly common, though not pre-
sistent and abdominal pains are sometimes
complained of. Either constipation or diarrhea may be present, with the former being
more common and urinary retention must be
watched for during the first four or five days.
Dizziness and irritability with pains in the
back and legs are often present with general
hyperesthesia and pain from deep pressure
near the spine. Photophobia sometimes exists. All these sensory symptoms are transient. An important diagnostic sign is a
course tremor, especially of the hands.

The child looks and acts sicker than the
amount of fever would indicate; he may act
drowsy but when aroused is irritable and
prefers to be left alone. The face may be
flushed, there is an anxious expression and
the pulse rate is rapid in proportion to the
fever.

The most important sign of involvement
of the nervous system is the unwillingness or
inability to bend the spine forward. When
the child is raised to a sitting position he
holds his back stiff, supports himself with
his hands behind him on the bed and complains when forced to bend forward. When

attempts are made to flex the neck forward
it is held rigid but generally is moved freely
from side to side. The patellar and other
deep reflexes are usually exaggerated in the
early stages and may be unequal sometimes.
The amount of meningeal irritation is shown
by the presence of such symptoms as headache, delirium, fever, muscle spasm, stiff
neck, positive Kernigs or Brudzinskis sign
and the number of cells found in the spinal
fluid.

When a sick child complains of headache,
and presents a stiff neck and spine with possibly a tremor, he should be looked upon as
a possible case of poliomyelitis and a spinal
puncture should be done. The fluid generally shows some increase in pressure and may
be perfectly clear or slightly hazy. The cell
count is increased to an average of 100 to 200
but may vary from 10 to 1200 and usually
returns to normal by the tenth to the fourteenth day. Albumen and globulin usually
show a moderate increase and the sugar content is normal or increased.

When muscular dysfunction comes on it
usually appears from the second to the fifth
day but may show up on the first day or even
after the tenth day. In most cases it reaches
its maximum within a day or two of its onset but in some instances it continues to
spread after this time. With the appearance
of muscular dysfunction the temperature
generally returns to normal in four to six
days but as long as there is fever there is
activity of the virus and possibility of extension of the muscular involvement.

The location of the muscular involvement
varies considerably in different epidemics but
in the majority of cases one or both legs are
involved. In the thigh there is usually spasm
of the hamstring group with later weakness
of the quadriceps femoris group; in the lower leg the gastroanemius group is commonly
spastic with weakness of the anterior peroneal group and resulting foot drop. In the
upper extremity the deltoid and shoulder girdle muscles are most commonly affected. The
anterior flexors of the neck are often found
to be weak, particularly the sternomastoids.

Respiratory difficulty may be due to (1)
thoracic cord involvement with dysfunction
of the intercostals, (2) cervical cord lesions
in the third and fourth segments with involvement of the diaphragm. If the diaphragm is completely affected, breathing is
entirely thoracic, the diaphragm descending
during expiration. (3) bulbar lesions may involve the vagus nuclei. Dyspnoea and cyanosis are marked and there are apt to be other
bulbar manifestations in the pharynx, larynx
and tongue. (4) the acute ascending so called
landrys type shows successive intercostal,
phrenic and bulbar involvement. (5) oc-

casionally patients may have pharyngeal paralysis resulting in marked respiratory difficulty because of excessive fatigue from the continual interference with respiration by unswallowed material in the pharynx or by actual aspiration of this material.

Bulbar paralysis involves one or more of the cranial nerves and because of the effects of this and the usually greater severity of the attack it is much more apt to be fatal. High fever with toxicity and prostration are common. In the usual epidemic some degree of bulbar involvement will show up in ten to thirty per cent of all cases.

The most common cranial nerve affected is the facial and when it is the only one involved, the patient is usually not very sick. More than one half of these clear up entirely. Involvement of the 3rd, 4th and 6th cranial nerves affecting the eye muscles are occasionally met with. About three fourths of the bulbar cases show some involvement of the muscles of swallowing and where respiratory paralysis goes with it the death rate is very high. Regurgitation of fluids through the nose is an early warning symptom. Following this, mucus may gather in the pharynx, swallowing may become impossible and coughing may become very weak. Bulbar nerve involvement is distinctly less apt to be permanent than cord paralysis so that in favorable cases without spinal cord involvement or respiratory involvement, particularly when only one side is affected, most patients will be able to swallow normally again in a week or ten days. One will see bulbar cases where no special cranial nerve seems to be involved but the cardiac respiratory and vasomotor centers are affected and early death follows. Death sometimes occurs as early as six hours after the onset but it more often comes after four or five days.

When poliomyelitis is suspected a lumbar puncture may be very helpful in confirming the diagnosis but repeated punctures are not indicated except in those unusual cases where there is evidence of excessive pressure. If the case is seen after the development of a typical paralysis and no meningitic symptoms are present, lumbar puncture is unnecessary.

Complete bed rest is indicated. It probably harms most patients to move them a great distance but this is often necessary in order to carry out proper hospitalization and treatment. It is sometimes desirable to give sedatives to induce sleep but one should be cautious about such measures when there is evidence of respiratory or bulbar paralysis. Pain, tenderness and muscle spasm are best relieved by hot applications.

The usual procedures recommended in the care of any sick child, such as administering fluids, a soft, high caloric diet and attention to elimination should be employed.

The respirator is needed for relief of respiratory embarassment due to intercostal or diaphragmatic paralysis without bulbar involvement. When the respiratory center is paralyzed the apparatus gives only temporary help and may even be harmful. Most cases with bulbar involvement are helped by lowering the head in order to better drain the mucus through the mouth and nose. Suction with a soft rubber tube is helpful and oxygen is often needed.

Treatment Of The Neuroses In General Practice*

HUGH M. GALBRAITH, M.D.

OKLAHOMA CITY, OKLAHOMA

Patients suffering from neuroses seem by general consent to form a major proportion of the average doctor's practice, general practitioner and specialist alike. Almost everyone suffering from organic disease at some time or another develops anxiety and functional disorders of various kinds which, if organic disease were not present, would be diagnosed as neurosis, and represents indeed a neurotic reaction to threats to one's physical integrity. And yet as one thumbs through medical journals one finds discussions on every disease process from alopecia to Zambesi fever with almost no reference to the human being who is doing the suffering. It is as though doctors felt that the living human body was a machine to be tinkered with when it was out of order and that the powerful emotions which distinguish the human organism from that of lower animals were considered to be of no consequence. The writer who attempts to approach the problem as though the word "scientific" were limited in its application to physics and chemistry, anatomy, pathology, physiology and the like.

When neuroses are discussed in the aver-

*Presented April 26 at Annual Meeting in Tulsa.

555

age medical journal, one too often finds people suffering from them dismissed lightly or even branded with uncomplimentary epithets. Walter Alvarez, writing recently in the Journal of the American Medical Association on "Diagnostic Time Savers[1]" said if a doctor followed a certain procedure "he can see in a few minutes that he is dealing with a scatterbrained neurotic, a constitutional inadequate, a fuss budget of a perfectionist or a psychopath." Again he says, "The patient is a fussy, opinionated person who is full of prejudices." One might be tempted to ask, "Who is— the patient or Dr. Alvarez?" The implication of the whole paper seems to be that once a diagnosis of neurosis is made the patient should be dismissed as a hopeless bore worthy only of contempt or as one whose difficulties are either an hereditary or a moral basis.

If this were the only way we expressed our hostility to the neurotic we would be on less vulnerable ground than we really are. In our lack of appreciation of the factors that enter into the formation of a neurosis and our emphasis on search for organic disease we subject neurotics to needless and often harmful (from the standpoint of treating a neurosis,) diagnostic procedures which serve merely to make the patient more nervous. And too often for inadequate reasons we perform operations on them which make the disease process more chronic. Every psychiatrist sees extreme examples of this tendency. One of my patients at 19 had had two submucous resections, two tonsillectomies, complete dental extraction, a cholecystectomy, an appendectomy and a complete colectomy. One may say with truth that an operation never cures a neurosis and usually serves to make it less amenable to more rational approaches.

The use of shock treatment in neurotics seems to fall in the same category. Shock treatment is of great value in some of the psychoses but I have never seen neurotics relieved by shock treatment for very long and I have frequently seen them made much worse. Too many reports of brain damage due to shock treatment have been made to make it safe for us to use this drastic method in patients whose rehabilitation can often be brought about by less severe and more rational methods.

The same can be said even more emphatically about frontal lobotomy. It is true that patients do not worry after a lobotomy. They couldn't possible do so, for the connection between the so-called center of emotion—the thalamus—and the seat of judgment—the frontal lobes—are severed. But there are some things worse than worry. After such an operation the capacity for ethical judgments is lost and the ability to

form emotional ties is destroyed, which makes the victims of the operation, in effect, vegetating animals to be tolerated with pity rather than loved for whatever favorable qualities they may formerly have possessed. Frontal lobotomy, in my opinion, should be used extremely sparingly and only on chronic psychotic patients of many years standing and whose behavior makes them menaces to the safety of fellow patients or attendants in their mental hospital.

Stanley Cobb in his most recent book[2] expresses a similar view. He says, "from the standpoint of therapy, radical excision of parts of the brain to relieve mental symptoms calls for careful consideration. Is the surgeon justified in depriving a patient of the most important part of his intellect in order to relieve him of emotional troubles? In the results as interpreted by the "psychosurgeons" themselves it is seen that they usually leave the patient lazy and undiscriminating. In other words they often take away the highest integration ("conscience" or superego," perhaps) in order to make the patient happier. In my opinion this is a justifiable procedure only when the patient is old and the prognosis hopeless. Specifically, I can only recommend the operation in rare instances in younger patients who show mental deterioration and neurological electroencephalorgraphic evidence of cerebral degeneration. To perform such an operation upon recoverable psychotic and neurotic states in people under sixty seems, to me, to be unjustified. I believe that practically all patients under sixty would refuse operation if compos mentis for a few moments so that they could be asked 'Would you rather suffer your present symptoms, perhaps for a period of years, or run a 50-50 risk of permanently losing your judgment?' So to advocate freely the cutting of the "worry cords" for chronic anxiety, is to be deprecated. The cure is much worse than the disease.

Anyone who has tried to understand neurotics knows that they suffer intensely. They do not enjoy their lot in life as they are so often accused. They come to the doctor seeking relief. When they are met with a nonsympathetic or hostile attitude and even told that there is nothing wrong with them and advised to stop worrying, to take a trip or to go away for a while, no one is relieved but the doctor. Rather, the doctor adds to the patient's desperation and it is small wonder that many seek aid from those whom we refer to as quacks but who treat them as welcome additions to their clientele. And when we, in desperate attempts to find organic pathology, subject them to needless and sometimes harmful diagnostic and operative procedures one can only marvel at their tenacious faith in us. Could this not be one , reason why there is now a strong movement to put us under government supervision and take away some of the responsibility and freedom we have enjoyed in the past? Human sufferers will not forever tolerate rebuff and abuse from those whom they justly expect relief.

It seems therefore appropriate that we should search for some reasons for our hostility toward these unfortunate people. One of the more important seems to stem from the fact that we teach so little psychiatry in medical schools. So much stress is laid on the diagnosis and treatment of organic diseases, in spite of the fact that many of them are rare and usually diagnosed accurately only by the specialist. Furthermore most of the psychiatry that is taught deals chiefly with the psychoses whose diagnosis is of little importance to the average doctor. His chief function in such cases is to determine that the patient is mentally ill so that he can send him to a psychiatric institution for confinement and treatment—and even a layman can do that. This is proven by the fact that, in Oklahoma County at least, there are no psychiatrists on the insanity board and the final judgment as to whether or not patients should be hospitalized is left in the hands of a judge who has had no medical education but who has said on occasion that since he has committed four thousand cases he considers himself a psychiatrist. And since there are few complaints who can dispute him?

The emphasis on the psychoses in teaching seems to be due to the fact that the teacher of psychiatry is usually a mental hospital official whose experience has been primarily with the psychoses so that his knowledge of the psychoses is greater than his knowledge of the neuroses. So this important field of the neuroses is grossly neglected and the graduating student is sent to his practice to discover he is entirely inadequately prepared to deal with patients who will form a major part of his practice. One cannot help being annoyed with patients whom one does not understand but whom one is expected to treat. And one cannot be blamed under the circumstances for overusing the methods which have been taught in medical school. Would not the remedy for this situation be to ignore more the rarer organic diseases and have more psychiatry taught by those with considerable experience in the treatment of neuroses?

Another reason for the arousing of hostility in the doctor toward the neurotic arises from the nature of the neuroses. As our understanding has increased we have found many discrepancies in our former beliefs regarding them. The theories of heredity and constitutional inadequacy have been largely exploded. Many physically handicapped persons have strong characters and neuroses appear in people whose bodies are thoroughly sound. The facts seem to be that we are all, as children, completely at the mercy of our environments. If we have loving, stable and wise parents and reasonably adequate living conditions as babies and children, without severely traumatic experiences, we develop good personalities. In so far as the opposite is true we develop more or less crippled personalities. This crippling arises out of intense cravings for the love which we failed to get in the formative years of our life with its resulting tendency toward hatred and resentment. This latter is not socially acceptable so we develop all sorts of devices to hide our hate not only from others but from ourselves. But the cravings, the guilt over feeling them and the hate of frustration persist and the symptoms of neurosis arise out of them. Since most of us do not have ideal childhoods we all have more or less neurosis. We are ashamed of our neurosis which we have pretty well hidden, so in order to protect ourselves from recognizing that we too are more or less neurotic we are prone to score who manifest symptoms of it more openly.

Further there is the matter of the expression of the patient's hate, and his guilt over his cravings and his hate. He expresses his hate in indirect ways and invites punishment to relieve his guilt. If we as doctors are not cognizant of these mechanisms we fall into the error of retaliating. If we know that behind the patient's disagreeable ways are intense cravings for love and understanding and that, if we can be tolerant and essentially sympathetic in our attitude, we can do much to alleviate his distress, we will have established a sound basis for treatment. Is it not better to try to understand the neurotic in terms of past history and present environmental difficulties, as he so frequently can be, than to drive him to the quack?

To be more specific then, the most important prerequisite in the therapeutic approach to the neuroses is emotional maturity. If the doctor is himself very neurotic he should not attempt to treat the neurotic. That is why the American Psychoanalytic Association requires of its members a successful therapeutic analysis before they are permitted to proceed to training courses and active therapy. Trainees who cannot be brought to a state of emotional maturity are not permitted to complete their training and to become members of the association. Maturity implies the capacity for assuming easily the role of the father. The neurotic is emotionally immature so he has many of the qualities of a child and needs a father substitute, the pyhsician, who can reassure him, and assist him to work out his problems. This father must not be easily aroused to anger or to sexual desire, for the love and understanding that he gives the neurotic must be that of a parent and not on a neurotic level. To yield either to anger or sexual desire is to defeat all success in treatment. The patient will involve tthe doctor in his neurosis if he can as an expression of his hostility so the sympathy must be objective, paternal.

With emotional maturity as a prerequisite the doctor will manifest a ready, but not maudlin, sympathy for his neurotic patient. He will inquire into the details of his early home life, whether there was fear of father or mother, overattachment to either parent, what his early attitude toward brothers or sisters was, what his capacity was for making friends in the community as a child, and many other details of his childhood. From this knowledge will come the capacity for determining how these childhood attitudes affect his present difficulties with his environment, why, in short, he cannot "make friends and influence people" to the degree necessary for happiness, and why he has to develop symptoms to win the attention he craves so much.

When the doctor recognizes the intensity of his patient's craving for sympathy, his real need for it, and the therapeutic success which often attends its administration he can approach the problem witth clearer understanding and more effective methods. He can, for example, recognize that the methods of the chiropractor and osteopath give the patient the personal attention he craves and prescribe massage and other physio-therapy or even learn to administer it himself if physiotherapists are not available. It makes the patient feel better so it should be used. Further it will enable him, with a clear conscience, to prescribe harmless medications, harmless doses of x-ray, and ultra violet light, at least until he can bring to bear on the problem more effective methods, if the procedure seems to make the patient feel better. The magic which patients unconsciously attribute to these procedures often helps to alleviate their distress. There is no real basis, then, to the feelings some of my colleagues have expressed to me that they feel like quacks for giving the patient something which makes him feel better but which they know has no pharmacological basis for the result obtained. Why should one feel guilty about administering harmless treatment as long as the patient feels better, especially as a temporary expedient until one can learn enough about the patient to use psychotherapy.

A powerful tool in the hands of the mature physician is confession with reassurance. The Catholic Church has long recognized the value of confession and doing penance and has designated "fathers" to act as the confessor, Protestants do not have this comforting outlet and often lack confidence in the tolerance or knowledge of their clergyman. Doctors can often bring about dramatic results by the use of this device if they can maintain an attitude of tolerance. The three following cases illustrate this.

CASE I

A 38 year old married woman came because of marked anxiety, shaking spells, crying, insomnia, fast pulse, palpitation and high blood pressure. She was the second of three rather widely spaced daughters and lived a lonely life on a farm, as a child, with an aloof, exacting father and a pessimistic mother. She became a graduate nurse and around 30 married a man several years younger. She enjoyed sex relations but often failed to attain organism and felt tense afterward. Several years before she suffered severe cramps and was given morphine and she had trouble getting off it. She had taken barbiturates off and on and feared addiction. She rested for several months after the birth of a baby because of exhaustion. For several years she had suffered tachycardia and was told that her blood pressure varied from 130 to 190 systolic. She felt anxious about this until a doctor told her that it was due to nervousness. She was told that her pituitary gland was not functioning properly. For several weeks she had been in bed most of the time because she felt exhausted and her heart beat rapidly. This followed a visit to her pessimistic mother.

She came into the office looking scared, cried much and talked breathlessly and rapidly. She said that she had been trying for years to get nerve enough to ask doctors about masturbation. She did it often and felt that it would ruin her health and drive her to insanity. Her most recent episode was associated with fears that her motther would disapprove of her if she knew about her "awful" habit. When reassured that masturbation was a common practice without evil consequences and that her "hypopituitarism" was without serious significance she showed marked relief. After five interviews in which added details were confessed she felt well enough to carry on her household duties without difficulty.

CASE 2

Another married woman became dramatically better after she had been reassured that some mild perversions she had been indulging in with her husband were commonplace experiences.

CASE 3

Still another, married and 55, who had been treated for gall bladder and heart trouble for several years because of pains in her epigastrium was relieved after a series of interviews which reassured her that she was not hopelessly a social outcast because she had carried on an affair with a married man, whom she loved, as an escape from a cruel and hated husband.

Another approach to patient's problems which often brings quick results is attention to details of their present situation and relating them to childhood attitudes. This makes for logical recommendations of changes in environmental situations. The final three cases demonstrate this principal.

CASE 4

A single woman in her late 20's complained of feelings of depression and inadequacy of such an intensity that she could not do her work properly and had to take frequent vacations from it. I learned that she had been reared in a prudish home and was now living with a prudish old maid aunt. She had carried on an affair with a man her aunt disapproved of so strongly that she broke off the affair. Moving into an apartment by herself and reassurance about her conduct brought about rapid recovery.

CASE 5

A 40 year old married man had taken a position of responsibility in which he was subjected to considerable criticism. He had taken more and more barbiturates and alcohol to relieve a persistent insomnia which came on about a year after he took the job. I learned that he had been reared in a home where a severe father induced a passive attitude; a sensitive nature and a fear of criticism. I put him in a hospital for a week, restored fluids and vitamins and withdrew all sedation. By that time he was sleeping well and felt better than he had for a long time. His sensitiveness was discussed with him and he agreed to accept a proferred job with less responsibility and to refrain from indulgence in barbiturates and alcohol. He called several weeks later to report that his troubles seemed to be over.

CASE 6

A 56 year old man, an accountant, had been given more and more duties over a period of years and had been given no vacations. He had no hobbies and prided himself on his ability to do more work than anyone else. He finally suffered acute exhaustion, with an accentuation of life l o n g obsessional thoughts, of a painful nature, and annoying compulsions. Very bad teeth were found and removed and he was advised to take a vacation. He resigned his position and, under encouragement, resumed some hobbies of collecting he had cultivated in his youth. After a month during which he returned to my office, chiefly for reassurance and sympathy, he was able to take a less exacting position and to carry on successfully.

In the brief time at my disposal I cannot begin to cover all of the possibilities of the broad subject of psychotherapy. I can only refer you to some very good textbooks on the subject which have been written recently. One objection which is often raised to the practice of psychotherapy by the general practitioner is that it takes too much time. My reply would be that if the doctor uses the approach outlined above he can gain helpful information and utilize attitudes toward the patient which will make him more effective in his treatment in relatively brief interviews. The cases I have described were used because prompt results were obtained and the effectivness of psychotherapy could be more easily demonstrated In most cases, however, much longer periods of time must elapse before relief is obtained. Therefore, frequent short interviews over a period of time can often be more effective than longer interviews over a period of a week or two. The knowledge the physician gains about his patients by such methods can be utilized for the benefit of the patient and the physician will gain much in the esteem of his patients. A doctor who makes his patient feel that he understands him is apt to be a successful doctor in every sense of the word.

SUMMARY

1. It is suggested that patients suffering from neuroses have been neglected by physicians not specializing in psychiatry.

2. Hostility, mostly unconscious, seems to have been expressed toward such patients by the use of uncomplimentary epithets in the literature, by harmful diagnostic and operative procedures in ordinary practice and by the use of shock treatment and frontal lobotomies among specialists.

3. Some reasons for this hostility are discussed.

4. The qualities necessary for the successful psychotherapist are outlined and a few procedures, with illustrative material, are described.

BIBLIOGRAPHY

1. Alvarez, Walter: "Diagnostic Time Savers" J.A.M.A. 122: 933 July 31, 1943.

2. Cobb, Stanley: Borderlands of Psychiatry. Cambridge Massachusetts Harvard University Press, pp. 69, 1943.

· THE PRESIDENT'S PAGE ·

The Council held its first meeting in the new Council Room at the Executive Office of the Association on the morning of Sunday, October 22, 1944, and took action which will likely prove to be a major step in the history of the Oklahoma State Medical Association. In the afternoon of the same day, the House of Delegates met in special session and accepted, by an overwhelming majority, the recommendation of the Council.

The report of the Committee, setting up a Prepaid Surgical and Obstetrical Plan on an indemnity basis, was adopted. This plan is the result of more than two years of untiring work of the Committee under the able leadership of Dr. John F. Burton. During this time they studied all plans now being operated in other states as well as the criticisms and suggestions of the members of our own Association. The complete text of the Committee's report will be found elsewhere in this issue of the Journal.

Dr. Burton's Committee has been discharged and the Council is now in the process of appointing a Board of Trustees to put the Plan into operation. This is no longer a theory—it is a fact. It is no longer a national problem so far as Oklahoma is concerned. It is an Oklahoma Plan which will be controlled by Oklahoma physicians for the benefit of their patients. I am personally glad that the debate is over and hope that, insofar as possible, every member of the Oklahoma State Medical Association will support the Plan to the utmost in an effort to offer to the public something whereby the citizens in the low income group will receive the best of medical care, and in a manner which will offset the encroachment of socialized or political medicine on the people of our State.

The Council also recommended and the House of Delegates approved, the legislative program as presented by the Committee on Public Policy. It consists of a law creating a Board of Health, a law to make it possible for the Basic Science Board to issue certificates of Registration in the Basic Sciences to those who were licensed to practice at the time of the passage of the Basic Science Law, and a law for an up-to-date medical examiner system to replace the antiquated Coroner's Law of Oklahoma. Each one of these laws is sorely needed and should have the unqualified support of every member of the Association. Your President and Executive Secretary hope to be able to visit each Councilor District between now and January 1, 1945, for the purpose of explaining this program in greater detail.

President.

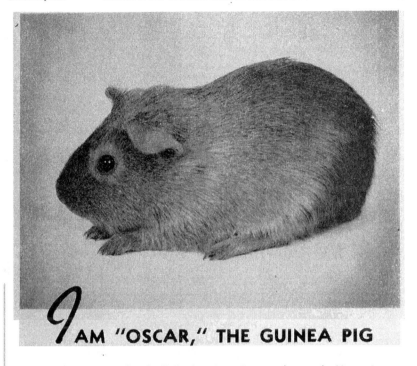
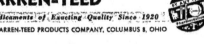

The JOURNAL Of The
OKLAHOMA STATE MEDICAL ASSOCIATION

EDITORIAL BOARD
L. J. MOORMAN, Oklahoma City, Editor-in-Chief

E. EUGENE RICE, Shawnee   BEN H. NICHOLSON, Oklahoma City

MR. PAUL H. FESLER, Oklahoma City, Business Manager

JANE FIRRELL TUCKER, Editorial Assistant

CONTRIBUTIONS: Articles accepted by this Journal for publication including those read at the annual meetings of the State Association are the sole property of this Journal.

The Editorial Department is not responsible for the opinions expressed in the original articles of contributors.

Manuscripts may be withdrawn by authors for publication elsewhere only upon the approval of the Editorial Board.

MANUSCRIPTS: Manuscripts should be typewritten, double-spaced, on white paper 8½ x 11 inches. The original copy, not the carbon copy, should be submitted.

Footnotes, bibliographies and legends for cuts should be typed on separate sheets in double space. Bibliography listing should follow this order: Name of author, title of article, name of periodical with volume, page and date of publication.

Manuscripts are accepted subject to the usual editorial revisions and with the understanding that they have not been published elsewhere.

NEWS: Local news of interest to the medical profession, changes of address, births, deaths and weddings will be gratefully received.

ADVERTISING: Advertising of articles, drugs or compounds unapproved by the Council on Pharmacy of the A.M.A. will not be accepted. Advertising rates will be supplied on application.

It is suggested that members of the State Association patronize our advertisers in preference to others.

SUBSCRIPTIONS: Failure to receive The Journal should call for immediate notification.

REPRINTS: Reprints of original articles will be supplied at actual cost provided request for them is attached to manuscripts or made in sufficient time before publication. Checks for reprints should be made payable to Industrial Printing Company, Oklahoma City.

Address all communications to THE JOURNAL OF THE OKLAHOMA STATE MEDICAL ASSOCIATION, 210 Plaza Court, Oklahoma City. (3)

OFFICIAL PUBLICATION OF THE OKLAHOMA STATE MEDICAL ASSOCIATION
Copyrighted November, 1944

EDITORIALS

MILITARY MEDICINE AT THE FRONT

In Ernie Pyle's new book "Brave Men'" Chapter Five is devoted to "Medics and Casualties." In the first part of this chapter the author states that, true to his record of being sick in every country he visited, he made a quick job of it in Sicily and landed in a clearing station, tent hospital of the 45th Division. The first regular hospital was fifteen miles back but he was kept on for diagnostic study and medical interest. What a graphic picture of the teaming life line and what a complimentary discourse about the soft-voiced, matter-of-fact, courageous Oklahoma boys from farms, ranches and small towns, including those in medicine and dentistry!

His closing remarks about the medics should make all doctors both humble and proud. "These men lived a rough and tumble life. They slept on the ground, worked ghastly hours, were sometimes under fire and handled the flow of wounded that would sicken and dishearten a person less immune to it. Time and again as I lay in my tent I hear wounded soldiers discussing among themselves the wonderful treatment that they had had at the hands of the medics.

They'll get little glory back home when it is all over but they had some recompense right there in the gratitude of men treated."

After perusal of an advanced copy, the writer dined with a young officer fresh from the front. He was enthusiastic about military medicine, praising the doctors and surgeons, "usually within 200 yards of the fighting front, ready to give the best of care."

The young soldier, waxing eloquent in commendation, soon turned to the subject of regimented medicine, saying the efficiency of medical care at the front causes "me to think that socialized medicine might be a good thing." When asked if he had followed military medicine back from the front where it becomes entangled in red tape, he admitted that further back there were more rules and regulations, more bulletins and blanks and a much less intimate relationship between patient and doctor with a waning of the warmth and sympathy so spontaneous in unregimented relationships. Supplementing this admission on his part, it was pointed out that military medicine is carried to the front on a purely voluntary basis by otherwise civilian doctors who are there in line of duty, prompted by love of their fellowmen and loyalty to the Stars and Stripes.

This comprehensive consideration of the question resulted in a change of viewpoint with an admission that perhaps we should cling to the time-tried plan of medical service.

But, this observation, coming from a University graduate, should cause us to wonder if many thousands of our good citizens are not employing the same line of thought with similar unwarranted conclusions. Please remember that there is no salvation in wondering—only by persistent working at the game of educating the public can we save the people from disaster and lift the onus from our shoulders.

1. Ernie Pyle: Brave Men. Henry Holt & Company. New York.

DIGILENCE

Shall we distribute the dole and destroy diligence or shall we encourage frugality and self respect by permitting people to work out their own salvation? Ralph Waldo Emerson, out of relative material poverty, spun untold psychological riches, consisting of intellectual superiority and spirtual serenity. He would have been staggered by the thought of 12 billion dollars for social security. There is a resounding message for our Nation in the following paragraph so long sequestered in his Journals[1]:

"The harvest will be better preserved and go farther, laid up in private bins, in each farmer's corn-barn, and each woman's basket, than if it were kept in national granaries. In like manner, an amount of money will go farther if expended by each man and woman for their own wants, and in the feeling that this is their all, than if expended by a great Steward, or National Commissioners of the Treasury. Take away from me the feeling that I must depend on myself, give me the least hint that I have good friends and backers there in reserve who will gladly help me, and instantly I relax my diligence."

1. Emerson, Ralph Waldo: The Heart of Emerson's Journals. Edited by Bliss Perry. Houghton Mifflin Company. Boston & New York. 1926.

A prominent French citizen in Paris had a very efficient butler who became infatuated with the Communist Party in France, attending all the meetings and often waxing enthusiastic in his praise of Communism—leading to some concern on the part of his employer. By and by it was noticed that he suddenly lost interest and ceased to attend the meetings. After some time had elapsed his employer ventured to inquire as to his lack of interest. The butler replied, "At one of the meetings figures were presented indicating that if all the money in France were equally distributed among the citizens, every individual would have 2,000 francs." After some hesitation he added, "And I already have 5,000!"

ADJUDICATION

In the light of what has happened to medicine and what may happen under the present socialistic trends, many doctors are wondering about the future welfare of the people. True to their principles, their education and medical traditions, doctors will continue to serve as best they can regardless of the handicaps imposed. But if there is some far away bar of justice for ultimate adjudication, God help those who take personal initative from the medical profession and obstruct the highways to medical achievements and the reward of merit.

SELLING THE PEOPLE DOWN THE RIVER, WE HOPE, UNWITTINGLY

The Governing Council of the American Public Health Association adopted a report favoring compulsory health insurance to be administered by the Federal Government. The United States Public Health Association was evolved through an effort on the part of physicians and public spirited citizens for the benefit of the people. A great service has been performed for which the American people should be forever grateful. But the time has come when the people must be prepared to protect themselves against the above recommendation. The following from an Editorial in the October 14 issue of the Journal of the American Medical Association reveals the essential features of the issue:

"The American Public Health Association has an obvious right to express itself on any subject related to the public health. The rejection by the majority group of the proposal for consultation with medical and dental leaders indicates the attitude that may be expected of them if they should have control of the Washington bureaucracy that would dominate American medicine should their ideas become effective. Perhaps this step in which these men had leadership will be useful in serving notice once more on the medical, dental, nursing, pharmaceutical and other professional groups as to the nature of the political manipulators in the fields of social security and public health whom the medical profession will be forced to combat."

May we modestly suggest that the people should be fully informed, in order that they may see in this dangerous trend the notice of their calamity under the regimented usurpation of their personal privileges. The price represents not only the loss of liberty in this sacred realm but double cost with the quality of service cut to a dangerous level. Every doctor in the United States should do his full duty by carrying the news of this menace directly to those who are most vitally concerned; to those who must pay the cost and suffer the loss—the American people. Doctors everywhere get busy, not in self defense but in behalf of humanity; in the spirit which animated those who made the American Public Health Association an instrument of mercy and protection for the American people. To avoid the seething estuary of bureaucratic calamity the time has come when the people must paddle upstream.

DAMNED IF WE DO — DAMNED IF WE DON'T

In a recent Editorial, attention was called to a relatively small percentage of our doctors who receive the Journal of the American Medical Association and the small chance of being broadly informed without it.

In the July 29 issue, the leading article is "Evolution in Medicine" by Ernest E. Irons, which might well be entitled "A Volley from Old Ironsides." Every member of the State Medical Association should read this timely discussion of some of the most significant problems confronting American medicine. In the September issue of Westchester Medical Bulletin, Westchester County, N.Y., there is an Editorial "Evolution versus Progress" criticizing Dr. Irons' position and raising controversial questions which further emphasize the seriousness of our present plight which is more ominous for the unsuspecting layman than for the doctor.

Again we insist that doctors are largely to blame for this situation because they have neglected the art of medicine and have failed to educate the people. We know that modern medicine represents five thousand years of Evolution and that any radical change spells devolution in its most damnable form. Dr. Irons discusses the Blue Cross Plan and the policies of oldline companies and advocates a broader coverage, especially through plans for voluntary insurance initiated by the doctors. Since medicine, concerning both laymen and doctors, is definitely in the hopper with the mill stones at the funnel, the plans sponsored by the doctors have the virtue of voluntary participation, preserving in some degree the "patient-doctor relationship" with its professional responsibilities.

Assuming that human nature is relatively static and that true medical education is incompatible with regimentation, it is natural for the busy doctor, when confronted with a blank he did not sponsor or anticipate, to throw up his hands and say "be damned if I do." For the average good doctor, any form of coercion, any unnecessary detail which diverts his attention from the patient's welfare, is anathema.

If the average good patient could be made to realize this and could be shown the devious, laborious course of medical evolution and what medicine in its present status means to the people of America, he would call the dogs off and let the doctors work out their salvation according to Hippocratic principles which are as humane as the teachings of Jesus Christ and yet as practical as modern science can make them.

OXYGEN IN PULMONARY CONDITIONS

Cecil K. Drinker[1] has recently reported certain observations on pulmonary physiology and the therapeutic use of oxygen. Drinker's observations are based upon many years of experimental work in what he terms mammalion physiology and his careful analysis of structural and physiological factors help to clarify the influence of pathology and to establish the value of oxygen therapy.

All good doctors know how vital pulmonary function is in the economy of the body and how dependent upon oxygen are all the cells of the body for the orderly performance of their functions. But, as Drinker so well points out, few doctors realize that, because of certain anatomic and physiological conditions in the lungs, "anoxia begets anoxia" and that the progressive effects may cause serious damage before the so-called indications for oxygen therapy appear. By calling attention to this fact, Drinker is performing a valuable service. It is unfortunate that this article cannot be brought to the attention of every practicing physician.

In summary, his discussion indicates that the therapeutic use of oxygen is too infrequent; that its administration is often delayed until the patient has suffered insurmountable handicaps, and that "the time to begin to use oxygen is before there is any certainty it is needed." In addition it should be remembered that sedatives, morphine being the best, requiring for dyspneic and painful conditions, depress the respiratory center and increase the danger of anoxia, but in the presence of oxygen therapy the administration of such sedatives is relatively safe and of great service to the patient.

1. Drinker, Cecil K.: The Application of Pulmonary Physiology to Therapeutic Procedures—With Special Reference to the Use of Oxygen. The New England Journal of Medicine. Vol. 231, No. 14. October 5, 1944.

Medicine and Freedom

With the French Revolution, which then convulsed Europe, came a radical change in social life all over Europe. Itself a horror, the Revolution gave freedom, and heralded great days for education, medicine, and science in our land. Many welcomed the change, glad that the spirit of progress inspired the world, and not knowing that the torch of freedom was to become an incendiary's brand. From these days sprang the greatest discoveries in science.—*Aberdeen Doctors, At Home and Abroad. Ella Hill Burton Rodger, page 42. William Blackwood & Sons. Edinburgh and London. 1913.*

ASSOCIATION ACTIVITIES

REPORT OF COMMITTEE ON PREPAID MEDICAL AND/OR SURGICAL SERVICE

(To be considered by House of Delegates, Sunday October 22, 1944).

At the meeting of the House of Delegates of the Oklahoma State Medical Association in Tulsa, April 25, 1944, the Prepaid Medical and/or Surgical Service Committee of the State Association was instructed to send out mimeographed copies of a proposed plan for prepaid medical and/or surgical care to the membership of the State Association including Service Members. Pursuant to that action, the Committee has carried out the order.

At this time, the Committee would like to report the results of the returned questionnaires.

	Active	Service	Total
ABSTRACTS MAILED	1,160	285	1,445
Answers—Yes	371	72	443
Answers—No	71	6	77
Undecided on Comment Only....	9		9
NO ANSWER	709	207	916

The Committee has gone over the various comments, suggestions and criticisms. As a result of the review, the Committee feels that the majority of the membership is in favor of some form of prepaid medical and/or surgical care plan. They do not favor the proposed plan in its entirety, and although there are various objections the main point of objection is in regard to the payment of fees.

In view of that fact and in the light of considerable additional information gathered in the interim from other states who have had similar plans, the Committee feels that it would like to recommend to the House of Delegates the following:

1. That the House of Delegates take definite action to establish a prepaid medical and/or surgical plan.
2. That the plan be organized under the existing insurance laws of the State of Oklahoma.
3. That the plan be a non-profit corporation.
4. That the plan shall recognize the age-old practice of free choice of Doctors of Medicine and free choice of approved hospitals.
5. That the payment of services be on an indemnity basis.
6. That this plan be incorporated and set up on a state-wide basis, but financing should be worked out by the Board of Trustees in such a manner that any participating county shall pay a pro rata share of capital in proportion to its membership as they are admitted to service.
7. That the Council of the Oklahoma State Medical Association select a Board of Trustees of 15 members, nine of whom shall be Doctors of Medicine and six of whom shall be laymen—these to serve as the original incorporators and who, with legal assistance, will set in force the plan. It is suggested that the term of office of these trustees should be staggered and they should be selected as nearly as possible with an idea of geographical distribution of the state.

MINUTES OF THE SPECIAL SESSION OF THE HOUSE OF DELEGATES October 22, 1944

A Special Session of the House of Delegates of the Oklahoma State Medical Association was called to order by the Speaker of the House, Dr. George H. Garrison,

Oklahoma City, in the Rose Room, Skirvin Hotel, Oklahoma City, Sunday, October 22, 1944, at 2:15 P.M.

Following the call to order, Dr. Garrison observed that the Credentials Committee had determined that a quorum was present, and further stated in his introductory remarks that the Special Meeting had been called in compliance with the provisions of the Constitution and By-Laws of the Association and that only the subjects mentioned in the call might be discussed; namely, Legislative Program and Report of Committee on Prepaid Medical and/or Surgical Service.

In compliance with the expressed feeling of the group that no members of the press be in attendance, the Speaker appointed the following as Sergeants at Arms: J. Hobson Veazey, M.D., Chairman; W. F. LaFon, M.D., Waynoka; W. S. Larrabee, M.D., Tulsa, and O. C. Standifer, M.D., Elk City.

At this time, the Speaker remarked that the legislative program as determined by the Committee on Public Policy would first be discussed.

Next, the Speaker introduced Mr. Fred Hansen, Assistant Attorney General.

Dr. John W. Shackelford, Oklahoma City, Chairman of the Committee on Public Health, was first recognized and presented the bill with reference to the establishment of a State Board of Health.

On motion by Dr. McLain Rogers, Clinton, seconded by Dr. J. M. Bonham, Hobart it was moved that the bill be adopted. Motion carried.

Following this action, the Speaker recognized Dr. J. D. Osborn, Frederick, Secretary of the Board of Examiners in Basic Sciences, who explained that at the time of the passage of the Basic Science Act in 1937 the "Grand-father Clause" granting permission for doctors to be issued basic science certificates giving them permission to reciprocate with another state to practice if they were licensed prior to 1937 had not been included in the original bill at the time of its enactment and that the purpose of the proposed amendment was to correct this defect. Dr. Osborn read the bill as prepared by the office of the Attorney General.

On motion by Dr. L. G. Kuyrkendall, McAlester, seconded by Dr. Finis W. Ewing, Muskogee, it was moved that the bill be sponsored. Motion carried.

Dr. W. Floyd Keller, Oklahoma City, was next recognized and briefly summarized the idea of a Medical Examiner system to replace the existing coroner law in Oklahoma and stated that it had been advantageous in states where it was in effect.

On motion by Dr. A. S. Risser, Blackwell, seconded by R. Q. Goodwin, Oklahoma City, it was moved that such a system be proposed. Motion carried.

Following this action, Dr. John F. Burton, Oklahoma City, Chairman of the Committee on Prepaid Medical and/or Surgical Service, presented the report of his committee recommending that the payment of fees be on an indemnity rather than on a service basis as heretofore recommended. Immediately following the reading of the report, Dr. Burton moved that the report be accepted.

Dr. A. S. Risser was recognized, seconded the motion, and spoke in behalf of the benefits of such a plan.

At this time, the Speaker recognized Dr. W. W. Cotton, Atoka, who was opposed to the plan if it were to be under the mechanical supervision of the Blue Cross Plan and who moved that the sale of the Prepaid Medical and Surgical Plan be put in the hands of a County Agent in each of the 77 counties, that the agent receive $1.50 per year for each new policy and that he receive $1.00 for each renewal in order that it might be taken to the people who needed it. Dr. Cotton's amendment to the original motion was seconded by Dr. O. H. Miller, Ada.

Following this action, the Speaker stated that discussion would be continued prior to voting on the amendment but that it would be considered in due time.

Discussion of the plan followed by those listed: Dr. V. C. Tisdal, Elk City; Dr. Finis W. Ewing, Muskogee; Dr. H. K. Speeed, Sayre; Dr. James Stevenson, Tulsa; Dr. McClain Rogers, Clinton; Dr. V. R. Hamble, Enid; Dr. Harry S. Stewart, Tulsa; Dr. Clinton Gallaher, Shawnee; Dr. G. E. Johnson, Ardmore; Dr. Sam A. McKeel, Ada; Dr. Tom Lowry, Oklahoma City; Dr. O. E. Templin, Alva; Dr. C. E. Northeutt, Ponca City, and Dr. W. S. Larrabee, Tulsa.

Questions concerning the plan were propounded by Dr. E. H. Shuller, McAlester; Dr. John A. Hayine, Durant; Dr. L. A. Mitchell, Stillwater; Dr. J. C. Matheney, Okmulgee; Dr. Harper Wright, Oklahoma City; Dr. Roscoe Walker, Pawhuska, and Dr. W. Pat Fite, Muskogee.

Dr. Burton further explained that the Delegates were voting on a principle and that the Board of Trustees would be responsible for working out the details. In response to further questions, it was pointed out that instituting such a plan would not be obligatory or any county and it would be applicable only to those counties who were anxious to put it into effect.

Mr. N. D. Helland, Director of the Blue Cross Plan, was also introduced by the Speaker and spoke in behalf of the plan pointing out the progress of Blue Cross during the past four years and observed that it was necessary to receive the cooperation of an interested group in a town before the hospitalization plan could be brought in and accepted by the citizenship. He also remarked that Blue Cross had been somewhat handicapped in its activities in some sections of the state due to the war.

The general consensus of opinion of the Delegates seemed to be that of approval of such a plan when they thoroughly understood the distinction between the collection of fees on an indemnity and service basis.

Following the above discussion, Dr. Cotton requested the *withdrawal* of his *amendment* with the consent of the second Dr. Miller. Dr. Miller acquiesced in the *withdrawal*.

Upon voting, the plan was adopted by a vote of 56 to 3.

At this time, the Speaker recognized Dr. C. R. Rountree, President of the Association, who remarked that, according to the vote of the House, the Council had been instructed to select a Board of Trustees consisting of 15 members—nine of whom were to be Doctors of Medicine and six of whom were to be laymen. The President further observed that in compliance with the action of the Council that it be recessed at the morning meeting until the action of the House had been determined that the Council would meet in the Green Room of the Skirvin Hotel immediately following adjournment.

On *motion* by Dr. W. S. Larrabee, *seconded by* Dr. W. W. Cotton, and *carried*, a motion for adjournment was adopted.

GEORGE H. GARRISON, Speaker

CRIPPLED CHILDRENS CLINIC TO BE HELD IN ALVA

On November 20, the Rotary-sponsored Crippled Children's Clinic will be held in Alva in the Stephenson-Traverse Clinic. Dr. O. E. Templin, Secretary of the Woods-Alfalfa, said "about 40 children went through the Clinic last year, and about that many are expected November 20." Children up to 21 years of age with physical handicaps may enter the Clinic, and if they are unable to pay for the treatment to follow, can make arrangements for admission to the Crippled Children's Hospital in Oklahoma City or in some other approved hospital.

Dr. C. R. Rountree and Dr. John F. Burton of Oklahoma City will be in Alva to make recommendations for the treatment of the children. Following the Clinic, Dr. Rountree and Dr. Burton will read papers for the meeting of the Woods-Alfalfa Medical Society. Joe Hamilton, Executive Secretary of the Crippled Children's Society and his Staff will be in attendance, also a number of physicians from Oklahoma City.

14th ANNUAL FALL CONFERENCE OKLAHOMA CITY CLINICAL SOCIETY

The Fourteenth Annual Conference of the Oklahoma City Clinical Society was held October 23-26 in Oklahoma City at the Biltmore Hotel. The meeting had the largest attendance of any previously held meeting of the Clinical Society, having a registration of 970. The programs were enthusiastically received and the physicians of the state and those from other states were high in their praise of the meeting. The following is taken from the article by D. H. O'Donoghue which appeared in the November issue of the Oklahoma County Bulletin:

"Our third wartime meeting and the fourteenth session was, I think, a complete success from the standpoint of enrollment. We had over a hundred more doctors register than at any previous meeting, along with a similar increase in other registrations. It is particularly gratifying to have so many register and attend the meeting. However, I believe that size alone is of secondary importance. Our goal has never been to have a large meeting, but rather to have a meeting at which there was presented a well-rounded program so that the registrants would feel it worth-while to attend the sessions. Careful check was kept of all the postgraduate symposia and always, without exception, the rooms would be full, a situation which has not always been present in the past. Of course, the big room was always well filled. It seemed to me that everyone who attended the meeting was anxious to actually hear the programs.

"I had the opportunity to talk to many of the exhibitors, and they, too, expressed their appreciation for the interest the local and visiting doctors showed in their various products. These exhibitors have the opportunity to attend many sessions and without exception, they were loud in their praise for the meeting of the Oklahoma City Clinical Society.

"Our guest speakers, again, expressed their surprise and pleasure at the lack of friction among the local men and their admiration for the general organization of the meeting."

UROLOGY AWARD

The American Urological Association offers an annual award 'not to exceed $500.00' for an essay (or essays) on the result of some specific clinical or laboratory research in Urology. The amount of the prize is based on the merits of the work presented, and if the Committee on Scientific Research deem none of the offerings worthy, no award will be made. Competitors shall be limited to residents in urology in recognized hospitals and to urologists who have been in such specific practice for not more than five years. All interested should write the Secretary for full particulars.

The selected essay (or essays) will appear on the program of the forthcoming June meeting of the American Urological Association.

Essays must be in the hands of the Secretary, Dr. Thomas D. Moore, 899 Madison Avenue, Memphis, Tennessee, on or before March 15, 1945.

Supplementary Roster

BECKHAM

ANDERSON, ROY W. .... *Elk City*

BLAINE

HARTSHORNE, WM. O. ....*Geary*
(member Seminole County Medical Society)

CADDO

ANDERSON, P. H. ....*Anadarko*
PATTERSON, F. L. JR. ....*Carnegie*

CANADIAN

WARREN, T. C. ....*Yukon*

CIMARRON

HALL, HARRY B. ....*Boise City*

CREEK

OAKES, C. G. ....*Sapulpa*

JOHNSTON

LOONEY, J. T. ....*Tishomingo*

KAY

ARMSTRONG, W. O. ....*Ponca City*
BEATTY, J. H. ....*Tonkawa*
BECKER, L. H. ....*Blackwell*
GHORMLEY, J. G. ....*Blackwell*
KINSINGER, R. R. ....*Blackwell*
McELROY, THOMAS ....*Ponca City*

MURRAY

DeLAY, W. D. ....*Sulphur*

OKLAHOMA

CRAWFORD, PAUL H. ....441 N. W. 12th
HYROOP, MURIEL ....Medical Arts Bldg.
JONES, N. A. ....Medical Arts Bldg.

OTTAWA

GILLESPIE, CLIFTON ....*Miami*
(member of Oklahoma County Medical Society)

PAWNEE

LeHEW, J. L. ....*Pawnee*

PAYNE

CLEVERDON, L. A. ....*Stillwater*
LARKIN, H. W. ....*Perkins*
(member Logan County Society)

POTTAWATOMIE

OWENS, J. N. JR. ....*Shawnee*

TULSA

CHILDS, D. B. ....1126 S. Boston

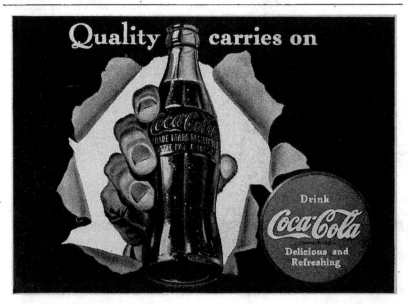

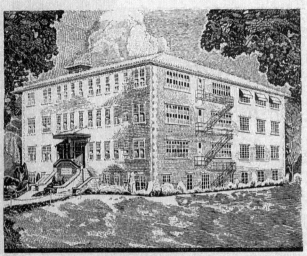

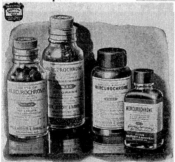
AMERICAN MEDICAL ASSOCIATION POINTS OUT WHAT TO EXPECT UNDER BUREAUCRATIC MEDICINE

Medical Leaders Not Consulted By A.P.H.A. Council Before Adopting Report Favoring Compulsory Health Plan, Journal Says.

The Governing Council of the American Public Health Association on October 4 adopted a report favoring in effect a federal plan of compulsory health insurance, without consultation with medical and dental leaders of the nation, despite a proposal to do so. This indicates, The Journal of the American Medical Association for October 14 declares, the attitude that may be expected of those committed to federal control of all matters in the health field if they should have control of the Washington bureaucracy that would dominate American medicine should their ideas become effective. The Journal says:

"At its annual meeting in New York, October 4, the Governing Council of the American Public Health Association adopted a report favoring in effect a federal plan of compulsory health insurance. . . This report, first prepared by a subcommittee, was approved after several amendments by the association's Committee on Administrative Practice. The proposed medical service would be supported by social insurance, supplemented by general taxation, or by general taxation alone.

"The ratification of the report as amended came after extended debate in which there was opposition to the adoption and publication of the report as a stated policy of the association. Those who opposed pointed out (a) that the administration of public health in the United States was by no means so universal or so generally adequate that public health departments in general were ready for this step, (b) that before the association placed itself publicly on record in the terms of this report there should be consultation with the most interested professional groups, particularly the American Medical Association and the American Dental Association, and (c) that the publication of the subcommittee report, its approval by the Committee on Administrative Practice and the call for adoption in the Governing Council occurred within less than thirty days elapsed time, although the subcommittee had been working on the report for a year.

"The motion to adopt the report was made at the October 2 meeting of the Governing Council and was extensively debated at that time. Action was postponed until the October 4 meeting. At that time an amendment was offered to the motion to adopt. This amendment called for the Governing Council to receive this portion of the report of the Committee on Administrative Practice and to refer it to the Executive Board of the American Public Health Association with instructions to confer with the Board of Trustees of the American Medical Association and with the American Dental Association in an attempt to arrive at a statement which these three great professional groups could support. The amendment was lost by a standing vote approximately three to one after a voice vote had left the chair in doubt. The Governing Council then proceeded to vote on a motion to adopt the report; this vote was 49 Aye and 14 No. The opposition to the adoption of the report was led by Drs. Walter A. Bierring, Past President of the American Medical Association, Haven Emerson and W. W. Bauer.

"Now what is the group that adopted this report? Of the 7,493 members of the American Public Health Association 1,571 are Fellows. Only Fellows have a right to vote for governing councilors; the vote is conducted by ballot given to each Fellow when he registers at the meeting; Fellows not in attendance do not have a vote. The Governing Council consists of approximately 100 members, of whom 30 are elected by vote of the Fellows,

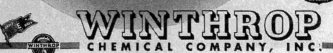

10 each year for three year terms; the rest of the members of the Governing Council hold membership by virtue of being section officers or representatives of affiliated (mostly state) public health associations. Members of the association other than Fellows can vote only on section affairs. The report on compulsory health insurance represents, therefore, the action of the subcommittee which prepared it, the Committee on Administrative Practice which approved it and the 49 members of the Governing Council who voted in its favor. Here is not a democratic practice in action; here is a shrewdly manipulated performance by full time public officials, economists, bureaucrats. Most of the names of those on the subcommittee are those of men long committed to federal compulsory sickness insurance and to federal control of all matters in the health field.

"The American Public Health Association has an obvious right to express itself on any subject related to the public health. The rejection by the majority group of the proposal for consultation with medical and dental leaders indicates the attitude that may be expected of them if they should have control of the Washington bureaucracy that would dominate American medicine should their ideas become effective. Perhaps this step in which these men had leadership will be useful in serving notice once more on the medical, dental, nursing, pharmaceutical and other professional groups as to the nature of the political manipulators in the fields of social security and public health whom the medical professions will be forced to combat."

BOOK REVIEWS

NEW AND UNOFFICIAL REMEDIES. 1944 Edition. Council on Pharmacy and Chemistry of the American Medical Association, Chicago.

The Council on Pharmacy and Chemistry of the American Medical Association has assumed an ever-increasing importance in the field of medicine. In accordance with their original purpose to "protect the public and medical profession against deception and objectionable advertising" as well as present the unbiased findings concerning the status of different drugs, the Council has published the 1944 Edition of New and Nonofficial Remedies. The present edition upholds the precedent of former editions in being a valuable and informative adjunct to rational therapeutics.

Chapters on the following subjects are included: Allergic Preparations, Analgesics and Antipyretics, Anesthetics, Anti-Infectives, Astringents and Caustics, Autonomic Drugs, Cardiovascular Agents, Central Nervous System Stimulants, Choleretics, Contraceptives, Diagnostic Aids, Diuretics, Ecbolics, Gastrointestinal Drugs, Hematics, Hormones and Synthetic Substitutes, Metabolic Agents, Parenteral Solutions, Pharmaceutic and Therapeutic Aids, Sedatives and Hypnotics, Serums and Vaccines, Vitamins and Vitamin Preparations for Prophylactic and Therapeutic Use.

Important revisions were made in the chapters concerning Barbituric Acid Derivatives; Estrogenic Substances; Parathyroid; Ovaries; Sulfonamide Compounds; and Vitamins, especially the sections on Vitamin B complex and Vitamin D.

Thirty-two drugs which appeared in the 1943 New and Nonofficial Remedies were omitted from the present edition because they conflicted with the rules governing the recognition of articles, or because of the lack of convincing evidence to demonstrate their continued eligibility.

Revision of statements were made regarding composition of 114 substances, and revisions concerning actions, uses or dosages of 13 other drugs were also included.—Arthur A. Hellbaum, Ph.D., M.D.

SUMMARY OF STATE LEGISLATION REQUIRING PREMARITAL AND PRENATAL EXAMINATIONS FOR VENEREAL DISEASE. Aneta E. Bowen and George Gould. Second Edition Revised to 1944 by George Gould. The American Social Hygiene Association. New York.

The second edition of this important monograph gives up-to-date information on this vital subject. It is significant that thirty states now require both bride and groom to have premarital examinations including a blood test for syphilis.

The amended California premarital law is recommended as a model for similar laws in other states not yet offering such protection for those contemplating matrimony.

This pamphlet is proving valuable to public health agencies and legislative committees in states where premarital examinations are being considered.

DR. COLWELL'S DAILY LOG FOR PHYSICIANS. A brief, simple, accurate financial record for the physician's desk. Colwell Publishing Company, Champaign, Illinois, 1944. Price $6.00.

Again Colwell's Daily Log is brought to our attention. Those who have made use of this valuable aid to the busy doctor will welcome the 1945 edition. Those who have not used it in the past will be interested in the system it presents.

Because of the War, many doctors must get along with inexperienced office help. This necessity makes this, almost foolproof method of bookkeeping more important than ever before.—Lewis J. Moorman, M.D.

Classified Advertisements

FOR SALE: 1 Spencer Microscope (fine adjustment on side) including Mechanical Stage and Carrying Case. Price—$115.00. For further information write Key 60, care of The Journal, 210 Plaza Court, Oklahoma City 3, Oklahoma.

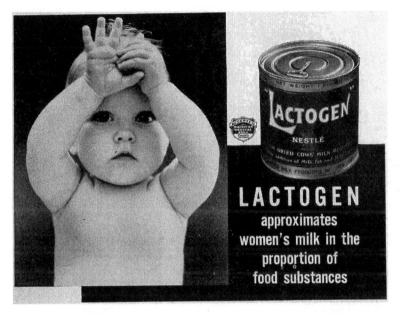

LACTOGEN
approximates women's milk in the proportion of food substances

THE cow's milk used for Lactogen is scientifically modified for infant feeding. This modification is effected by the addition of milk fat and milk sugar in definite proportions. When Lactogen is properly diluted with water it results in a formula containing the food substances—fat, carbohydrate, protein, and ash—in approximately the same proportion as they exist in woman's milk.

One level tablespoon of LACTOGEN dissolved in 2 ounces of water (warm, previously boiled) makes 2 onces of LACTOGEN formula yielding 20 calories per ounce.

No advertising or feeding directions, except to physicians. For feeding directions and prescription blanks, send your professional blank to "Lactogen Dept."

"My own belief is, as already stated, that the average well baby thrives best on artificial foods in which the relations of the fat, sugar, and protein in the mixture are similar to those in human milk."
John Lovett Morse, A. M., M. D.
Clinical Pediatrics, p. 156.

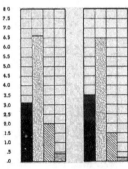

MOTHER'S MILK   DILUTED LACTOGEN

Fat   Carb.   Protein   Ash

NESTLÉ'S MILK PRODUCTS, INC.
155 EAST 44TH ST., NEW YORK, N. Y.

★ FIGHTIN' TALK ★

Ordered to active duty: LT. RENE GABRIEL GERARD, Chickasha; LT. PAUL DAVID MACRORY, Bethany.

Promoted from Lieutenant to Captain; CLAUDE BYRON KNIGHT, Wewoka: from Captain to Major; RALPH MARTIN ALLEY, Shawnee; from Major to Lieutenant Colonel; JOHN EDWIN McDONALD, Tulsa.

Seen at Oklahoma City Clinical Society Meeting

As you all probably know by this time, the Oklahoma City Clinical Society had their annual meeting at the Biltmore Hotel, Oklahoma City from October 23 to 26. It was a wonderful meeting and was thoroughly enjoyed, in every phase, by all those in attendance. The following doctors who are now in the service were in attendance:

MAJOR G. S. INGALLS, Stroud, who is now Chief of Neuropsychiatry at the Borden General Hospital in Chickasha.

CAPTAIN PHILIP G. TULLIUS, Oklahoma City, graduate of Oklahoma '42, is now stationed at Camp Maxey, Texas. Previously, Captain Tullius was stationed in Coral Gables, Florida.

CAPTAIN R. R. COATES, Oklahoma City, Class of '37, has spent the past several months in Australia. Very recently he has returned to the United States and is in Oklahoma City awaiting reassignment.

LT. JOE COLEY, USNR, Oklahoma City, is now stationed at the Naval Hospital in Norman. Lt. Coley has been in Norman for several months having previously served quite some time in the Southwest Pacific.

CAPTAIN MARK H. DONOVAN, Oklahoma City, is home on an emergency furlough, having spent the past eighteen months in Trinidad.

CAPTAIN SAM R. FRYER, Oklahoma City, Class of '33, is now stationed in McCook, Nebraska.

CAPTAIN J. R. HUGGINS, Oklahoma City, Class of '33, is recuperating at the Borden General Hospital from wounds received in New Guinea.

CAPTAIN WEBBER W. MERRELL, Guthrie, who was previously reported missing in action, is back in the States now and is a patient at Borden General, recovering from wounds received while serving in the European Theater.

MAJOR M. P. PROSSER, Norman, Class of '35, is Chief of Neuropsychiatry at Camp Gruber, Oklahoma.

LT. GEORGE TALLANT, USNR, Walters, Class of '36, is stationed at the Naval Gunnery School in Purcell.

COMDR. D. G. WILLARD, Norman, Class of '29, has returned from the South Pacific and has been stationed at the Naval Hospital in his home town—Norman.

Major Lively Appointed Air Surgeon

The following release has been received from the Fifth Air Service:

"Fifth Air Force, Southwest Pacific: MAJOR CLAUDE E. LIVELY, husband of Mrs. Virginia Lively, McAlester, has been appointed Air Surgeon of a Fifth Air Service Command depot in the Southwest Pacific, and the advanced echelon of the Fifth Air Service Area Command.

"Receiving his Bachelor of Science degree in Pharmacy at the University of Oklahoma in 1930, Major Lively entered the School of Medicine and graduated in 1934. He served his internship at Wesley Hospital in Oklahoma City before taking up practice, interrupting his service in 1941 to enter the Armed Forces."

MAJOR E. C. MURRAY, Ada, who recently returned from duty overseas has been assigned to Selfridge Field, Michigan.

MAJOR HARL D. MANSUR, JR., Oklahoma City, is with the Air Forces in India and has recently been promoted from Captain.

CAPTAIN CARSON L. OGLESBEE, Dewey, has returned to the States after duty with the 45th Division and is now stationed with a Coast Artillery Battery a Ft. Miles, Delaware.

Captain Donovan Home on Emergency Furlough

CAPTAIN MARK H. DONOVAN, Oklahoma City, has been stationed at a station hospital in Trinidad for the past eighteen months. He is now home on an emergency furlough occasioned by the death of his father, D. E. Donovan of Oklahoma City.

Captain Donovan studied tropical diseases at Walter Reed Hospital before going overseas and says that his work has been largely in that field. He is a graduate of Notre Dame and St. Louis University, and also did some work at the University of Oklahoma. He will report back to Trinidad when his leave here is up.

LT. (sg) JOHN A. CUNNINGHAM has reported to Pensacola, Florida where he will be stationed at the Naval Base. Lt. Cunningham returned in May after 22 months in the Southwest Pacific and has been stationed at the Naval Hospital in Norman.

Enid Doctor Retires from Army

After a long and interesting Army career, LT. COL. ROSCOE C. BAKER, Enid, has retired from the Armed Forces at the age of 62. He began his military career in 1901 as a member of the First Oklahoma regiment, forerunner of the present national guard, and served as a lieutenant in the medical corps in 1918 during the first World War.

Col. Baker is known as the "physician who attended the birth of the 189th." In 1922 he became regimental surgeon and held the post continuously until he left the division the day before Pearl Harbor. He helped organize it as a representative of his regiment. After leaving the 45th, he opened the medical division of the Army Induction Station in Tulsa in 1942. Later he set up the hospital at the Lordsburg, New Mexico prisoner of war camp.

He began his private practice in Granite, later moving to Arcadia, then to Enid. He was retired recently at Brooks General Hospital, San Antonio, Texas, after being hospitalized for several months there and at McCluskey General Hospital, Temple, Texas.

LT. RUFUS GOODWIN, Oklahoma City, with his wife and son, was a recent visitor in Oklahoma City at the home of his parents Dr. and Mrs. R. Q. Goodwin. Lt. Goodwin is stationed at Fort Hamilton station hospital near Brooklyn, New York.

The following is an excerpt from an article written by Lt. Ralph H. Major for the Kansas City Star. Lt. Major is the son of Dr. Ralph H. Major of the University of Kansas School of Medicine who was a speaker at the recent conference of the Oklahoma City Clinical Society. Lt. Major is a former member of the Kansas City Star's Staff and left Yale University to join the armed forces. As the following will disclose, he was one of the first to land in Italy.

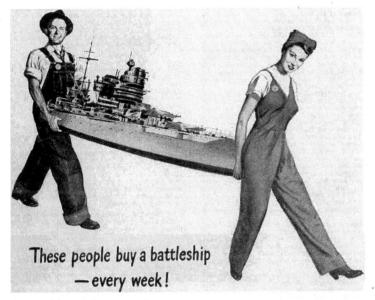

These people buy a battleship
— every week!

Meet John S..........and Mary D.........

John works at an electronics plant on Long Island, and makes $85 a week. Almost 16% of it goes into War Bonds.

Mary has been driving rivets into bombers at an airplane plant on the West Coast. She makes $55 a week, and puts 14% of it into War Bonds.

John and Mary are typical of more than 27 million Americans on the Payroll Savings Plan who, every single month, put half a BILLION dollars into War Bonds. That's enough to buy one of those hundred-million-dollar battleships every week, with enough money for an aircraft carrier and three or four cruisers left over.

In addition, John and Mary and the other people on the Payroll Plan have been among the biggest buyers of *extra* Bonds in every War Loan Drive.

They've financed a good share of our war effort all by themselves, and they've tucked away billions of dollars in savings that are going to come in mighty handy for both them and their country later on.

When this war is won, and we start giving credit where credit is due, don't forget John and Mary. After the fighting men, they deserve a place at the top. They've earned it.

You've backed the attack—now speed the victory!

Oklahoma State Medical Association

"We were impressed by the completely cool-deportment of the American troops, but especially by the initial bravery of the medical aid men who landed with the first wave and within several hours had complete installations set up and functioning.

"CAPTAIN RALPH S. PHELAN, Waurika (graduate Class of '39), a soft-spoken doctor whose practice had been among the tribes in the Oklahoma Indian territory, led the first company aid men ashore to establish temporary medical stations in the sand. Covered with sand which had stuck to his sea-soaked shirt and slacks, CAPTAIN PHELAN was directing the evacuation of casualties from the front line itself.

"An enlarged fox-hole, above which flew a Red Cross flag improvised from dressings and red paint, was the first United States army medical unit to set up. Most of the casualties suffered in the first few waves were taken back to the convoy vessels aboard the landing craft which debarked the combat troops.

"First of two evacuation hospitals to be landed under fire, an outfit of doctors and enlisted men from the Michael Reese hospital, Chicago, unit was landed with their entire equipment intact, and today began installing their tents and operating sections. The nurses of the unit are expected to arrive tomorrow, the earliest date that nurses have been landed in enemy territory after the first attack.

" . . . The first medical battalion to pitch their tents and go to work picked the sheltering columns of the Temple of Neptune for their headquarters and hospital zone.

"We figured our Red Cross, and these historical monuments, would make us practically immune from air attack," said Major Jay W. Pickens of Cleburne, Texas, the commanding officer. Major Pickens had established his 'office' in the temple itself, while the huge ward tents were put up between the Temple of Neptune and the Temple of Ceres.

"Among the modern conveniences which function beside the ruined temples are portable operating tables, washing apparatus complete with foot-pedal dispensers, and a collapsible folding-screen operating room."

JOURNAL RECEIVES FIRST MEDICAL REPORT FROM A NAZI LIBERATED NATION

A. M. A. Journal Gets First Communication from Regular Correspondent in Belgium Since Germany Occupied the Country

· Gratitude for the liberation of Belgium by the Allies and amazement at the organization or war surgery that has been built up at the front by the Allied armies is expressed by the regular correspondent in Belgium for The Journal of the American Medical Association in the first communication received from him since Germany occupied the country. In the October 28 issue of The Journal he says:

"The people of Belgium deeply appreciate the liberation of our country by the Allies. They have shown their patriotic enthusiasm for the cause of liberation and their admiration for your army. We, the Belgium physicians, wish to express also our deep gratitude to your country and our admiration for your army. We are now able to see for ourselves on our reconquered soil the amazing organization of war surgery that has been built up by the Allies at the front. Because of our experience with the hospitals during the war of 1914-1918 we can appreciate the progress achieved in the care of the wounded, and we propose to learn from contact with your medical officers the advances in war surgery that have given such good results in this war.

"I wish to write a few words regarding our experiences during the occupation; The practice of all Belgian physicians was regulated by a dictatorial order which had many arbitrary rules(for authorization to practice, location of physicians and similar matters). Fortunately these regulations were received generally with inertia, and 90 per cent of physicians continued practicing without openly protesting against the regulations suffering vexation, to be sure, but practically ignoring their existence.

"As for the Belgian medical press, two journals continued to be published, one in Flemish and one in French. Some of the material of medical journals which was suppressed by the invaders was provisionally published by the International Office of Medico-Military publications in the Archives medicales Belges from May 10, 1940. We never could obtain any medical literature except from Germany. All papers were suppressed by the invaders. The literature that we received consisted of medical items from Swiss journals sent to us in envelops as if they were letters.

"The nightmare is over now. The medical profession and the rest of the country are ready to resume their normal place in the world."

Freedom Has Many Blessings*

The United Nations are fighting for freedom for many different reasons. One of the most unique reasons was brought out by one of our smaller allies, the Nagas of Assam and North Burma. Known as headhunters, it took something concrete to sway them to our side.

With these people hostile to us, our efforts in Burma would have been less effective. The American medical profession played a great part in helping win the confidence of the Nagas by doing its job of caring for the sick and wounded.

The Nagas were afflicted with sores which ate to the bone and were considered incurable by these tough little people. The American doctors went about treating this common sore with sulfa drugs and in a short time the sores disappeared miraculously. Their King Peter was cured of blindness through the removal of cataracts in both eyes.

It didn't take any more to convince this ally that our cause was for their good. The Nagas played an important part in helping push the Ledo Road through to completion.

This is another victory for the American doctor who works and achieves under a free enterprise system, which is the backbone of a free nation.

If the Naga people knew about the plans in this country to socialize medicine and destroy our free American doctor, they would think we were very stupid indeed.

*Industrial News Review. Herald, Shawnee, Oklahoma. October 12, 1944.

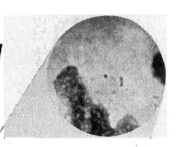
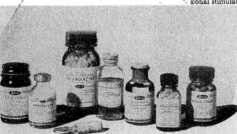

ALL GOOD DOCTORS LIVE IN PATIENT'S HEARTS*

In looking backward, one of our cherished memories is that of the family doctor. When he came to visit a sick child in the family circle his appearance was like throwing up a window shade to let the sun come in. No matter how sick the child had been she suddenly seemed to grow better in the presence of that personality, radiant with kindly feeling. In his advice and prescription there was perfect confidence for as we realized, his enthusiasm for his calling and his dedication to it were absolute.

Several times through the years the name of the doctor has changed, but with little alteration in personality. Always there has been a skill achieved by study and striving, a warm goodwill, a fine poise and a selfless devotion to the art of healing both mind and body. Always, too, there has been something in the very presence of the doctor to relieve suspense and cast out fear.

It is in a time such as this when hundreds of doctors come to our town to learn from one another that we are reminded of our dependence upon the medical profession and the priceless service it can give. In the lives of many of us there may have been hours when the doctor has meant more to us than another human soul. But how few of us are as thoughful of the doctor as we should be and as appreciative of his or her services!

Who among us realize how hard a good doctor's life is, especially in these days when one physician is trying to do the work of three or four. Thousands of doctors, weary after the day's work never go to bed in calm expectation of unbroken night's rest. Holidays and family feasts and Sunday rest are seldom for them. Their bills are the last to be paid—few among them are efficient collectors. But if they do not earn very much money, and many excellent doctors do not, they do find rich satisfaction in the realization that they relieve pain and terror, that they assist in bringing new life into the world and that again and again they snatch the sick and the wounded from the clutches of death.

Of all professions unless it be that of the clergy, medicine follows closest to the teachings of Christianity, for it knows no nationality, race or creed. To foe as well as friend the spirit of the Great Physician ministers impartially. Hundreds of our doctors and surgeons give care as tender to the sick and wounded of the enemy as to our own soldiers, sailors and airmen.

Doctors like nurses, chaplains and other non-combatants have left home, family and friends to go to strange places and brave the discomfort, the fatigue and peril of war. Some have given their lives for the causes for which we fight.

With every gain comes some loss. As medicine has become more highly specialized there has been less time and opportunity for doctors to develop with their patients those close personal ties that existed between a family and a physician in a day when one doctor had to treat all ills.

But if patients have had to relinquish some measure of that personal and priest-like ministration they are receiving in compensation the benefits of amazing progress in technical training.

*Edith Johnson. Oklahoma City Times. October 25, 1944.

A Doctor's Prayer

Teach me, dear Lord, that the hypertrophy of the head is more deadly than the hypertrophy of the heart, that the hyper-acidity of unforgiveness is more distressing than the "heart burn" of an ulcer.

Help me to live so that I can lie down and sleep each night, with a clear conscience, without a bromide or barbiturate, and unhaunted by the faces of those I have charged fees.

Grant, I beseech Thee, the power to focus my eyes on the distant goal of Heaven; eyes undimmed by the

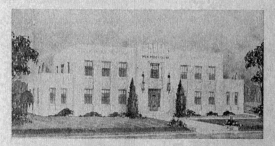

BEING a stable, organic iodide, NEO-IOPAX may be used with greater safety than other types of iodine preparations in all age groups. Because of its optimal iodine content and its rapid excretion in high concentration, diagnostic films may be obtained within five minutes after injection. NEO-IOPAX is usually well tolerated both by intravenous injection and retrograde administration.

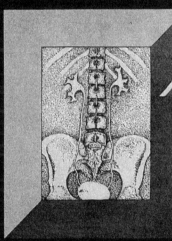

Neo-Jopax

IN INTRAVENOUS
UROGRAPHY

IN RETROGRADE
PYELOGRAPHY

SOLUTION NEO-IOPAX: Crystal-clear solution of disodium N-methyl-3, 5-diiodo-chelidamate in 50% and 75% concentration.

COMBINATION economy package of 50% solution containing both 20 cc. ampules and 10 cc. ampules: also 75% solution in ampules of 20 cc. or 10 cc.

SCHERING CORPORATION · BLOOMFIELD · N.J.

blurring myopia of fame or fortune. Keep my ears alert to the call of duty, undefeated by the clinking of polluted dollars.

Guide my mind and hand as I administer healing potions to suffering patients; help me to remember that the hypodermic needles should be tempered with the therapy of sympathy; the tonics enhanced by the stimulant of kindness; the transfusions aided by the nourishment of tenderness.

And then, when the last patient has been comforted, when the stethoscope, journals, and books have been laid aside, may my last call be Thy call, as I rest in the peace which Thou only can send. Amen—(Los Angeles County Bulletin).

Medical School Notes

Dr. Ernest Lachman attended the Joint Meeting of the American Roentgen Ray Society and the Radiological Society in Chicago from September 24 to 29 and took the Refresher Course which was given in conjunction with the meeting.

Dr. Louis A. Turley, Professor Emeritus of Pathology, recently presented to the Library of the School of Medicine a doctor's saddle bag given him by Dr. Nancy Campbell of the United States Indian Service. This was used in the Rio Ariba country, New Mexico, in the period "between the horse and buggy." As the saddle bag stands, it is a grip. However, by releasing the straps on either end, the bag is divided into two parts which hung over the skirt of the saddle.

At the same time the saddle bag was donated, Dr. Turley also gave the Library some phlebolances and other surgical instruments used in the early 19th century donated by Paul Sanger, M.D., Class of '31.

Among the books recently received at the Medical School Library are the following: Barach, A. L., Principles and Practices of Inhalational Therapy—1944; Bargen, J. A., Modern Management of Colitis—1943; Downes, R. M., Medical Ethics—1942; Draper, George, et al., Human Constitution in Clinical Medicine—1944; Edelstein, Ludwig, Hippocratic Oath, Text, Translation and Interpretation—1943; Hunt, J. M., Personality and the Behavior Disorders (2 vol.)—1944; Lewin, Phillip, Backache and Sciatic Neuritis—1943; Massler, Maury and Schour, Isaac, Atlas of the Mouth and Adjacent Parts in Health and Disease—1944; Moschcowitz, Eli, Vascular Sclerosis—1942; Osler, Sir William, Principles and Practice of Medicine (15th Edition)—1944; Piney, A., Sternal Puncture (2nd Edition)—1944, Samuels, S. S., Peripheral Vascular Diseases (Angiology)—1943; Seiffert, Gustav, Virus Diseases in Man, Animal and Plant—1944; Simmons, J. S. and Gentzkow, C. Laboratory Methods of the U. S. Army (5th Edition)—1944; Stieglitz, E. J., Geriatric Medicine—1943; Urbach, Erich, Allergy—1943; Watson-Jones, R., Fractures and Joint Injuries (3rd Edition—2 vol.)—1943; Willius, F. A., Cardic Clinics—1941; Yater, W. M., Fundamentals of Internal Medicine. (2nd Edition)—1944.

Registration for the first semester of the 1944-45 school year took place on September 22 and 23. Class work began Monday, September 25. Seventy-six freshmen were admitted. There are sixty-eight students in the Sophomore Class, seventy in the Junior Class, and seventy-two in the Senior Class. There are also two special students and one graduate student making a grand total of 289 students enrolled in the School of Medicine at the present time.

Of this total number, 168 students are under the Army Specialized Training Program, 73 students are under the Navy V-12 Program, and 48 are on civilian status. Of the 51 civilians 13 are women.

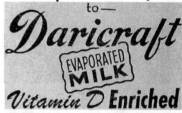
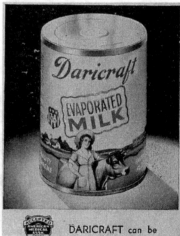

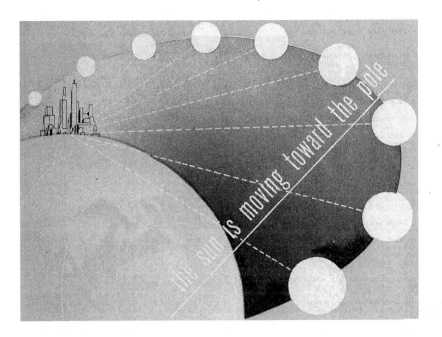

the sun is moving toward the pole

and with it, the benefits to your patients of solar ultraviolet,

source of vitamin D.

'It has been calculated that in the temperate latitude, exposure during the whole day in Winter would be required to be effective, and that in many parts of that zone no effective radiation occurs after 3 p.m. in Winter."*

However, there is an easy as well as economical method of assuring an adequate intake at all times of vitamin D together with its close partner in Nature—vitamin A.

WHITE'S COD LIVER OIL CONCENTRATE

contains the natural vitamins of time-proved cod liver oil, in concentrated potency, free from excess oily bulk.

A single tablet or two drops of the Liquid provides the vitamin A and D potency of a teaspoonful of cod liver oil**—and with very notable economy. Liquid, Tablet and Capsule dosage forms.

Ethically promoted—not advertised to the laity. White Laboratories, Inc., Pharmaceutical Manufacturers, Newark 7, N.J.

*Youmans, J. B.: Nutritional Deficiencies, Lippincott, New York, 1941.   **U. S. P. Minimum Requirements.

White's PRESCRIPTION *vitamins*

Now enrolled in the School of Nursing are 169 students plus 40 affiliates.

The Oklahoma Society of Medical Technologists held their Annual Convention on October 7 and 8 at the University of Oklahoma School of Medicine. Mrs. Marie Gard Clark, President, presided at the meetings. The program included the following papers;

Use of Penicillin in the Laboratory—Lt. Robert Finkelstein, U.S.A.M.C., Station Hospital, Fort Sill, Oklahoma.

Routine Bacteriological Detection of Gonococci in the Public Health Laboratory—H. L. Spencer, M. T.

Demonstration and Discussion of the Mazzini Test—Miss Catherine Harris, Chief Serologist, and Miss Egie Brisben, Assistant Serologist, State Health Department.

Film—"To the Ladies," presented by Captain Susan M. Fatherty, WAC Commanding Officer, Oklahoma WAC Recruiting District.

The Status of Laboratory Personnel in Hospitals of Oklahoma with Announcement of Commonwealth Scholarships available for Technologists training—Dr. F. R. Hassler, Director of Laboratories, State Health Department.

The Rh Factor and its Relation to Erythroblastosis—Dr. J. M. Parrish, Oklahoma City.

The Rh Blood Factor from the Standpoint of the Surgeon, Obstetrician and Gynecologist—Lt. Comdr. Victor F. Woldman, (MC) USNR, Naval Training School—Y, Stillwater, Oklahoma.

The annual banquet was held in the Crystal Room of the Skirvin Hotel with Dr. Howard C. Hopps, Professor of Pathology of the School of Medicine, as Toastmaster. Dr. Aute Richards, Director of the School of Applied Biology, University of Oklahoma, gave an address on "Growing Pains of a Profession."

Hints for Sickroom Visitors

. . . A few simple "Do's" and "Dont's" that will help the patient you are visiting . . .

Good Etiquette and Good Sense . . . in a Sickroom

Don't stay too long . . . a patient tires quickly. Thirty minutes may be only half an hour to you . . . and half a year to one in pain.

Be cheerful . . . not just artificially "cheery." There's a difference.

And be natural . . . not doleful. Tact is more precious than gold in a sickroom.

Talk quietly, comfortably, about things of interest to your friend, news, gossip of home and people. Keep away from topics that can bring worry or distress.

Do not leave it to the patient to "entertain" you . . . you're not the one who's sick. If your visit becomes awkward or strained . . . don't stay. Sit where the patient can see you without twisting or straining . . . preferably at one side of the foot of the bed.

Never sit on the bed . . . the patient has troubles enough already.

One or two visitors at a time is best. Larger numbers increase the nervous strain. The patient is here to rest and recover . . . not to attend a convention.

Show sympathy . . . not pity. Again, there's a difference. Sympathy supports . . . pity humiliates. No one wants mere pity.

If you are worried about the patient . . . try not to show it. Assume that he will soon be well. The patient may know better . . . but hope and faith have astonishing curative powers. Your attitude can help.

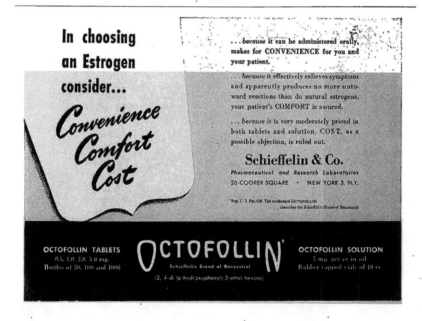

'Particularly valuable'

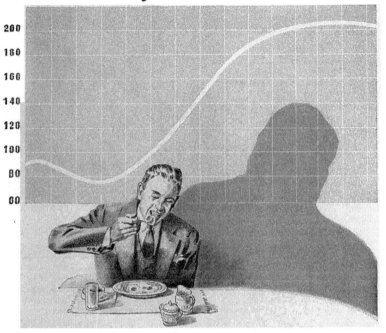

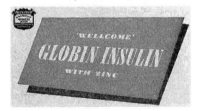

Don't keep referring to his pain and illness. He wants to forget them if he can.

It generally is better to leave children under 14 at home (a State Board of Health ruling forbids any visitors under 12 on the maternity floor). Their high-spirited energy and innocent restlessness can be very wearing.

If you bring flowers, remember that potted plants or small bouquets are more welcome than lavish arm-fuls (especially in wartime when nurses need six hands) and less heavy cloying fragrance.

And if you bring books, select them carefully. They should fit the patient's tastes and state of mind. And don't forget . . . a 3 pound book is no bargin to one who must read in bed.

Smoking in a semi-private room may be objectionable to other patients. If you ask, they are apt to deny that it bothers them even though it does.

Visitors in semi-private rooms must obviously be asked to leave when any patient in the room is to be given treatment.

Don't visit a sickroom if you have a cold . . . or if your condition can jeopardize the patient's health. If in doubt . . . DON'T.

And if you don't visit the patient when he's well . . . don't push yourself upon him when he's sick. A note or flowers will express your sympathy more appropriately.

Please understand that these are SUGGESTIONS only . . . not RULES. No rules can take the place of common sense and tact in comforting the sick. We offer them from our long experience because we know that you are as anxious as we are to help speed the patient's recovery. For your thoughtful cooperation . . . thank you.—*Reprinted.*

$34,000 in War Bonds as Prizes

$34,000 in War Bonds as Prizes will be given for the best art works by physicians, memorializing the medical profession's "Courage and Devotion Beyond the Call of Duty" (in war and in peace).

This prize contest is open to any physician member of the American Physicians Art Association, including medical officers in the armed forces of the United States and Canada.

Full information available on request of the sponsor, Mead Johnson & Co., Evansville, Ind., U.S.A.

Origin of Medicine

The origin of medicine, hidden in the mist of ages, carries us back to the old home story of the world, and is more or less interesting to all of us. The physician is with us from the cradle to the grave, and the primitive doctor of old history may have his modern representative.—*Aberdeen Doctors—At Home and Abroad. Ella Hill Burton Rodger. Page A. William Blackwood & Sons. Edinburgh and London.* 1913.

Abercrombie on Diet

He ordered people to eat three ounces of food three times a day, without drinking. A patient having confided to Sir Astley (Cooper) his entire belief in Mr. Abernethy's regimen, his rival cruelly said: "I will faithfully recount to you the dinner he ate himself yesterday at the Freemason's Tavern, where I sat down next to him. He took turtle-soup and punch, venison, champagne, pastry, and cheese; and now, he said, 'Waiter, bring me a glass of brown stout'." The patient indignantly cried, "How could I have been such a fool as to starve myself!"—*Aberdeen Doctors, At Home and Abroad,* pp. 116-117. *Ella Hill Burton Rodger. William Blackwood and Sons. Edinburgh and London.* 1913.

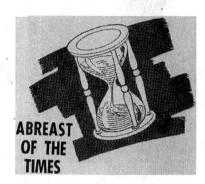

ABREAST OF THE TIMES

The action of Estrogenic Hormone is specific. It's use is suggested for control of menopausal symptoms, treatment of senile vaginitis, gonorrheal vaginitis, infantile conditions, also nausea and vomiting of pregnancy.

**ESTROGENIC
HORMONE
U. S. S. P. CO.**

is the naturally occurring hormone. It is not a synthetic preparation.

U.S.S.P. CO. supplies standardized preparations of Estrogenic Hormone in oil solution and aqueous suspension in all practical concentrations in single and multiple dose containers.

Available at Leading Pharmacies,

Write for Literature   OK 11-44

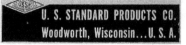

U. S. STANDARD PRODUCTS CO.
Woodworth, Wisconsin...U. S. A.

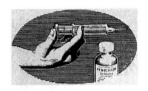

• OBITUARIES •

Cephas John Wells. M.D.
1865-1944

Dr. Cephas J. Wells, Bartlesville, died at his home on September 9 of congestive heart failure. He was born in Michigan in 1865, leaving Michigan to go to Kentucky where he attended the Louisville Medical College, graduate in 1894. From Kentucky, Dr. Wells moved to Grove, Oklahoma where he practised until 1918. After spending two years in Hillsdale County, Michigan, he returned to Oklahoma where he located in Bartlesville.

Dr. Wells was a member of the Washington-Nowata County Medical Society, the Oklahoma State Medical Association and the American Medical Association.

M. M. DeArman. M.D.
1878-1944

On Saturday, November 4, Dr. M. M. DeArman of Miami, died at a Columbus, Ohio, hospital after an illness of several weeks.

Dr. DeArman graduated in 1901 from the University of Tennessee College of Medicine at Memphis. For many years he practiced in Miami and became a leading civic figure. Dr. DeArman was a former mayor and president of the Security Bank and Trust Company of Miami. He was a member of the Ottawa County Medical Society, the Oklahoma State Medical Association and the American Medical Association.

Surviving Dr. DeArman are his widow and two sisters, Mrs. Elbert Hurst, Oklahoma City, and Mrs. Mattie Hudson, Wellington, Texas.

DeLoss Wallace. M.D.
1903-1944

Dr. DeLoss Wallace, formerly of Ada, died at his home in Monte Vista. Colorado. On October 23, Dr. Wallace, his wife and two children, Shirley Jean, 8, and Carlos, 7, were asphyxiated by fumes from a coal furnace in their home.

Dr. Wallace was born at Cedarvale, Kansas. He was a graduate of the University of Oklahoma School of Medicine, Class of 1934, and took his internship at St. Mary's Hospital, Denver. For a year following his internship, Dr. Wallace practiced in Ada, moving then to Colorado where he was practicing at the time of his death. He was a member of the Colorado Medical Association.

Dr. Wallace is survived by his mother, Mrs. Mary J. Wallace, Oklahoma City, four sisters and four brothers. Mrs. Wallace is survived by her parents, Mr. and Mrs. L. Zachary, Cement, three sisters and a brother.

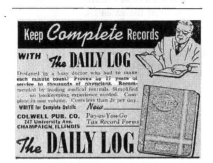
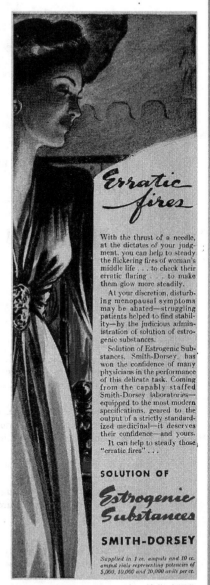

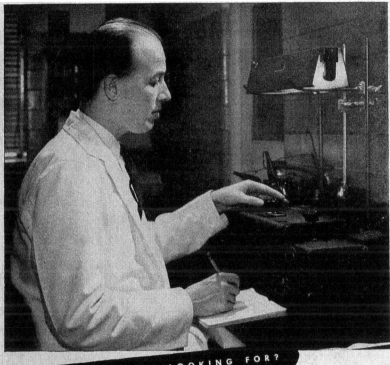

THE IMPORTANCE OF HEALTH
TO VICTORY
BY ROBERT CARSE
Ensign, U. S. M. C.

Up inside the Arctic Circle at Murmansk where we fought the Nazis day and night, the men of my convoy learned from the valiant Russian people that there is absolutely no difference between those at the front and those behind it. The safety of one, we found, depends upon the safety of all, and the health of a nation as a whole is as vital in war as arms.

Returning to the United States on leave from active service, I have been informed that tuberculosis is still the Number One Killer during the most productive years of life, from 15 to 45, among those on the home front. In very simple terms—terms that every American should know and understand — tuberculosis took approximately 145,000 lives in the first 31 months after Pearl Harbor. Deaths among the armed forces for this same period, according to a recent estimate, were about 57,000.

One out of every 100 men entering the armed services examined for tuberculosis was disqualified because of this disease in some stage. Thirty out of every 100 men disqualified for tuberculosis had the disease in a clinically active form. Figures from mass X-ray surveys among industrial workers indicate that a somewhat higher percentage of active cases is found because more of the persons so engaged are in the older age groups.

This is the condition existing on the American home front in the year of the great assault upon Europe, in the year when every man and woman who is active and fit is desperately needed, and the demands of the armed services are daily stripping industry more and more to fill our fighting ranks.

Here is nothing but a sheer and criminal waste. For no one need die with the disease today. It can be prevented and can be cured. Diagnosis and treatment for it are proved procedures.

According to the figures of the National Tuberculosis Association, whose Christmas Seal Campaign appeal is again being made to you, the tuberculosis death rate has been reduced 75 per cent in the last 40 years of struggle against the disease. But the obvious fact remains that the fight must continue until the disease is completely conquered.

Your sons, your brothers and your husbands who are serving overseas have seen in the countries they have freed from our enemies the awful effects of malnutrition, lack of clothing, lack of sanitation and medical care. They dream endlessly of returning home to you, but returning to a healthy and happy people, free at least of this disease from which, if treated correctly, one can recover.

Education has been the chief weapon used to gain all past victories against

tuberculosis. Education must continue to be the chief weapon. Last year, tuberculosis killed 50,000 people in this country; that means one person every nine minutes. It is estimated that over half a million people in the United States have tuberculosis, and of these only half are known cases. The remaining half must be located. They are losing their health, perhaps thei rlives, and, all unconsciously, holding back the war effort and impeding the victory.

Buy, buy all you can of Christmas Seals and you will help reach them. You will help stop the march of the White Plague that has already taken so many lives.

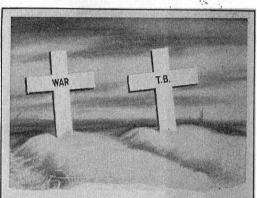

TWINS OF DEATH

HAND IN HAND go War and Tuberculosis — the dread disease that since Pearl Harbor has exacted a toll of 145,000 civilians.

Wartime conditions — worry, overwork, abnormal eating and housing — are the *allies* of TB.

Yet Tuberculosis can be controlled. The annual sale of Christmas Seals has helped cut the death rate by 75%!

But the current death rate shows that the battle is *far from won* — that your dollars are needed now, urgently.

Please, send in your contribution today.

BUY CHRISTMAS
SEALS!

The National, State and Local Tuberculosis Associations in the United States

In the Management of
Severe Third-Degree Burns

much has been learned through the unfortunate occurrence
of the Cocoanut Grove fire at Boston. The numerous reports
in the medical press emphasize the need for large amounts
of dietary protein of adequate biologic value, given as
early as possible.* Meat is one of man's main sources
of protein that can be eaten with relish several times
daily in goodly quantities; its proteins are of highest
quality, and it contributes to the satisfaction of
the greatly increased vitamin requirements as well.

*"All the patients with ten per cent of surface area, or more,
involved in third-degree burns became serious nutritional
problems. . . . All patients were started on high protein, high
vitamin diets. . . . This diet contained 140 Gm. of protein."
(Clowes, G. H. A., Jr.; Lund, C. C., and Levenson, S. M.: The
Surface Treatment of Burns, Ann. Surg. 118:761[Nov.]1943.)

". . . at least from 200 to 300 grams of protein is needed for
replacement alone. One must give the patient as much food
as he can take . . . give him a good protein, one that contains
all of the essential amino acids." (Elman, R.: Physiologic
Problems of Burns, J. Missouri M. A. 41:1 [Jan.] 1944.)

The Seal of Acceptance denotes
that the nutritional statements
made in this advertisement are
acceptable to the Council on
Foods and Nutrition of the
American Medical Association.

AMERICAN MEAT INSTITUTE
MAIN OFFICE, CHICAGO... MEMBERS THROUGHOUT THE UNITED STATES

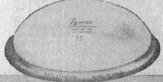
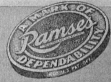

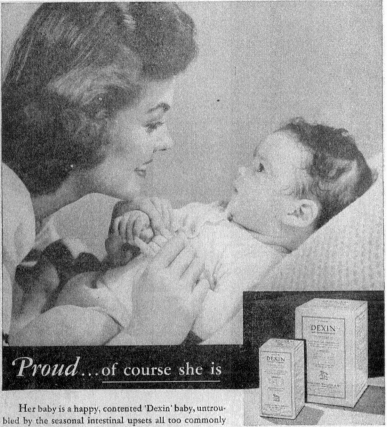

Proud...of course she is

Her baby is a happy, contented 'Dexin' baby, untroubled by the seasonal intestinal upsets all too commonly associated with **excessive carbohydrate fermentation.**

When 'Dexin', a high dextrin carbohydrate, is used as the milk modifier, infants are notably free from intestinal fermentative reactions. 'Dexin' reduces the possibility of distention, colic and diarrhea.

'Dexin' formulas are easily digested. The high dextrin content favors soft milk-curd formation. 'Dexin' is readily soluble in hot or cold milk.   Dexin reg. trademark

Literature on request

'Dexin' does make a difference

COMPOSITION

Dextrins	. . . 75%	Mineral Ash	. 0.25%
Maltose	. . . 24%	Moisture	. . 0.75%

Available carbohydrate 99% 115 calories per ounce
6 level packed tablespoonfuls equal 1 ounce

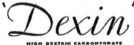

HIGH DEXTRIN CARBOHYDRATE

BURROUGH WELLCOME & CO. (U. S. A.) INC., 9-11 East 41st Street, New York 17, N. Y.

OFFICERS OF COUNTY SOCIETIES, 1944

★

COUNTY	PRESIDENT	SECRETARY	MEETING TIME
Alfalfa	H. E. Huston, Cherokee	L. T. Lancaster, Cherokee	Last Tues. each Second Month
Atoka-Coal	R. C. Henry, Coalgate	J. S. Fulton, Atoka	
Beckham	G. H. Stagner, Erick	O. C. Standifer, Elk City	Second Tuesday
Blaine	L. R. Kirby, Okeene	W. F. Griffin, Watonga	
Bryan	John T. Wharton, Durant	W. K. Haynie, Durant	Second Tuesday
Caddo	F. L. Patterson, Carnegie	C. B. Sullivan, Carnegie	
Canadian	P. F. Herod, El Reno	A. L. Johnson, El Reno	Subject to call
Carter	F. W. Boadway, Ardmore	H. A. Higgins, Ardmore	
Cherokee	P. H. Medearis, Tahlequah	W. M. Wood, Tahlequah	First Tuesday
Choctaw		E. A. Johnson, Hugo	
Cleveland	F. T. Gastineau, Norman	Iva S. Merritt, Norman	Thursday nights
Comanche	George L. Berry, Lawton	Howard Angus, Lawton	
Cotton	A. B. Holstead, Temple	Mollie F. Scism, Walters	Third Friday
Craig	Lloyd H. McPike, Vinita	J. M. McMillan, Vinita	
Creek	J. E. Hollis, Bristow	F. H. Sisler, Bristow	
Custer	F. R. Vieregg, Clinton	C. J. Alexander, Clinton	Third Thursday
Garfield	Julian Feild, Enid	John R. Walker, Enid	Fourth Thursday
Garvin	T. F. Gross, Lindsay	John R. Callaway, Pauls Valley	Wednesday before Third Thursday
Grady	Walter J. Baze, Chickasha	Roy E. Emanuel, Chickasha	Third Thursday
Grant	I. V. Hardy, Medford		
Greer	R. W. Lewis, Granite	J. B. Hollis, Mangum	
Harmon	W. G. Husband, Hollis	R. H. Lynch, Hollis	First Wednesday
Haskell	William Carson, Keota	N. K. Williams, McCurtain	
Hughes	Wm. L. Taylor, Holdenville	Imogene Mayfield, Holdenville	First Friday
Jackson	C. G. Spears, Altus	E. A. Abernethy, Altus	Last Monday
Jefferson	F. M. Edwards, Ringling		Second Monday
Kay	J. Holland Howe, Ponca City	G. H. Yeary, Newkirk	Second Thursday
Kingfisher	A. O. Meredith, Kingfisher	H. Violet Sturgeon, Hennessey	
Kiowa	J. William Finch, Hobart	William Bernell, Hobart	
LeFlore	Neeson Rolfe, Poteau	Rush L. Wright, Poteau	
Lincoln	W. B. Davis, Stroud	Carl H. Bailey, Stroud	First Wednesday
Logan	William C. Miller, Guthrie	J. L. LeHew, Jr., Guthrie	Last Tuesday
Marshall	J. L. Holland, Madill	J. F. York, Madill	
Mayes	Ralph V. Smith, Pryor	Paul B. Cameron, Pryor	
McClain	W. C. McCurdy, Sr., Purcell	W. C. McCurdy, Jr., Purcell	
McCurtain	A. W. Clarkson, Valliant	N. L. Barker, Broken Bow	Fourth Tuesday
McIntosh	Luster I. Jacobs, Hanna	Wm. A. Tolleson, Eufaula	First Thursday
Murray	P. V. Annadown, Sulphur	J. A. Wrenn, Sulphur	Second Tuesday
Muskogee-Seqnoyah Wagoner	H. A. Scott, Muskogee	D. Evelyn Miller, Muskogee	First Monday
Noble	C. H. Cooke, Perry	J. W. Francis, Perry	
Okfuskee	C. M. Cochran, Okemah	M. L. Whitney, Okemah	Second Monday
Oklahoma	W. E. Eastland, Oklahoma City	E. R. Musick, Oklahoma City	Fourth Tuesday
Okmulgee	S. B. Leslie, Okmulgee	J. C. Matheney, Okmulgee	Second Monday
Osage	C. R. Welrich, Pawhuska	George K. Hemphill, Pawhuska	Second Monday
Ottawa	Walter Kerr, Picher	B. W. Shelton, Miami	Third Thursday
Pawnee	E. T. Robinson, Cleveland	R. L. Browning, Pawnee	
Payne	H. C. Manning, Cushing	J. W. Martin, Cushing	Third Thursday
Pittsburg	P. T. Powell, McAlester	W. H. Kaeiser, McAlester	Third Friday
Pontotoc	A. R. Sugg, Ada	R. H. Mayes, Ada	First Wednesday
Pottawatomie	E. Eugene Rice, Shawnee	Clinton Gallaher, Shawnee	First and Third Saturday
Pushmataha	John S. Lawson, Clayton	B. M. Huckabay, Antlers	
Rogers	R. C. Meloy, Claremore	Chas. L. Caldwell, Chelsea	First Monday
Seminole	J. T. Price, Seminole	Mack I. Shanholtz, Wewoka	Third Wednesday
Stephens	W. K. Walker, Marlow	Wallis S. Ivy, Duncan	
Texas	R. G. Obermiller, Texhoma	Morris Smith, Guymon	
Tillman	C. C. Allen, Frederick	O. G. Bacon, Frederick	
Tulsa	Ralph A. McGill, Tulsa	E. O. Johnson, Tulsa	Second and Fourth Monday
Washington-Nowata	K. D. Davis, Nowata	J. V. Atkey, Bartlesville	Second Wednesday
Washita	A. S. Neal, Cordell	James F. McMurRy, Sentinel	
Woods	Ishmael F. Stephenson, Alva	Oscar E. Templin, Alva	Last Tuesday Odd Months
Woodward	H. Walker, Buffalo	C. W. Tedrowe, Woodward	Second Thursday

*(Serving in Armed Forces)

THE JOURNAL
OF THE
OKLAHOMA STATE MEDICAL ASSOCIATION

VOLUME XXXVII	OKLAHOMA CITY, OKLAHOMA, DECEMBER, 1944	NUMBER 12

Endocarditis[*]

RALPH H. MAJOR, M. D.

*Department of Internal Medicine, The
University of Kansas School
of Medicine*

KANSAS CITY, KANSAS

Only in our generation has the clinical and pathological picture of subacute bacterial endocarditis been clearly portrayed. Many masters in the fields of pathology and of clinical medicine must have encountered this disease in the course of their work, yet for centuries they failed to grasp clearly its essential pathological and clinical features.

According to Laennec, the first description of endocarditis was that of Lazare Riviere, professor of medicine at Montpellier. Riviere described a patient who consulted him in 1646 complaining of palpitation of the heart and showing a very irregular pulse. The patient died two months after coming under the care of Riviere, and at autopsy "round caruncles similar in substance to the lungs were found in the left ventricle of the heart, which resembled a cluster of hazelnuts and filled up the entrance to the aorta, which I think to have caused the defect of the pulse in the arteries." While the description lacks much in clarity and no mention is made of the heart valves, a caruncle resembling a cluster of hazelnuts and filling up the entrance into the aorta, very probably was a verrucous vegetation on the aortic valve. Some sixty years later Giovanni Maria Lancisi in his *De subitaneis mortis* (1707), written on account of the panic in Rome at the great number of sudden deaths, described clearly valvular vegetations.

Morgagni, the father of pathological anatomy, described several cases of endocarditis. A relatively fresh endocarditis was seen in one patient, some six and thirty years of age,

*Delivered at the Fourteenth Annual Conference of Oklahoma City Clinical Society, Wednesday, October 25, 1944.

who showed at autopsy protuberant excrescences on his heart valves which "might be very easily pull'd away by the fingers and by the nails." His later remark that "These excrescences being taken away, the substance of the valves remain'd, but was contracted and deficient" confirms this diagnosis and suggests a recent endocarditis on a previously damaged valve. His description of the spleen which "had on the external surface some thick adipose ramifications, as it were, if our eyes were to be believ'd; but the substance of them was a tendinous firmness, and even of a middle nature betwixt a cartilage and a ligament" certainly suggests an infarction of the spleen, so common in subacute bacterial endocarditis. 'Though this pioneer saw endocarditis, much ground had to be broken by his successors before endocarditis became a clear-cut entity, separable into the acute, subacute, and chronic varieties.

Edward Sandifort in his *Observations Anatomico-pathologicae,* published at Leyden in 1777, described vegetative endocarditis and illustrated the condition with excellent drawings, as did Matthew Baillie, whose *Morbid Anatomy* was published in London in 1793.

Corvisart in his *Essai sur les maladies et les lesions organiques du coeur,* published in 1806, devotes a section to "vegetations of the semilunar valves." Corvisart describes "true excrescences or soft vegetations . . . the nature of which is entirely unknown' 'and notes that they resemble venereal warts, which led him to suspect a possible syphilitic origin. Corvisart's famous pupil Laennec, in his *De l'auscultation mediate,* published in 1819, discusses in Chapter XVI "Vegetations which develop on the valves and the walls of the cavities of the heart." Later French treatises on disease of the heart, such as Bertin and Bouillaud's *Traite des maladies du coeur,* published in 1824, describe vegetations on the heart valves with illustrative histories and autopsy protocols.

Bouillaud later, in 1835, published his excellent *Traite clinique des maladies du coeur* and wrote extensively on the relationship between rheumatic fever and heart disease. "He was," notes Herrick, "the first accurately to describe the endocardium (the name is his) ; the first to conceive of this membrane as the seat of an inflammation, which he called endocarditis, and the first clearly to describe the stages of this inflammation." His book introduced the terms "endocardium" and "endocarditis" into medical nomenclature.

One of the earliest, if not the earliest, descriptions of endocarditis with embolism is from the pen of Rudolf Virchow and was published in the first volume of Virchow's Archiv in 1847. The pathological summary was "thickening and narrowing of the mitral valve, fibrous softening coagulum on the same. Infarcts in the cerebral artery, left femoral artery and right iliac artery. Hemorrhagic infarctions of the spleen."

Five years later, in 1852, William Senhouse Kirkes published one of the earliest and clearest descriptions of chronic endocarditis with embolism. This paper had the title, "On Some of the Principal Effects Resulting from the Detachment of Fibrinous Deposits from the Interior of the Heart and their Mixture with the Circulating Blood."

Virchow, in 1856, in his classic studies on embolism, emphasized the importance of endocarditis in the production of emboli. In this paper he also describes a case of endocarditis with emboli in the pulmonary vein, the emboli showing under the microscope "innumerable vibrions."

In 1869, Winge demonstrated before the Medical Society of Christiania, a case of ulcerative endocarditis with embolism of the lungs, kidneys, and spleen. He noted "on the aortic valves greyish, feltlike masses resembling thrombi, the size of a pea to that of a bean, scraped off, leaving a rough ulcerated endocardium beneath." Under the microscope the thrombus-like masses "proved with moderate enlargement to be a fine felt of fibrinous threads." When the higher power was employed "these threads were clearly crisscrossed bodies or round granules . . ."—the first description of bacteria in endocardial lesions.

Osler gave a very concise yet comprehensive picture of malignant endocarditis in his Gulstonian lectures of 1885. He stressed the frequency with which the disease attacked

valves previously damaged and states that this was true in three-fourths of his Montreal cases. He discussed very fully the clinical picture of the disease and the pathological findings, noting that "micrococci are constant elements in the vegetations."

Heubner in 1899 described five cases of long-continued fever lasting from three to nine months, all of which showed endocarditis with splenic infarctions at autopsy. The same year marked the appearance of Lenhartz' book *Die Septischen Erkrankungen* which formed one volume of Nothnagel's well-known *Spezielle Pathologie und Therapie.* In this work Lenhartz described acute endocarditis due to the staphylococcus, streptococcus, pneumococcus and gonococcus, and also discussed in detail chronic endocarditis. Lenhartz pointed out that acute streptococcic endocarditis occurs in patients who are extremely ill, show a high irregular temperature with frequent chills, run an acute stormy course, and is usually due to the "ordinary streptococcus." In chronic streptococcic endocarditis by contrast, the onset was often gradual, the course of the disease was milder, petechiae were usually present, infarctions in the spleen and kidneys were common, and cerebral complications such as aphasia and paralysis were sometimes noted. The organism found in the blood cultures of these patients was not the "ordinary" streptococcus but "a delicate, fine streptococcus which is characterized by its slower growth, by the formation of a greenish zone about the individual colonies . . . and is not virulent for animals."

Schottmuller in 1903 stressed the fact that the "ordinary" streptococcus when grown on blood agar produced hemolysis while the "small" streptococcus described by Lenhartz, grew with the production of a greenish pigment. For this reason he named the organism Streptococcus *mitior seu viridans* (milder or green growing streptococcus). He stressed the importance of the green growing streptococcus in the etiology of chronic and subacute endocarditis. In subsequent articles he emphasized the fact that this type of endocarditis due to the streptococcus *mitior seu vididans* was a definite clinical entity which he called Endocarditis *lenta.* This contribution of Schottmuller is a classic on the subject of endocarditis and following his work, the terms Streptococcus *hemolyticus* and Streptococcus *viridans* become well-known both in clinical medicine and in bacteriology.

American interest in subacute bacterial endocarditis dates largely from the publication of Libman and Celler's classic paper in 1910. These authors studied forty-three cases of subacute endocarditis and described in detail the type of organism isolated. Since the publication of these papers, the American literature alone on the subject of subacute bacterial endocarditis has grown to large proportions, which bears witness not only to the increased interest in this disease but also to its growing clinical importance. Several excellent analytical reviews of subacute bacterial endocarditis have been written during the past two decades. Outstanding among these is the review of George Blumer which appeared in 1923.

There is unfortunately little statistical data concerning the frequency of this disease. The earlier writers regarded the disease as relatively rare, although as long ago as 1899, Ebstein wrote that "Chronic cases of ulcerative malignant endocarditis are much more frequent than has formerly been supposed." From this period we frequently find the opinion expressed that the disease is not uncommon and its frequency underestimated. Horder found it to occur about once in every two hundred ward patients while Cotton describes a frequency of eight per cent in soldiers invalided for chronic valvular disease. In our medical clinic fifty cases occurred in 15,382 admissions, a percentage of .33.

The age of the patients suffering from subacute endocarditis is of some interest. Blumer in the study of 317 cases found 36 per cent between the ages of 21 and 30, and 27 per cent between the ages of 31 and 40, which is in substantial agreement with Horder's figure of 50 per cent and Blumer's figure of 56 per cent for this age group. Our youngest patient was eleven, our oldest 65 years of age. I have personal knowledge of one patient of 80 succumbing to a typical subacute bacterial endocarditis. The great majority of cases are between the ages of 20 and 40. The difference between the frequency with which the two sexes are involved is slight. Some observers found a preponderance of males, other of females. In one experience the difference is so slight as to be of no significance.

The micro-organism responsible for subacute bacterial endocarditis in the overwhelming number of cases is the streptococcus first carefully studied by Schottmuller and named by him the S. viridans because it produced a greenish pigment when grown on blood agar. According to Libman's studies, this organism is responsible for 95 per cent of his cases while 5 per cent were due to B. influenzae. While in the literature there are scattered reports of isolated cases due to various organisms, yet subacute bacterial endocarditis is practically always synonymous with infection by the S. viridans. In our series of 50 cases it was the only organism isolated. While chronic endocarditis may be caused occasionally by the gonococcus or the

pneumococcus or the M. melitensis (and we have seen examples of these), these diseases have a distinct entity and for the purpose of defining a disease entity it seems best to exclude them from consideration. While all continued fevers are not due to typhoid fever, yet typhoid fever is caused by the typhoid bacillus. Since subacute bacterial endocarditis as a clinical entity is caused by the S. viridans, other types should perhaps be called pneumococcus endocarditis or gonococcal endocarditis just as we differentiate epidemic meningococcic meningitis from pneumococcic or tuberculous meningitis. In some respects the term "endocarditis lenta," introduced by Schottmuller to designate a specific disease entity caused by the S. viridans, is preferable to the more embracing term "subacute bacterial endocarditis."

The first attempt to differentiate the different strains of streptococci was made by Andrews and Horder in 1906. They showed that these strains differ in their ability to ferment carbohydrates with the production of acid. They classified them in four groups: S. pyogenes, S. salivarius, S. anginosus and S. fecalis. Many cultures of S. viridans with which we have worked have been further classified as S. salivarius, S. anginosus and S. fecalis. This classification has been attacked by later observations on the grounds that the ability of the streptococcus to attack carbohydrates varies from time to time. In our clinic, however, continued and painstaking study of our cultures of S. viridans have usually permitted a definite identification of the organisms as belonging to one of these three groups.

Lancefield more recently has proposed a classification of streptococci based on agglutination with immune sera.

Among the seventeen different names in English, French, German and Italian which have been employed to describe this disease, there is an interesting term "Schleichende Endocarditis" or "Sneaking Endocarditis." This term is especially appropriate in describing the onset of this disease.

In the majority of cases, the disease begins insidiously, almost unnoticed by the patient who cannot fix very accurately the exact date when he began to feel badly. Often he consults the physician complaining of weakness, loss of strength or lack of endurance. He may have lost weight, had slight fever, noticed chilly sensations or fleeting pains in his joints. Loss of appetite is common, and backache is often an early symptom. Palpitation of the heart, dyspnea and pains in the chest are frequent.

While in most cases the onset is "sneaking," some cases begin with a dramatic suddenness. Several of our patients insisted they were "as well as usual" until one day a sudden hemiplegia appeared. One patient stated he was well until seized with sudden pain in the leg which proved to be an embolism of the popliteal artery. In other patients the disease may appear abruptly with chills and fever, or may develop immediately after an attack of acute arthritis, or after an abortion.

When first seen by the physician, the patient usually shows some daily elevation of temperature, and an examination of his heart shows murmurs at the mitral or aortic area and often at both areas. Petechiae in the conjunctivae often appear early in the disease and hemorrhages in the retina are at times seen rarely although often a later manifestation. Similarly, definite enlargement of the spleen appears early in some patients.

Patients with subacute bacterial endocarditis do not as a rule show very high elevations of temperature, and maximum rarely exceeds 103° F. There are, however, many exceptions. Some patients have severe chills associated with such marked fluctuations of temperature that their charts resemble that of a patient with malaria.

When viewed in retrospect, the course of the disease is progressively downward. Yet this may not be apparent at the moment, since these patients, in the early stages, may live for weeks with but little change in their condition and even show periods of marked temporary improvement. In the early stages of this disease the patient's symptoms seem so slight and his condition so good that it is often difficult to convince the patient's friends and relatives that the disease is serious and usually fatal. As the disease progresses, the patient slowly loses weight, the appetite fails, and anemia which may not have been marked in the beginning becomes more pronounced, the fever tends to rise higher, and petechiae become more numerous. Although these patients lose weight steadily as a rule throughout their illness, yet cachexia is not a common finding and some patients appear well nourished on the final day of their illness. The blood picture in this disease is that of a secondary anemia, the red blood count gradually diminishing but rarely going below 2,000,000 per cu. mm. The lowest red blood seen in our series was 1,840,000 with 28 per cent (4.3 grams) hemoglobin. The first count recorded on this patient was 3,650,000 with 65 per cent (10 grams) hemoglobin. A moderate leukocytosis is the rule in subacute endocarditis.

The duration of the disease varies between wide limits due to the virulence of the organism, the resistance of the individual, the condition of the heart at the onset of the illness and the frequency and location of the emboli. Blumer found that death occurred between the third and the end of the eighth month, in the cases he studied. The average duration of our cases was six months, one patient living 15 months, three living 12 months and five living 10 months.

Osler in 1908 described a lesion, since known as Osler nodes. They consist of painful, reddish thickening from 1 to 1.5 centimeters in the pads of the fingers which often appear in corps and may last a few hours or several days. Osler found them in seven of his ten cases, a much higher incidence than that observed by anyone else. "Splinter hemorrhages," which are small hemorrhages under the finger resembling splinters, are seen from time to time. Clubbed fingers are seen not infrequently and may appear while the patient is under observation.

Spontaneous recovery from subacute bacterial endocarditis is extremely rare. Schottmuller in 1903 reported one case of endocarditis lenta which recovered. Billings states that he saw three cases recover. Libman saw four recoveries in 150 cases, Horder saw one recovery in 150 cases, while Thayer saw no recovery in 200 cases. A large number of observers have never seen a case recover. Libman, in a review of 1,000 cases enumerated twelve recoveries or 1.2 per cent. Three per cent is the most favorable incidence of spontaneous recovery observed by any author.

Two reports in the literature are unique. In 1915, Ollie, Graham and Detweiler reported 23 cases from whose blood Streptococcus *viridans* was isolated. The patients had heart murmurs, none of them had petechiae although one showed painful subcutaneous nodules, four had a leukocytosis, six showed signs of nephritis. The patients were re-examined ten years later. All the patients showed cardiac murmurs except two, one who had never shown a murmur and another patient who had shown a mitral systolic murmur in 1912, which had disappeared.

A similar series was reported in 1920 by Salus from Funke's Clinic in Prague. Salus reported that he had seen 18 cases of Streptococcus viridans bacteriemia which recovered and were working a year and a half later. He believed they had suffered from a mild form of endocarditis which he called endocarditis lenta benigna.

Many different drugs have been recommended in subacute bacterial endocarditis. The multiplicity of those recommended is good evidence of their lack of effect. Various silver salts, optochin, gentian violet, quinine and arsenic have been employed. Capps was at one time hopeful but cautious in regard to the results from treatment with sodium cacodylate, but later expressed much skepticism regarding its value.

With the introduction of sulfonamides into medicine, it was natural that their effects on subacute bacterial endocarditis should be studied. Blumer in 1941 expressed the following opinions upon the value of the sulfonamides in the treatment of endocarditis. He stated that a study of these cases "leads me to the pessimistic conclusion that the occasional recoveries under sulfamide treatment can be explained on the basis of spontaneous recovery." Other writers, however, are less pessimistic.

Lichtman and Bierman in 1941, after a review of the literature, found that 198 cases of subacute infectious endocarditis had been treated with sulfonamides and that 12 patients, or six per cent, recovered. In cases where fever therapy was combined with sulfonamides, these authors reported 88 cases treated, with 14 or 16 per cent recoveries. Smith, Sauls and Stone in 1942 found 35 authentic instances of cure in subacute bacterial endocarditis after sulfonamide therapy. They reported 15 cases with two cures. Since the introduction of sulfonamides, 19 cases of subacute bacterial endocarditis have been treated with sulfonamides in our clinic with eight cures. Seven of these patients are alive and well today; the eighth died of cardiac disease and showed a healed endocarditis.

In contrast to these findings, Herill and Brown of the Mayo Clinic stated that they treated 91 patients with sulfonamides and did not see a single recovery.

It is obvious that the sulfonamides, or at least the compounds employed to date, are not the therapeutic answer to subacute bacterial endocarditis. However, it is the only method of treatment until recently that has any cures to its credit. The different results reported in the literature may depend upon the dosage employed, the difference in virulence of the strain of S. viridans encountered, or what is more important, in our opinion, the stage of the disease at which the sulfonamides are employed. In four of our recoveries, sulfonamide treatment was instituted within one month after the onset of the disease. It would seem reasonable to assume that the sulfonamide therapy would be more effective when vegetations were small than when they had formed large cauliflower-like excrescences. In all our cases which recovered, except two, the organism isolated was the S. salivarius type of S. viridans.

There is, as yet, no reliable indication as to the choice of the sulfonamide employed. The majority of the cases cured were treated with sulfapyridine. Sulfathiazole and sulfadiazine, however, seem to be just as effective and in too many cases just as ineffective as sulfapyridine.

The average dose of the sulfonamides should probably be between four and eight grams in 24 hours. Much larger doses have been employed. Dick described a patient who received 40 grams of sodium sulfadiazine intravenously at a single dose. The patient developed marked signs of renal insufficiency but eventually recovered, both from the kidney complications and from the endocarditis. In two instances we have given sodium sulfadiazine intravenously, in doses from 15 to 30 grams and repeated the dose two or three times weekly. The patients showed evidence of kidney damage immediately after the injection but no alarming symptoms developed. Neither patient recovered, although these large doses with resulting sulfadiazine blood values of 50 to 90 mg. per 100 cc. produced a definite reduction in the number of streptococci in the circulating blood. Such dosage is however, unquestionably dangerous and in the light of our present knowledge should not be employed except as a last resort and only where there is no obvious kidney damage present. One of our recent patients who has now been well for one year took 10 grams of sulfamerazine daily for two months, with no bad effects.

Kelson and White in 1939 reported a series of seven patients with subacute endocarditis, treated with a combination of heparin and sulfapyridine. The heparin was employed with the idea that it might prevent the deposit of fresh fibrin and in that way assist the sulfapyridine in combating the organisms. Three recoveries were reported. Freidman later described two patients treated by this method with no result. This method Blumer states "should, I believe, be abandoned. There is, so far as I can discover, no evidence that heparin can dissolve thrombi, and following this treatment there are being reported an increasing number of deaths from subarachmoid, cerebral and cerebellar hemorrhages."

In our own experience the best results from sulfonamide therapy may be expected when it is employed as soon as possible after the diagnosis has been established. We have seen but one patient recover when the therapy was applied later than one month after the onset of the illness. Theoretically, it would seem that the drug would be most effective when the vegetations were small and not covered by large masses of fibrin. It has been shown experimentally by Friedman that the permeability of a fibrin-platelet mass to sulfanilamide and sulfapyridine is limited. These experiments are in accord with the clinical observation that patients with subacute bacterial endocarditis after treatment with sulfonamides often show a marked reduction in the number of streptococci in the circulating blood or even a sterilization of the blood stream for a period, without, however, healing the endocarditis.

It is difficult to speak confidently of prophylaxis in subacute bacterial endocarditis since the predisposing causes and the actual portal of entry of the infection are so commonly unknown. However, there are a few facts at our disposal from which we may learn important lessons.

In the overwhelming majority of cases the infection is engrafted upon a diseased heart valve or upon a congenital heart lesion. Individuals with old valvular defects, or congenital heart disease, should be watched with extreme care in any acute infection such as acute tonsilitis, pharyngitis, mastoiditis, endocervicitis or influenza. If the patient does not recover promptly, he should be watched carefully as a suspect case of endocarditis. An early diagnosis with prompt sulfonamide therapy may produce a brilliant therapeutic success.

The frequency with which S. *viridans* is found in pulpitis and apical disease of the teeth calls for prompt and radical treatment of such infections in individuals with valvular or congenital heart disease. Since the evidence is clear that some cases of subacute bacterial endocarditis develop soon after dental extractions, all persons with valvular or congenital heart disease should receive sulfonamide therapy before and after such extractions. The sulfonamides may be administered by mouth in daily doses of four grams of sulfapyridine, sulfathiazole or sulfadiazine two days before and two days after dental extractions. In addition, the sulfonamides in the form of powder may be dropped into the root socket.

A continued emphasis on the relationship between valvular disease, congenital heart disease and subacute bacterial endocarditis will in time lead to earlier diagnosis and more successful therapy.

The recent introduction of penicillin into our therapeutic armamentarium lead naturally to its employment in the treatment of endocarditis. Early reports were uniformly discouraging, a later one conspicuously encouraging. Personally, I have treated only one patient with penicillin. He received both penicillin and sulfamerazine, and is well six months later.

As we look back over the history of subacute bacterial endocarditis, we note that this disease has been sharply differentiated as a clinical entity for 45 years. For some 40 years investigators described its clinical course, studied its bacteriology and, with few exceptions, stressed its high mortality and the futility of treatment. Today we must admit that the percentage of recovery remains low and that the complete therapeutic answer has not been found. Yet we can surely take heart in the fact that more progress in treatment has been made in the past five years than in the previous forty, and that up to date the therapeutic possibilities of some 4,000 sulfonamide compounds remain to be explored, not to mention penicillin-like substances and derivatives. In the future we may look on subacute bacterial endocarditis with the same equanimity with which we now regard lobar pneumonia and epidemic meningitis, provided the diagnosis is made early.

BIBLIOGRAPHY

Andrewes, F. W. and Horder, T. J.: A Study of the Streptococci Pathogenic for Man. Lancet, 1906 II: 708, 775, 852.

Baillie, Matthew: The Morbid Anatomy of Some of the Most Important Parts of the Human Body, First American Edition. Barber & Southwick, Albany. 1795, p. 19.

Blumer, George: Remarks on Subacute Bacterial Endocarditis. West. J. Surg. Ob. & Gyn., XLIX: 406. 1941.

Blumer, George: Subacute Bacterial Endocarditis, Medicine, II: 105. 1923.

Bouilland, J. B.: Nouvelles recherches sur le rheumatisme articulaire, Paris, 1836.

Dick, George F.: Subacute Bacterial Endocarditis, Recovery Following Intravenous Sodium Sulfadiazine, J.A.M.A., CXX: 24. 1942.

Friedman, Myer: Use of Sulfanilamide and Sulfapyridine in Therapy of Subacute Bacterial Endocarditis, Arch. Int. Med., LXVII: 921. 1941.

Friedman, Myer, Latz, L. N. and Howell, K.: Experimental Endocarditis Due to Streptococcus Viridans, Arch. Int. Med., LXI: 95. 1938.

Helberg, Hjalmar: Ein Fall von Endocarditis ulcerosa puerperalis mit Pilzbildungen im Herzen (Mycosis endocardii) Virchows Arch. F. Path. Anat., LVI: 407. 1872.

Herrick, James B.: A Short History of Cardiology, Springfield, Thomas, 1942.

Libman, E.: A Study of the Endocardial Lesions of Subacute Bacterial Endocarditis, Am. J. M. Sc., CXLIV: 313. 1912.

Libman, E. and Celler, H. L.: The Etiology of Subacute Infective Endocarditis, Am. J. M. Sc., CXL: 516. 1910.

Lichtman, S. S. and Bierman, William: Subacute Bacterial Endocarditis: Present Status, J.A.M.A., CXV: 286. 1941.

Major, Ralph H.: Clinical and Bacteriological Studies on Endocarditis Lenta, Bull. Johns Hopkins Hosp., XXIII: 326. 1912.

Major, Ralph H.: The Effect of Sulphanilamide Compounds on Endocarditis, Am. J. M. Sc., CXCIX: 759. 1940.

Major, Ralph H. and Leger, Lee: Recovery from Subacute Infectious Endocarditis Following Prontosil Therapy, J.A.M.A., CXI: 1919. 1938.

Morgagni, John Baptist: The Seat and Causes of Distases Translated by Benjamin Alexander, London, 1769, Book II, Letter XXIV, Article 18, p. 730.

Oille, John A., Graham, Duncan, and Detweiler, H. K.: Streptococcus Bacteremia in Endocarditis, J.A.M.A., LXV:1159, 1915.

Oille, John A., Graham, Duncan and Detweiler, H. K.: Further Report on a Series of Recovered Cases of Subacute Bacterial Endocarditis, Trans. Assoc. Am. Phys., XXXIX: 227. 1924.

Riviere, Lazare: Opera, omnia Venice Viezziri, 1723, p. 526

Schottmuller, H.: Endocarditis Lenta, Munchen. Med. Wchnschn, 617, 697. 1910.

Schottmuller, H.: Die Artunterscheidung der fur den Menschen pathogenen Streptokokken durch Blutagar, Munchen. Med. Wchnschr, 1: 849, 909. 1903.

Smith, Carter, Sauls, H. Cliff and Stone, Charles F.: Subacute Bacterial Endocarditis due to Streptococcus Viridans, J.A.M.A., CXIX: 478. 1943.

Virchow, Rudolf: Ueber die akute Entzundung der Arterien, schaftlichen Medicin, Frankfurt, Meidinger, 1856, p. 705.

Virchow, Rudolf: Ueber die akuate Entzundung der Arterien, Virchows Arch. f. Path. Anat. Physiolog. und Klin. Med., I: 272. 1847.

Intestinal Obstruction In Childhood *

E. EUGENE RICE, M.D.
SHAWNEE, OKLAHOMA

Intestinal obstructions in children present problems that are not found in adults, and conditions which require early and adequate diagnosis if the life of the child is to be saved.

Obstructions of the intestine of the child may be classified as follows:

I. Mechanical

A. Intrinsic
1. Atresias and stenosis, due to errors of development
2. Enteric Cysts
3. Intussusceptions
4. Strictures, either tuberculous or enteric
5. Foreign bodies
6. Neoplasms
B. Extrinsic
1. Mal-rotation and Non-rotation of intestine
2. Peritoneal bands and hernias
3. Volvulus
4. Inflammatory masses, abscesses, tumors
5. Meckel's diverticulum, with cyst or ulcer

Probably the most practical method of classifying obstructions in the young, is to consider them from the age of occurrence.

The earliest cause of obstruction is the congential type, which is usually of the intrinsic variety, and due to failure of fetal development. Atresia, which is a complete obstruction of the bowel, or stenosis, which is a partial obliteration of the lumen of the bowel, are due to the failure of re-establishment of the lumen of the intestine during early fetal development.

The most common site of such a defect is in the terminal bowel involving the anus, or the rectum, and, fortunately, this is the area that is more amendable to treatment, while the next more frequent site is the duodenum.

Another type of intrinsic development error presents the intra - intestinal leaflets, either partial or complete, or complete absence of portions of the intestines or duplication of portions of the alimentary tract.

An accurate anatomical diagnosis may not be possible, but the symptoms of intestinal obstructions are usually very definite.

*Presented before the Annual State Meeting, April 26, 1944, Tulsa.

Congenital intestinal obstruction of the new-born should be considered when the infant begins to vomit persistently soon after birth. The vomitus at first contains swallowed amniotic fluid, mucus, and any colostrum, water, or milk that the child may have ingested, soon becoming bile stained, the vomiting projectile in character. Dehydration, loss of weight, and rapid malnutrition soon develop. Immediate examination and a diagnosis as accurately as possible of the probable site of the lesion should be made.

The anus and rectum should be examined and explored for signs of atresia or stenosis, and if found normal, a lesion higher up is suspected. A flat x-ray film of the abdomen will show an abnormal pattern of distended loops of bowel. A barium enema, or barium by mouth, may be indicated and necessary, for diagnosis.

Immediate exploratory laparotomy should be done, and an attempt made to relieve the obstruction. If the lesion involves the anus, it is often possible to reconstruct or open the anal orifice. Should there be a complete absence of the anus, or rectum, the operation indicated, is a colostomy. Lesions of the upper intestinal tract should be explored, and an attempt made at an anastomosis, rather than an enterostomy, as infants do not tolerate this type of surgery.

CONGENITAL HYPERTROPHIC PYLORIC STENOSIS

Congenital hypertrophic pyloric stenosis is the most common lesion causing intestinal obstruction during the first few weeks of life. This condition is usually encountered more frequently in males in the first born, and in the breast-fed, which have developed normally until the third to eighth week of life. At this time the child begins to vomit. The vomitus consists of the food just taken, and is of the usual type. Soon the vomiting becomes projectile, and the child vomits more than it has taken during the feeding, as some of the water and previous feedings has remained in its stomach. The vomitus is never bile-stained, which helps to differentiate the lesion from one occurring below the ampulla of Vater. Soon there is a failure of normal bowel movement, a marked loss of weight, dehydration, and malnutrition. Peristolic waves are visible over the stomach area. In most cases a tumor is palpable in the area of the pylorus.

An adequate early diagnosis of the condition present prevents a normal, healthy baby from becoming greatly dehydrated and malnourished, and offers excellent response to surgery. It is probably advisable to attempt medical treatment of the condition if it is not too severe, which usually consists of small, frequent feedings, with the use of atropine. If the response to the regime is not prompt and adequate, surgery offers a prompt cure of this condition.

The operation of choice is the Rhamstedt-Fredet procedure. An upper right rectus or mid-line incision is made with exposure and delivery of the pyloric tumor into the wound. A longitudinal incision extending through all the muscle fibers of the pyloric ring down to the pyloric mucosa, is made, care being taken that all the fibers are incised, the mucosa not damaged, and there is strict hemostasis. The omentum is sutured over the incised area, and the abdomen closed in the usual manner. Fluids by mouth can be started within a few hours after operation, and a small quantity of water, breast milk, or formula taken, and in a few days the child is back on its regular diet.

INTUSSUSCEPTION

Intussusception is essentially a pediatric disease, and by far the commonest cause of intestinal obstruction in infants. It is one of the few diseases of childhood where a few hours' delay in diagnosis may influence the prognosis so much.

The majority of cases occur in well-nourished infants. Seventy-five per cent occur during the first year of life, males predominating two to one. The on-set of this condition is usually very dramatic. There is usually no history of previous intestinal disturbances, where, without apparent cause, a normal, healthy child cries out, draws up its legs in pain, and shows signs of shock, becoming cold and clammy, with a sub-normal temperature. The episodes recur periodically, and soon the child vomits, and continues to vomit periodically, with the attacks of crying. The bowel movements which have previously been normal may, early in the disease continue to appear normal, but soon become scant, with mucus, and often blood in them.

As the disease advances, the sub-normal temperature may rise above normal. A palpable tumor can be felt in practically all cases. This mass is sausage-shaped, usually found above the umbilicus, usually movable, and may, or may not be tender. Rectal examination should be made in all cases, and at times a mass may be felt rectally, and in

practically all cases blood-stained mucus is revealed on the examining finger. Any type of intussusception may occur in children, but by far the most frequent is the ileocecal. Non-surgical methods rarely give adequate reduction of the intussusception. Attempts by the use of enemas or air injections may reduce the lesion in some cases. Laparotomy is indicated in the greater majority of cases, and should be done early before dehydration and intoxication becomes apparent. In most cases the condition can be reduced with ease if the lesion has not been present over a long period of time, and little swelling has taken place. Mechanical removal of one portion of the bowel from the other is adequate without attempt at immobilization of any portion of the bowel. In the late cases intestinal resection may be necessary.

FOREIGN BODIES

Foreign bodies in the alimentary tract of children are not uncommon, as the child will often swallow objects that will cause obstruction, and if they are not passed spontaneously, may need intervention for their removal.

NEOPLASMS AND STRICTURES

Neoplasms and strictures of inflammatory intrinsic nature are rare in children, but must be considered in a differential diagnosis. The extrinsic type of obstructions in children is more unusual than in adults.

PERITONEAL BANDS AND HERNIAS

Peritoneal bands are due, usually, to some congenital abnormality, most often found in the upper abdomen which may cause obstruction by external pressure on the intestine. Hernias are not often found in the very young sufficient to cause obstruction, as the hernial ring is usually pliable and adequate so that strangulation of the intestine does not usually occur.

MAL-ROTATION

Mal-rotation or non-rotations of the intestine are usually due to failure of the midgut loop to return from the umbilical cord during the first few weeks of fetal life, and often produces congenital hernia into the cord. There may be an incomplete or abnormal rotation upon its return with the duodenocolic isthmus remaining narrow, and with the restraining force missing, there is a marked tendency to the occurrence of torsion or volvulus.

VOLVULUS

The symptoms of volvulus are usually found in older children past one year of age, and is characterized by the cardinal symptoms of obstruction, namely, abdominal pains, constipation, or obstipation, nausea and vomiting. The lesion is usually characterized by sudden on-set, with early symptoms of shock, followed by an increase in the temperature and blood count. Often the anatomical diagnosis is obscure until laparotomy is performed.

MECKEL'S DIVERTICULUM, WITH CYST OR ULCER

Meckel's diverticulum is not infrequently the site of an intestinal obstruction. There may be an acute inflammation of the diverticulum resembling acute appendicitis, with the symptoms of inflammatory obstruction.

Cysts of Meckel's diverticulum, although uncommon, do occur, and bleeding ulcers in the diverticulum may be a cause of the abdominal symptoms.

ACUTE APPENDICITIS

Acute appendicitis is the most common inflammatory lesion occurring in children.

This condition should always be considered in any child, particularly those past two or three years of age where there is any evidence of inflammatory or obstructive symptoms in the abdomen. Unlike young adults, the symptoms in children are not always typical, particularly when seen early. Frequently there is a predominance of one or more symptoms. Vomiting is often greatly exaggerated early in this disease, and may be difficult to differentiate from the vomiting occurring with intestinal obstruction.

Constipation is usually very common and persistent in acute appendicitis. The temperature in children is usually markedly elevated during the initial stage, and there is an early increase in the leucocyte and polymorphonuclear cells. Appendiceal abcess results frequently in neglected cases of acute appendicitis, and is very frequently a cause of inflammatory obstruction.

A history of an acute attack is important, and associated with the finding of rigidity, tenderness, and a palpable mass in the right lower quadrant is sufficient to make a diagnosis of inflammatory obstruction.

There are a few important generalizations that are characteristic of congenital obstructions in children.

1. There is an exceedingly high mortality rate due to the delay in establishing the correct diagnosis which is in direct proportion to the age of the child.

2. Persistent vomiting occurring shortly after birth in infancy, or during infancy, should make one suspicious of an intestinal abnormality. Errors of rotation, do not present manifestations of obstruction until later in life when some such complication as volvulus occurs, while intrinsic defects present immediate obstructive symptoms.

3. Accurate and anatomical diagnosis is seldom possible, but the evidence of obstruction is often definite and indicates the necessity for surgery.

4. Operation offers the only satisfactory method of treatment, and the surgeon must be able to recognize the abnormality and correct it in the most direct and gentle manner. Children tolerate dehydration very poorly, and should never be operated on until it is overcome, and it should be remembered that normal fluid balance cannot be maintained satisfactorily until the obstruction is relieved.

Aids in diagnosis are:

(a) Persistent vomiting of bile indicates a lesion below the ampulla of Vater, and non-bile stained fluid above that area.

(b) A flat film over the abdomen showing an abnormal pattern of distended loops of bowel, with the small bowel predominately on the right suggests the presence of an error in rotation.

(c) Radio opaque material is apparently safe, and if necessary, may offer valuable information.

The treatment of intestinal obstructions in children like obstructions in adults, in the majority of cases, is surgical. Although children stand surgery remarkably well, there are certain important factors that should be borne in mind, and certain preoperative conditions which should be met.

The preoperative and postoperative care are very important, and should be under the direction of a pediatrician, or other qualified person. The importance of giving fluids before and after the operation cannot be stressed too strongly. The results of an operation depend often on how thoroughly this is carried out. Enough fluids in the form of five per cent glucose in normal saline, or Ringer's Solution, should be given to combat dehydration and acidosis, and if necessary, citrated blood should be given. The important thing to remember is that the child should be in the best possible condition before going to the operating room. Body heat should always be maintained by external applications of heat, and the pain should be controlled by the simplest forms of sedatives.

In conclusion, an early adequate diagnosis of intestinal obstruction in children is essential where delay in diagnosis may greatly affect the outcome. With adequate preoperative care, and adequate fluids in combination with early, gentle, adequate surgery, means that the obstruction can be relieved, acidosis prevented, and the life of the child saved.

BIBLIOGRAPHY

1. Lewis, Dean: Practice of Surgery, Vol. VII, Chap. 7, 1-46.
2. Glover, Donald M. and Hamann, Carl A.: Intestinal

Obstruction in the Newborn due to Congenital Anomalies, Ohio State Medical Journal, 36: 833 (August) 1940.

3. Duckett, J. W.: Intestinal Obstruction in the Newborn, Annals of Surgery, 116: 321 (September) 1942.

4. Flynn, J. G.: Hypertrophic Pyloric Stenosis in Infants, A result of Birth Injury, Texas State Journal of Medicine 37: 367, (September) 1941.

5. Williams, Howard: The Surgical Treatment of Congenital Pyloric Stenosis of Infancy: A Review of 400 cases, Medical Journal of Australia, 1: 303 (March 14) 1942.

6. Marinacci, Sertorio: Hypertrophic Stenosis in the Newborn, Extramucasal Pylorotomy, Il Policlinico (sez. prat.) 46: 1826, (October 16) 1939.

7. Bombardier, J. B.: Hypertrophic Stenosis of the Pylorus, L' Union Medicale du Canada, 71: 589, (June) 1942.

8. Bellini, O.: Congenital Stenosis of the Jejunum of a High Degree in an Infant of 14 Months, Cured by Intestinal Resection, Il Polichnico, (sez .chir.) 46: 417 (September 15) 1939.

9. Rosenblum, Philip: Intussusception, III, Medical Journal, 74: 309 (October) 1938.

10. Ireland, Jay: Treatment of Intussusception, Archives of Surgery, 43: 418 (September) 1941.

11. Goldman, Lawrence and Elman, Robert: Spontaneous Reduction of Acute Intussusception in Children, American Journal of Surgery, 49: 259 (August) 1940.

12. Carley, A. W.: Diagnosis of the Acute Surgical Abdomen in Children, Ohio State Medical Journal, 35: 1056 (October) 1939.

13. Chaffin, Lawrence: Surgical Emergencies during Childhood Caused by Meckel's Diverticulum, Annals of Surgery 113: 47, (January) 1941.

No Doubt Coronary

Working from eight in the morning till sometimes near midnight, Dr. Abercrombie found time to write in his carriage, and when he started from home by mistake without a light, wrote his notes in the dark. Little is known about this great doctor's daily life—he who was so careful of others' lives being, we are told, nobly careless of his own. One who spoke of him as a "living epistle," thought Dr. Abercrombie, like an epistle of St. John, "pure, profound, and illuminated with the spirituality of heaven." He died suddenly, of an unusual form of heart complaint, in November, 1894, while his carriage stood at his door in York Place, at ten in the morning, waiting for him to go his rounds. In his portraits he appears as a fine-looking man, of strong features, with a remarkably pleasing expression of face, serene and happy. His pleasant look, as that of one lifted above all care, was said to be distinctly beautiful as he lay in his coffin. A medallion is carved upon his gravestone, which is said to be a remarkably good likeness of this Christian gentleman and physician, whose riches never caused him to forget his duty to suffering humanity.—*Aberdeen Doctors, At Home and Abroad, page 113. Ella Hill Burton Rodger. William Blackwood and Sons. Edinburgh and London.* 1913.

Peptic Ulcers and Allied Conditions*

JAMES C. CAIN, LT. COL. M.C.

CAMP GRUBER, OKLAHOMA

One of the most common symptoms experienced by man is that of so-called "Dyspepsia." Unfortunately, too often the busy physician, in desperation, labels those cases as "peptic ulcers" 'and begins a somewhat unsuccessful ulcer diet. In the army, the medical officer has an excellent opportunity to practice almost ideal medicine as far as the diagnosis of gastro-intestinal diseases is concerned. Patients with symptoms related to the gastro-intestinal system are thoroughly studied by gastro-intestinal, gall bladder and colon roentgenology. Procotoscopic examinations and laboratory procedures are used when indicated.

The symptoms arising from the gastro-intestinal tract are frequent, often quite vague, and due to a host of etiological factors. The gastro-intestinal tract has three primary functions: motor, secretory, and absorptive. It is quite obvious that if any of these functions are seriously interferred with, the patient will have distress of some type. Many factors may interfere with one or more of these primary functions. Ulcers, new growths, bacterial infections, and parasite infestations are examples of the numerous factors that may influence mechanically and

*Delivered at the Annual State Meeting in Tulsa, April 26, 1944.

functionally the actions of the digestive tract. It is known that symptoms from the gastro-intestinal tract may be caused reflexly by gall bladder disease, heart disease, urinary tract disease, conditions involving the brain, and toxicity from various diseases. Disturbance of the secretory function is noted in various types of choronic gastritis, pernicious anemia, and many of the vitamin deficiencies. Probably the greatest single factor that disturbs the functions of the gastro-intestinal tract is psychogenic in character. It would be futile to try to discuss in detail all the factors that disturb the digestive tract. An attempt will be made to differentiate a few of the most common conditions that cause abdominal distress and to offer some suggestions as to aids in determining the significance of certain symptoms.

During 1943 a total of 122 patients with duodenal ulcers and 11 with gastric ulcers were seen at our hospital. One hundred and one of the patients with duodenal and nine of the patients with gastric ulcers had symptoms prior to entering the military service. Two cases of chronic hypertrophic antral gastritis were diagnosed. A gastroscope was not available, and undoubtedly some cases of chronic gastritis were not diagnosed. Because of the age group involved, these were probably very few. Only one case of allergic gastritis was encountered. Two cases of carcinoma of the stomach were found during the past year. Both of these were in patients over the age of fifty. Some soldiers had psychoneurosis with disabling major psychosomatic gastro-intestinal complaints. A detailed discussion of the manner in which the diagnosis of psychoneurosis was made is obviously beyond the scope of this paper. In this series of cases all patients were carefully studied by Moorman P. Prosser, Major, Medical Corps and his Staff on the Neuropsychiatric Section. A detailed personality study and a careful psychiatric evaluation were made in each case. Many patients who were not psychoneurotics complained of psychosomatic gastro-intestinal symptoms, but these cases were not included in this study. Table No 1 shows a comparison of our statistics with those found at the Medical Clinic of the University of Pennsylvania Hospital[1].

TABLE I

CAUSES OF CHRONIC GASTRO-INTESTINAL SYMPTOMS

Disease	Number of Cases *	Percent of Cases *	Number of Cases **	Percent of Cases **
Gall Bladder Disease	14	3.2	787	30.9
Duodenal Ulcer	122	28.1	624	24.5
Functional Disease ***	280	64.9	642	25.2
Chronic Gastritis	3	0.7	123	4.8
Stomach Ulcer	11	2.5	105	4.3
Stomach Cancer	2	0.4	102	4.0
Duodenitis	1	0.2	99	3.9
Appendicitis	0	0	60	2.4
TOTAL	433	100.0	2542	100.0

*Cases admitted to this hospital.

**From Miller, T. Grier "The Cause of Indigestion and Their Recognition."

The New England Journal of Medicine 224, pp. 537-540. March 27, 1941.

***Includes functional diseases of both the upper and lower gastrointestinal tract.

There are a number of typical syndromes that might be briefly summarized. The peptic ulcers are divided into two classes, those involving the stomach and those involving the duodenum. It cannot be emphasized too strenuously that the duodenal ulcer and the gastric ulcer are two entirely different diseases, and their significance and prognosis are entirely different. The patient with a duodenal ulcer usually lives a tense, perhaps unhappy life with distress in the spring and fall of the year. His pain occurs between meals and wakes him at night. He lives a long profitable life, and frequently he makes quite a success. The only danger to his life is that the ulcer may give rise to perforation, obstruction, or hemorrhage.

The gastric ulcer, although usually described in textbooks as a fairly classical syndrome, did not present any typical symptoms in our group. Several patients showed the typical "food-comfort-pain-comfort rhythm" with gnawing, dull, high epigastric pain slightly to the left of the midline, with frequent vomiting and gaseous distress; but the inconsistency of the syndrome is probably its most characteristic feature. It was not difficult to distinguish the gastric ulcer from the duodenal ulcer. Most of the patients with gastric ulcers were severe psychoneurotics, and the additional roentgenological evidence of an ulcer usually came as a complete surprise. It is of great importance to remember that the psychoneurotic patient may also have organic disease. The gastric ulcer is often acute or subacute and can be cured by adequate treatment in a relatively short time. In our series of eleven gastric ulcers, seven were located in the prepyloric area, three on the lesser curvature, and one on the greater curvature. The gastric ulcer may be complicated by obstruction, hemorrhage or perforation, but the major concern is that the so-called gastric ulcer may be a carcinoma. Allen and Welch[2], in their series found 100 per cent of the ulcers in the greater curvature and 65 per cent of the ulcers in the prepyloric area to be malignant. Because of the possibility of malignancy the gastric ulcer becomes an emergency, and the greatest of care must be exerted to be sure of the diagnosis. Our policy is to repeat the roentgenogram on these men each week while keeping them on a rigid diet consisting primarily of milk and cream with either alkaline powders or aluminum hydroxide. We transfer patients that do not recover in 3 to 5 weeks to a hospital where a gastroscopic examination m a y be done. If the lesion is in the prepyloric area or on the greater curvature, operative intervention may be necessary.

Gall bladder disease has been encountered in only 14 patients during the past year. Of this group only three patients had cholelithiasis. The typical syndrome of recurrent attacks of excruciating right upper quadrant pain with radiation to the angle of the right scapula, fever, chill, nausea, vomiting, and later jaundice was rarely encountered. This combination of symptoms was considered as diagnostic of common duct stone, requiring surgical investigation. The other 11 patients showed a non-functioning gall bladder by x-ray, with rather vague symptoms of nausea, vomiting, belching, fat intolerance, and right upper quadrant pain with tenderness. Frank jaundice was rare in the cholecystitis without stones, but these patients usually had a high normal or slightly elevated icterus index. Operative procedures in cholecystitis without stones were not considered indicated. All of these patients were treated by a conservative medical routine with satisfactory results. It is interesting that although 348 cholecystrograms were made, only 14 showed evidence suggestive of gall bladder disease. This is in district contradiction to statistics so frequently quoted from other sources. Dr. Miller[1] in his series of 2,542 cases of dyspepsia studied at the Medical Clinic of the University of Pennsylvania Hospital, found 30.9 per cent due to gall bladder disease. The obvious answer is that our patients are of a younger age group and are males. Here again the greatest problem is to differentiate organic gall bladder disease from psychosmatic abdominal distress.

The irritable colon syndrome, while probably only a synonym of anxiety psychoneurosis, should constantly be remembered. This syndrome usually occurs in a thin, fearful, restless, apprehensive individual. He complains of numerous vague symptoms such as nausea, belching, distension, excessive flatulence, and irregular bowel action. There may be diarrhea ranging from 10 to 20 stools a day or only one or two liquid stools immediately after meals or when excited. The stools often show excessive amounts of mucus but seldom have visible blood. Constipation may be a symptom. Dull, boring, aching lower abdominal pain is present, and a tender contracted colon can frequently be palpated. The patients usually show other evidence of psychoneurosis such as nervousness, insomnia, fatigability, and vasomotor reactions. It is our policy to diagnose each such case as a psychoneurosis of an anxiety type rather than to dignify this syndrome with a specific name such as irritable colon.

From the above brief discussion of a few of the fairly classical syndromes it is obvious that the gastro-interologist's chief diagnostic problem is eliminating psychogenic conditions. To recognize that the patient with a duodenal ulcer, a gastric ulcer, or gall bladder disease may also have a severe psychoneurosis, is of paramount importance. The question arises, did the patient have organic disease prior to or as a result of psychoneurosis. The only method of accurate diagnosis is through a detailed, thorough, and systematic history. The diagnosis of psychoneurosis must be made with great care. It requires prolonged observation and a detailed personality and psychiatric evaluation. At this hospital, cases suspected of having a psychoneurosis are transferred to the neuropsychiatric section and carefully studied. Although practically all psychoneurotic patients have psychosomatic complaints, not all patients with psychosomatic complaints fulfill the pattern necessary for a diagnosis of psychoneurosis. We insist that the diagnosis of psychoneurosis be a positive diagnosis and not merely a diagnosis of exclusion. Leading questions must be carefully avoided. Many patients with gastro-intestinal complaints subconsciously try to please the physician and will agree to symptoms suggested in a leading manner. The patient must tell his own story with enough questions asked to keep him on the subject. After this, specific questions may be asked. A detailed past-history, family history and social history are obtained. A brief personality and psychiatric study is made by the gastroenterology section and all questionable cases of psychoneurosis or of patients suffering from psychosomatic symptoms are transferred to the neuropsychiatric section for detailed study. Our policy is to use the following outline in the study of individuals complaining of chronic gastrointestinal symptoms:

1. Chief complaints.
2. Onset:
   a. Exact date of original attack.
   b. Onset of original attack and following attacks.
   c. Factors existing during and prior to each attack.
      (1) Emotional
      (2) Physical
3. Description of Complaints:
   a. Description of pain, eg., sharp, dull, tearing, aching, boring, throbbing, burning, nauseating, etc.
   b. Accurate location of the pain by outlining it with one finger on the skin.
   c. Superficial or deep pain.
   d. Extent and transmission of the pain.
   e. Degree of disability caused by the pain.
4. Occurance:
   a. Continuous, periodic, or intermittent.
   b. Description of a typical day.
   c. Relation of symptoms to defecation, passing of flatus, belching, and vomiting.
   d. When last completely free of symptoms.
5. Precipitating factors:
   a. Food. Specific foods that cause symptoms.
   b. Hunger.
   c. Physical factors.
   d. Nervous factors.
6. Relief:
   a. Alkalies, milk, amphyjel.
   b. Food—name specific food.
   c. Defecating or passing flatus.
   d. Vomiting or belching.
   e. Aspirin or morphine sulphate.

7. Association symptoms:
   a. Nausea, vomiting, belching, pyrosis, borborygmus, bloating, flatulence, constipation, diarrhea (Describe character of stool) dysphagia, jaundice, hemorrhage, tenderness, residual soreness, visable peristalsis and tumefaction.

8. Progression:
   a. Change in character of complaints.
   b. Effect of treatment, medical or surgical or both.

The importance of an accurate detailed history cannot be over emphasized for only in this manner can a logical diagnosis be reached.

Unfortunately in the army one encounters a problem not found in civilian practice except possibly in compensation industrial cases. Soldiers are away from home and their loved ones. They are performing duties foreign to those they have been trained for since youth, and they are homesick and unhappy. Often they are forced to perform physical feats of a very tiring, boring, and frequently dangerous character. Their financial compensation is slight in comparison to that received by civilians. With this background, the subconscious desire to get well and leave the protection and comfort of the hospital may be minimal. It is very important to keep patients with vague gastro-intestinal complaints out of the hospital and study them thoroughly as out patients. In our experience, psychosomatic complaints are very contagious. It might be well to emphasize that we are actually dealing with psychosomatic complaints and not malingering. Malingering is rarely seen. One of the fundamental factors in treatment of the psychoneurotic is to alter the individual's undesirable situation to one that is acceptable to him. This is obviously impossible in many cases in the army.

It might be of interest to mention a few symptoms frequently encountered and discuss briefly their significance. As has been noted by many investigators, pain of a burning nature is rarely organic. If the pain is constant for days or weeks without remission, it is practically always functional. Pain that flits from one location to another is seldom of importance. Surprisingly enough, duodenal ulcers seldom cause pain on awakening in the morning. The location of the pain from gastro-intestinal lesions is important. Characteristically the pain of a duodenal ulcer is in the mid epigastric area approximately five centimeters above the umbilicus with some tendency to be slightly to the left of the midline. The pain of the gastric ulcer is often higher in the epigastric region and slightly to the right of the mid-line. Usually when the peptic ulcer is complicated by hemorrhage, the patient becomes relatively free from pain. Not infrequently gastric and duodenal ulcers will perforate or hemorrhage without the patient having any previous warning symptoms suggestive of a peptic ulcer. The gastro-jejunal ulcer pain is usually in the mid-umbilical region with some tendency to be more to the left. Small bowel lesions refer their pain to the umbilical region. Colon pain tends to be referred along the course of a colon and to the region below the umbilicus. Vomiting is a frequent symptom of both functional and organic gastro-intestinal disease. Vomiting that occurs immediately after eating and that is precipitated by almost any type of food is usually functional. This is particularly true in the daily after breakfast vomiting that has been present for years without loss of weight. Care must be exercised to rule out esophageal stricture and diaphragmatic hernia. It is helpful to remember that cancers in young individuals are usually of a high degree of malignancy and lead to rapid cachexia and an early fatal outcome. If a young man has had gastro-intestinal symptoms for over a year without showing definite evidence of physical deterioration, malignancy probably does not exist.

DISCUSSION

ARTHUR W. WHITE, M.D.

Lt. Colonel Cain has given us quite a comprehensive discussion, but in order to stay within the time limit given me, I will confine my remarks to a restricted phase of the subject, that of development and diagnosis as found in civilian practice. I do, however, wish to endorse what Colonel Cain said as to the multiplicity of indirect causes and to the changes found in the chemistry and physiology of the upper digestive tract, due to various diseases. On the other hand I beg leave to take with the statement that peptic ulcer in the stomach is a widely different disease from that of duodenal ulcer. The same basic condition produces a peptic ulcer regardless of the point at which there is a breaking down of the mucosa.

It has long been accepted by the unbaised student that the corrosive or irritating action of the hydrochloric acid is the immediate cause as well as the continuing cause of ulcer. Wagenstein,[3] in 1942, reported producing all of the ulcer types in dogs by the continuous use of Histidine, refuting the statement frequently made that hydrochloric acid has no bearing on the ulcer question and re-enforcing the proposition first advocated by Sippy, and the premise on which most successful treatment has been carried out for several years. Recently it has been emphasized, notably in the teachings of Lehey, "that pylorospasm is the most prominent factor, but there is such an interdependency between the pylorus and the glandular function of the stomach that this is, in most cases another form of expression.

To one who has had an opportunity to observe the action of the pylorus in its relation to the hydrochloric acid content, in any great number of instances, it is obvious that while there are extra-gastric influences on the pyloric action and antral muscles, the neutralization of the hydrochloric acid sooner or later brings a complete relaxation of the pylorus in at least 80 per cent of cases. Having a like influence on the normal as well as the ulcer affected stomach.

In the normal stomach the ratio between the ingredients of the gastric juice is constant, while in the ulcer type of patient there is always an imbalance, except possibly at those times at which the patient is entering the quiescent stage following a spring or fall exacerbation of symptoms, i. e., after the subsidence of symptoms. The hydrochloric acid being out of the normal ratio and showing either a relative or absolute increase, or both. Further, the normal period of digestion is approximately five hours, at the end of which time, in the normal stomach there is found practically no free hydrochloric acid. In the ulcer type, however, there is found an amount of hydrochloric acid equal to or greater than that found in the same case at the height of digestion, i. e., one hour after a carbohydrate meal. In other words there is a definite tendency to a continuing secretion of digestive juice during the twenty-four hours and not limited to the normal digestive period, a condition found often before a defect can be demonstrated, this to my mind is the crucial factor, as was shown by Wagenstein. Hypersecretion, especially noted in the latter part of the day or during the night, while not so constant, is also an important consideration.

The symptoms from this type of trouble should be obvious, however, it is a notable fact that often there are not characteristic symptoms. We are reminded of the great number of healed ulcers found at autopsies, there having been no symptoms during life to make one think of ulcer; of the number of cases in which the first evidence was hemorrhage or perforation; again, of the number of cases which present more or less classical symptoms when no ulcer could be demonstrated at the operating table. So that a careful correlation of all of the possible evidences obtainable is necessary to arrive at a dependable conclusion.

Pain, the most outstanding symptom, when present, may be one of two types and the analysis of this symptom is of most importance. Chemical distress, often referred to as ulcer pain is undoubtedly what the above term implies and is associated with the chemical state of the stomach. This type of pain occurs at a time distant from the ingestion of a meal. The threshold being determined by the height of hydrochloric acid secretion, although the presence of an ulcer seems to lower that threshold. A different type of pain, appearing during or immediately after a meal, is of mechanical origin and does not occur except in an advanced state of distruction of the mucosa.

Palmer and Heinz in m o s t conclusive studies of the manner in which pain arises, the site of origin, and to the nature of the stimulus, found, "That ulcer pain arises from the site of the lesion and is not dependent on the pylorospasm, gastrospasm, or intragastric pressure, but on the presence of a stimulus acting on the pain producing mechanism in the region of the ulcer—and that the increased irritability depends on the continued action of acid gastric juice; conversely, desensitization may be produced by continued neutralization of the hydrochloric acid. The action of the stimulus may be mechanical due to the peristaltic traction, or chemical due to the highly acid chyme, but in either case the action of the stimulus is probably exerted directly on the nerves rendered hyper-irritable resulting from the destructive action of the acid gastric juice."

All peptic ulcers are found on or near the lesser curvature of the stomach or in the pylorus, or the duodenum. Any ulcer having the appearance of peptic ulcer occurring on the greater curvature is not a peptic ulcer, but is malignant, luetic or traumatic. The blood supply in this region and inferior gastric arteries, the branches taking on a cork-screw course in the walls of the stomach so that the upright position brings about more interference with the blood supply of the affected area by changing the position of the stomach. Again, interference, which may be due to pressure or position, with the emptying of the duodenum plays a definite part in bringing about a disturbance of the gastric secretions, in addition to an increased exposure of the duodenum to the corrosive action of its contents. It has been impressed upon me that a determination of the position of the duodenum is an important factor, this can only be done by the use of the fluoroscope.

The x-ray is of great value as one of the procedures in obtaining information as to the condition of the stomach following the plan developed particularly by Akerlund and Berg, i. e., the mucosal relief technique. The fluoroscope is of special value, as muscular action is not registered in films and the duodenum is rarely seen on a film. Further, the defect in an ulcer may not be so situated as to be exposed to the film when taken in the ordinary position.

SUMMARY

1. Attention was directed to the frequency with which functional factors caused abdominal distress among soldiers.

2. The importance of a detailed, systematic, accurate history was emphasized.

3. The significance of certain common symptoms was discussed.

BIBLIOGRAPHY

1. Miller, T. Grier: The Causes of Indigestion and Their Recognition. New England Journal of Medicine, 224, pp. 537-540. 1941.

2. Allen, A. W. & Welch, C. E.: Gastric Ulcer—The Significance of this Diagnosis and its Relationship to Cancer. Annals of Surgery, 122, pp. 339-343. 1940.

3. Reported at College of Physicians Meeting, February, 1942.

4. Palmer, W. L.: Journal of the A.M.A., Vol. 119, No. 15. August 8, 1942.

5. Archives of Internal Medicine, Vol. 53, page 269. February, 1934.

Psychiatry In Oklahoma--Historical Aspect[*]

CARL T. STEEN, M.D.

NORMAN, OKLAHOMA

For the purpose of this article the whole of the territory now embraced in the State of Oklahoma has been considered, and all of those people residing within this territory concerning whom a history could be obtained will be discussed. The subject will be taken up as nearly chronologically as possible. While the history embraces a time period of slightly more than a hundred years and begins after many other communities had well established systems for the care of their mentally afflicted citizens, still it is interesting and very well worth recording. It has seemed justifiable to depart from the strictly historical in a few instances to give an insight into the environment and line of thought of the times as development proceeded.

EARLY DIFFICULTIES

In earlier times mystery and superstition, especially among the Indians, added to the difficulty of travel and lack of hospital facilities, made the lot of the insane person extremely doleful. All imagineable forms of primitive restraint were employed and treatment was necessarily likewise primitive.

The Federal government, as long as it was guardian of the Indians, made an effort in extreme cases to aid in the care of their insane. Accordingly we find as our earliest recorded account a bill rendered for services as follows:

"The United States to To Ke o tack (a Sac woman) Dr. July 1st to keeping, feeding and taking care of Nah to an a che

[*]Delivered at the Annual State Meeting in Tulsa, April 26, 1944.

ke (a Fox Indian) who was insane, 30 days until his death at the rate of $1 (sic) per day—$30.00."

The Sac woman was paid on July 25, 1854 and acknowledged receipt.

The Indian agents of pre-statehood days were quite often hard pressed in their efforts to hospitalize their psychotic wards. The states to the north and east, Kansas, Iowa and Missouri, as well as private hospitals of that region, were frequently requested to provide hospital facilities. These requests were in most instances denied for various reasons, usually because they were unable to take non-resident patients.

Among the tribes inhabiting this region and needing assistance were the Sac and Fox and Shawnees; the Cheyennes, Arapahoes and Conchos from near El Reno and Anadarko; the Pawnees and Poncas[2]. The Choctaws had a pension system in 1888, providing for the payment of $50.00 for the relief of the crippled, blind and idiotic, at the discretion of the court[3]. The Cherokees also had a similar system which was discarded in 1875.

HOME FOR THE DEAF, DUMB, BLIND AND INSANE

The Cherokees, recognizing the extreme need of the situation, in 1872 began plans for establishing an asylum near Tahlequah, but made no distinction between the needs of the different types of patients and so placed the deaf, dumb, blind and insane in one category. This earliest of organized hospitals in the now State of Oklahoma, began functioning in March of 1877, having been constructed with funds received from sale of land in the "Kansas Strip[4]." The little haven was beset by many trials, among them financial loads, inexperience of personnel, and some degree of politics. It continued to function until 1908, when its insane were removed to Norman.

THE NON-CITIZEN INSANE

Not only were the Indians beset, but there were quite a few white people within their territory who were insane. Dew M. Wisdom, Agent, had in 1897, stated that the number was approximately 200. Among them were ten or twelve bad cases of incurable insane, whom he could only recommend to the charity of friends, although they needed the care of the government. The letters he received indicated that the condition of the insane, if incorporated in a report would present a harrowing picture of sorrow that would make the "very stones cry out for pity."

One method of caring for these individuals was to charge them with crime and turn them o v e r to the Department of Justice, which in turn sent them to Washington to Saint Elizabeths' Hospital. There was no authority for the restraint of insane persons. After considerable delay, the Secretary of the Interior was authorized to make arrangements for the care and support of the insane persons in the Indian Territory by an act approved April 28, 1904. The Shawnee Herald of January 20, 1905, had this article headed: "Car Load of Crazy Persons Being Taken from Muskogee to a St. Louis Institution." "The first car load of insane persons ever taken out of the Indian Territory left here yesterday over the Missouri, Kansas and Texas, for St. Louis. The patients were in charge of D. H. Kelsey, Chief Clerk to Indian Inspector Wright. They will be taken to St. Vincent's Institution for the insane at St. Louis, which has a special contract to care for white insane persons of the Indian Territory." This arrangement lasted for four years only, by which time statehood had arrived, November 16, 1907, and the non-citizen had become a citizen and entitled to the haven of a state hospital.

CANTON ASYLUM FOR INSANE INDIANS

As only one of the Indian Tribes had elected to build an asylum, the Federal Government established in,1898 an asylum for insane Indians at Canton, South Dakota, in the heart of the Indian Country of that region, but to which Indians of this locality were eligible. Dr. R. H. Hummer, Superintendent of the Asylum, in 1912 reported that of 126 patients admitted since 1898, 27 were from Oklahoma, probably more than from any other state[5].

Dr. Emil Kraepelin visited the institution about 1927, and told Dr. Humner that there was no record of a single case of general paralysis of the insane among the Indians (and other aboriginal races.) Dr. Humner was inclined to doubt this because he had knowledge of two cases in which this clinical diagnosis had been made[7]. The last appropriation for this institution was for the year ending June 30, 1933[8]. Following this the patients and records were sent to St. Elizabeths' Hospital, Washington, and on the records of our present state hospitals are the names of many who had been at Canton.

OAK LAWN RETREAT — JACKSONVILLE, ILLINOIS

The Territory of Oklahoma, created under the "Organic Act" on May 2, 1890[9], took as its first step towards care of the insane, the signing of a contract with Dr. G. C. McFarland, of Jacksonville, Illinois. This agreement, made November 5, 1891, by Governor George W. Steele, was in effect until 1895, and provided among other things for the payment of $300.00 per patient per year, Dr. McFarland to pay for transportation of the patients, the Territory to pay the officers' transportation expenses. The expense, however, seemed to be such a burden to the young Territory that agitation began to return these patients home. The fruit of this agitation was the formation of a company by Oklahoma City business men, who in 1895, made a contract to keep them at the same rate per annum as the Oak Lawn people.

NORMAN SANITARIUM COMPANY

High Gate Female College, first college to be opened in Oklahoma Territory, a Methodist School located just east of Norman, was established in 1890, but before it had gone far on its way the State University was opened, September 15, 1892, "Tuition free, full corps professors, use of a library and apparatus from the first" and by 1894 the college was abandoned[10]. The Oklahoma Sanitarium Company secured the building, having made a three year contract from March 5, 1895, at a rate of $300.00 per annum.[11]

The first patient recorded at Norman was June 15, 1895. On July 26, 108 patients arrived from Jacksonville, Ill.[12] Dr. T. S. Galbraith, of Indiana, was then first manager. Dr. Threadgill, the first superintendent, according to Daily Oklahoman of April 30, 1898, contracted for the care of all insane Indians in the United States, and accordingly six were brought from South Dakota. In 1901 there had been admitted twelve others, from Indian Territory. The Governor was to appoint three physicians who were to make quarterly trips to the Sanitarium, to inspect and to pass upon dismissals[13]. In 1903 the

Sanitarium Company contracted to keep a part of the insane convicts returned from the state prison at Lansing, Kansas.[41]

The Sanitarium Company was to remain in action until its properties were purchased by the State on July 1, 1915,[15] since which time it has been the Central Oklahoma State Hospital. As was to be expected, the charge of graft, corruption, cruelty and mismanagement was frequently heard. As an example, Miss Kate Barnard, in the Oklahoman of January 9, 1910, was quoted as saying that "Hell has reigned here twenty years undisturbed. In the light of the unparalleled and appalling conditions found, my first suggestion is that an immediate change be made in the head of that institution." The Lawton Constitution of March 30, 1905, stated that the "Sanitarium Company is making a profit of $37,000.00 annually out of the Territorial Insane Contract. This is the greatest graft in the Territory, and the politicians interested in it will not be quick to turn loose."

VETERANS' WARDS

In 1923 the Soldiers' Relief Commission sponsored a state built separate ward for soldiers of all wars to be located at Central Oklahoma State Hospital. Several other units have been added.[16]

McALESTER ANNEX

An appropriation for constructing on state-owned land, a hospital located near but not within the walls of the state penitentiary at McAlester was approved May 24, 1937. Capacity of the hospital was to be 180 beds, one wing of the structure to be reserved for the poor and indigent of the state and the other for the prisoners of the State penitentiary[17]. After some discussion it was decided that the State could better be served by housing some of its elderly men from the state hospitals there and so 250 men patients from Supply, Vinita and Norman were removed to that place in 1939.[18]

WESTERN OKLAHOMA STATE HOSPITAL

The establishment and occupation of the Hospital at Fort Supply, in Woodward County, was attended with considerable expenditure of time and effort. The United States had on February 8, 1899, proffered the Fort Supply Military Reservation to Oklahoma for the purpose of using it as an asylum for its insane[19]. Because of its inacessibility said some, the state of disrepair said others, and the desire to wait for statehood by still others, the matter went along until the Seventh Legislature accepted the donation, made an appropriation for repairs and a small amount of work was done. However, the law provided that the hospital was to be located as soon as a railroad should reach Supply.

The Eighth Territorial Legislature repealed the above law and passed an act providing for the removal of the asylum from Norman to Supply as soon as the buildings were repaired and proper arrangements made for transfer. Another hitch here occurred. The Legislature had made provision that no new buildings were to be located during 1905-06, and the Sanitarium Company promptly opposed the repairs and improvements as they were so extensive as to violate this provision. Judge Hainer sustained the contention of the company and the Territory appealed the case.

Statehood came November 16, 1907, and the First State Legislature appropriated funds for repairs to buildings and maintenance of an estimated 600 patients at $120.00 per annum.[20]

Four hundred patients were sent on May 18, 1908,[21] from Norman, and at Miss Barnard's first visit in October she reported the buildings already overcrowded. Dr. E. G. Newell was then superintendent, Dr. W. W. Rucks, assistant physician. Tangier, the nearest railroad point, was twelve miles away, and coal and supplies were hauled by wagon, but by September of 1911, the road was building through[22]. The continued growth of this institution has been rapid, with its ups and downs about similar to those of other public institutions, and now the records show that it has been under one superintendent for about ten years, Dr. John L. Day.

EASTERN OKLAHOMA HOSPITAL

The need for a hospital supplying the eastern part of the state was of course early recognized and plans were completed in 1909, when on March 27, an appropriation was made for building and equipping of the East Oklahoma Hospital for the Insane.[23] On the same date, House Bill 242 located this institution at Vinita, in Craig County, conditioned upon Vinita's deeding to the State 160 acres of land and supplying artesian water. Before the building warrants could be sold, appropriations for more land were made.

The Hospital was opened January 28, 1913, upon the receipt of 300 patients from Norman, with Dr. F. M. Adams, as superintendent. This institution was the first in the state to have been planned for the purpose of caring for the insane. The plans for the hospital were copies of those used in the construction of the hospital at Madison, Indiana[24].

In 1918 Dr. Adams reported that the question of help was his most serious one; that his mechanical department was a training school for mechanics, because as soon as a man learned some of the work he left for a better job. He again called attention to the abuse of sending aged, infirm and pauper patients to the State Hospitals.[25]

The hospitals at Supply and Vinita had, until 1915, been governed by a board of trustees. On April 30 of that year, these boards were abolished and their duties assigned to the State Board of Public Affairs. A lunacy commission was created, consisting of the State Commissioner of Health, as ex-officio chairman, the Chairman of the State Board of Affairs, and the superintendent of the hospitals at Supply, Vinita and Norman. This commission was to have general supervision of policy, and to formulate and adopt a permanent plan and system for the proper care and treatment of the insane[26].

The Lunacy Law of 1917,[27] is practically the same as that under which we are today working. It had one provision—that the counties be responsible for the expense of keeping public patients—which met serious opposition and was later declared "in conflict with Article 21 of the Constitution of Oklahoma, and void, and for that reason the judgment of the trial court must be reversed."[28]

NORTHERN OKLAHOMA HOSPITAL

The Eufaula Independent Journal, of September 9, 1910, had this to say: "The State Institute for the Feeble Minded is now ready to receive patients as provided by law. - - - Address Dr. Frank D. Davis, Superintendent. - - - ." This institution had been established March 27, 1909. It was a greatly needed institution, but one now through force of necessity, not performing its original assignment. It was founded for the purpose of receiving and training feeble minded boys up to the age of fourteen, and girls and women up to the age of forty-five. Epileptic patients were also admitted. In 1935, the name was changed to Northern Oklahoma Hospital and its function as a state hospital began. It seems almost tragic that with our extreme need for such an institution as originally planned here, that the state has been forced to use it for other purposes.

DUKE SANITARIUM

The earliest mental hospital established by an individual was that of Dr. John W. Duke, at Guthrie in 1908. Upon the death of Dr. Duke in 1920, Dr. C. B. Hill, a former superintendent at Supply, took charge. Throughout the life of the institution, or until 1936-1937, Miss Bertha Bishop was associated very closely as nurse, business manager and supervisor. Miss Barnard gave the institution a very good report.

OKLAHOMA REHABILITATION AND INDUSTRIAL INSTITUTE

A noble experiment, but conceived in haste, and carried forward without the aid of trained personnel, this institution lasted from 1923 to 1925, at which time the patients were sent to Fort Supply. It was located near Fort Reno, in a building formerly used by the Masons as a home for the aged. The Darlington Indian Agency was earlier located here. The Institution was founded "as a state hospital, as a house of refuge, and rehabilitation home for all persons addicted to the use of any drug, chemical, or other deleterious substances, or addicted to any other self-debauching habit or practice . . ." The Board of Lunaticm Inquirendem of each County was vested with authority as to whom should be received[29]. The site is now occupied by the State Quail Hatchery.

OAKWOOD SANITARIUM

In 1931, at Tulsa, Dr. Ned R. Smith established his Oakwood Sanitarium, at first as a clinic. This institution is several miles out of Tulsa, near Sand Springs, and answered a rather pressing need for a private hospital in that locality. This hospital handled most any type of psychosis as well as some of the year, addictions. This institution grew year by year, so that there were several buildings in which the most up-to-date treatment was given, including occupational therapy and physio-therapy.

HOSPITAL FOR COLORED

At one time the building of a separate ward for the colored insane of the State was considered at Vinita, but for some reason this was not carried out and as all the colored patients had been sent to the State Hospital at Norman, the colored population had reached almost 600 patients. In 1931, a hospital for these patients was established at Taft, in Muskogee County, but the hospital was not completed and the patients were not moved there until 1934, at which time 591 patients were moved in April and June.

This, of course, was a move that had been needed for many years and fortunately one of the members of the original staff, Dr. E. P. Henry, is now superintendent. At the present time this is the only State hospital with adequate space for its patients.

COYNE CAMPBELL CLINIC AND HOSPITAL

We find in 1939, another private clinic and hospital being established at Oklahoma City under the direction of Dr. Coyne Campbell, which thus gave two of the larger cities of the State a clearing place for their insane.

In these private establishments many patients can be treated and gotten back into civilian pursuits, without the trouble and annoyance of being committed to State hospitals. In this way particularly is the State served by such institutions.

JAMES A. WILLIE CLINIC AND HOSPITAL

In 1942 Dr. James A. Willie established a hospital and later a clinic at Oklahoma City, thus adding one more private institution for amelioration of the mentally ill.

The history of the insane of Oklahoma sounds more or less colorless and commonplace when limited to dates and towns and appropriations, but in the records of each institution there is much of warm, human interest, some red hot political maneuvering, some of sordid self interest, and some grimly humorous. One would be inclined to entertain a hopeless feeling with reference to the situation were it not for the knowledge that so many of the patients committed to these various institutions are salvaged and put back into normal economic and social service. One phase of this should be particularly noted. Since World War II began the drain upon the professional staffs, as well as upon other trained personnel, soon reached such proportions that it was found necessary to begin the employment of patients as attendants. This experiment was attended with many misgivings, and while it has many drawbacks and uncertainties, it has been a life saver and it now appears that it would have been impossible to get along without this source of man power.

It is doubtless possible that there are and have been institutions for the care of the insane, or near-insane which deserve to be, but have not been included here. But available is not sufficient to warrant their inclusion. I refer to such institutions as the Dr. McKanna Sanitarium for drug addictions as an example. This located in Oklahoma City and for many years was quite well known. Such institutions probably saved quite a bit of money for the State and at a time when saving was more important than now.

BIBLIOGRAPHY

1. Indian Archives: Historical Building, Oklahoma City, Okla.
2. Indian Archives: Historical Building, Oklahoma City, Okla.
3. Philip's Collection: Choctaw Ink Laws. University of Oklahoma, Norman, Okla.
4. Philip's Collection: Choctaw Ink Laws. University of Oklahoma, Norman, Okla.
5. Philip's Collection: Indian Affairs Report. University of Oklahoma, Norman, Okla.
6. Proceedings of Medico Psychological Association. May 14, 1912.
7. Dr. Hummer: Personal communication.
8. Congress, Seventy-Second: Session I, Chapter 125.
9. Smith Bill: No. 895.
10. Kinchen, Oscar H.: Chronicles of Oklahoma, Vol. xiv, No. 3. September, 1936.
11. Daily Oklahoman: Sunday, January 13, 1895.
12. Hospital Records.
13. Legislature, Fifth Regular Session Territorial: Chapter 3.
14. Purcell Register. October 2, 1903.
15. Session Laws, Joint Resolution, No. 35. 1915.
16. Session Laws: Chapter 165, H.B. 141. 1923.
17. House Bill 504, Chapter 26.
18. Hospital Records.
19. Department of Interior: Annual Report, Vol. 30, p. 84.
20. Commissioner of Charities and Correction; First Report.
21. Hospital Records.
22. Dr. Newell's Report to State Commissioner of Charities and Corrections.
23. Session Laws, Chapter 3, Article XXII, H.B. 535.
24. Third Report Commissioner Charities and Corrections.
25. Sixth Biennial Report Comissioner Charities and Corrections.
26. Sesion Laws, Chapter 275, Sections 1 and 2. 1915.
27. Session Laws, Chapter 75, Sections 1 and 2. 1915.
28. Board of Commissioners of Loan County, Versus State, ex rel. Short, Attorney General (No. 17411).
29. Senate Bill 885. Session Laws. 1923.

The Value of Knowledge

Ralph Waldo Emerson made the following observation while on the way to Europe in search of health.

Past Gibraltor, January 25, 1833

If the sea teaches any lesson, it thunders this through the throat of all its winds, 'That there is no knowledge that is not valuable.' How I envied my fellow passenger who yesterday had knowledge and nerve enough to prescribe for the sailor's sore throat, and this morning to bleed him. In this little balloon of ours, so far from the human family and their sages and colleges and manu-factories, every accomplishment, every natural or acquired talent, every piece of information is some time in request.—*The Heart of Emerson's Journals, page 64. Houghton Mifflin Company. Boston and New York.*

Cullen's Advice to His Son

Every doctor who has a son in medicine or in business might do well to pass this on. "Study your trade eagerly; decline no labour; recommend yourself by briskness and diligence; bear hardships with patience and resolution; be obliging to everybody, whether above or below you; and hold up your head, both in a literal and figurative sense." Dr. Cullen who was Professor of the Practice of Medicine at the University of Edinburgh, materially influenced medical education in America. Largely due to the face of Cullen in medicine and the Monros in Anatomy, the medical department became so popular it had 900 students in 1810.

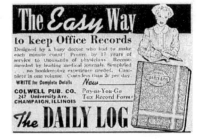

• THE PRESIDENT'S PAGE •

Someone has said: "Give the people light and they will find the way." This may not be the exact quotation, but it will serve to bring out the point I have in mind.

For the past month your President and Executive Secretary, accompanied by a very capable corps of co-workers have been meeting with each Councilor District for the purpose of explaining to the membership the program of the Association.

Dr. V. C. Tisdal, Chairman of the Public Policy Committee, assisted by Dr. John W. Shackelford, Dr. Floyd Keller and Dr. J. D. Osborn, have discussed the proposed legislative program. Dr. Tom Lowry, Dean of the School of Medicine, has explained the aims and objectives of the Post-War Planning Committee and the budget of the Medical School. Dr. John F. Burton has interpreted the Prepaid Surgical and Obstetrical Plan.

These meetings have been well received and some interesting discussion has followed. It is our hope that, through these meetings, each member may become fully informed on these subjects as well as all others pertaining to the affairs of the State Association. If, at any time, any member wishes to ask a question or would like additional information, the State Association will be anxious to cooperate. It is urged that every interested doctor get busy and use his individual influence to see that these problems are solved in a way that will reflect credit and respect for organized medicine. The Legislative Program should be brought to the attention of your Representatives and Senators.

The proposed laws, in our opinion, are for the betterment of the people of the State of Oklahoma. We are asking nothing for ourselves but are doing our utmost to improve the health and welfare of the public.

Thank you for your keen interest and whole-hearted support. Wishing you a Merry Christmas and a very Happy New Year, I am,

Sincerely,

President.

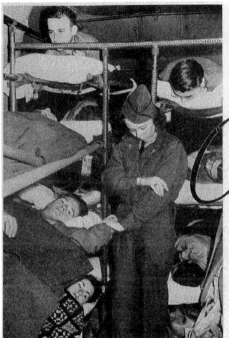

Liberator Express transporting wounded. Interior outfitted with movable litters. Information transmitted with the photo does not tell whether woman in the lowest bunk on left is a WAC or a nurse. (Army Air Force picture)

Casualties?

YES!

But not for long! Scientific research, convenient hospitalization plus modern transportation will soon convert most of these casualties into well, able-bodied men.

Warren-Teed pharmaceuticals are manufactured with keen regard for every advancement in science and research.

The JOURNAL Of The
OKLAHOMA STATE MEDICAL ASSOCIATION

EDITORIAL BOARD

L. J. MOORMAN, Oklahoma City, Editor-in-Chief

E. EUGENE RICE, Shawnee   BEN H. NICHOLSON, Oklahoma City

MR. PAUL H. FESLER, Oklahoma City, Business Manager

JANE FIRRELL TUCKER, Editorial Assistant

CONTRIBUTIONS: Articles accepted by this Journal for publication including those read at the annual meetings of the State Association are the sole property of this Journal.

The Editorial Department is not responsible for the opinions expressed in the original articles of contributors.

Manuscripts may be withdrawn by authors for publication elsewhere only upon the approval of the Editorial Board.

MANUSCRIPTS: Manuscripts should be typewritten, double-spaced, on white paper 8½ x 11 inches. The original copy, not the carbon copy, should be submitted.

Footnotes, bibliographies and legends for cuts should be typed on separate sheets in double space. Bibliography listing should follow this order: Name of author, title of article, name of periodical with volume, page and date of publication.

Manuscripts are accepted subject to the usual editorial revisions and with the understanding that they have not been published elsewhere.

NEWS: Local news of interest to the medical profession, changes of address, births, deaths and weddings will be gratefully received.

ADVERTISING: Advertising of articles, drugs or compounds unapproved by the Council on Pharmacy of the A.M.A. will not be accepted. Advertising rates will be supplied on application.

It is suggested that members of the State Association patronize our advertisers in preference to others.

SUBSCRIPTIONS: Failure to receive The Journal should call for immediate notification.

REPRINTS: Reprints of original articles will be supplied at actual cost provided request for them is attached to manuscripts or made in sufficient time before publication. Checks for reprints should be made payable to Industrial Printing Company, Oklahoma City.

Address all communications to THE JOURNAL OF THE OKLAHOMA STATE MEDICAL ASSOCIATION, 210 Plaza Court, Oklahoma City. (3)

OFFICIAL PUBLICATION OF THE OKLAHOMA STATE MEDICAL ASSOCIATION

Copyrighted December, 1944

EDITORIALS

ACCELERATION WITHOUT DUE CONSIDERATION

Editorials in the August and September issues of Surgery, Gynecology and Obstetrics and in the November 2 issue of The New England Journal of Medicine present facts of great significance.

Evarts A. Graham, in the August issue of Surgery, Gynecology and Obstetrics, calls attention to the evils of the accelerated program in medical schools and sounds a warning against the belief that streamlined medical education with only nine months hospital training can put doctors in the line of duty capable of maintaining the high standards reached by members of the profession who received four years medical education under the direction of the medical profession with one to three full years of hospital training and for some sufficient special training to achieve certification by The American Boards. Clearly, government control of medical education represents a long step backward. Both medics and casualties will pay at the front and parents and loved ones at home will feel the loss.

By way of clarification we quote from Graham's editorial: "The Army has recognized the importance of (such) qualifications . . . by giving a certain amount of preferential consideration to the members of the College and particularly to those who hold certificates of the American Board. . . .

"This splendid plan, however, . . . has been scrapped by the War and Navy Departments. Laymen . . . have dictated what may be given in a premedical course, have streamlined the medical course itself and have practically destroyed the resident system of training. Many medical officers will now enter the army to serve in battalion aid stations and in other places demanding a knowledge of surgery whose maximum graduate hospital experience has been nine months of a rotating intern service with perhaps only two months in surgery. Is this the kind of medical officer the armed forces wants? Pity the wounded if it is! "Let us imagine a group of surgeons with the authority to prescribe the education of line officers, be they Army or Navy. Would they wreck West Point and Annapolis? Would they reduce their facilities by 30 or 50 per cent at the same time that they increase the number of the students? Would they reduce the period of training of artillery officers or submarine commanders to an amount which could not possibly make them efficient? It seems unlikely that they would. . . .

"Is the medical officer of less value than the line officer? The General Staff may think so, but we know full well that a modern army could not function at all without its medical department. . . .

"Although the Surgeon General . . . is no longer a member of the General Staff, the Army must appreciate the value of the medical officers because it wants so many of them even if they are only half-baked. In fact much of the present difficulty arises because of the large number wanted. At the outbreak of the present war we were told that the army needed 6.5 medical officers for each 1000 men in the Army. . . .

. "The demand for so large a number of medical officers is the fundamental cause of the disruption of the prewar efficient plan for their education. . . . Shall we send our men into battle with Civil War muskets if the supply of modern arms is deficient. Of course not. Anybody can see how ridiculous and murderous a half-baked medical officer can be.

"Is it necessary that this large number of medical officers be provided. If it is then everybody will be glad to make the best of it. The armies of other countries have not been furnished with anything like so high a proportion of medical officers. The British, the Australian, and the Canadian armies, for example, get along with a proportion only a little more than half of what is felt necessary by our armed forces; and the quality of the work done is excellent. . . . Is not this demand for so many medical officers an unjustifiable extravagence for which there is no demonstrated need?

"These remarks have been directed at the evil effects upon the medical officers themselves caused by the disruption of the only plan for developing properly trained surgeons which has ever been found to work. A similar editorial could be written on the disaster to the civilian population. Are we to go backward a quarter of a century and to surrender to our two great allies the enviable position in medicine which this country occupied before the war? The British Commonwealth and Russia have not found it necessary to disrupt their medical education to anything like the extent which we have been forced to do. As a result we may find ourselves a poor third in medicine in the postwar world. Is it necessary? I know of no convincing evidence that it is. But nothing will be done to remedy the situation unless the medical profession itself, the only body capable of understanding how a medical officer should be educated, speaks its mind loud enough for Congress and the President to hear. Reduce the 6.5 ratio to a reasonable one and much of the basis for the wrecking of our medical education will disappear. The 9-9-9 plan will not train surgeons and will not provide competent surgical officers. Still less will the nine months' rotating internship. That plan would be scrapped and in its place a reasonable program for the training of medical officers should be substituted immediately after a proper inventory of the real needs of the armed services has been made. . . . "

The three editorials referred to above point to the fact that lay rather than medical direction renders the Surgeon General and the medical officers impotent in the matter of organization and the number of medical officers required. They are under the Control of the General Staff. All over-worked doctors on the home front should urge their Congressmen to see that medicine in the Army is placed under the direction of medical personnel rather than the General Staff. Also that the government grip on medical education be replaced by the system which has worked so well in the past.

Finally all patients, their families and friends should be informed as to what goes on when the government takes full charge of medicine anytime, anywhere. Horace said, "Neither the gods nor the booksellers shelves tolerate mediocrity in poetry." We feel that medicine is more important than poetry, and that the people are more concerned than the gods.

"I WAS SICK AND YE VISITED ME"

As we go to press with the last issue of The Journal for 1944, our hearts are saddened by five additional obituaries, making a total of 32 for the year. This represents an increase of ten over last year's toll. Perhaps homefront casualties account for this in-increase.

Because of the spirit which animates the service of doctors high and low and the genuine gratitude of patients rich or poor, we are glad to make this column the mouthpiece for many who otherwise would remain inarticulate. Let us read from *The Doctor of the Old School* while with bowed heads we stand before the grave of William MacLure:

"Friends of Drumtochty, it would not be right that we should part in silence and no man say what is in every heart. We have buried the remains of one that served this Glen with a devotion that has known no reserve, and a kindness that never failed, for more than forty five years. . . . If it be your pleasure, I shall erect a cross above his grave, and shall ask my old friend and companion, Dr. Davidson, your minister, to choose the text to be inscribed."

"We thank you, Lord Kilspindie," said the doctor, "I choose this for his text:"

"Greater love hath no man that this, that a man lay down his life for his friends."

WHAT OF THE FUTURE

Without a careful scrutiny of the past, a look at the world today with the potential striking power in the war of tomorrow, would discourage the spirit of medical progress. Naturally, the soul of the serious minded doctor silently assails the seat of reason with disturbing questions. Is it really worthwhile to continue the sleepless, critical pursuit of life saving, and health preserving gifts of science which mean the conservation of manpower for War consumption. Is the prospect of merciful salvage of war casualties a sufficient incentive for medical progress? Should not the cause of humanity hold a higher and more productive motive toward which medicine might strive!

But in comprehensive retrospect we find that the casualties from the arrow, propelled by a bent stick strung with the gut of an innocent animal, gave rise to one of the earliest

expressions of the "primal sympathy of man for man." Here we have the rudiments of medicine, the germinal concept which has motivated medical evolution. Also worthy of note is the fact that, in the past, disease has been mightier than war. Until the future becomes more definitive let us be chastened but not deterred by the silent questions. We must keep abreast with, if not ahead of scientific development in other fields of endeavor.

HAVE WE REACHED THE CLIMACTERIC IN SCIENCE

In the war between man and man it is the unpredictable Vergeltungswaffe Zwei — V2, which runs ahead of its sound waves, and lands among unsuspecting human beings with a gigantic explosion. The cycle of the swift catastrophic phenomina is instantaneous and only those beyond the zone of destruction live to hear the posthumous swish of this hellish instrument of human depravity. Our serenity may be partially recovered when we turn to a consideration of science in the war between man and deadly bacteria. The climax in the latter is reached in chemotherapy, where a few well directed doses carefully administered and physiologically propelled, may result in wholesale destruction of a low form of life in order to save a higher form.

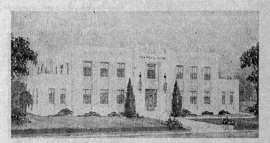

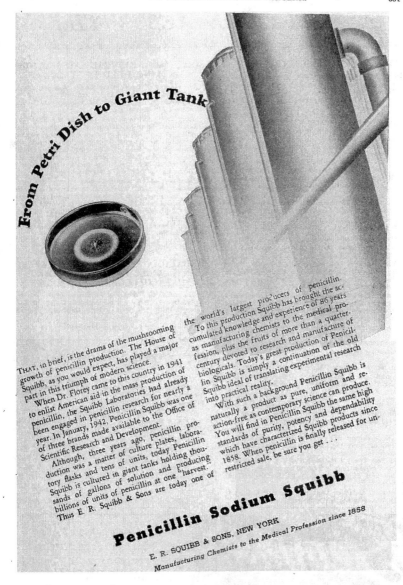

ASSOCIATION ACTIVITIES

COUNCILOR DISTRICT MEETINGS

District No. 5—Chickasha, Okla. December 1, 1944

This meeting was called by the Councilor of the District. The day before the meeting we were advised of the death of Dr. J. I. Hollingsworth, Councilor. After consulting with several of the Secretaries of the Counties of the District, it was decided that he would prefer that the meeting be held as planned.

Those present were: Dr. C. R. Rountree, President of the Association; Dean Tom Lowry, University of Oklahoma School of Medicine; Dr. John Shackelford, State Health Department; W. F. Keller, Oklahoma City; Mr. Paul Fesler, Executive Secretary of the Association. The meeting was called to order by President Rountree.

Dr. Rountree requested that those present stand for a moment in memory of Dr. Hollingsworth.

It was explained that the purpose of the meeting was to familiarize the members with the activities of the Association, especially the legislative program as follows:

1. The proposed Board of Health.
2. The Coroner's Bill.
3. The amendment to the Basic Science Law.
4. The appropriation for the Medical School.

Dr. Shackelford explained the new Board of Health Bill. The Coroner's Law was explained by Dr. Keller and Dr. Lowry told of the Post War Planning Program and also the Medical School. President Rountree explained the Prepaid Surgical and Obstetrical Plan.

Following the explanations, questions were answered relative to the activities of the State Association. Those present were requested to support the legislation and to contact their legislators.

Suggestions for candidates to succeed Dr. Hollingsworth as Councilor were requested. Dr. Patterson of Duncan was nominated.

The meeting adjourned.

District No. 2—Hobart, Oklahoma—December 2, 1944

The meeting was called by J. William Finch, M.D., Councilor of the District. Those present were: Dr. C. R. Rountree, President of the Association; Dr. J. D. Osborn, Secretary of the State Board of Medical Examiners; Dr. W. F. Keller, Oklahoma City; Dr. V. C. Tisdal, Elk City; Dr. John Shackelford, State Health Department; Dean Tom Lowry, University School of Medicine.

The Basic Science Bill was explained by Dr. Osborn; Dr. Keller explained the Coroner's Bill; Dr. Tisdal and Dr. Shackelford discussed the Board of Health Bill; and Dr. Tom Lowry told the members of the Post War Planning Program for the training of returning servicemen and also of the appropriation for the Medical School.

After some discussion those present voted to support the officers and committee in the legislative program.

SOUTHERN MEDICAL ASSOCIATION MEETING HELD IN ST. LOUIS

The meeting of the Southern Medical Association held in St. Louis, November 14-17, was well attended by several Oklahoma physicians. The meeting was the Association's 38th annual session.

Many timely messages were given by the Army and Navy doctors covering the many tropical diseases that may be brought back by the service men. It was pointed out that all members of the medical profession in the entire south should be on their guard against tropical diseases, notably, filiaria, malaria of a recurrent type and tick fever. It was urged that great attention should be given the ills of the discharged soldier.

Various uses of penicillin were discussed as were other new phases of medicine. Some of the papers given were "The Progress of Medicine" by the retiring president, Dr. James A. Ryan; "The Nutrition of the Body" by Dr. William J. Dardy, International Health Division, Rockefeller Foundation; "New Horizons in Medicine," by Col. Howard A. Rusk; and "Navy Medicine in the War" by Rear Adm. Luther Sheldon.

The next meeting will be held in New Orleans.

OKLAHOMA PHYSICIANS ACCEPTED INTO FELLOWSHIP IN THE AMERICAN COLLEGE OF SURGEONS

The following Oklahoma Physicians have been accepted into Fellowship in the American College of Surgeons in 1944: Dr. Harry C. Ford, Oklahoma City; Dr. Lloyd H. McPike, Vinita.

Blue Cross Reports

The following tabulation shows the division of the $208,420.96 that has been paid by Blue Cross to 108 hospitals in the State of Oklahoma during the first nine months of 1944:

Board and Room	125,176.20
Operating Room	21,517.90
Delivery Room	3,467.00
Nursery	2,681.40
Facilities for Circumcision	308.50
Flat Rate Maternity	797.50
Drugs	9,623.25
Special Diets	2,710.73
Surgical Dressings	3,213.53
Total 108 hospitals	$208,420.96

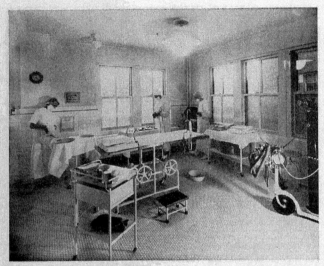

★ FIGHTIN' TALK ★

Ordered to active duty: LT. ORVILLE DAVIS, Cushing; LT. HAROLD LEROY BEDDO, Tulsa; LT. WILLIAM BEST THOMPSON, Clinton; LT. JACK W. MYERS, El Reno.

LT. COLONEL ELTON LEHEW, Pawnee, Class of '30, has recently been promoted from Major.

MAJOR EVANS E. TALLEY, Enid, is serving in the Southwest Pacific and has been stationed there with an evacuation hospital unit for the last fifteen months. Recently Major Talley was promoted from the rank of Captain. He left Enid for duty in August, 1942.

The following excerpts are taken from a letter received in the office from LT. COL. GEORGE H. KIMBALL, Oklahoma City, Class of '26. Lt. Col. Kimball is serving "somewhere in the Southwest Pacific."

"Our boys are the Champions of the area in baseball—lost the championship of the basket ball league because of an injury to one of the players just before the last game. We have a good softball team among the officers. I play left field and am the best!

"The hospital mortality rate is so low that you wouldn't believe it. Our doctors act as consultants to other installations in various departments. Also we give a great many lectures to other groups on the treatment of battle casualties. Soon we hope to send you some pictures, figures, and news of some citations for the unit.

"I acted as C.O. for a while. Am still Chief of Surgery and I believe I enjoy life more as that than as C.O.

"So far as eating goes, we have a fine mess here. We have about 20 acres in garden so we get green stuff to augment the army rations.

"Things in general are going well out our way. The so-called young men in the hospital staff are developing in a commendable manner. There are some master surgeons in the making out here."

MAJOR S. E. FRANKLIN, Broken Arrow and Tulsa, is now serving as Chief of Orthopedic Service of a Station Hospital on Guadalcanal.

LT. COL. GEORGE S. BOZALIS, Class of '35, has been awarded the bronze star and recommended for the Legion of Merit for his work while with an evacuation hospital in France. The citation sets out that the enviable accomplishments of the unit may be attributed in great measure to Lt. Col. Bozalis' superior professional ability and his loyal and untiring devotion to duty during operations in France.

After graduating from the University of Oklahoma in 1935, Colonel Bozalis served his internship in St. Louis. He is a member of the Missouri State Medical Association.

COLONEL JAMES T. HUGHES, from Tennessee, former Instructor of Pediatrics of the Postgraduate Course in Oklahoma in 1940-41, has recently been promoted from Lt. Colonel to the rank of Colonel. He is serving with a station hospital in Italy.

MAJOR JAMES S. PETTY, Guthrie, has recently been assigned to a station hospital in India as Chief of Medicine. He is Senior Officer of the station. Major Petty graduated from the University of Oklahoma School of Medicine in 1935 and was practicing in Guthrie before he entered the armed forces.

CAPTAIN F. C. LATTIMORE, Kingfisher, Class of '32, writes from 'somewhere in France' where he is stationed with an 'Air Evacuation Holding Unit.' He states that he has had the opportunity to see the end results of some excellent surgery. He sends his regards to all.

LT. COMDR. W. D. HOOVER, Tulsa, Class of '33, has just returned from almost eighteen months duty in the South Pacific and has been assigned duty at the Dispensary at the U. S. Naval Air Station in Glenview, Illinois.

Lt. COL. JAMES H. HAMMOND, Tulsa, writes from his station overseas: "Have been with this outfit for about one and a half years through all its ultra and secret phases.

"Now it's no secret that Japan can be bombed and that our boys here are doing a good job.

"Haven't seen much of any of you since September, 1940 when I was picked up with the 45th Division from the office of Dr. Braswell, Tulsa."

LT. COL. W. G. DUNNINGTON, Lawton, has been in France since September 1. Before going overseas he was with his Medical Battalion at Ford Ord and Camp Breckenridge. In July, 1943 he returned from Panama after being there a year and a half.

CAPTAIN L. P. SMITH, Marlow, says, by V-Mail, "I am now with this general hospital and have been for the past two and a half months. Enjoy my work but would sure like to get back to Oklahoma. Am on the Surgical Service and keep quite busy. Only Oklahoman in the hospital!"

LT. COMDR. HOWARD L. PUCKETT, Stillwater, has just returned after three years active duty with the Navy in the South Pacific and is now stationed at the naval hospital in Norman. On October 27, Lt. Comdr. Puckett spoke to the American Red Cross Chapter Clinic in Stillwater, at which 18 Oklahoma Counties were represented. Comdr. Puckett stated that "the Red Cross was the foremost, in fact, almost the only non-military organization that gave us assistance overseas in New Zealand, at Tarawa, at Saipan and in Hawaii.'' He further stated that many thousands of surgical dressings being made by Red Cross volunteers were used on ''thousands of the wounded in battle, where time was too precious for cutting and making them. Much suffering, and even lives, were saved by having these battle dressings at hand,'' said Comdr. Puckett.

DIARY OF A BATTLE SURGEON

A British surgeon, who followed closely on the heels of the Allied troops when they landed on D-Day, describes the care and precision of surgery on the battlefield. Extracts from his diary were given in a BBC broadcast. The first part which follows deals with the experiences of one of the writer's colleagues.

Surgery on D-Day

At 9:30 A.M. on D-Day they arrived off the beach and two hours after the first assault had gone in they landed and clamored laboriously up the beach in the rear of the troops, but only just in the rear. The surgeon, his anesthetist and two theater orderlies set up a suitable shelter to act as an operating theater. In front of him were Germans, beside him were Germans and behind him were Germans. In fact, they occupied houses between him and the shore for the next five days.

Miraculous Achievements of a Small Staff

In the next twenty-four hours he worked without ceasing. During that time he learned much and he saw the treachery and bestiality of war. During that twenty-four hours of continuous surgery he operated on nineteen cases, nineteen serious cases. A wonderful achievement: twenty-four hours continuous operating under the ordinary tension of a civilian operating theater would be some ordeal. But here it was no ordinary tension. Consider the conditions of that theater which was being run by two men only. One of these, a sergeant, assisted the surgeon with each case which left the other man to do all the many necessary jobs in a working theater, the sterilization, the preparation of instruments, the cleansing and the preparation of the patient, and so on.

Now in most civilian theaters three nurses are detailed to do all these tasks, and they have plenty of room and cover to work in. The anesthetist also had to do double duty for there was no resuscitation officer. He would anesthetize each patient and then, when the patient was well under, after first making sure that his condition was good, he would fix the anesthetic mask and start giving blood transfusions. He succeeded in getting up thirty-five transfusions during that time.

Rest After Nineteen Operations

After the nineteenth operation, they went to bed or rather they found a suitable hollow to lie down in. The work had not ceased but they just could not go on any longer. For the surgeon could scarcely keep his eyes open and the anesthetist was half doped with his own anesthetic.

"The Biggest Shock in My Life"

In the second extract the writer reviews his own experiences showing how promptly our wounded are seen by surgeons.

A day or so later, I was introduced to battle surgery when I was sent out on a surgical team to help at another hospital. It was about the biggest shock I have had in my life.

At 8:00 P.M. we reached the operating theater, a tent in which there were two operating tables connected to another tent where those wounded next for operations lie waiting their turn. Your first case had multiple wounds. Some fine man you don't know. You cut out the first wound, you cut out the second. You come to the third wound, and you would strike a hemorrhage deep in the wound and wonder whether you will be able to stop it. You are lucky. You do stop it and you bandage

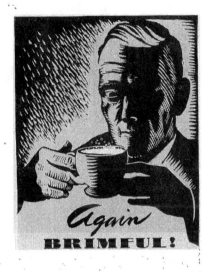

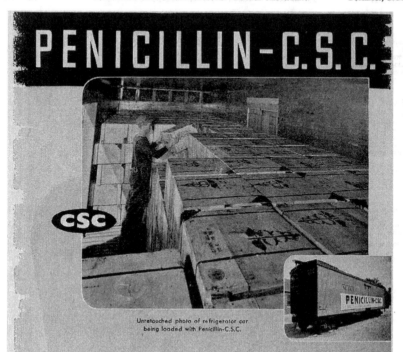

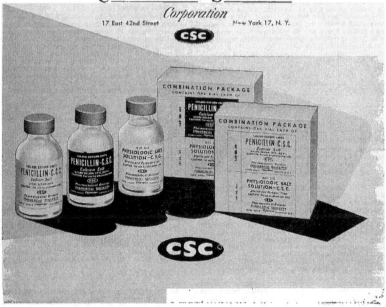

the wounds up. You feel a little tired and wonder what will happen to this fellow. You will not see him again, for he will be evacuated in the morning.

The next patient is on the table. He is not very well. He has an abdominal wound. You have to be quick and so you pull yourself together and fight with time. You are relieved, and so is the anesthetist when you have got him out again. You both want to sit down and smoke for a while, but there is another patient on the table, some one else you have never seen before and will never see again who needs an amputation.

"On and On Until Light Comes"

So it goes on. In the middle of the night somebody says: "What about tea," You are weary to death, morally and physically, but the tea does a lot of good. So you go through to the waiting tent to see how things are getting along. There were ten patients waiting when you started and now there are fifteen—fifteen men bearing their wounds with amazing patience, accepting the pain as part of themselves, just as a woman accepts her labor. You go back to work, and go on and on, until at last light comes. Then you can go to bed, only to fight for sleep against visions of wounded men, only to get up in a few hours time and start all over again. That is what battle surgery is like when first you meet it. It numbs your mind.

I personally found that I approached the operating tent with dread, that I only needed to hear the hum of the electric light generators or the roar of the sterilizers to feel a little sick, but it passes off in time, and custom revives the mind. You begin to think, and think scientifically. You watch your surgery improve and interest returns.

Visible Results

Actually it was about the 70th case that I had done since landing that really revived me. The man was paralyzed from his trunk downward, and had a wound at the bottom of his neck at the back. At the end of the deep penetration this formed, I could feel a piece of metal stuck between the two vertobrae. By the greatest good fortune I was able to withdraw it. It must have been lying against the spinal cord without severing it, for during the next few days I was able to watch the patient, evacuation being impossible, and his sensation was gradually returning. That case was, in a way, salvation to me, for witnessing the improvement gave more meaning to all the other surgery I was doing on cases which were evacuated too rapidly for me to see the outcome of my work.

Medical School Notes

Dr. A. A. Hellbaum, Professor of Pharmacology, represented the University of Oklahoma School of Medicine at the meeting of the Association of American Medical Colleges held in Detroit, Michigan, October 23 to 27.

Dr. Wann Langston has been promoted from Professor of Clinical Medicine to Professor of Medicine and Chairman of the Department of Medicine. This appointment become effective September 1, 1944.

Dr. Howard G. Glass has been appointed Instructor in Pharmacology. He received his B. S. Degree in 1932 from the University of Illinois, his M.S. Degree from Northwestern University in 1935, and his Ph.D. Degree from the University of Chicago in 1942. Dr. Glass was previously employed as Research Assistant in the Department of Pharmacy at the University of Chicago.

Dr. Nathaniel A. Jones, who was appointed Assistant Director of the Admitting and Out-Patient Departments at the University of Oklahoma Hospitals, October 1, 1944, died of a heart attack November 15.

Among the books recently received at the Medical School Library are the following: Grinker, R. R. and Spiegel, J. P.; War Neuroses in North Africa—1943: Heilmeyer, Ludwig; Spectrophotometry in Medicine—1943: Ishihara, Shinobu; Tests for colour blindness—9th ed., 1944: James, N. R.; Regional Analgesia for Intra abdominal Surgery—1943; McMurray, T. P.; Practice of Orthopaedic Surgery—2nd ed., 1943; May, C. H.; Manual of Diseases of the Eye—18th ed., 1943: Medical Annual (International)—1944: Modern Medicine Annual, 1943-1944: Oberling, Charles; Riddle of Cancer—1944: Ogilvie, R. F.; Pathological Histology—2nd ed., 1943: Simmons, J. S. et al.; Global Epidemiology—1944: Smedley-Maclean; Metabolism of Fat—1943: Stunkard, H. W., et al. Parasitic Diseases and American Participation in War—1943: Trail, R. R., et al.; Mass Miniature Radiography—1943: Vitamins and Hormones, v. 2., 1944: Wilkinson, M. C.; Non-Pulmonary Tuberculosis—1942: Wilson, S.A.K.; Neurology Edited by A. N. Bruce. 2 vols., 1940.

Dr. H. A. Shoemaker, Assistant Dean, has been a patient in the University Hospital since October 13, as a result of injuries received in an automobile accident.

BOOK REVIEWS

MEDICAL CARE OF THE DISCHARGED HOSPITAL PATIENT. Forde Jensen, M.D., Instructor of Medicine, Syracuse University College of Medicine; H. G. Weiskotten, M.D., Dean and Professor of Pathology, Syracuse University College of Medicine; Margaret A. Thomas, M. A. The Commonwealth Fund, New York. 1944. 94 pages. Price, $1.00.

The question of the care of the chronically ill patient is studied by the Commonwealth Fund at the Syracuse University in contemplation of extending their activities in urban centers over the whole United States. They have sudied the care of the discharged patient and find that with extramural supervision by certain medical, health and welfare services they could cut the hospitalization costs to one third and release more hospital beds for the acutely ill. This study was predicated on the fact that 90 per cent of the hospital costs were for convalescent and chronically ill which could receive better care in their own homes when under aforesaid supervision. Where there are funds and agencies for so doing this is a very practical solution for our overcrowded hospitals. It does not attempt to solve the problem of the decimation of help at home and these agencies servicing them during war time conditions.

This brochure should be of especial interest to those interested in community health. The set-up they have had, however, is not applicable to all urban centers throughout the country. It is another step, however, leading towards socialized medicine.—Lea A. Riely, M.D.

Classified Advertisements

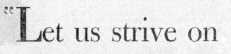

• OBITUARIES •

J. I. Hollingsworth. M. D.
1879-1944

Dr. J. I. Hollingsworth died at his home in Waurika on November 30 after a short illness.

Dr. Hollingsworth was a pioneer physician in the State, entering practice in Muskogee in 1912. In 1916 he moved to Douglas, Arizona where he remained until 1921 at which time he returned to Muskogee and joined Dr. H. T. Ballantine and the late Doctors Sessler Hoss and H. C. Rogers. Dr. Hollingsworth also became City Physician of Muskogee and held that post from 1921 to 1924. In 1925 he went to the Philippine Islands where he was connected with a sugar company as physician. Returning to the United States in 1927, he entered a partnership in directing a hospital in Waurika with which he was still connected at the time of his death.

Dr. Hollingsworth was Councilor of District No. 5 of the Oklahoma State Medical Association. He was very active in organized medicine and his untiring efforts for its advancement will long be remembered.

Survivors include his widow, Mrs. Inez Hollingsworth of the home; two sisters, Mrs. Ida Cobb of Muskogee and Mrs. Beulah Gilmore of Tyler, Texas, and two nephews, H. H. Hollingsworth, manager of the Locke Seed Company in Muskogee, who was with him at the time of his death, and Robert Hollingsworth of Chicago, Ill. Services were held at Waurika Saturday, December 2, with burial there.

W. T. Huddleston. M.D.
1867-1944

Dr. W. T. Huddleston died Thursday, November 30, at his home in Konawa following a three weeks' illness.

After graduating from Vanderbilt University School of Medicine in Nashville, Tennessee, in 1895, Dr. Huddleston went to Sulphur Springs, Arkansas. In 1910, he moved to Seminole County and practiced in Konawa until the time of his death.

Dr. Huddleston was a 32nd degree Mason, belonging to the Consistary at Guthrie and the India Shrine Temple at Oklahoma City. He was a member of the Seminole County Medical Society, the Oklahoma State Medical Association and the American Medical Association.

Surviving Dr. Huddleston are his wife, one son, W. E. Huddleston of Seminole, two daughters, Mrs. Irene McIntyre of Konawa and Mrs. T. R. Wilson of Bartlesville, a brother, three half-brothers and two half-sisters. Services were held in the Methodist Church at Konawa and burial was in the Konawa cemetery.

T. M. Aderhold, M.D.
1871-1944

Dr. T. M. Aderhold, retired El Reno physician, died September 7 in a Dallas hospital. Although in poor health for several years, Dr. Aderhold did not retire from active practice until 1938.

A native of Georgia, Dr. Aderhold graduated from the North West University Medical School in Chicago in 1901. After his graduation he served 18 months as an American Red Cross doctor in the Boer War in South Africa. Upon his return he served internship in Augustanta Hospital, St. Mary's and Dr. Lee's Maternity Center. In 1904 he moved to Ziegler, Illinois where he practiced until coming to El Reno in 1909. Dr. Aderhold purchased the interest of the late Dr. Fred H. Clark in the El Reno Sanitarium and thus became associated with the late Dr. J. A. Hatchett. In 1920 Dr. Aderhold purchased Dr. Hatchett's interest in the institution and from then

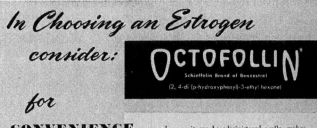

until his retirement he was its manager as well as conducting his private practice.

Active in civic affairs, Dr. Aderhold was a charter member and past president of the El Reno Lions Club and past president of the El Reno Chamber of Commerce. He was a member of the First Presbyterian Church, the Masonic Blue Lodge and the Ascension Commandery, Knights Templar, as well as a 32nd degree Scottish Rite Mason. He was a Fellow of the American College of Surgeons, a member of the Oklahoma Academy of Science, the Oklahoma State Medical Association and the American Medical Association.

Surviving are his wife, three daughthers, one son and three grandchildren.

David W. Connally, M.D.
1871-1944

Dr. David W. Connally died at his home in Antlers after several months' illness.

Dr. Connally attended the Gate City Medical College in Dallas, Texas, graduating in 1907. After his graduation he came to Oklahoma where he began practice in Antlers. Dr. Connally became prominent in civic affairs and held the high esteem of his community and state. He was a member of the Methodist Church and was a 32nd degree Mason. He was a member of the Oklahoma State Medical Association and the American Medical Association.

Surviving Dr. Connally are his wife and several nieces and nephews.

N. A. Jones, M.D.
1915-1944

Dr. N. A. Jones, Oklahoma City, died suddenly on November 18 of a heart attack. He had been in ill health more than a year, having been discharged from the Army because of his physical condition.

Dr. Jones received his preliminary education at the University of Oklahoma, going then to Baylor College of Medicine in Dallas, where he graduated in 1940. He then served a year internship in the Toledo Hospital in Toledo, Ohio. In 1941, Dr. Jones joined the Army Medical Corps and began service with the rank of Captain. He served two years in Arizona, New Mexico and California and was given a medical discharge due to his heart condition in the autumn of 1943. After his discharge, Dr. Jones came to Oklahoma City where he was associated with the Douglas Aircraft Workers Clinic for nine months. He then entered private practice in the Medical Arts Building, Oklahoma City.

Besides his degree in Medicine, Dr. Jones held a degree in electrical engineering.

Surviving Dr. Jones are his parents Mr. and Mrs. Cecil F. Jones of Tulsa. Funeral services and burial were held in Tulsa.

American Adaptability

The American people have taken to a good many fast going things since Ralph Waldo Emerson learned to ride on the cars.

Baltimore, Barnum's Hotel
January 7, 1843

Here to-day from Philadelphia. The railroad, which was but a toy coach the other day, is now a dowdy, lumbering country wagon. . . The Americans take to the little contrivance as if it were the cradle in which they were born.

New York, February 7

Dreamlike traveling on the railroad. The towns through which I pass between Philadelphia and New York make no distinct impression. They are like pictures on a wall. The more, that you can read all the way in a car a French novel—*The Heart of Emerson's Journals, page 194. Houghton Mifflin Company, Boston and New York.*

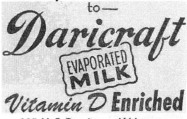
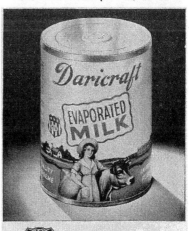

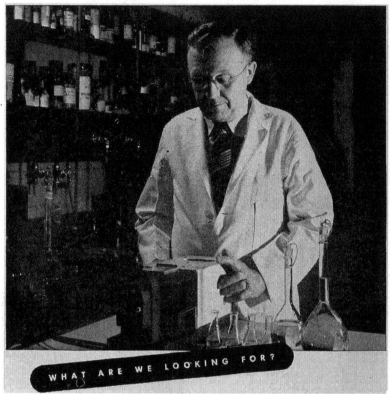

WHAT ARE WE LOOKING FOR?

In research on the sulfa drugs we are investigating the long list of possible chemical analogues of sulfanilamide . . . seeking compounds of greater effectiveness and less toxicity. But our studies go far deeper than that . . . we are inquiring into the interference of various substances with the action of sulfonamide drugs, for through a knowledge of the mechanics of these inhibitory agents we hope, in turn, to learn more about the action of the sulfas, and thus throw new light on this important field of chemotherapy.

PARKE, DAVIS & COMPANY • DETROIT 32, MICHIGAN

XXXVII   Index To Contents   1944

The use of the index will be greatly facilitated by remembering that articles are often listed under more than one head. Scientific articles may be found under both the name of the author and the various phases of the subject discussed. Editorials, Book Reviews and Obituaries are listed under the special headings as well as alphabetically.

KEY TO ABBREVIATIONS

(S)—Scientific articles
(A)—Association Activities
(E)—Editorials
(SP)—Special Article
(pic)—Picture

(br)—Book Review
(MW)—Medicine at War
(abs)—Abstract
(R)—Resolution
(o)—Obituary

(rep)—Reprint

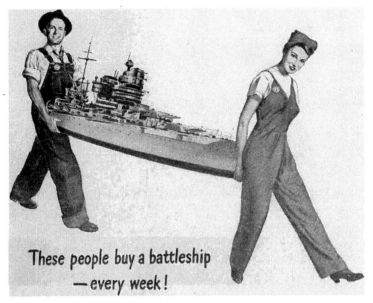

These people buy a battleship
— every week!

Meet John S..........and Mary D........

John works at an electronics plant on Long Island, and makes $85 a week. Almost 16% of it goes into War Bonds.

Mary has been driving rivets into bombers at an airplane plant on the West Coast. She makes $55 a week, and puts 14% of it into War Bonds.

John and Mary are typical of more than 27 million Americans on the Payroll Savings Plan who, every single month, put half a BILLION dollars into War Bonds. That's enough to buy one of those hundred-million-dollar battleships every week, with enough money for an aircraft carrier and three or four cruisers left over.

In addition, John and Mary and the other people on the Payroll Plan have been among the biggest buyers of *extra* Bonds in every War Loan Drive.

They've financed a good share of our war effort all by themselves, and they've tucked away billions of dollars in savings that are going to come in mighty handy for both them and their country later on.

When this war is won, and we start giving credit where credit is due, don't forget John and Mary. After the fighting men, they deserve a place at the top. They've earned it.

You've backed the attack—now speed the victory!

Oklahoma State Medical Association

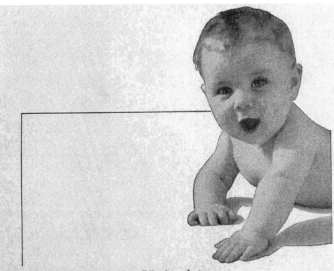

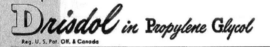

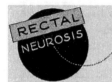

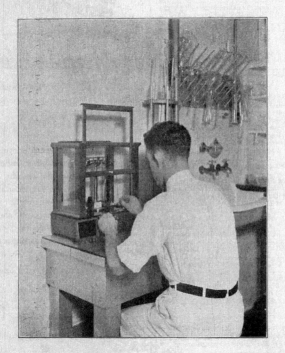

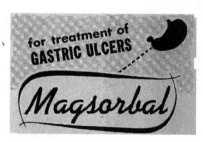
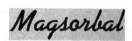

Being a stable, organic iodide, NEO-IOPAX may be used with greater safety than other types of iodine preparations in all age groups. Because of its optimal iodine content and its rapid excretion in high concentration, diagnostic films may be obtained within five minutes after injection. NEO-IOPAX is usually well tolerated both by intravenous injection and retrograde administration.

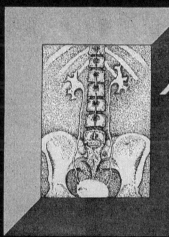

Neo-Iopax

IN INTRAVENOUS
UROGRAPHY

IN RETROGRADE
PYELOGRAPHY

SOLUTION NEO-IOPAX: Crystal-clear solution of disodium N-methyl-3,5-diiodo-chelidamate in 50% and 75% concentration.

COMBINATION economy package of 50% solution containing both 20 cc. ampules and 10 cc. ampules: also 75% solution in ampules of 20 cc. or 10 cc.

SCHERING CORPORATION · BLOOMFIELD · N.J.

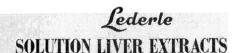

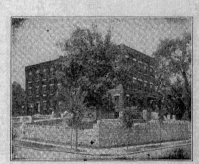

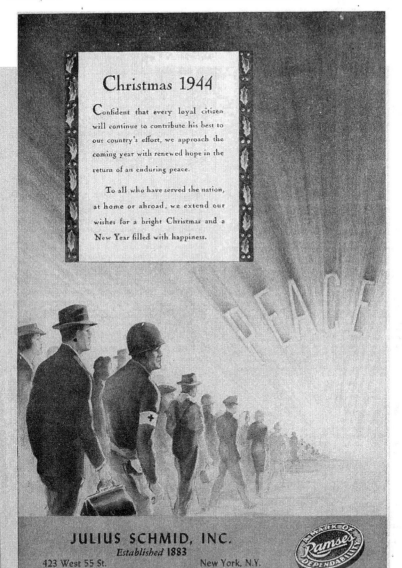

Sustained TIMED
diabetic control

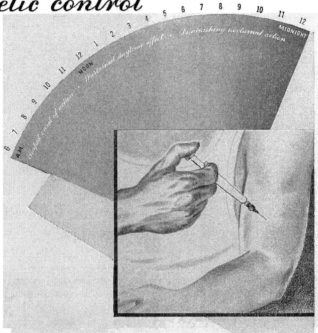

'Wellcome' Globin Insulin with Zinc is a distinct new aid to the physician seeking an effective method of controlling a particular patient's hyperglycemia. Injected an hour before breakfast, it is timed for the day's normal activities. Action is prompt initially, concentrated during daytime hours, diminished during the night.

'Wellcome' Globin Insulin with Zinc is a clear solution and, in its freedom from allergenic properties, is comparable to regular insulin. It is accepted by the Council on Pharmacy and Chemistry, American Medical Association, and was developed in the Wellcome Research Laboratories, Tuckahoe, New York. U. S. Pat. No. 2,161,198. Available in vials of 10 cc., 80 units in 1 cc.   'Wellcome' Trademark Registered

Comprehensive booklet "GLOBIN INSULIN" sent on request.

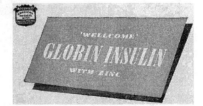

BURROUGHS WELLCOME & CO., (U. S. A.) INC.
9-11 East 41st Street, New York 17, New York

Vesalius

The Belgium anatomist Vesahus was a grand tradition to the Scottish student of medicine in the eighteenth century, but the Dutch school chiefly influenced him through Boerhaave of Leyden and his pupil Van Swieten. Scottish students flocked in numbers to Leyden, where Boerhaave was professor of medicine and had a world-wide reputation. They had the greatest veneration for their teacher, and bore away with them a lifetime belief in his greatness.—*Aberdeen Doctors—At Home and Abroad. Ella Hill Burton Rodger. Page 29. William Blackwood & Sons. Edinburgh and London. 1913.*

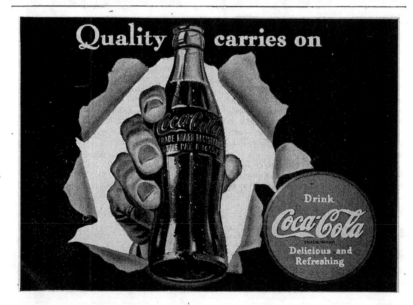

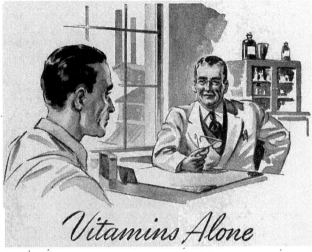
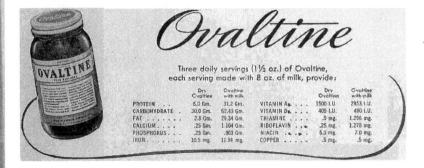

OFFICERS OF COUNTY SOCIETIES, 1944

★

COUNTY	PRESIDENT	SECRETARY	MEETING TIME
Alfalfa	H. E. Huston, Cherokee	L. T. Lancaster, Cherokee	Last Tues. each Second Month
Atoka-Coal	R. C. Henry, Coalgate	J. S. Fulton, Atoka	
Beckham	G. H. Stagner, Erick	O. C. Standifer, Elk City	Second Tuesday
Blaine	L. R. Kirby, Okeene	W. F. Griffin, Watonga	
Bryan	John T. Wharton, Durant	W. K. Haynie, Durant	Second Tuesday
Caddo	F. L. Patterson, Carnegie	C. B. Sullivan, Carnegie	
Canadian	P. F. Herod, El Reno	A. L. Johnson, El Reno	Subject to call
Carter	F. W. Boadway, Ardmore	H. A. Higgins, Ardmore	
Cherokee	P. H. Medearis, Tahlequah	W. M. Wood, Tahlequah	First Tuesday
Choctaw		E. A. Johnson, Hugo	
Cleveland	F. T. Gastineau, Norman	Iva S. Merritt, Norman	Thursday nights
Comanche	George L. Berry, Lawton	Howard Angus, Lawton	
Cotton	A. B. Holstead, Temple	Mollie F. Seism, Walters	Third Friday
Craig	Lloyd H. McPike, Vinita	J. M. McMillan, Vinita	
Creek	J. E. Hollis, Bristow	F. H. Sisler, Bristow	
Custer	F. R. Vieregg, Clinton	C. J. Alexander, Clinton	Third Thursday
Garfield	Julian Feild, Enid	John R. Walker, Enid	Fourth Thursday
Garvin	T. F. Gross, Lindsay	John R. Callaway, Pauls Valley	Wednesday before Third Thursday
Grady	Walter J. Baze, Chickasha	Roy E. Emanuel, Chickasha	Third Thursday
Grant	L. V. Hardy, Medford		
Greer	R. W. Lewis, Granite	J. B. Hollis, Mangum	
Harmon	W. G. Husband, Hollis	R. H. Lynch, Hollis	First Wednesday
Haskell	William Carson, Keota	N. K. Williams, McCurtain	
Hughes	Wm. L. Taylor, Holdenville	Imogene Mayfield, Holdenville	First Friday
Jackson	C. G. Spears, Altus	E. A. Abernethy, Altus	Last Monday
Jefferson	F. M. Edwards, Ringling		Second Monday
Kay	J. Holland Howe, Ponca City	G. H. Yeary, Newkirk	Second Thursday
Kingfisher	A. O. Meredith, Kingfisher	H. Violet Sturgeon, Hennessey	
Kiowa	J. William Finch, Hobart	William Bernell, Hobart	
LeFlore	Neeson Rolle, Poteau	Rush L. Wright, Poteau	
Lincoln	W. B. Davis, Stroud	Carl H. Bailey, Stroud	First Wednesday
Logan	William C. Miller, Guthrie	J. L. LeHew, Jr., Guthrie	Last Tuesday
Marshall	J. L. Holland, Madill	J. F. York, Madill	
Mayes	Ralph V. Smith, Pryor	Paul B. Cameron, Pryor	
McClain	W. C. McCurdy, Sr., Purcell	W. C. McCurdy, Jr., Purcell	
McCurtain	A. W. Clarkson, Valliant	N. L. Barker, Brokeu Bow	Fourth Tuesday
McIntosh	Lester I. Jacobs, Hanna	Wm. A. Tolleson, Eufaula	First Thursday
Murray	P. V. Annadown, Sulphur	J. A. Wrenn, Sulphur	Second Tuesday
Muskogee-Sequoyah Wagoner	H. A. Scott, Muskogee	D. Evelyn Miller, Muskogee	First Monday
Noble	C. H. Cooke, Perry	J. W. Francis, Perry	
Okfuskee	C. M. Cochran, Okemah	M. L. Whitney, Okemah	Second Monday
Oklahoma	W. E. Eastland, Oklahoma City	E. R. Musick, Oklahoma City	Fourth Tuesday
Okmulgee	S. B. Leslie, Okmulgee	J. C. Matheney, Okmulgee	Second Monday
Osage	C. R. Weirich, Pawhuska	George E. Hemphill, Pawhuska	Second Monday
Ottawa	Walter Kerr, Picher	B. W. Shelton, Miami	Third Thursday
Pawnee	E. T. Robinson, Cleveland	R. L. Browning, Pawnee	
Payne	H. C. Manning, Cushing	J. W. Martin, Cushing	Third Thursday
Pittsburg	P. T. Powell, McAlester	W. H. Kaeiser, McAlester	Third Friday
Pontotoc	A. R. Sugg, Ada	R. H. Mayes, Ada	First Wednesday
Pottawatomie	E. Eugene Rice, Shawnee	Clinton Gallaher, Shawnee	First and Third Saturday
Pushmataha	John S. Lawson, Clayton	B. M. Huckabay, Antlers	
Rogers	R. C. Meloy, Claremore	Chas. L. Caldwell, Chelsea	First Monday
Seminole	J. T. Price, Seminole	Mack I. Shanholtz, Wewoka	Third Wednesday
Stephens	W. K. Walker, Marlow	Wallis S. Ivy, Duncan	
Texas	R. G. Obermiller, Texhoma	Morris Smith, Guymon	
Tillman	C. C. Allen, Frederick	O. G. Bacon Frederick	
Tulsa	Ralph A. McGill, Tulsa	E. O. Johnson, Tulsa	Second and Fourth Monday
Washington-Nowata	K. D. Davis, Nowata	J. V. Athey, Bartlesville	Second Wednesday
Washita	A. S. Neal, Cordell	James F. McMurry, Sentinel	
Woods	Ishmael F. Stephenson, Alva	Oscar E. Templin, Alva	Last Tuesday Odd Months
Woodward	H. Walker, Buffalo	C. W. Tedrowe, Woodward	Second Thursday

*(Serving in Armed Forces)

ROSTER

Oklahoma State Medical
Association

1944

ROSTER

Oklahoma State Medical Association

1944

(*Members are listed according to the County of their residence.*)
(**Indicates the member is serving in the Armed Forces.*)

ALFALFA

*BEATY, C. SAM ....Cherokee
DOUGAN, A. L. ....Carmen
    (member Woods County Medical Society)
*DUNNINGTON, W. G. ....Cherokee
HALE, FORREST ....Cherokee
HARRIS, G. G. ....Helena
HUSTON, H. E. ....Cherokee
LANCASTER, L. T. ....Cherokee
*PARSONS, JACK F. ....Cherokee
STEPHENSON, WALTER L. ....Aline
    (member Woods County Medical Society)
WEBER, A. G. ....Goltry

ATOKA

BRIGGS, T. H. ....Atoka
COTTON, W. W. ....Atoka
DALE, CHARLES D. ....Atoka
FULTON, J. S. ....Atoka
HUNTLEY, H. C. ....Atoka

BEAVER

BENJEGERDES, THEODORE D. ....Beaver
    (member Woods County Medical Society)
McGREW, EDWIN A. ....Beaver
    (member Woods County Medical Society)

BECKHAM

BAKER, L. V. ....Elk City
*DEVANNEY, P. J. ....Sayre
KILPATRICK, E. S. ....Elk City
*LEVICK, J. E. ....Elk City
McCREERY, R. C. ....Erick
McGRATH, T. J. ....Sayre
MURRAY, F. L. ....Elk City
PHILLIPS, G. W. ....Sayre
*SLABAUGH, R. M. ....Sayre
SPEED, H. K. ....Sayre
SPENCE, W. P. ....Sayre
STAGNER, G. H. ....Erick
STANDIFER, O. C. ....Elk City
TISDAL, V. C. ....Elk City

BLAINE

ANDERSON, H. R. ....Watonga
*BOHLMAN, W. F. ....Watonga
COX, A. K. ....Watonga
CURTIN, VIRGINIA OLSON ....Watonga
GRIFFIN, W. F. ....Watonga
KIRBY, L. R. ....Okeene
MILLIGAN, E. F. ....Geary
ROGERS, C. L. ....Canton
STOUGH, D. F., JR. ....Geary
STOUGH, D. F., SR. (honorary) ....Geary
    (member Canadian County Medical Society)

BRYAN

*BAKER, A. T. ....Durant
BLOUNT, W. T. ....Durant
CAIN, P. L. (honorary) ....Albany
COCHRAN, R. L. ....Caddo
*COKER, B. B. ....Durant
COLWICK, J. T. ....Durant
COLWICK, O. J. ....Durant
DICKEY, R. P. ....Caddo
HAYNIE, JOHN A. ....Durant
HAYNIE, W. KEILLER ....Durant
HYDE, W. A. ....Durant

McCALIB, D. C. ....Colbert
MOORE, CHARLES F. ....Durant
MOORE, W. L. ....Bokchito
NICHOLS, JONAT ....Durant
PRICE, CHARLES G. ....Durant
SAWYER, R. E. ....Durant
SIZEMORE, PAUL ....Durant
TONEY, S. M. ....Bennington
WANN, C. E. (honorary) ....Albany
WEBB, JAMES P. ....Durant
WELLS, A. J. ....Calera
WHARTON, J. T. ....Durant

CADDO

BENWARD, JOHN H. ....1034 N. E. Grand Ave.,
                                            Portland, Oregon
CAMPBELL, GEORGE C. ....Anadarko
DIXON, W. L. ....Cement
HASLAM, G. E. ....Anadarko
HENKE, J. R. ....Hydro
INMAN, E. L. ....Apache
JOHNSTON, R. E. ....Anadarko
KERLEY, W. O. ....Anadarko
*LYONS, MASON R. ....Anadarko
McMILLAN, C. B. ....Gracemont
PATTERSON, FRED L. ....Carnegie
PUTNAM, W. B. ....Carnegie
ROGERS, F. W. ....Carnegie
SULLIVAN, CLARENCE B. ....Carnegie
WRIGHT, PRESTON ....Anadarko

CANADIAN

ADERHOLD, THOMAS M. (honorary) ....El Reno
BROWN, HADLEY C. ....El Reno
CATTO, W. B. ....El Reno
*CRADEN, PAUL J. ....El Reno
DEVER, HARVEY K. ....El Reno
GOODMAN, GEORGE L. ....Yukon
HARTSHORNE, WM. O. ....Geary
    (member Seminole County Medical Society)
HEROD, PHILIP F. ....El Reno
JOHNSON, ALPHA L. ....El Reno
LAWTON, W. P. ....El Reno
MYERS, PIRL B. ....El Reno
NEUMANN, MILTON A. ....Okarche
PHELPS, JOSEPH T. ....El Reno
PHELPS, MALCOM E. ....El Reno
RICHARDSON, D. P. ....Union City
RILEY, JAMES T. ....El Reno
TOMKINS, J. E. ....Yukon

CARTER

BARKER, E. R. ....Healdton
BOADWAY, F. W. ....Ardmore
CANADA, J. C. ....Ardmore
*CANTRELL, D. E., JR. ....Healdton
CANTRELL, D. E., SR. ....Healdton
CANTRELL, EMMA JEAN ....Healdton
*CARLOCK, J. HOYLE ....Ardmore
COX, J. L. ....Ardmore
DAVIS, EDWARD F. ....Ardmore
GILLESPIE, L. D. ....Ardmore
*GORDON, J. M. ....Ardmore
HARDY, WALTER ....Ardmore
HATHAWAY, W. G. ....Lone Grove
HIGGINS, H. A. ....Ardmore
JACKSON, T. J. ....Ardmore

JOHNSON, C. A. ....Wilson
JOHNSON, G. E. ....Ardmore
JOHNSON, WALTER ....Ardmore
KETCHERSID, J. W. ....Ardmore
MEAD, W. W. ....Ardmore
MOTE, W. R. ....Ardmore
*MOXLEY, JOE N. ....Ardmore
*PERRY, FRED T. ....Healdton
**POLLOCK, JOHN R. ....Ardmore
*REID, ROGER ....Ardmore
*STONE, S. N. ....Ardmore
SULLIVAN, R. C. ....Ardmore
VEAZEY, J. HOBSON ....Ardmore
*VEAZEY, LYMAN C. ....Ardmore
**Deceased June 28, 1944.

CHEROKEE

ALLISON, J. S. ....Tahlequah
BAINES, SWARTZ ....Tahlequah
*GRAY, JAMES K. ....Tahlequah
HINES, S. J. T. ....Tahlequah
MASTERS, H. A. ....Tahlequah
*McINTOSH, R. K., JR. ....Tahlequah
MEDEARIS, P. H. ....Tahlequah
WOOD, W. M. ....Tahlequah

CHOCTAW

GEE, ROBERT L. ....Hugo
GREGG, O. R. ....Hugo
**HALE, C. H. ....Boswell
JOHNSON, E. A. ....Hugo
SWITZER, FRED D. ....Hugo
**Deceased April 27, 1944.

CLEVELAND

ATKINS, W. H. ....Norman
BERRY, CURTIS ....Norman
BRAKE, CHARLES A. ....Norman
*BUFFINGTON, F. C. ....Norman
CARROLL, W. B. ....Norman
GASTINEAU, F. T. ....Norman
GRIFFIN, D. W. ....Norman
HADDOCK, J. L. ....Norman
*HADDOCK PHIL ....Norman
*HOOD, J. O. ....Norman
HOWELL, O. E. ....Norman
LAMBERT, J. B. ....Lexington
*LOY, WILLIAM A. ....Norman
MAYFIELD, W. T. ....Norman
MERRITT, IVA S. ....Norman
NEILSEN, GERTRUDE ....Norman
*PROSSER, MOORMAN P. ....Norman
*RAYBURN, CHARLES R. ....Norman
*REICHERT, R. J. ....Moore
RIEGER, J. A. ....Norman
SCHMIDT, ELEONORA L. ....Norman
STEEN, C. T. ....Norman
STEPHENS, E. F. ....Norman
WICKHAM, M. M. ....Norman
WILEY, G. A. ....Norman
*WILLARD, D. G. ....Norman
WOODSON, O. M. ....Norman

COAL

CLARK, J. B. ....Coalgate
CODY, ROBERT D. ....Centrahoma
HENRY, R. C. ....Coalgate
HIPES, J. J. ....Coalgate

COMANCHE

ANGUS, DONALD A. ....Lawton
ANGUS, H. A. ....Lawton
ANGUS, HOWARD ....Lawton
ANTONY, JOSEPH T. ....Lawton
BARBER, GEORGE S. ....Lawton
BERRY, G. L. ....Lawton
COLE, WILLIAM C. ....Lawton
DOWNING, GERALD G. ....Lawton
DUNLAP, ERNEST B. ....Lawton
FERGUSON, LAWRENCE W. ....Lawton
FOX, FRED T. ....Lawton

GOOCH, L. T. ....Lawton
HAMMOND, FRED W. ....Lawton
HATHAWAY, EUEL P. ....Lawton
JOYCE, CHARLES W. ....Fletcher
KNEE, L. C. ....Lawton
LEWIS, W. F. ....Lawton
MARTIN, CHESLEY M. ....Elgin
MASON, W. J. ....Lawton
PARSONS, O. L. ....Lawton

COTTON

BAKER, G. W. ....Walters
SCISM, MOLLIE F. ....Walters
*TALLANT, GEORGE A. ....Walters
*VAN METER, R. M. ....Walters

CRAIG

ADAMS, F. M. ....Vinita
*BRADSHAW, J. O. ....Welch
CHUMLEY, C. P. ....Vinita
*DARROUGH, J. B. ....Vinita
FAUST, HUGH H. ....Vinita
HAYS, P. L. ....Vinita
HERRON, A. W. ....Vinita
LEHMER, ELIZABETH E ....Vinita
MARKS, W. R. ....Vinita
MAXWELL, THOMAS M. ....Vinita
McMILLAN J. M. ....Vinita
McPIKE, LLOYD H. ....Vinita
SANGER, PAUL G. ....Vinita

CREEK

**BISBEE, W. G. ....Bristow
COPPEDGE, O. C. ....Bristow
*COPPEDGE, O. N. ....Bristow
COPPEDGE, O. S. ....Depew
*COWART, O. H. ....Bristow
CROSTON, GEORGE C. ....Sapulpa
*CURRY, J. F. ....Sapulpa
HAAS, H. R. ....Sapulpa
HOLLIS, J. E. ....Bristow
JOSEPH, PHILIP G. ....Sapulpa
KING, E. W. ....Bristow
LAMPTON, J. B. ....Sapulpa
LEWIS, P .K. ....Sapulpa
LONGMIRE, W. P., JR. ....Johns Hopkins Hospital,
                                Baltimore, Maryland
LONGMIRE, W. P., SR. ....Sapulpa
McDONALD, C. R. ....Mannford
*MOTE, PAUL ....Sapulpa
*PICKHARDT, W. L. ....Sapulpa
REESE, C. B. ....Sapulpa
REYNOLDS, S. W. ....Drumright
SISLER, FRANK H. ....Bristow
*SISLER, FRANK H., JR. ....Bristow
STARR, O. W. ....Drumright
WHARTON, J. L. ....Depew
**Deceased March 17, 1944.

CUSTER

ALEXANDER, C. J. ....Clinton
ASHER, JAMES O. ....Clinton
BISHOP, H. H. ....Clinton
BOYD, T. A. ....Weatherford
BRUNDAGE, BERT T. ....Thomas
**BULLOCK, BERNARD ....Clinton
CUNNINGHAM, C. B. ....Clinton
*CUSHMAN, H. R. ....Clinton
DEPUTY, ROSS ....Clinton
DOLER, C. ....Clinton
FRIZZELL, J. T. (honorary) ....Clinton
GAEDE, D. ....Weatherford
GOSSOM, K. D. ....Clinton
*HINSHAW, J. R. ....Butler
*KENNEDY, LOUIS ....Clinton
LAIN, W. B. ....Clinton
LAMB, ELLIS ....Clinton
*LINGENFELTER, PAUL B. ....Clinton
McBURNEY, C. H. ....Clinton
*PAULSON, ALVIN W. ....Clinton

ROGERS, McLAIN _____Clinton
RUHL, N. E. _____Weatherford
SMITH, WILLARD H. _____Clinton
STOLL, A. A. _____Clinton
*TISDAL, WILLIAM C. _____Clinton
VIEREGG, F. R. _____Clinton
*WILLIAMS, GORDON _____Weatherford
*WOOD, J. GUILD _____Weatherford
**Deceased June 10, 1944.

DELAWARE

WALKER, C. F. _____Grove
(member Ottawa County Medical Society)

DEWEY

LOYD. E. M. _____Taloga
(member Custer County Medical Society)
MABRY, W. L. _____Leedey
(member Beckham County Medical Society)
SEBA, W. E. _____Leedey
(member Beckham County Medical Society)
VINCENT, D. W. _____Vici
(member Woodward County Medical Society)

ELLIS

BEAM, J. P _____Arnett
(member Woodward County Medical Society)
*DUBE, PAUL H. _____Shattuck
(member Woodward County Medical Society)
*NEWMAN, FLOYD _____Shattuck
(member Woodward County Medical Society)
NEWMAN, M. HASKELL _____Shattuck
(member Woodward County Medical Society)
NEWMAN, O. O. _____Shattuck
(member Woodward County Medical Society)
NEWMAN, ROY _____Shattuck
(member Woodward County Medical Society)

GARFIELD

*BAKER, R. C. _____Enid
BITTING, B. T. _____Enid
BONHAM, KENNETH W. _____Enid
*CHAMBERS, E. EVANS _____Enid
CHAMPLIN, PAUL R. _____Enid
*CORDONNIER, BYRON J. _____Enid
COTTON, LEE W. (honorary) _____Enid
DUFFY, FRANCIS M. _____Enid
FEILD, JULIAN _____Enid
FRANCISCO, GLENN _____Enid
HALL, R. L. _____Enid
HAMBLE, V. R. _____Enid
HARRIS, D. S. _____Drummond
*HINSON, BRUCE B. _____Enid
HOPKINS, P. W. _____Enid
HUDSON, F. A. _____Enid
HUDSON, HARRY H. _____Enid
*JACOBS, RAYMOND C. _____Enid
McEVOY, S. H. _____Enid
*MERCER, WENDELL J. _____Enid
METSCHER, ALFRED J. _____Enid
*NEILSON, W. P _____Enid
*NEWELL, W. B., JR. _____Enid
NEWELL, W. B., SR _____Enid
REMPEL, PAUL H. _____Enid
RHODES, W. H. _____Enid
*ROBERTS, C. J. _____Enid
ROBERTS, D. D. _____Enid
*ROSS, GEORGE _____Enid
ROSS, HOPE _____Enid
SHEETS, MARION E. _____Enid
*TALLEY, EVANS E. _____Enid
VANDEVER, H. F. _____Enid
WALKER, JOHN R. _____Enid
WATSON, JOHN M. _____Enid
WILKINS, A. E. _____Covington
WILSON, GEORGE S. _____Enid

GARVIN

ALEXANDER, ROBERT M. _____Paoli
CALLAWAY, JOHN R. _____Pauls Valley
GREENING, WILLIAM P. _____Pauls Valley

GROSS, T. F. _____Lindsay
JOHNSON, GALVIN L. _____Pauls Valley
*LINDSEY, RAY H. _____Pauls Valley
MONROE, HUGH H. _____Pauls Valley
ROBBERSON, MARVIN E. _____Wynnewood
ROBBERSON, MORTON E. _____Wynnewood
SHI, AUGUSTIN H. _____Stratford
SHIRLEY, EDWARD T. _____Pauls Valley
SULLIVAN, CLEVE L. _____Elmore City

GRADY

*BAZE, ROY E. _____Chickasha
BAZE, WALTER J. _____Chickasha
BONNELL, W. L. _____Chickasha
BOON, U. C. _____Chickasha
*BYNUM, W. TURNER _____Chickasha
COOK, W. H. _____Chickasha
DOWNEY, D. S. _____Chickasha
EMANUEL, LEWIS E. _____Chickasha
EMANUEL, ROY E. _____Chickasha
GOODRICH, E. E. _____Chickasha
HENNINGS, A. E. _____Tuttle
*JOYCE, FRANK T. _____Chickasha
LEEDS, A. B. _____Chickasha
*LITTLE, AARON C. _____Minco
LIVERMORE, W. H. (honorary) _____Chickasha
MASON, REBECCA H. _____Chickasha
McCLURE, H. M. _____Chickasha
MITCHELL, C. P. _____Chickasha
PYLE, OSCAR S. _____Chickasha
RENEGAR, J. F. _____Tuttle
*SCHUBERT, H. A. _____Chickasha
WOODS, LEWIS E. _____Chickasha

GRANT

HARDY, I. V. _____Medford
SHANNON, H. R. _____Pondcreek
(member Garfield County Medical Society)

GREER

**CHERRY, G. P. (honorary) _____Mangum
HOLLIS, J. B. _____Mangum
LANSDEN, J. B. _____Granite
LEWIS, R. W. _____Granite
LOWE, J. T. _____Mangum
PEARSON, LEE E. _____Mangum
POER, E. M. _____Mangum
*RUDE, JOE C. _____Mangum
**Deceased May 21, 1944.

HARMON

HUSBAND, W. G. _____Hollis
LYNCH, R. H. _____Hollis
RAY, W. T. (honorary) _____Gould
STREET, O. J. _____Gould
YEARGAN, W. M. _____Hollis

HARPER

CAMP, EARL (honorary) _____Buffalo
(member Woodward County Medical Society)
HILL, H. K. _____Laverne
(member Woodward County Medical Society)
*PIERSON, DWIGHT _____Buffalo
(member Woodward County Medical Society)
WALKER, HARDIN _____Buffalo
(member Woodward County Medical Society)
WINCHELL, F. Z. _____Buffalo
(member Woodward County Medical Society)

HASKELL

CARSON, WILLIAM S. _____Keota
RUMLEY, J. C. _____Stigler
THOMPSON, W. A. _____Stigler
WILLIAMS, N. K. _____McCurtain

HUGHES

DAVENPORT, A. L. _____Holdenville
FLOYD, W. E. _____Holdenville
GEORGE, L. J. _____Stuart
(member Pittsburg County Medical Society)
HAMILTON, S. H. _____Non

HICKS, C. A. ...._Holdenville_
HOWELL, H. A. ...._Holdenville_
*JOHNSTON, L. A. S. ...._Holdenville_
*KERNEK, CLYDE ...._Holdenville_
KERNEK, PAUL ...._Holdenville_
MAYFIELD, IMOGENE ...._Holdenville_
MORRIS, C. H. ...._Wetumka_
*MUNAL, JOHN ...._Holdenville_
PRYOR, V. W. ...._Holdenville_
*SHAW, JAMES F. ...._Wetumka_
**TAYLOR, W. L. ...._Holdenville_
WALLACE, C. S. ...._Holdenville_
**_Deceased April 16, 1944._

JACKSON

ABERNETHY, E. A. ...._Altus_
*ALLGOOD, J. M. ...._Altus_
CROW, E. S. ...._Olustee_
*FOX, R. H. ...._Altus_
*HOLT, W. D. ...._Altus_
IRBY, J. P. ...._Altus_
MABRY, E. W. ...._Altus_
McCONNELL, L. H. ...._Altus_
McFADIN, J. S. ...._Altus_
REID, JOHN R. ...._Altus_
SPEARS, C. G. ...._Altus_
STULTS, J. S. (_honorary_) ...._Altus_
TAYLOR, R. Z. ...._Blair_

JEFFERSON

ANDERSKOWSKI, W. T. ...._Ryan_
COLLINS, D. B. ...._Wewrika_
DERR, J. I. ...._Wewrika_
EDWARDS, F. M. ...._Ringling_
HOLLINGSWORTH, J. L. ...._Wewrika_
MAUPIN, C. M. ...._Wewrika_
**WADE, L. L. ...._Ryan_
YEATS, H. WESLEY ...._Ringling_
**_Deceased April 1, 1944._

JOHNSTON

RAINES, S. W. ...._Wapanucka_
(_member Bryan County Medical Society_)

KAY

ARRENDELL, C. W. ...._Ponca City_
CLIFT, MERL ...._Blackwell_
*CURRY, JOHN R. ...._Blackwell_
GARDNER, C. C. ...._Ponca City_
GIBSON, R. B. ...._Ponca City_
*GORDON, D. M. ...._Ponca City_
GOWEY, H. O. ...._Newkirk_
*HARMS, EDWIN M. ...._Blackwell_
HOWE, J. HOLLAND ...._Ponca City_
*KENNEDY, VIRGIL ...._Newkirk_
KINNAMAN, JOSEPH H. ...._Ponca City_
*KREGER, G. S. ...._Tonkawa_
KREGER, J. RUSSELL ...._Tonkawa_
MALL, W. W. ...._Ponca City_
MATHEWS, DEWEY ...._Tonkawa_
MILLER, D. W. ...._Blackwell_
*MOHLER, ELDON C. ...._Ponca City_
MOORE, G. C. ...._Ponca City_
*MORGAN, L. S. ...._Ponca City_
*NEAL, L. G. ...._Ponca City_
NIEMANN, G. H. ...._Ponca City_
NORTHCUTT, C. E. ...._Ponca City_
NUCKOLS, A. S. ...._Ponca City_
RISSER, A. S. ...._Blackwell_
RISSER, PHILIP C. ...._Blackwell_
VANCE, L. C. ...._Ponca City_
WAGGONER, E. E. ...._Tonkawa_
WAGNER, J. C. ...._Ponca City_
WALKER, I. D. ...._Tonkawa_
*WHITE, M. S. ...._Blackwell_
*WRIGHT, L. I. ...._Blackwell_
YEARY, G. H. ...._Newkirk_

KINGFISHER

DIXON, A. ...._Hennessey_

GOSE, C. O. ...._Hennessey_
HODGSON, C. M. ...._Kingfisher_
*LATTIMORE, F. C. ...._Kingfisher_
MEREDITH, A. O. ...._Kingfisher_
PENDLETON, JOHN W. ...._Kingfisher_
STURGEON, H. VIOLET ...._Hennessey_
*TAYLOR, JOHN R. ...._Kingfisher_
TOWNSEND, B. I. ...._Hennessey_

KIOWA

BERNELL, WILLIAM ...._Hobart_
BONHAM, J. M. ...._Hobart_
BRAUN, J. P. ...._Hobart_
FINCH, J. WILLIAM ...._Hobart_
HATHAWAY, A. H. ...._Mountain View_
MOORE, J. H. ...._Hobart_
PRESTON, C. R. ...._Mountain Park_
WATKINS, B. H. ...._Trementina, N. M._

LATIMER

BOOTH, G. R. ...._Wilburton_
(_member Le Flore County Medical Society_)

LE FLORE

BAKER, F. P. ...._Talihina_
BEVILL, S. D. ...._Poteau_
COLLINS, E. L. ...._Panama_
DEAN, S. C. ...._Howe_
FAIR, E. N. ...._Heavener_
GILLIAM, WILLIAM C. ...._Spiro_
MINOR, R. W. ...._Spiro_
MIXON, A. M. ...._Spiro_
ROLLE, NEESON ...._Poteau_
*SHIPPEY, W. L. ...._Poteau_
WOODSON, E. M. ...._Poteau_
WRIGHT, R. L. ...._Poteau_

LINCOLN

ADAMS, J. W. ...._Chandler_
BAILEY, CARL H. ...._Stroud_
BROWN, R. A. ...._Prague_
(_member Pottawatomie County Medical Society_)
BURLESON, NED ...._Prague_
DAVIS, W. B. ...._Stroud_
ERWIN, PARA ...._Wellston_
HURLBUT, E. T. ...._Meeker_
MARSHALL, A. M. ...._Chandler_
NICKELL, U. E. ...._Davenport_
NORWOOD, F. H. ...._Prague_
ROBERTSON, C. W. ...._Chandler_
ROLLINS, J. S. ...._Prague_

LOGAN

BARKER, PAULINE ...._Guthrie_
BUSSEY, H. N. ...._Mulhall_
CORNWELL, N. L. ...._Coyle_
GARDNER, P. B. ...._Guthrie_
GRAY, DAN F. ...._Guthrie_
HAHN, L. A. ...._Guthrie_
HILL, C. B. ...._Guthrie_
LEHEW, J. L. JR. ...._Guthrie_
MILLER, W. C. ...._Guthrie_
PETTY, C. S. ...._Guthrie_
*PETTY, JAMES S. ...._Guthrie_
REDING, ANTHONY C. ...._Coyle_
RINGROSE, R. F. ...._Guthrie_
*RITZHAUPT, LOUIS H. ...._Guthrie_
SOUTER, J. E. ...._Guthrie_

LOVE

*LAWSON, PAT ...._Marietta_
(_member Carter County Medical Society_)
LOONEY, M. D. ...._Marietta_
(_member Carter County Medical Society_)

MAJOR

McCROSKIE, M. R. ...._Fairview_
(_member Garfield County Medical Society_)
RYAN, ROBERT O. ...._Fairview_
(_member Garfield County Medical Society_)
SPECHT, ELSIE ...._Fairview_
(_member Garfield County Medical Society_)

MARSHALL

COOK, ODIS A. _____Madill
HOLLAND, JOHN LEE _____Madill
YORK, JOSEPH F. _____Madill

MAYES

CAMERON, PAUL B. _____Pryor
HERRINGTON, V. D. _____Pryor
MORROW, B. L. _____Salina
RUTHERFORD, S. C. _____Locust Grove
SMITH, R. V. _____Pryor
WERLING, E. H. _____Pryor
WHITE, L. C. _____Adair

McCLAIN

COCHRANE, J. E. _____Byars
DAVIS, S. C. _____Blanchard
KOLB, I. N. _____Blanchard
McCURDY, W. C., JR. _____Purcell
McCURDY, W. C., SR. _____Purcell
ROYSTER, R. L. _____Purcell

McCURTAIN

BARKER, N. L. _____Broken Bow
CLARKSON, A. W. _____Valliant
KELLEAM, E. A. _____Wright City
McBRAYER, WILLIAM H. _____Haworth
MORELAND, J. T. _____Idabel
MORELAND, W. A. _____Idabel
OLIVER, R. B. _____Idabel
SHERRILL, R. H. _____Broken Bow
WILLIAMS, R. D. _____Idabel
WILLIAMS, W. W. _____Idabel

McINTOSH

BAKER, J. HOWARD _____Eufaula
FIRST, F. R. _____Checotah
JACOBS, LUSTER I. _____Hanna
LITTLE, DANIEL E. _____Eufaula
*STONER, RAYMOND W. _____Checotah
TOLLESON, WILLIAM A. _____Eufaula
WOOD, JAMES L. _____Eufaula

MURRAY

ANNADOWN, P. V. _____Sulphur
RUDELL, W. P. _____Sulphur
WRENN, J. A. _____Sulphur

MUSKOGEE

BALLANTINE, H. T. _____Muskogee
BRUTON, L. D. _____Muskogee
COACHMAN, E. H. _____Muskogee
*DORWART, F. G. _____Muskogee
*DOYLE, W. H. _____Muskogee
EARNEST, A. N. _____Muskogee
ELKINS, MARVIN _____Muskogee
EWING, FINIS W. _____Muskogee
FITE, E. HALSELL _____Muskogee
FITE, W. PAT _____Muskogee
FULLENWIDER, C. M. _____Muskogee
GEE, L. E. _____Muskogee
(member LeFlore County Medical Society)
HAMM, SILAS G. _____Haskell
*HOLCOMBE, R. N. _____Muskogee
JOHNSON, S. E. _____Muskogee
KLASS, O. C. _____Muskogee
KUPKA, JOHN F. _____Haskell
McALISTER, L. S. _____Muskogee
*McINNIS, J. T. _____Muskogee
MILLER, D. EVELYN _____Muskogee
MOBLEY, A. L. _____Albuquerque, N. M.
*NEELY, SHADE D. _____Muskogee
OLDHAM, I. B. _____Muskogee
RAFTER, JOHN R. _____Muskogee
*REYNOLDS, JOHN H. _____Muskogee
ROGERS, ISAAC W. _____Muskogee
*SCHNOEBELEN, RENE E. _____Muskogee
SCOTT, H. A. _____Muskogee
STARK, W. W. _____Muskogee
(member Okmulgee County Medical Society)
THOMPSON, M. K. _____Muskogee

*WEAVER, W. N. _____Muskogee
WHITE, CHARLES ED _____Muskogee
WHITE, J. HUTCHINGS _____Muskogee
*WOLFE, I. C. _____Muskogee
*WOODBURN, J. TINDER _____Muskogee

NOBLE

COLDIRON, D. F. _____Perry
COOKE, C. H. _____Perry
DRIVER, JESSE W. _____Perry
*EVANS, A. M. _____Perry
FRANCIS, J. W. _____Perry
HEISS, J. E. _____Perry
RENFROW, T. F. _____Billings

NOWATA

DAVIS, KIEFFER D. _____Nowata
KURTZ, R. L. _____Nowata
LANG, S. A. _____Nowata
ROBERTS, S. P. _____Nowata
SCOTT, M. B. _____Delaware

OKFUSKEE

COCHRAN, C. M. _____Okemah
JENKINS, W. P. _____Okemah
LUCAS, A. C. _____Castle
MELTON, A. S. _____Okemah
**PEMBERTON, J. M. _____Okemah
PRESTON, J. R. _____Weleetka
SPICKARD, L. J. _____Okemah
WHITNEY, M. L. _____Okemah
**Deceased February 21, 1944.

OKLAHOMA

ABSHIER, A. BROOKS _____1200 N. Walker
ADAMS, ROBERT H._____515 N. W. 11th St.
AKIN, ROBERT H. _____400 N. W. 10th St.
ALFORD, J. M. _____Medical Arts Bldg.
ALLEN, E. P. _____1200 N. Walker
*ALLEN, GEORGE T. _____1200 N. Walker
ANDREWS, LEILA E. _____1200 N. Walker
*APPLETON, M. M. _____400 N. W. 10th St.
*AYCOCK, BYRON W. _____301 N. W. 12th St.
BAILEY, FRANK M. _____1219 N. W. 21st St.
*BAILEY, W. H. _____301 N. W. 12th St.
BAKER, MARGUERITE M. _____1200 N. E. 63rd St.
BALYEAT, RAY M. _____1200 N. Walker
*BARB, T. J. _____318 S. W. 25th St.
BARKER, C. E. _____1200 N. Walker
BARRY, GEORGE N. _____Medical Arts Bldg.
*BATCHELOR, JOHN J. _____Medical Arts Bldg.
*BATTENFIELD, JOHN Y. _____State Health Dept.
BAUM, E. ELDON _____Perrine Bldg.
BAYLOR, R. A. _____400 N. W. 10th St.
*BEDNAR, GERALD _____Medical Arts Bldg.
*BELL, AUSTIN H. _____301 N. W. 12th St.
BELL, J. T. _____3400 N. Eastern Ave.
BERRY CHARLES N. _____Medical Arts Bldg.
*BINDER, HAROLD J. _____628 N. W. 21st St.
BINKLEY, J. G. _____Medical Arts Bldg.
*BIRGE, JACK P. _____204 N. Robinson St.
BLACHLY, CHARLES D. _____2752 N. W. 18th St.
BLACHLY, LUCILE SPIRE _____605 N. W. 10th St.
BOATRIGHT, LLOYD C. _____Perrine Bldg.
BOGGS, NATHAN _____Perrine Bldg.
*BOLEND, REX _____Medical Arts Bldg.
BONDURANT, C. P. _____Medical Arts Bldg.
BONHAM, WILLIAM L. _____Medical Arts Bldg.
*BORDER, CLINTON L. _____American Nat'l Bldg.
*BORECKY, GEORGE L. _____204 N. Robinson St.
BRADLEY, H. C. _____Perrine Bldg.
*BRANHAM, D. W. _____Medical Arts Bldg.
BREWER, A. M. _____521 N. W. 10th St.
*BRIGHTWELL, RICHARD J. ___1230 N. W. 41st St.
*BROWN, GERSTER W. _____Medical Arts Bldg.
BRUNDAGE, C. L. _____1200 N. Walker
BURKE, R. M. _____Medical Arts Bldg.
BURTON, JOHN F. _____1200 N. Walker
BUTLER, H. W. _____1200 N. Walker
CAILEY, LEO F. _____Medical Arts Bldg.
CAMPBELL, COYNE H. _____131 N. E. 4th St.

CAMPBELL, J. MOORE, III ....Medical Arts Bldg.
CANNON, J. M. ....210½ W. Commerce St.
CATES, ALBERT M. (honorary) ...2733 N. E. 20th St.
CAVINESS, J. J. ....Medical Arts Bldg.
*CHAFFIN, ZALE ....Municipal Bldg.
*CHARNEY, L. H. ....Medical Arts Bldg.
CLARK, ANSON L. ....Medical Arts Bldg.
*CLARK, JOHN V. ....1706 S. E. 29 St.
CLARK, LEMON ....Medical Arts Bldg.
CLARK, RALPH O. ....1706 S. E. 29th St
CLOUDMAN, H. H. ....Medical Arts Bldg.
CLYMER, C. E. ....Medical Arts Bldg.
COLEY, A. J. (honorary) ....Hightower Bldg.
*COLEY, JOE H. ....105 N. Hudson St.
COOPER, F. MANEY ....Medical Arts Bldg.
COSTON, TULLOS O. ......Medical Arts Bldg.
COTTEN, DAISY V. H. .....807 N. W. 23rd St.
CRICK, L. E. ....Britton
DANIELS, HARRY A. .....610 N. W. 9th St.
DERSCH, WALTER H. .....Medical Arts Bldg.
DEUPREE, HARRY L. ......Medical Arts Bldg.
*DEVANNEY, LOUIS R. ....1200 N. Walker
DICKSON, GREEN K. ......2124 Carey Place
DILL, FRANCIS E. ....Medical Arts Bldg.
DOUDNA, HUBERT E. ......800 N. E.13 th St.
DOWDY, THOMAS W. ......Medical Arts Bldg.
*DRUMMOND, N. ROBERT ....Medical Arts Bldg.
DUDLEY, ALBERTA W. ......First Nat'l. Bldg.
**EARLY, RALPH O. ....Medical Arts Bldg.
EASTLAND, WILLIAM E. .....Medical Arts Bldg.
ELEY, N. PRICE ....400 N. W. 10th St.
*EMENHISER, LEE K. ....Medical Arts Bldg.
EPLEY, C. O. ....1200 N. Walker
ERWIN, FRANTZ B. ....Medical Arts Bldg.
ESKRIDGE, J. B., JR. ....1200 N. Walker
FAGIN, HERMAN ....Nat'l Aid Life Bldg.
FARIS, BRUNEL D. ....Medical Arts Bldg.
FARNAM, LARRY M. ....1200 N. Walker
FELTS, GEORGE R. ....625½ N. W. 10th St.
FERGUSON, E. GORDON ......Medical Arts Bldg.
FISHMAN, C. J. ....132 N. W. 4th St.
FLEETWOOD, D. H. ....Edmond
FLESHER, THOMAS H. ....Edmond
*FOERSTER, HERVEY A. ....Medical Arts Bldg.
*FORD, HARRY C. ....Medical Arts Bldg.
FRIERSON, S. E. ....Medical Arts Bldg.
*FRYER, SAM R. ....119 N. W. 5th St.
*FULTON, C. C. ....Medical Arts Bldg.
FULTON, GEORGE ....American Nat'l Bldg.
GALBRAITH, HUGH M. ....First Nat'l Bldg.
GALLAGER, C. A. ....610 N. W. 9th St.
GARRISON, GEORGE H. ......1200 N. Walker
GEE, O. J. ....Medical Arts Bldg.
*GIBBS, ALLEN G ....Apco Tower
*GINGLES, R. H. ....State Health Dept.
GLISMANN, M. B. ....1021 N. Lee
GLOMSET, JOHN L. ....1200 N. Walker
GOLDFAIN, E. ....228 N. W. 13th St.
GOODHUE, WILLIAM W. .....521 N. W. 11th St.
GOODWIN, R. Q. ....Medical Arts Bldg.
GRAENING, P. K. ....605 N. W. 10th St.
GRAHAM, A. T. ....26 S. W. 25th St.
GRAY, FLOYD ....1200 N. Walker
HACKLER, JOHN F. ....801 N. E. 13th St.
HALL, CLARK H. ....Medical Arts Bldg.
HAMMONDS, O. O. ....623 N. E. 18th St.
HARBISON, FRANK ....510 N. W. 12th St.
HARBISON, J. E. ....510 N. W. 12th St.
HARRIS, HENRY W. ....1200 N. Walker
HARRIS, J. M. ....Midwest City
(member Pittsburg County Medical Society)
*HARRISON, LYNN H. ....510 N. W. 12th St.
HASKETT, PAUL E. ....Hales Bldg.
HASSLER, F. R. ....State Health Dept.
HASSLER, GRACE C. ....Medical Arts Bldg.
HAYES, BASIL A. ....625 N. W. 10th St.
*HAZEL, ONIS G. ....1200 N. Walker
HEATLEY, JOHN E. ....Medical Arts Bldg.
*HERRMANN, JESS D. ....Medical Arts Bldg.
HETHERINGTON, A. J. ....2014 Gatewood
HICKS, FRED B. ....Medical Arts Bldg.
*HIGHLAND, J. B. ....634 N. E. 13th St.
HIRSHFIELD, A. C. ....Medical Arts Bldg
*HOLLINGSWORTH, C. E. .....Medical Arts Bldg.
HOLLIS, LYNN E. ....830 N. E. 21st St.
(member Harmon County Medical Society)
*HOOD, F. REDDING ....1200 N. Walker
*HOWARD, ROBERT B. ....1200 N. Walker
HOWARD, R. M. ....1200 N. Walker
HUFF, RHEBA L. ....1200 N. Walker
*HUGGINS, J. R. ....2225 Exchange Ave.
HULL, WAYNE M. ....1200 N. Walker
HUNTER, GEORGE ....County Court House
*HYROOP, GILBERT L. ....Medical Arts Bldg.
*ISHMAEL, WILLIAM K. ......605 N. W. 10th St.
JACKSON, A. R. ....2528½ S. Robinson
JACOBS, MINARD F. ....Medical Arts Bldg.
JANCO, LEON ....10 W. Park
JETER, HUGH ....1200 N. Walker
JOBE, VIRGIL E. ....1213 N. Hudson
JONES, HUGH ....Medical Arts Bldg.
KELLER, W. FLOYD ....Medical Arts Bldg.
KELSO, JOSEPH W. ....Medical Arts Bldg.
KELTZ, BERT F. ....Medical Arts Bldg.
KENNEDY, JULIAN J. ....Douglas Aircraft Co.
KERNODLE, STRATTON E. ....First Nat'l Bldg.
KILLEEN, EMMET R. ....521 N. W. 11th St.
*KIMBALL, GEORGE H. ....Medical Arts Bldg.
*KUHN, JOHN F. ....Medical Arts Bldg.
*KURZNER, MEYER ....1200 N. Walker
LACHMANN, ERNST ....801 N. E. 13th St.
LAIN, E. S. ....Medical Arts Bldg.
LAMB, JOHN H. ....Medical Arts Bldg.
LAMBKE, PHIL M. ....105 N. W. 23rd St.
LAMOTTE, GEORGE A. ....Colcord Bldg.
LANGSTON, WANN ....Medical Arts Bldg.
*LEMON, CECIL W. ....Medical Arts Bldg.
LENEY, FANNIE LOU ....1200 N. Walker
LEONARD, C. E. ....131 N. E. 4th St.
LEVY, BERTHA M. ....1200 N. Walker
LEWIS, A. R. ....Hightower Bldg.
*LINDSTROM, W. C. ....Medical Arts Bldg.
LINGENFELTER, F. M. ......1200 N. Walker
*LITTLE, JOHN R. ....Apco Tower
LONG, LEROY D. ....Medical Arts Bldg.
LONG, WENDELL ....Medical Arts Bldg.
LOVE, R. S. ....Perrine Bldg.
LOWRY, TOM ....1200 N. Walker
LOY, C. F. ....400 N. W. 10th St.
LUTON, JAMES P. ....Medical Arts Bldg.
LYON, JAMES I. ....Edmond
MACDONALD, J. C. ....301 N. W. 12th St.
*MACKEY, ABNER ....901 N. W. 13th St.
MARGO, ELIAS ....605 N. W. 10th St.
*MARIL, JOSEPH J. ....Medical Arts Bldg.
*MARTIN, HOWARD C. ....204 N. Robinson St.
MARTIN, J. T. ....200 N. W. 14th St.
MASTERSON, MAUDE M. .....Medical Arts Bldg.
MATHEWS, GRADY F. ....State Health Dept.
(member Cherokee County Medical Society)
*MATTHEWS, SANFORD ....400 N. W. 10th St.
McBRIDE, EARL D. ....605 N. W. 10th St.
*McCLURE, WILLIAM C. ......1200 N. Walker
McGEE, J. P. ....1200 N. Walker
McHENRY, L. CHESTER ......Medical Arts Bldg.
McKINNEY, MILAN F. ....Medical Arts Bldg.
McNEILL, P. M. ....Medical Arts Bldg.
MECHLING, GEORGE S. ......1200 N. Walker
*MELVIN, JAMES H. ....First Nat'l Bldg.
MESSENBAUGH, J. F. ....Medical Arts Bldg.
*MESSINGER, R. P. ....807 N. W. 23rd St.
*MILES, W. H. ....1200 N. Walker
*MILLER, NESBITT L. ....Medical Arts Bldg.
MILLS, R. C. ....Hightower
MOOR, H. D. ....800 N. E. 13th St.
MOORE, B. H. ....Perrine Bldg.
MOORE, C. D. ....Perrine Bldg.
MOORE, ELLIS ....Medical Arts Bldg.

MOORMAN, FLOYD ....1200 N. Walker.
MOORMAN, LEWIS J. ....1200 N. Walker
MORGAN, C. A. ....First Nat'l Bldg.
MORLEDGE, WALKER ....1200 N. Walker
MORRISON, H. C. ....807 N. W. 23rd St.
MOTH, M. V. ....American Nat'l Bldg.
*MULVEY, BERT E. ....Medical Arts Bldg.
MURDOCH, L. H. ....Medical Arts Bldg.
  (member Blaine County Medical Society)
*MURDOCH, RAYMOND L. ....Medical Arts Bldg.
MUSICK, E. R. ....Medical Arts Bldg.
MUSICK, VERN H. ....Medical Arts Bldg.
MUSSIL, W. M. ....Medical Arts Bldg.
MYERS, RALPH E. ....1200 N. Walker
NAGLE, PATRICK S. ....1021 N. Lee
NEEL, ROY L. ....Medical Arts Bldg.
*NEFF, EVERETT B. ....1200 N. Walker
NICHOLSON, BEN H. ....301 N. W. 12th St.
*NOELL, ROBERT L. ....Medical Arts Bldg.
O'DONOGHUE, D. H. ....Medical Arts Bldg.
O'LEARY, CHARLES M. ....Medical Arts Bldg.
PARRISH, J. M., JR. ....1200 N. Walker
PAULUS, D. D. ....301 N. W. 12th St.
PAYTE, J. I. ....2429 Aurora Court
PENICK, GRIDER ....Colcord Bldg.
PHELPS, A. S. ....Medical Arts Bldg.
PINE, JOHN S. ....Medical Arts Bldg.
POINTS, THOMAS C. ....1200 N. Walker
*POOLE, WARREN B. ....521 N. W. 11th St.
POSTELLE, J. M. (honorary) ....Box 2586
  Portland, Oregon
POUNDERS, CARROLL M. ....1200 N. Walker
PRICE, JOEL S. ....1200 N. Walker
PUCKETT, CARL ....22 W. 6th St.
  (member Mayes County Medical Society)
RANDEL, HARVEY O. ....Medical Arts Bldg.
RECK, JOHN A. ....Colcord Bldg.
*RECORDS, JOHN W. ....301 N. W. 12th St.
REED, HORACE ....1200 N. Walker
REED, JAMES R. ....Medical Arts Bldg.
REEVES, C. L. ....400 N. W. 10th St.
REICHMANN, RUTH S. ....124 N. W. 15th St.
RICE, PAUL B. ....800 N. E. 13th St.
*RICKS, J. R. ....1200 N. Walker
RIELY, LEA A. ....Medical Arts Bldg.
RILEY, J. W. ....119 N. W. 5th St.
ROBINSON, J. H. ....301 N. W. 12th St.
RODDY, JOHN A. ....Apco Tower
ROGERS, GERALD ....1200 N. Walker
ROUNTREE, C. R. ....1200 N. Walker
*ROYCE, OWEN, JR. ....800 N. E. 13th St.
*RUCKS, W. W., JR. ....301 N. W. 12th St.
RUCKS, W. W., SR. ....301 N. W. 12th St.
RUSSO, PETER E. ....Medical Arts Bldg.
*SADLER, LEROY H. ....1200 N. Walker
SALOMON, A. L. ....1200 N. Walker
*SANGER, F. A. ....Key Bldg.
SANGER, F. M. ....Perrine Bldg.
SANGER, WINNIE M. ....Perrine Bldg.
*SANGER, W. W. ....301 N. W. 12th St.
*SEBA, CHESTER R. ....1200 N. Walker
SEBRING, MILTON H. ....Apco Tower
*SELL, L. STANLEY ....Medical Arts Bldg.
SERWER, MILTON J. ....1200 N. Walker
*SEWELL, DAN R. ....400 N. W. 10th St.
SHACKELFORD, JOHN W. ....State Health Dept.
SHAVER, S. R. ....Medical Arts Bldg.
SHELBY, HUDSON S. ....Hales Bldg.
SHELTON, J. W. ....Hightower Bldg.
SHEPPARD, MARY S. ....1200 N. Walker
*SHIRCLIFF, E. E., JR. ....128 N. W. 14th St.
*SHORBE, HOWARD B. ....605 N. W. 10th St.
*SMITH, CHARLES A. ....717 N. Robinson St.
SMITH, DELBERT G. ....First Nat'l Bldg.
SMITH, EDWARD N. ....400 N. W. 10th St.
SMITH, L. L. ....229 S. W. 29th St.
SMITH, RALPH A. ....443½ N. W. 23rd St.
*SNOW, J. B. ....1200 N. Walker
STANBRO, GREGORY E. ....Medical Arts Bldg.

STARRY, L. J. ....1200 N. Walker
STILLWELL, R. J. ....American Nat'l Bldg.
STOUT, MARVIN E. ....209 N. W. 13th St.
*STRADER, S. E. ....105 N. Hudson St.
*STRECKER, WILLIAM E. ....Medical Arts Bldg.
SULLIVAN, ELIJAH E. ....Medical Arts Bldg.
TABOR, GEORGE R. (honorary) ....First Nat'l Bldg.
*TACKETT, ORVILLE H. ....3424 N. W. 19th St.
TAYLOR, CHARLES B. ....Medical Arts Bldg.
*TAYLOR, JIM M. ....Medical Arts Bldg.
TAYLOR, WILLIAM M. ....625½ N. W. 10th St.
THOMPSON, WAYMAN J. ....1200 N. Walker
*TOOL, DONOVAN ....Edmond
TOWNSEND, CARY W. ....Medical Arts Bldg.
TRENT, ROBERT I. ....Medical Arts Bldg.
TURNER, HENRY H. ....1200 N. Walker
*VAHLBERG, E. R. ....First Nat'l Bldg.
VON WEDEL, CURT ....610 N. W. 9th St.
WAILS, T. G. ....Medical Arts Bldg.
*WAINWRIGHT, TOM L. ....Medical Arts Bldg.
*WATSON, I. NEWTON ....Edmond
WATSON, O. ALTON ....1200 N. Walker
WATSON, R. D. ....Britton
WEIR, MARSHALL W. ....Apco Tower
WELLS, EVA ....Medical Arts Bldg.
WELLS, LOIS LYON ....1200 N. Walker
WELLS, W. W. ....Medical Arts Bldg.
WEST, W. K. ....1200 N. Walker
WESTFALL, L. M. ....Medical Arts Bldg.
WHITE, ARTHUR W. ....Medical Arts Bldg.
WHITE, OSCAR ....1200 N. Walker
WHITE, PHIL E. ....Perrine Bldg.
*WILDMAN, S. F. ....Medical Arts Bldg.
WILKINS, HARRY ....Medical Arts Bldg.
WILLIAMS, BYRON E. ....204 Plaza Court
WILLIAMS, LEONARD C. ....1200 N. Walker
WILLIAMSON, W. H. ....128 N. W. 14th St.
WILLIE, JAMES A. ....218 N. W. 7th St.
WILSON, KENNETH J. ....Medical Arts Bldg.
*WITTEN, HAROLD B. ....Harrah
*WOLFF, JOHN POWERS ....1200 N. Walker
WOODWARD, NEIL W. ....1200 N. Walker
WRIGHT, HARPER ....318 S. W. 25th St.
*YEAKEL, EARL L. ....306 N. Robinson
YOUNG, A. M., III ....Medical Arts Bldg.
**Deceased June 6, 1944

OKMULGEE

ALEXANDER, LIN ....Okmulgee
*ALEXANDER, R. L. ....Okmulgee
BOLLINGER, I. W. ....Henryetta
BOSWELL, H. D. ....Henryetta
CARLOSS, T. C. ....Morris
CARNELL, M. D. ....Okmulgee
*COTTERAL, J. R. ....Henryetta
EDWARDS, J. G. ....Okmulgee
HAYNES, W. M. ....Henryetta
HOLMES, A. R. ....Henryetta
HUDSON, W. S. ....Okmulgee
KILPATRICK, G. A. ....Henryetta
*LESLIE, S. B., JR. ....Okmulgee
LESLIE, S. B., SR. ....Okmulgee
MABEN, CHARLES S. ....Okmulgee
MATHENEY, J. C. ....Okmulgee
McCALEB, PHILIP ....Morris
McCAULEY, D. W. ....Okmulgee
McKINNEY, G. Y. ....Henryetta
MING, L. M. ....Okmulgee
MITCHENER, W. C. ....Okmulgee
PETER, M. L. ....Okmulgee
RAINS, HUGH L. ....Okmulgee
RODDA, E. D. ....Okmulgee
SIMPSON, N. N. (honorary) ....Henryetta
*SMITH, C. E. ....Henryetta
*TRACEWELL, GEORGE L. ....Okmulgee
VERNON, W. C. ....Okmulgee
WATSON, F. S. ....Okmulgee

OSAGE

AARON, WILLIAM H. ....Pawhuska
ALEXANDER, E. T. ....Barnsdall
*DALY, JOHN F. ....Pawhuska
DOZIER, BARCLAY E. ....Shidler
GUILD, CARL H. ....Shidler
HEMPHILL, GEORGE K. ....Pawhuska
*HEMPHILL, PAUL H. ....Pawhuska
KARASEK, MATTHEW ....Shidler
KEYES, E. C. ....Hominy
LIPE, EVERETT N. ....Fairfax
*RAGAN, T. A. ....Fairfax
*SMITH, R. O. ....Hominy
SULLIVAN, B. F. ....Barnsdall
WALKER, G. I. ....Hominy
WALKER, ROSCOE ....Pawhuska
WEIRICH, COLIN REID ....Pawhuska
WILLIAMS, CLAUDE W. ....Pawhuska
WORTEN, DIVONIS ....Pawhuska

OTTAWA

*AISENSTADT, E. ALBERT ....Picher
BARRY, J. R. ....Picher
*BISHOP, CALMES ....Picher
BUTLER, V. V. ....Picher
CANNON, R. F. ....Miami
*CHESNUT, W. G. ....Miami
COLVERT, GEORGE W. ....Miami
CONNELL, M. A. ....Picher
CORNELL, DON D. ....Picher
CRAIG, J. W. ....Miami
CUNNINGHAM, P. J. ....Miami
DeARMAN, M. M. ....Miami
DeTAR, GEORGE A. ....Miami
GRAHAM, REX M. ....Miami
HAMPTON, J. B. ....Miami
HETHERINGTON, L. P. ....Miami
HUGHES, A. R. ....Miami
JACOBY, J. SHERWOOD ....Commerce
KERR, WALTER C. H. ....Picher
LANNING, J. M. ....Picher
McNAUGHTON, G. P. ....Miami
*MURRAY, A. V. ....Picher
PRATT, T. W. ....Miami
RALSTON, BENJAMIN W. ....Commerce
RITCHEY, H. C. ....Picher
RUSSELL, RICHARD ....Picher
SANGER, WALTER B. ....Picher
*SAYLES, W. JACKSON ....Miami
SHELTON, B. WRIGHT ....Miami
SIEVER, CHARLES M. ....Picher
STAPLES, J. H. L. ....Afton
WORMINGTON, F. L. ....Miami

PAWNEE

BROWNING, R. L. ....Pawnee
HADDOX, CHARLES H. ....Pawnee
ROBINSON, E. T. ....Cleveland
SADDORIS, M. L. ....Cleveland
SPAULDING, H. B. ....Ralston

PAYNE

*BASSETT, CLIFFORD M. ....Cushing
*DAVIDSON, W. N. ....Cushing
DAVIS, BENJAMIN ....Cushing
FRIEDEMANN, PAUL W. ....Stillwater
*FRY, POWELL E. ....Stillwater
HOLBROOK, R. W. (honorary) ....Perkins
JENKINS, H. B. ....Stillwater
LEATHEROCK, R. E. ....Cushing
LOVE, T. A. ....Ripley
MANNING, H. C. ....Cushing
MARTIN, E. O. ....Cushing
*MARTIN, JAMES D. ....Cushing
MARTIN, JOHN F. ....Stillwater
MARTIN, JOHN W. ....Cushing
MITCHELL, L. A. ....Stillwater
MOORE, CLIFFORD W. ....Stillwater
OEHLSCHLAGER, F. KEITH ....Yale
*PUCKETT, HOWARD L. ....Stillwater
*ROBERTS, R. E. ....Stillwater
SEXTON, C. E. (honorary) ....Stillwater
SILVERTHORN, LOUIS E. ....Stillwater
SMITH, A. B. ....Stillwater
SMITH, HASKELL ....Stillwater
WAGGONER, ROY E. ....Stillwater
WEBER, ROXIE A. ....Stillwater
*WILHITE, L. R. ....Perkins

PITTSBURG

*BARTHELD, FLOYD T. ....McAlester
BAUM, FRANK J. ....McAlester
DAKIL, LOUIS N. ....McAlester
DORROUGH, JOE ....Haileyville
ELLIS, H. A. ....Kiowa
*GREENBERGER, EDWARD D. ....McAlester
KAEISER, WILLIAM H. ....McAlester
*KLOTZ, WILLIAM ....McAlester
KUYRKENDALL, L. C. ....McAlester
*LEVINE, JULIUS ....McAlester
*LIVELY, C. E. ....McAlester
McCARLEY, T. H. ....McAlester
MILLER, FRANK A. ....Hartshorne
*MILLS, C. K. ....McAlester
MUNN, JESSE A. ....McAlester
PARK, JOHN F. ....McAlester
PEMBERTON, R. K. ....McAlester
POWELL, PAUL T. ....McAlester
RICE, O. W. ....McAlester
SAMES, W. W. ....Hartshorne
SHULLER, E. H. ....McAlester
SPRINKLE, D. L. ....McAlester
STOUGH, A. R. ....McAlester
VAN CLEAVE, WM. E. ....McAlester
WAIT, WILLIAM C. ....McAlester
WILLIAMS, C. O. ....McAlester
WILLOUR, L. S. ....McAlester
WILSON, HERBERT A. ....McAlester

PONTOTOC

*BIGLER, IVAN ....Ada
BRECO, J. G. ....Ada
BRYDIA, CATHERINE T. ....Ada
BURNS, S. L. ....Stonewall
*CHEATWOOD, W. R. ....Ada
COWLING, ROBERT E. ....Ada
CUMMINGS, I. L. ....Ada
*CUNNINGHAM, JOHN A. ....Ada
DEAN, W. F. ....Ada
GULLATT, ENNIS M. ....Ada
LANE, WILSON H. ....Ada
LEWIS, E. F. ....Ada
LEWIS, M. L. ....Ada
MAYES, R. H. ....Ada
McBRIDE, OLLIE ....Ada
*McDONALD, GLEN ....Ada
McKEEL, SAM A. ....Ada
MILLER, O. H. ....Ada
*MOREY, J. B. ....Ada
*MUNTZ, E. R. ....Ada
*MURRAY, E. C. ....Ada
NEEDHAM, C. F. ....Ada
*PADBERG, E. D. ....Ada
PETERSON, WILLIAM G. ....Ada
RICHEY, S. M. (honorary) ....Ada
   (member Tulsa County Medical Society)
ROSS, S. P. (honorary) ....Ada
SEABORN, T. L. ....Ada
SUGG, ALFRED R. ....Ada
*WEBSTER, HARRELL ....Ada
WEBSTER, M. M. ....Ada
WELBORN, O. E. ....Ada

POTTAWATOMIE

APPLEWHITE, G. H. ....Shawnee
BAKER, M. A. ....Shawnee
BALL, W. A. ....Wanette
BAXTER, GEORGE S. ....Shawnee
BAXTER, JACK W. ....Shawnee
BYRUM, J. M. ....Shawnee
CAMPBELL, H. G. ....Tecumseh
CARSON, F. L. ....Shawnee
CARSON, JOHN M. ....Shawnee
CULBERTSON, R. R. ....Maud
GALLAHER, CLINTON ....Shawnee
*GALLAHER, PAUL ....Shawnee
GALLAHER, W. M. ....Shawnee
HAYGOOD, CHARLES W. ....Shawnee
HILL, R. M. C. (honorary) ....McLoud
*HUGHES, H. E. ....Shawnee
HUGHES, J. E. ....Shawnee
KAYLER, R. C. ....McLoud
KEEN, FRANK M. ....Shawnee
MATHEWS, W. F. ....Tecumseh
McFARLING, A. C. ....Shawnee
MULLINS, WILLIAM B. ....Shawnee
NEWLIN, FRANCES P. ....Shawnee
PARAMORE, C. F. ....Shawnee
RICE, E. EUGENE ....Shawnee
ROWLAND, T. D. ....Shawnee
WALKER, J. A. ....Shawnee
WILLIAMS, ALPHA McADAMS ....Shawnee
YOUNG, C. C. ....Shawnee

PUSHMATAHA

CONNALLY, D. W. ....Antlers
HUCKABAY, B. M. ....Antlers
LAWSON, JOHN S. ....Clayton
PATTERSON, E. S. ....Antlers

ROGER MILLS

CARY, W. S. ....Reydon
  (member Beckham County Medical Society)
HENRY, J. WORRALL ....Cheyenne
  (member Beckham County Medical Society)

ROGERS

ANDERSON, F. A. ....Claremore
*ANDERSON, P. S. ....Claremore
*ANDERSON, W. D. ....Claremore
BESON, CLYDE W. ....Claremore
*BIGLER, E. E. ....Claremore
CALDWELL, C. L. ....Chelsea
COLLINS, B. F. ....Claremore
*HOWARD, W. A. ....Chelsea
JENNINGS, K. D. ....Chelsea
MACRAE, DONALD H. ....Claremore
MELINGER, ROY J. ....Claremore
MELOY, R. C. ....Claremore
*NELSON, D. C. ....Claremore
WALLER, GEORGE D. ....Claremore

SEMINOLE

CHAMBERS, CLAUDE S. ....Seminole
*DEATON, Q. N. ....Wewoka
*FELTS, CLIFTON ....Seminole
GIESEN, A. F. ....Radford, Va.
GRIMES, JOHN P. ....Wewoka
HARBER, J. N. (honorary) ....Phoenix, Ariz.
HUDDLESTON, W. T. ....Konawa
JONES, W. E. ....Seminole
*KNIGHT, CLAUDE B. ....Wewoka
*LYONS, D. J. ....Seminole
*LYTLE, WILLIAM R. ....Seminole
McGOVERN, J. D. ....Wewoka
MOSHER, D. D. ....Seminole
PACE, L. R. ....Seminole
PRICE, J. T. ....Seminole
REEDER, H. M. ....Konawa
*RIPPY, O. M. ....Seminole
SHANHOLTZ, MACK I. ....Wewoka

STEPHENS, A. B. ....Seminole
*TERRY, JOHN B. ....Seminole
TURLINGTON, M. M. ....Seminole
VAN SANDT, GUY B. ....Wewoka
VAN SANDT, MAX M. ....Wewoka
WALKER, A. A. ....Wewoka
WILLIAMS, J. CLAY ....Wewoka
WRIGHT, H. L. ....Konawa

SEQUOYAH

MORROW, JOHN A. ....Sallisaw
NEWLIN, WILLIAM H. ....Sallisaw

STEPHENS

BERRY, THOMAS ....Duncan
IVY, WALLIS S. ....Duncan
*KING, E. G. ....Duncan
LINDLEY, E. C. ....Duncan
LINDLEY, E. H. ....Duncan
McCLAIN, W. Z. ....Marlow
McMAHAN, A. M. ....Duncan
PATTERSON, J. L. ....Duncan
RICHARDSON, R. W. ....Duncan
*SMITH, L. P. ....Marlow
TALLEY, C. N. ....Marlow
THOMASSON, E. B. ....Duncan
WALKER, W. K. ....Marlow
*WATERS, CLAUDE B. ....Duncan
WEEDN, ALTON J. ....Duncan

TEXAS

BLACKMER, L. G. ....Hooker
*BLUE, JOHNNY A. ....Guymon
HAYES, R. B. ....Guymon
LEE, DANIEL S. ....Guymon
OBERMILLER, R. G. ....Texhoma
RUDE, EVELYN ....Guymon
  (member Seminole County Medical Society)
SMITH, MORRIS ....Guymon

TILLMAN

ALLEN, C. C. ....Frederick
ARRINGTON, J. E. ....Frederick
BACON, O. G. ....Frederick
*BOX, O. H., JR. ....Grandfield
CALVERT, HOWARD A. ....Frederick
CHILDERS, J. E. ....Tipton
COLLIER, E. K. ....Tipton
*FISHER, ROY L. ....Frederick
FOSHEE, W. C. ....Grandfield
*FRY, F. P. ....Frederick
FUQUA, W. A. ....Grandfield
MILLER, W. R. ....Frederick
OSBORN, J. D. ....Frederick
SPURGEON, T. F. ....Frederick

TULSA

ADAMS, R. M. ....521 N. Boulder
*AKINS, J. O. ....Medical Arts Bldg.
ALLEN, V. K. ....Medical Arts Bldg.
ARMSTRONG, O. C. ....Medical Arts Bldg.
ATCHLEY, R. Q. ....507 S. Cincinnati
ATKINS, PAUL N. ....Medical Arts Bldg.
BARHAM, J. H. ....Daniels Bldg.
BEESLEY, W. W. (honorary) ....1733 S. Lewis
*BEST, RALPH L. ....Medical Arts Bldg.
BEYER, J. WALTER ....McBirney Bldg.
BILLINGTON, J. JEFF ....Medical Arts Bldg.
BIRNBAUM, WILLIAM ....915 S. Cincinnati
BLACK, HAROLD J. ....Medical Arts Bldg.
*BOONE, W. B. ....2112 W. 41st St.
BRADFIELD, S. J. ....Medical Arts Bldg.
*BRANLEY, B. L. ....Medical Arts Bldg.
BRASWELL, JAMES C. ....Medical Arts Bldg.
*BROCKSMITH, H. A. ....Medical Arts Bldg.
BROGDEN, J. C. ....Medical Arts Bldg.
BROOKSHIRE, J. E. (honorary) ....409 S. Boulder
BROWN, PAUL R. (honorary) ....1614 E. 35th St.
BROWNE, HENRY S. ....Medical Arts Bldg.
BRYAN, W. J., JR. ....Medical Arts Bldg.
CALHOUN, C. E. ....Sand Springs
CALHOUN, W. H. ....Medical Arts Bldg.

CARNEY, A. B. ....915 S. Cincinnati
CHALMERS, J. S. ....Sand Springs
CHARBONNET, P. N. ....Oklahoma Bldg.
CHILDS, J. W. ....Medical Arts Bldg.
CLINTON, FRED S. (honorary) 230 E. Woodward Blvd.
CLULOW, GEORGE H. ....1307 S. Main
COHENOUR, E. L. ....Medical Arts Bldg.
COOK, W. ALBERT ....Medical Arts Bldg.
COULTER, T. B. ....Medical Arts Bldg.
CRANE, DONALD V. ....Medical Arts Bldg.
CRAWFORD, WILLIAM S. .Nat'l Bank of Tulsa Bldg.
DAILY, R. E. ....Bixby
DAVIS, A. H. ....Medical Arts Bldg.
DAVIS, GEORGE M. ....Bixby
*DAVIS, T. H. ....Medical Arts Bldg.
DEAN, W. A. ....Medical Arts Bldg.
*DENNY, E. RANKIN ....Medical Arts Bldg.
*EADS, CHARLES H. ....Medical Arts Bldg.
*EDWARDS, D. L. ....Philcade
*EDWARDS, JOHN ....Medical Arts Bldg.
ETHERTON, MONTE C. ....10-A S. Lewis
EVANS, HUGH J. ....Medical Arts Bldg.
*EWELL, WILLIAM C. ....1307 S. Main
FARRIS, H. LEE ....Medical Arts Bldg.
FLACK, F. L. ....Nat'l Bank of Tulsa Bldg.
FLANAGAN, O. A. ....912 S. Boulder
FORD, H. W. ....915 S. Cincinnati
*FORD, RICHARD D. ....Braniff Bldg.
FORRY, W. W. ....Bixby
FRANKLIN, ONIS ....Broken Arrow
*FRANKLIN, S. E ....Broken Arrow
FULCHER, JOSEPH ....Medical Arts Bldg.
FUNK, ROBERT E. ....Medical Arts Bldg.
GARRETT, D. L. ....Medical Arts Bldg.
**GILBERT, J. B. ....Nat'l Mutual Bldg.
GLASS, FRED A. ....Medical Arts Bldg.
GODDARD, R. K. ....Skiatook
GOODMAN, SAMUEL ....Medical Arts Bldg.
GORRELL, J. F. ....Medical Arts Bldg.
GRAHAM, HUGH C. ....1307 S. Main
*GREEN, HARRY ....Medical Arts Bldg.
GROSSHART, PAUL ....Medical Arts Bldg.
HALL, G. H. (honorary) ....2235 E. 24th St.
*HAMMOND, JAMES H. ....Medical Arts Bldg.
HARALSON, C. H. ....Medical Arts Bldg.
*HARDMAN, T. J. ....Medical Arts Bldg.
HARRIS, BUNN ....Jenks
HART, MABEL M. ....1228 S. Boulder
HART, M. O. ....1228 S. Boulder
HAYS, LUVERN ....Medical Arts Bldg.
HENDERSON, F. W. ....Medical Arts Bldg.
HENLEY, MARVIN D. ....Medical Arts Bldg.
*HENRY, G. H. ....Medical Arts Bldg.
HILL, O. L. ....915 S. Cincinnati
HOKE, C. C. ....Philtower Bldg.
HOOPER, J. S. (honorary) ....1645 S. Boston
*HOOVER, W. D. ....511 S. Boston
HOTZ, CARL J. ....Springer Clinic
HOUSER, M. A. ....McBirney Bldg.
HUBER, W. A. ....Medical Arts Bldg.
HUDSON, DAVID V. ....21 N. Cincinnati
HUDSON, MARGARET G. ....1759 S. Victor
HUMPHREY, B. H ....Sperry
HUTCHISON, A. ....Bixby
HYATT, E. G. ....Springer Clinic
JOHNSON, E. O. ....Medical Arts Bldg.
JOHNSON, R. R. ....Sand Springs
JONES, ELLIS ....Medical Arts Bldg.
JONES, WILLIAM M. ....915 S. Cincinnati
KEMMERLY, H. P. ....Medical Arts Bldg.
*KORNBLEE, A. T. ....1307 S. Main
KRAMER, ALLEN C. ....Medical Arts Bldg.
LARRABEE, W. S. ....Medical Arts Bldg.
LAYTON, O. E. ....Collinsville
*LEE, J. K. ....Medical Arts Bldg.
LeMASTER, D. W ....Medical Arts Bldg.
LHEVINE, MORRIS B. ....Medical Arts Bldg.
LONEY, W. R. R. ....Medical Arts Bldg.
LOWE, J. O. ....915 S. Cincinnati

*LUSK, EARL M. ....915 S. Cincinnati
LYNCH, THOMAS J. ....Philcade Bldg.
MacDONALD, D. M. ....1739 S. Utica
MacKENZIE, IAN ....Medical Arts Bldg.
MARGOLIN, BERTHE ....1568 S. Yorktown Place
MARKLAND, J. D. ....Medical Arts Bldg.
*MATT, JOHN G. ....1304 E. 20th St.
MAYGINNES, P. H. ....Palace Bldg.
MAZZARELLA, VINCENT ....1701 S. St. Louis
*McDONALD, J. E. ....Medical Arts Bldg.
McGILL, RALPH A. ....Medical Arts Bldg.
McKELLAR, MALCOLM M. ....Springer Clinic
McQUAKER, MOLLY ....1552 E. 17th Place
MILLER, GEORGE H. ....Atlas Life Bldg.
MINER, JAMES L. ....Medical Arts Bldg.
MISHLER, D. L. ....Springer Clinic
*MITCHELL, T. H. ....Nat'l Bank of Tulsa Bldg.
MOHRMAN, S. S. ....Daniels Bldg.
*MUNDING, L. A. ....Medical Arts Bldg.
MURDOCK, H. D. ....Medical Arts Bldg.
MURRAY, P. G. ....Medical Arts Bldg.
MURRAY, SILAS ....Medical Arts Bldg.
NEAL, JAMES H. ....1944 N. Denver Place
NELSON, FRANK J. ....Medical Arts Bldg.
NELSON, F. L. ....Atlas Life Bldg.
NELSON, I. A. ....Medical Arts Bldg.
NELSON, IRON H. ....Medical Arts Bldg.
NELSON, M. O. ....Medical Arts Bldg.
NESBITT, E. P. ....Medical Arts Bldg.
NESBITT, P. P. ....Medical Arts Bldg.
NORTHRUP, L. C. ....1307 S. Main
*ORR, HERBERT ....1307 S. Main
OSBORN, GEORGE R. ....Medical Arts Bldg.
PAVY, C. A ....Medical Arts Bldg.
PEDEN, JAMES C. ....Medical Arts Bldg.
*PERRY, FRED J. ....Atlas Life Bldg.
PERRY, HUGH ....Atlas Life Bldg.
PERRY, JOHN C. ....Medical Arts Bldg.
PIGFORD, A. W. ....Medical Arts Bldg.
*PIGFORD, R. C. ....Medical Arts Bldg.
*PITTMAN, COLE D. ....Broken Arrow
*POLLOCK, SIMON ....Tulsa
*PORTER, H. H. ....Medical Arts Bldg.
PRESSON, L. C. ....1948 N. Main
PRICE, H. P. ....Medical Arts Bldg.
RAMEY, CLYDE ....Palace Bldg.
*RAY, R. G. ....915 S. Cincinnati
REESE, K. C. ....Medical Arts Bldg.
REYNOLDS, E. W. ....915 S. Cincinnati
REYNOLDS, JAMES L. (honorary) ...402 W. 2nd. St.
RHODES, R. E. L. ....Medical Arts Bldg.
RILEY, NOLAN C. ....915 S. Cincinnati
ROBERTS, T. R. ....Wright Bldg.
ROBINSON, F. P. ....915 S. Cincinnati
ROBINSON, LILLIAN H. ....915 S. Cincinnati
ROGERS, J. W. ....Medical Arts Bldg.
ROTH, A. W. (honorary) ....1616 S. Peoria Ave.
RUPRECHT, H. A. ....Springer Clinic
RUPRECHT, MARCELLA ....Springer Clinic
RUSHING, F. E. ....Medical Arts Bldg.
RUSSELL, G. R. ....Springer Clinic
SCHRECK, PHILIP M. ....Medical Arts Bldg.
*SCHWARTZ, H. N. ....Medical Arts Bldg.
SEARLE, M. J. ....Medical Arts Bldg.
SHAPIRO, DAVID ....Atlas Life Bldg.
SHEPARD, R. M. ....Medical Arts Bldg.
*SHEPARD, S. C. ....Medical Arts Bldg.
SHERWOOD, R. G. ....14 Court Arcade
*SHIPP, J. D. ....Medical Arts Bldg.
SHOWMAN, W. A. ....Medical Arts Bldg.
SIMPSON, CARL F. ....Medical Arts Bldg.
*SINCLAIR, F. D. ....Springer Clinic
SIPPEL, MARY EDNA ....1542 E. 15th St.
SISLER, WADE ....Mercy Hospital
SMITH, D. O. ....Springer Clinic
SMITH, NED D. ....Medical Arts Bldg.
*SMITH, ROY L. ....Medical Arts Bldg.
SMITH, RURIC N. ....Medical Arts Bldg.
SMITH, W. O. ....Stanolind Bldg.

*SPANN, LOGAN A. ....Braniff Bldg.
*SPOTTSWOOD, MAURICE D. ....Medical Arts Bldg.
SPRINGER, M. P. ....Springer Clinic
STALLINGS, T. W. ....724 S. Elgin St.
STANLEY, M. V. ....904 N. Denver
STEVENSON, JAMES ....Medical Arts Bldg.
STEWART, H. B. ....2500 E. 27th St.
*STUART, C. G. ....Tulsa
*STUART, FRANK A. ....Nat'l Mutual Bldg.
STUART, LEON H. ....Medical Arts Bldg.
SUMMERS, C. S. ....Daniels Bldg.
SWANSON, K. F. ....Springer Clinic
*THOMPSON, OLIVER H. ....1737 E. 30th St.
TRAINOR, W. J. ....Medical Arts Bldg.
*TURNBOW, W. R. ....Medical Arts Bldg.
UNDERWOOD, DAVID J. ....Medical Arts Bldg.
UNDERWOOD, F. L. ....Medical Arts Bldg.
UNGERMAN, A. H. ....Medical Arts Bldg.
VENABLE, S. C. ....602 S. Cheyenne
WALKER, WILLIAM A. ....Kennedy Bldg.
WALL, GREGORY A. (honorary) ....1159 N. Cheyenne
WALLACE, J. E. ....Medical Arts Bldg.
WARD, BEN W. ....Wright Bldg.
*WENDEL, WILLIAM E. ....915 S. Cincinnati
*WHITE, ERIC M. ....Medical Arts Bldg.
WHITE, N. S. ....Medical Arts Bldg.
WILEY, A. RAY ....Medical Arts Bldg.
WILLIAMS, THEO S. ....Medical Arts Bldg.
WITCHER, R. B. ....Medical Arts Bldg.
*WOLFF, EUGENE G. ....St. John's Hospital
WOODSON, FRED E. ....Medical Arts Bldg.
*YANDELL, HAYES R. ....Medical Arts Bldg.
ZINK, ROY ....Daniels Bldg.
**Deceased July 6, 1944.

WAGONER

DIVINE, D. G. ....Wagoner
JOBLIN, W. R. ....Porter
PLUNKETT, J. H. ....Wagoner
RIDDLE, H. K. ....Coweta

WASHINGTON

ATHEY, J. V. ....Bartlesville
BEECHWOOD, E. E. ....Bartlesville
CHAMBERLIN, E. M. ....Bartlesville
CRAWFORD, HORACE G. ....Bartlesville
**CRAWFORD, JOHN E. ....Bartlesville
DORSHEIMER, G. V. ....Dewey
*ETTER, FORREST S. ....Bartlesville
GENTRY, RAYMOND C. ....Bartlesville
GREEN, OTTO I. ....Bartlesville
HUDSON, L. D. ....Dewey
KINGMAN, W. H. (honorary) ....Bartlesville
LeBLANC, WILLIAM ....Ochelata
PARKS, SETH M. ....Bartlesville
REWERTS, FRED C. ....Bartlesville
*RUCKER, RALPH W. ....Bartlesville
SHIPMAN, WILLIAM H. ....Bartlesville
SMITH, JOSEPH G. ....Bartlesville
SOMERVILLE, O. S. ....Bartlesville
STAVER, BENJAMIN F. ....Bartlesville
TORREY, JOHN P. ....Bartlesville

VANSANT, J. P. ....Dewey
WEBER, HENRY C. ....Bartlesville
WEBER, SHERWELL G. ....Bartlesville
WELLS, CEPHAS J. ....Bartlesville
WELLS, THOMAS ....Bartlesville
*WORD, LEE B. ....Bartlesville
**Deceased March 19, 1944.

WASHITA

ADAMS, ALLEN C. ....Cordell
BENNETT, D. W. ....Sentinel
BUNGARDT, A. H. ....Cordell
*DARNELL, E. E. ....Colony
FREEMAN, W. H. (honorary) ....Sentinel
    (member Kiowa County Medical Society)
HARMS, J. H. (honorary) ....Newton, Kansas
JONES, J. P. (honorary) ....Dill
*LIVINGSTON, L. G. ....Cordell
McMURRY, JAMES F. ....Sentinel
NEAL, A. S. ....Cordell
*STOWERS, AUBREY E. ....Sentinel
TRACY, C. M. ....Sentinel
WEAVER, E. S. ....Cordell
WEBER, A. ....Bessie

WOODS

ENSOR, DANIEL B. ....Hopeton
GRANTHAN, ELIZABETH (honorary) ....Alva
LaFON, WILLIAM F. ....Waynoka
*ROYER, CHARLES A. ....Alva
*SIMON, JOHN F. ....Alva
SIMON, WILLIAM E. ....Alva
STEPHENSON, ISHMAEL F. ....Alva
TEMPLIN, OSCAR E. ....Alva
TRAVERSE, C. A. ....Alva

WOODWARD

DARWIN, D. W. ....Woodward
DAY, JOHN L. ....Supply
*DUER, JOE L. ....Woodward
*ENGLAND, MYRON ....Woodward
HUMPHREY, J. H. ....Mooreland
JOHNSON, H. L. ....Supply
**KING, FRANK M. ....Woodward
LEACHMAN, THAD C. ....Woodward
MITCHELL, CLARENCE ....Supply
ORRICK, GEORGE W. ....Supply
PEARSON, GLENN A. ....Woodward
PIERSON, ORRA A. ....Woodward
*RUTHERFORD, V. M. ....Woodward
TEDROWE, C. W. ....Woodward
TRIPLETT, T. BURKE ....Mooreland
WILLIAMS, C. E. ....Woodward
**Deceased January 10, 1944.

ASSOCIATE MEMBERS

ALLEY, R. M., M. D. ....Shawnee
GILLICK, DAVID, M. D. ....Shawnee
HANSEN, FRED, MR. ....Oklahoma City
MOLLICA, S. G., M. D. ....Muskogee
MYERS, DAVID A., M. D. ....San Francisco, Cal.
TURLEY, LOUIS A., PH. D. ....Oklahoma City

VOL. XXXVII

December, 1944

NUMBER 12

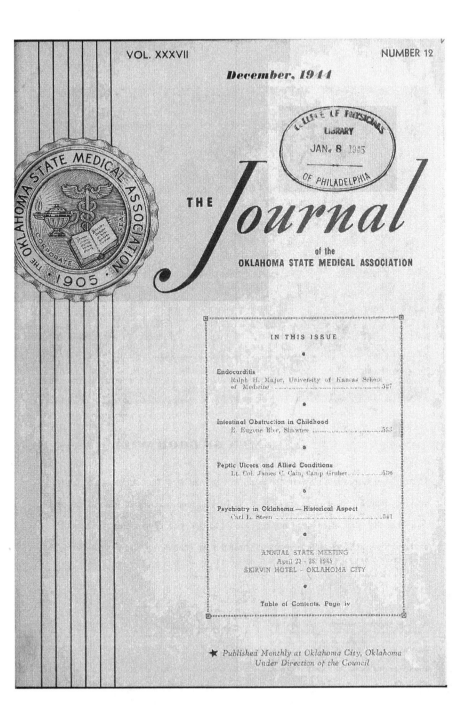

THE *Journal*

of the
OKLAHOMA STATE MEDICAL ASSOCIATION

★ *Published Monthly at Oklahoma City, Oklahoma
Under Direction of the Council*

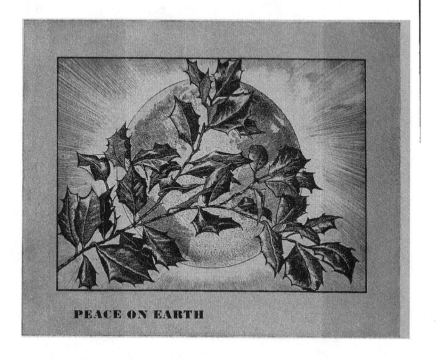

PEACE ON EARTH

...TO MEN OF GOOD WILL

That all men everywhere may breathe again as free men ☆ ☆ That suffering and oppression may vanish forever from the earth ☆ ☆ That all men may regain their self-respect ☆ ☆ That the labor of all men may be devoted to the good of mankind ☆ ☆ That the pain and the hurt of all men be mercifully healed ☆ ☆ That all may live in peace forever!

We, men and women of Wyeth...as one voice, make this wish. To the doctors and nurses in our Army and Navy in the far corners of the earth; to our doctors and nurses at home; to our druggists; we at Wyeth are proud to have been of service. Proud and honored to have received our third Army-Navy "E". To you, men and women of mercy—our hand and our utmost support at all times.

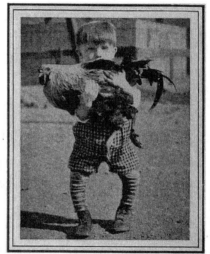

The rooster's legs are straight.

The boy's are not.

The rooster got plenty of vitamin D.

Fortunately, extreme cases of rickets such as the one above illustrated
are comparatively rare nowadays, due to the widespread prophylactic use of vitamin D recommended by the medical profession.

One of the surest and easiest means of routinely administering vitamin D (and vitamin A)
to children is MEAD'S OLEUM PERCOMORPHUM WITH OTHER FISH-LIVER
OILS AND VIOSTEROL. Supplied in 10-cc. and 50-cc. bottles. Also supplied in bottles
of 50 and 250 capsules. Council Accepted. All Mead Products Are Council Accepted. Mead
Johnson & Company, Evansville 21, Ind., U.S.A.

FOR HOSPITALIZED PATIENTS

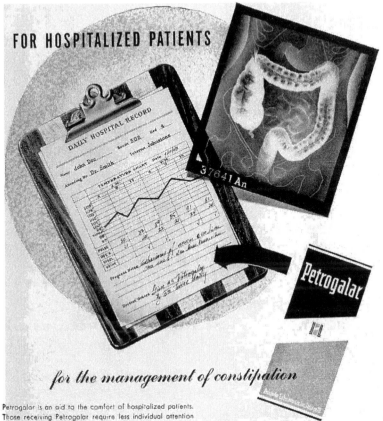

for the management of constipation

Petrogalar is an aid to the comfort of hospitalized patients. Those receiving Petrogalar require less individual attention and fewer visits from busy internes and nurses. Petrogalar relieves nurses of the extra burden of having to change bed linens and sleeping garments as a result of "leakage" sometimes caused by plain mineral oil.

The special 10⅔ ounce Petrogalar Hospital Dispensing Unit allows the physician complete control over the administration of a routine laxative during confinement.

Years of professional use have established Petrogalar as a reliable, efficacious aid for the restoration and maintenance of comfortable bowel action.

PETROGALAR LABORATORIES, INC., CHICAGO, ILLINOIS
Copyright 1943, by Petrogalar Laboratories, Inc.

DIVISION *Wyeth* INCORPORATED

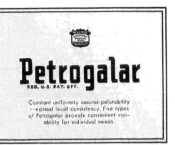

Petrogalar
REG. U.S. PAT. OFF.

Constant uniformity assures palatability
—normal fecal consistency. Five types
of Petrogalar provide convenient variability for individual needs.

Petrogalar is an aqueous suspension of pure mineral oil each 100 cc. of which contains 65 cc pure mineral oil suspended in an aqueous jelly.

The rooster's legs are straight.

The boy's are not.

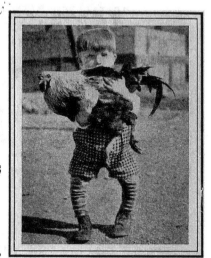

The rooster got plenty of vitamin D.

Fortunately, extreme cases of rickets such as the one above illustrated are comparatively rare nowadays, due to the widespread prophylactic use of vitamin D recommended by the medical profession.

One of the surest and easiest means of routinely administering vitamin D (and vitamin A) to children is MEAD'S OLEUM PERCOMORPHUM WITH OTHER FISH-LIVER OILS AND VIOSTEROL. Supplied in 10-cc. and 50-cc. bottles. Council Accepted. All Mead Products Are Council Accepted. Mead Johnson & Company, Evansville 21, Ind., U.S.A.

This Book is due on the last date stamped
below.   No further preliminary notice
will be sent.   Requests for renewals must
be made on or before the date of expiration.

DUE	RETURNED
APR 4 - 1947	APR 10 1947
JUL 10 1951.	JUL 3 - 1951
JUN 27 1956	
Aug 31, 1957	

www.ingramcontent.com/pod-product-compliance
Lightning Source LLC
Chambersburg PA
CBHW071353050326

40689CB00010B/1629